PSYCHIATRY

volume 1

The Personality Disorders and Neuroses

Psychiatry Series

PSYCHIATRY

volume one

The Personality Disorders and Neuroses

Arnold M. Cooper, MD

Professor and Associate Chairman for Education
Department of Psychiatry
Cornell University Medical College
Director of Training
Payne Whitney Clinic
The New York Hospital
New York, New York

Allen J. Frances, MD

Professor of Psychiatry
Cornell University Medical College
Director, Outpatient Department
Payne Whitney Clinic
The New York Hospital
New York, New York

Michael H. Sacks, MD

Associate Professor of Psychiatry
Cornell University Medical College
Chief, Inpatient Unit
Payne Whitney Clinic
The New York Hospital
New York, New York

BASIC BOOKS, INC., PUBLISHERS
New York

J.B. LIPPINCOTT COMPANY
Philadelphia
London   Mexico City   New York   St. Louis   São Paulo   Sydney

PUBLISHER'S NOTE

The six volumes of this series comprise a work also published in a three-volume set entitled *Psychiatry*, which is available in a loose-leaf format that is updated annually and carries the ISBN 0-397-50686-4.

Each of the six volumes has its individual ISBN. The ISBN for the six-volume set is 0-397-50685-6.

Acquisitions Editor: William Burgower
Sponsoring Editor: Rene Boudreau
Production Supervisor: June Eberharter
Looseleaf Coordinator: Shirley Kuhn
Indexer: Tony Greenberg, MD
Compositor: Bi-Comp, Incorporated
Printer and Binder: The Murray Printing Company

DRUG DOSAGE

The authors and publisher have exerted every effort to ensure that drug selection and dosage set forth in this text are in accord with current recommendations and practice at the time of publication. However, in view of ongoing research, changes in government regulations, and the constant flow of information relating to drug therapy and drug reactions, the reader is urged to check the package insert for each drug for any change in indications and dosage and for added warnings and precautions. This is particularly important when the recommended agent is a new or infrequently employed drug.

6 5 4 3 2 1

Library of Congress Cataloging-in-Publication Data
The Personality disorders and neuroses.
  (Psychiatry Series: Michels, Robert, Chairman, Editorial Board;
Cavenar, Jesse O, Jr, Editor; v. 1)
   Also published as part of: Psychiatry.
   Includes bibliographies and index.
   1. Personality, Disorders of. 2. Neuroses.
I. Cooper, Arnold M. II. Frances, Allen, 1942–
III. Sacks, Michael H. IV. Psychiatry (Philadelphia,
Pa.: 1985) V. Series: Psychiatry series (New York,
N.Y.: 1986) ; v. 1. [DNLM: 1. Neurotic Disorders.
2. Personality Disorders. WM 100 P9885 v. 1]
RC554.P47 1986   616.85′82   86-10546
ISBN 0-397-50810-7 (Lippincott)

Contents
Volume 1

Personality Disorders

Neurosis

Other Disorders

Sexual Disorders

Arnold M. Cooper, Allen Frances, and Michael Sacks

The Psychoanalytic Model

The development of psychoanalysis has been largely the work of one man, Sigmund Freud. Freud was primarily responsible for the major propositions of psychoanalytic theory, most of the early clinical findings, and the organization of the psychoanalytic movement that spread his teachings. Although today there are a number of variants of psychoanalysis, they share fundamental hypotheses and observations rooted deeply in clinical experience. Psychoanalysis encompasses three related but different activities: (1) a method of research into mental activity based on observations made under special conditions, emphasizing free association; (2) a theory of human behavior; and (3) a method of psychotherapy designed particularly for the treatment of symptom and character neuroses.

Only the psychoanalytic observational methods and theory of behavior are discussed in this chapter; psychoanalytic treatment is covered elsewhere in this volume. During the past century Freud's revolutionary view of human behavior has become so deeply ingrained in Western thought that the extent to which psychoanalytic concepts are accepted in our ordinary understanding of persons is often forgotten. The methods Freud developed have helped to explain a wide range of human behaviors: from the most trivial (*e.g.*, slips of the tongue) to the most momentous; from pathologic to clearly normal behaviors; from the development of sexuality to the development of creativity; and from alert, waking behavior to the sleeping behavior of dreams. No human endeavor is exempt from psychoanalytic efforts at understanding, and many have clearly been enriched by this effort.

The Basic Hypotheses

Psychoanalysis has developed a set of basic propositions that help to define the field:

Psychic determinism. Mental events are not random but rather result from antecedent causes. Cause and effect relationships are as important in understanding mental events as they are for physical events. The concept of psychic determinism is essential for claiming the mind as a field for orderly scientific study.

The dynamic unconscious. There are important feelings, thoughts, and desires that remain out of awareness and cannot be brought to awareness by an ordinary effort of will and yet serve as major sources of motivation and determinants of behavior. Freud believed that the discovery of the dynamic unconscious, with its implication that humans are not the conscious masters of their fate, was the third great narcissistic wound to humanity; the first was the Copernican discovery that the Earth is not the center of the universe; the second was the Darwinian discovery that humans are descendants of other animals.

The motivational point of view. Behavior arises out of wishes or needs inherent in the constitutional makeup of the human organism (in psychoanalytic theory these are organized around drives); the mind is propelled to work by the "pressure" of the drives for their satisfaction and is, therefore, capable of spontaneous activity, not only reactive to stimuli. The compass for directing motivation is provided by the pleasure–unpleasure principle leading toward activities that provide gratification and away from those that provide pain.

Psychic conflict. At any given moment, the behavior (state of the mind) of an individual is a result of conflicting desires or of conflicts of desire and prohibition, which, through defenses and compromises, lead to the expressed behavior.

The genetic point of view. All behavior can be understood in terms of the individual history of the epigenetic stages of development, determined by the nature of the developing drives and psychic structures and their interactions with the environment. Any behavior is part of a continuum of events extending back to earliest infancy. The genetic point of view refers to internalized psychic reality of the individual and may not accord with actual events as perceived by an outside observer.

The social and adaptive points of view. A human is born with constitutional preadaptations to the human social environment, and all behaviors reflect the series of hierarchical adaptations to the changing ''reality'' demands during the course of development. Motivations are created by the cultural environment as well as by the drives.

The principle of multiple function. Any mental action serves to gratify multiple demands of different needs and mental agencies.

These propositions provide different modes of exploring the meaning of any psychic event and include hypotheses derived from biological (drive), environmental, and learning (developmental) perspectives.

The Historical Context

Even the most innovative genius is rooted in his epoch, and his ideas form part of the historical continuum. Before Freud came to be the discoverer and inventor of psychoanalysis, he was already a highly skilled neurologist and had conducted basic research in squid neurones and clinical research in aphasia and hysteria. He was a young and successful practitioner of neurology in Vienna, educated in the classical tradition, and very much a part of the high culture of his time. A few of the major influences on Freud's thinking are mentioned below.

The dominant scientific mode of Freud's era was the so-called school of Helmholtz. The program of this scientific movement was to reduce all physiology to physics and chemistry and to demonstrate that any complex phenomenon could be understood in terms of simpler atomistic units. The theories tended to be mechanistic as well as reductionistic; they viewed the organism as a machine that is fully comprehensible in terms of the workings of its parts. The metaphor of the complicated clockwork mechanism was dominant.

Darwin's influence is evident in Freud's views of the evolution of complex, advanced organizations out of primitive, simple beginnings. Freud's concern with first causes, the relationship of phylogeny and ontogeny, and the adaptations of instinct and behavior to environment all rested on the ideas of Darwin. Darwin's studies on the expression of emotions in animals and humans clearly presaged Freud's rooting of psychology in evolutionary biology and his interest in the instinctual patterning of complex human behaviors.

It is clear that many of Freud's ideas concerning the nature of motivation and unconscious conflict were related to the philosophy of his times, particularly to Nietzsche and Schopenhauer.

Freud frequently acknowledged the priority of the artist in having discerned and described behaviors that he was attempting to explain systematically. He was especially enraptured with the classics and with Shakespeare and Goethe, and several writers have suggested that Goethe's essay ''On Nature'' was crucial for determining Freud's scientific mode.[1]

Freud believed that his Jewishness was an important part of his creative inspiration. The emphasis on the importance of the word, the constant search for meanings behind text (the Talmudic method), and the sense of isolation from the mainstream that allowed pursuit of unpopular ideas were undoubtedly significant for Freud.

The Victorian era, although outwardly marked by sexual repression, was accompanied by a subterranean, powerful interest in sex and sexual perversion.[2,3] It was, perhaps, inevitable that in this climate Freud should perceive that sex must be an essential, although disclaimed element in the formation of thought and character.

There are now many biographies of Freud that attempt to explain the personal characteristics that allowed him to become the discoverer of psychoanalysis.[4,5] Of the many ideas that have been advanced, a few points merit special attention. Freud combined the deepest interest in literature and the humanities with the most thorough training in the advanced neuroscience of his time. Because of his financial needs, Freud had been unable to continue his fulltime scientific career and had become a practicing neurologist. This forced him away from laboratory observation and led him to apply his scientific talent to solve a major clinical problem of the time—hysteria. His private practice brought him patients of the upper and middle class who were intelligent, educated and potentially creative, introspective, and psychologically minded. He had studied with Charcot and Janet and was familiar with the experimental work in hypnosis and suggestion. Freud's background fitted him, perhaps uniquely, for seeing human meaning in what he could simultaneously consider to be biological events.

Freud's personal characteristics included dogged curiosity in the pursuit of deeper meanings. He was willing to reveal aspects of his own unconscious and to conduct a self-analysis for the sake of understanding his own neurosis. He was also courageous, putting forth unpopular ideas that endangered his economic well-being and subjected him to the wrath of the academic community. Freud used ideas with extraordinary boldness, borrowing from neurology, anthropology, embryology, and literature to make a coherent picture of the mind. He had been a favored eldest son and at an early age saw himself as a "conquistador" who would make his mark, whether it was to be in literature, basic science, or clinical research. Freud had extraordinary personal power and charisma. He attracted brilliant and devoted followers, eager to advance the work of psychoanalysis.

The Early Clinical Discoveries

The early work of Josef Breuer and Freud, published in "Studies on Hysteria,"[6] revealed that hysterical patients, urged or permitted to speak all their thoughts, regularly related their hysterical symptoms to traumatic life events that had aroused painful thoughts and feelings, and which the patient had shut out of awareness. Freud found that these traumatic experiences regularly involved some form of sexual excitation that the patient shamefully or guiltily kept out of consciousness. The therapeutic task was to reconnect the isolated (unconscious) thoughts with the ongoing conscious train of the ego's activities.

Freud described this method of reconnection as follows:

We found, to our great surprise at first, that *each individual hysterical symptom immediately and permanently disappeared when we had succeeded in bringing clearly to light the memory of the event by which it was provoked and in arousing its accompanying affect, and when the patient had described that event in the greatest possible detail and had put the affect into words.*

He and Breuer attempted to explain why the "cathartic" method works by their statement that

it brings to an end the operative force of the idea which was not abreacted in the first instance, by allowing its strangulated affect to find a way out through speech; and it subjects it to associative correction by introducing it into normal consciousness (under light hypnosis) or by removing it through the physician's suggestion, as is done in somnambulism accompanied by amnesia.

Freud went on to discover that not only hysterical but also obsessional symptoms seemed to be responsive to the cathartic method and also that the method was more complex than the usual hypnotic technique indicated. It was at this point that he became interested in "analytic" rather than cathartic methods. In the final chapter of "Studies in Hysteria" he outlined the major clinical observations describing his psychoanalytic method. He stated, "the procedure is laborious and time consuming for the physician. It presupposes great interest in psychological happenings, but personal concern for the patients as well." Freud described the importance of knowing not only the immediate traumatic event but the need to conduct an "*analysis*," tracing in detail the preceding and surrounding circumstances that contributed to making the event traumatic.

Freud next described the concept of *resistance*. He stated:

this insistence [the demand that the patient produce memories related to the symptoms] involved effort on my part and so suggested the idea that I had to overcome a resistance, the situation led me at once to the theory that *by means of my psychical work I had to overcome a psychical force in the patients which was opposed to the pathogenic ideas becoming conscious (being remembered).*

It was but a brief further step for him now to develop the idea of *defense:*

I recognized a universal characteristic of such ideas [those that were pathogenic, forgotten, and out of consciousness]: they were all of a distressing nature, calculated to rouse the affects of shame, of self-reproach and of psychical pain, and the feeling of being harmed; they were all of a kind that one would prefer not to have experienced, that one would rather forget. From all this there arose, as it were automatically, the thought of *defense* . . . The patient's ego had been approached by an idea which proved to be incompatible, which provoked on the part of the ego a repelling force of which the purpose was defense against this incompatible idea. This defense was in fact successful. The idea in question was forced out of consciousness and out of memory.

The resistance to recall was the same force that had driven the repellent ideas out of memory when they first arose.

Freud gave a description of *free association* as he then understood it.

The task of the therapist, therefore, lies in overcoming by his psychical work this resistance to association. He does this in the first place by "insisting," by making use of psychical compulsion to direct the patients' attention to the ideational traces of which he is in search . . . It should not be forgotten, however, that it is always a question here of a *quantitative* comparison, of a struggle between motive forces of different degrees of strength or intensity . . . He is not to keep it (images or thoughts) to himself because he may happen to think it is not what is wanted, not the right thing, or because it would be too disagreeable for him to say it. There is to be no criticism of it, no reticence, either for emotional reasons or because it is judged unimportant. Only in this manner can we find what we are in search of, but in this matter we shall find it infallibly.

Freud next gave an early view of the psychoanalytic tasks of *interpretation and reconstruction:*

If, now, I could make it appear probable that the idea had become pathogenic precisely as a result of its expulsion and repression, the chain would seem complete . . . Thus a psychical force, aversion on the part of the ego, had originally driven the pathogenic idea out of association and was now opposing its return to memory. The hysterical patient's "not knowing" was, in fact a "not wanting to know"—a not wanting which might be to a greater or less extent conscious. The task of the therapist, therefore, lies in overcoming by his psychical work this resistance to association.

Sometimes this procedure, starting from where the patient's waking retrospection breaks off, points the further path through memories of which he has remained aware; sometimes it draws attention to connections which have been forgotten; sometimes it calls up and arranges recollections which have been withdrawn from association for many years but which can still be recognized as recollections; and sometimes, finally, at the climax of its achievement in the way of reproductive thinking, it causes thoughts to emerge which the patient will never recognize as his own, which he never "remembers," although he admits that the context calls for them inexorably, and while he becomes convinced that it is precisely these ideas that are leading to the conclusion of the analysis and the removal of his symptoms.

It is important to note that Freud is explaining psychological symptoms entirely in psychological terms of everyday life—shame, disgust, guilt, conflicting wishes, and self-defense against repugnant ideas. The "dynamic unconscious" is vividly described.

Freud described *how the analyst listens.* He stated:

But if we examine with a critical eye the account that the patient has given us without much trouble or resistance, we shall quite infallibly discover gaps and imperfections in it. At one point the train of thought will be visibly interrupted and patched up by the patient as best he may, with a turn of speech or an inadequate explanation; at another point we come upon a motive which would have to be described as a feeble one in a normal person. The patient will not recognize these deficiencies when his attention is drawn to them. But the physician will be right in looking behind the weakspots for an approach to the material in the deeper layers and in hoping that he will discover precisely there the connecting threads for which he is seeking with the pressure procedure. Accordingly, we say to the patient: "You are mistaken; what you are putting forward can have nothing to do with the present subject. We must expect to come upon something else here, and this will occur to you. . ."

Freud also gave a description of *transference:*

I have already indicated the important part played by the figure of the physician in creating motives to defeat the psychical force or resistance. In not a few cases, especially with women, and where it is a question of elucidating erotic trains of thought, the patient's co-operation becomes a personal sacrifice, which must be compensated by some substitute for love. The trouble taken by the physician and his friendliness have to suffice for such a substitute. If, now, this relation of the patient to the physician is disturbed, her co-operativeness fails, too; when the physician tries to investigate the next pathological idea, the patient is held up by an intervening consciousness of the complaints against the physician that had been accumulating in her.

In discussing when this obstacle arises, he says,

"the patient is frightened at finding that she is transferring onto the figure of the physician the distressing ideas which arise from the content of the analysis. This is a frequent, and indeed in some analyses a regular, occurrence. Transference onto the physician takes place through a *false connection.*"

Finally, Freud has given a clear description of the origins of neurotic symptoms and, by implication, of neurotic character styles. An early traumatic experience is reawakened by a later traumatic event that threatens the patient with fear, shame, guilt, or disgust as the unwanted memories threaten to become conscious. In an effort to avoid these painful states, the patient *represses* the unacceptable memories and institutes maladaptive defenses (symptoms, distortions of memory or perception) to ensure against their becoming conscious.

In an extraordinary burst of creative energy, Freud had by 1895 described a major portion of the technical elements related to psychoanalysis—the technique of free association, the concept of the dynamic unconscious, the experience of intrapsychic conflict over wishes and their attendant guilt and shame, the phenomenon of resistance, the defense that is constructed to protect against the recognition of the wish and the experience of the guilt, the role of interpretation, the appearance of transference, and a theory of neurosogenesis. These discoveries were essentially clinical, that is observational, with little in the way of theory. These clinical roots of psychoanalysis have been solidly confirmed during the many decades since Freud's original description.

The Structure of Psychoanalytic Theory

Having discovered the basic elements of the psychoanalytic situation, the dynamic unconscious and psychic conflict, Freud set out to create a complete scientific theory of the mind. His original, and

never fully abandoned intention, as revealed in the posthumously published "Project" of 1895,[7] was to root this theory in the advanced neurophysiology of his time. As he realized this was not yet possible, he rededicated himself to the task of constructing a *psychological* theory of the mind and wrote two of his major works: "The Interpretation of Dreams"[8] and "Three Essays on Sexuality."[9] It is beyond the scope of this chapter to attempt a detailed description of these works. Rather, only a few of the important conclusions and some of their consequences are mentioned.

Freud's solution to the riddle of the meaning of dreams provided him with the opportunity to demonstrate that the crucial findings of his earlier work with hysteria (unconscious wishes, intrapsychic conflict, infantile trauma) were not only present in pathologic conditions but were also a regular part of universal human experience; in fact, they were basic to understanding all behavior.

Freud's theory of dreams was an anchoring point not only for his concepts of neurosogenesis but also for his important theories of creativity. One cannot do justice to that theory in this brief description, but it can be emphasized that, for Freud, dreams were the psychological, mental device by which the sleeping individual maintained his sleeping state against the anxieties aroused by infantile, sexual, or aggressive wishes that arose during sleep. It was Freud's view that some events of the prior day (the day residue) had established unconscious connection with and had activated repressed infantile wishes. Under conditions of the weakened attention of the ego during sleep, the aroused desires sought access to consciousness. These infantile wishes are unacceptable to the more mature ego because of their sexual and aggressive content, and their potential eruption into consciousness threatens sleep. Therefore, the ego resistances are mustered to maintain repression. Under usual conditions the dreamer maintains sleep because the now-anxious ego exerts "censorship" to convert the dream wishes into disguised visual contents that represent a compromise formation. On the one hand, the *manifest* dream (the dream as dreamed) might seem meaningless and random and harmless; and on the other the *latent* content, the underlying wishes, are given expression in the form of symbols and sequences whose meanings are disguised. Freud gave the name "primary process" to the nature of thought under the conditions of being unconscious. In contrast to the logical, conscious thought of "secondary process," primary process is marked by a disregard of logical rules, absence of the sense of time (past and present are melded), absence of negation, immediate gratification, mutuality of opposites (no and yes lose distinction), representation of the whole by a part (a breast is a mother), and the use of such mental mechanisms as condensation (representing several meanings in a single image), and displacement (attaching affect derived from one situation to a different one). Primary process represents the continuation in the unconscious of the mode of thought of the infant and young child; it is a normal aspect of the mind and crucial for the understanding of symbol formation in literature, art, and culture, as well as in dreams. In fact, most conscious mental activity may be viewed as a compromise formation resulting from unconscious wishes and the defenses against them, which permit disguised, attenuated forms of those wishes to reach consciousness.

The "Interpretation of Dreams," one of the great works of Western culture, powerfully influenced the way a human views himself in his world. All actions are multiply determined, the past is always part of our present, and our conscious aims provide partial representation of the actual goals toward which we are driven unwillingly by unconscious forces. Current research on the physiology and neurochemistry of sleep are complementary rather than contradictory to the explanations offered by Freud.

The "Three Essays on Sexuality" represented Freud's attempt to explain the origin and nature of the infantile wishes that were so crucial in his view of mental functioning. Freud's original claim that neurosis was caused by the trauma of a childhood seduction collapsed after he gathered further data, both from patients and self-analysis, that suggested that many reported seductions were products of imagination. This crucial finding presented Freud with a crisis, during which he contemplated giving up his psychological work. But Freud had a special gift for capitalizing on what seemed to be reverses. He soon realized that in disproving his former theory, he had come on new data that provided even more interesting possibilities—that these imagined sexual events of childhood had been imagined precisely because they represented the child's desires (*i.e.*, they were imagined wish fulfillments).

Influenced by the work of Darwin, Freud then took a further step and suggested that wishing is the psychological representation of biologically organized drives, originating in the evolutionarily determined constitution of the human organism. He postulated that every individual has an inborn developmental sequence of sexual stages and that neurosis occurs because of excessive frustration or premature gratification or excessive strength of the instinct at any one of these stages. In collaboration with Abraham, he described oral, anal, phallic, and genital phases of development. The energy of the sexual instinct, in the course of development focused initially on the mouth, later the anus, then at the phallus or clitoris, and finally achieved maturity at the genitals, where the aim is union with another person. The drive at each stage has specific aims and object (*e.g.*, the aim of the oral drive is sucking and its object is some appropriate part of the body, preferably the nipple), and the drive creates a tension in the organism that is relieved by carrying out the appropriate phase-specific activity. Although each phase consisted of both core instinctual wish and a characteristic psychic organization, Freud's emphasis at this time was on the innate sequence of drive development.

The hypothesis turned out to be enormously fruitful in the interpretation of dreams, neurosis, and normal behavior. It provided the bridge from infantile behaviors to complex adult behaviors and character traits. For example, Freud was able to derive aspects of the obsessional personality from the responses of the infant during the anal phase of development, as he is confronted with the prospect of giving up pleasures associated with the retention or expulsion of feces, with consequent guilty anger at his educators. The outcome of this "battle of the pot" can be the development of retentive or obedient defensive reaction formations (excessive neatness, obstinacy, and parsimony) or the persistence of defiant expulsions.

Sexual development culminates in the Oedipus complex, a drive-determined sequence in human development in which the child sexually desires the parent of the opposite sex and wishes for the elimination of the parent of the same sex. The Oedipus complex was for Freud "the nuclear complex of the neuroses,"[9] the time that the child recognizes a full world of objects, including the father as well as the mother, and is confronted by the full power of external threat and internal superego to give up unacceptable sexual and aggressive wishes. Freud, writing of the male child, concluded that castration anxiety was regularly aroused by the powerful desires of the Oedipus complex because of the fear that the father would angrily retaliate for the son's desire to be rid of him. It is this castration anxiety, internalized in one's own unconscious as a punitive superego, that ensures adherence to social morality.

These propositions concerning the origin and nature of the sexual drives and their role in mental life were organized by Freud into the *libido theory*. This is an experience-distant theory that was a part of Freud's program to construct a metapsychology, a high level of general theory, from which specific findings of psychoanalysis could be derived. Freud postulated a sexual energy, libido, that was the source of all psychological actions. In later years he added a second drive, aggression, and considered that derivatives of libido and aggression motivated all actions. In the libido theory, neurotic symptoms are traced to excessive frustrations and gratifications met by inborn sexual instincts in interaction with the environment of early childhood (most especially in relationships within the family). Excessive gratification at any stage (either because of constitutional or environmental factors) might promote fixation at that stage. Excessive frustration at any stage might promote regression to an earlier stage. Failures of psychosexual development toward mature genitality result in excessive amounts of the more primitive oral, anal, or phallic libido. These are discharged directly in the oral, anal, or phallic perversions, are defended against through neurotic symptoms or character traits, or are sublimated. Direct expression of infantile genital libidinal instincts is inhibited by the prohibitions and repressions occasioned by the incest taboo that accompanies resolution of the Oedipus complex. Freud observed that all earlier stages of development represent modes of psychic organization to which individuals may *regress* under adaptive stress. For example, the toilet-trained child may begin to soil again when a new sibling arrives, threatening his bond to his mother. *Regression* is a universal capacity occurring under normal and pathologic circumstances.

Today many analysts would regard the libido theory as a useful metaphor and would not give heed to the quantitative, energic aspect to which Freud gave so much attention. Nonetheless, the theory fostered discoveries connecting adult character traits to childhood experience and revealing the unconscious wishes and fears behind conscious symptoms. Many analysts today also prefer to see the developmental expression of drives as more interwoven with their objects, rather than pursuing an innate course of independent development. This issue will be discussed in the section on object relations theory. A general tendency in psychoanalytic theory has been to give increasing attention to the perceived reality of the environment of development (psychic reality) and to give less heed to the innate instinctual course of development. Hartmann and others have pointed out that the infant is born preadapted to "an average expectable environment," and the drives depend, for their development, on appropriate cues and stimuli from that environment.

THE TOPOGRAPHIC MODEL OF PSYCHIC CONFLICT

Freud, in his early work, divided the mind into conscious, unconscious (actively repressed), and preconscious (out of awareness, but available on the focus of attention). This *topographic* model of the mind emphasized the distinction between conscious and unconscious (repressed) mental contents, regarding this distinction as the central guiding principle for the understanding of intrapsychic conflict. The self-preservative instincts of the conscious ego struggle to prevent the "dangerous" access to consciousness of repressed, unacceptable thoughts and feelings, thereby avoiding guilt, shame, and fear of punishment. All the varied mechanisms of defense are called into action by the ego to achieve this goal. From the point of view of the topographic model, the aim of analysis is to make the unconscious conscious, thereby permitting a cognitive and affective reassessment of residual infantile wishes and fears, since unconscious thoughts and feelings are inaccessible to learning and new experience. Freud regarded his discovery of the characteristics of the dynamic unconscious as one of his most important and original contributions.

THE STRUCTURAL MODEL OF PSYCHIC CONFLICT

As Freud progressed in his researches, he realized that many of the ego resistances and defenses against unconscious wishes were themselves unconscious, as were certain self-punitive tendencies. This blurring of the content distinction between conscious and unconscious led to the development of the *structural model*.

This is the convenient grouping of mental functions into three agencies of the mind (id, ego, superego) distinguished by different origins, purposes, and modes of operation. The id describes the instinctual determinants of behavior, the libidinal and aggressive wishes. The ego refers to the executive agency of the mind, controlling the regulatory functions of defense, affect and impulse modulation, reality testing, and synthesis and mediation among the varying demands of id, superego, and the external world in order to preserve the organism's well-being. The superego refers to the agency of conscience that sets internalized standards, inspires guilt and shame when these are not achieved, and provides pride and satisfaction when they are. The id is inborn and only minimally subject to the influence of experience. Both the ego and superego have inborn constituents but are much shaped by experience. The id remains unconscious and is known only through its derivatives. The ego and superego have both conscious and unconscious components.

This tripartite structural model has proved enormously useful in delineating the components of intrapsychic conflict and in fostering the exploration of these different psychic functions. Although the understanding of the id was the aim of early psychoanalytic investigations, beginning with Freud's "Inhibitions, Symptoms and Anxiety,"[10] the focus shifted toward elucidating the ego and superego and their regulatory functions. From the structural point of view, the aim of analysis is that "where id was, there shall ego be."

By this point in his researches, Freud had developed a simple, elegant, and clinically useful model of unconscious conflict and he proceeded to find an extraordinarily wide application for it in the understanding of neurotic and psychotic symptoms, dreams, character, the psychopathology of everyday life, jokes, works of art, myths, fairy tales, religions, and anthropology.

Contemporary Models of Psychoanalysis

The basic model of psychoanalysis has inspired numerous thinkers to develop special elaborations of the theory in an effort to account better for the ever-increasing quantity and complexity of analytic information. The different modern models tend to vary mainly in giving different emphases to instinct, ego-regulatory mechanism, the role of object relations, the place of external reality, the nature of the self, or the inherent health or neuroticism of the "normal" person. This chapter cannot attempt to do justice to all the workers who have proposed important new ideas in psychoanalysis. Furthermore, the work of those who began with Freud and went on to form alternate and competing schools, most notably Jung and Adler will be omitted.

An effort at a comprehensive history of psychoanalysis would, of course, give prominent mention to these and other figures. The justification for omitting them, apart from the unyielding constraints of space, is the belief that the major ideas of many of these schools have been incorporated into the corpus of "mainstream" psychoanalysis, although often without adequate acknowledgment of the sources of the ideas. There are, of course, important remaining differences among the separate schools, and anyone interested in tracing the history of ideas within psychoanalysis, or wishing a more detailed view of the work of those omitted here, may be referred to the excellent works of Ellenberger,[11] Havens,[12] Wyss,[13] or Munroe.[14]

THE EGO PSYCHOLOGICAL MODEL

The predominant version of psychoanalysis in the United States has been the ego psychological point of view. Beginning with *The Ego and the Id*[15] and greatly enriched by the many new ideas in *Inhibitions, Symptoms and Anxiety,* major interest in psychoanalytic theory and technique began to shift from a focus on the stages and expressions of drive development to the modes by which the ego established its controlling and regulatory functions over the "mental apparatus." Two works, *The Ego and the Mechanisms of Defense,*[16] by Anna Freud, and *Ego Psychology and the Problem of Adaptation*[17] by Hartmann, contributed enormously to the development of ego psychology.

The ego psychological view emphasizes that the ego's mastery and modulation of id demands and superego prohibitions is an essential shaper of personality characteristics and the only point of access to unconscious wishes and defensive mental processes. Any modifications of psychic structure and changes in the relative strengths of drives and defenses will come about through the mediating influence of the ego, since the latter is the only portion of the psyche in communication with the external world. Anna Freud in her work emphasized the central role of defensive processes in shaping behavior.

In "Inhibitions, Symptoms and Anxiety," Freud had clearly described the role of the mechanisms of defense; the ego, threatened by the anticipation of a danger situation, responds with an anxiety signal (a subliminal dose of the feared danger) and upon this signal initiates defense mechanisms (such as regression, denial, reaction-formation, projection, isolation, and conversion) intended to ward off the danger. This entire process occurs outside of awareness; the most successful defenses proceed silently, altering perception and behavior so that the danger situation will become neither conscious nor actual. Freud described a developmental sequence of prototypal danger situations that throughout life would be the occasions for the signal of anxiety: (1) fear of separation (*i.e.,* loss of the mother); (2) fear of the loss of the mother's love (*i.e.,* fear of the mother's anger and disapproval); (3) fear of castration (*i.e.,* fear of the father's retaliation for the sexual and aggressive wishes of the Oedipus complex); and (4) fear of the loss of the superego's love (*i.e.,* fear of the punitive inner conscience and its demand for guilt and punishment if now internalized standards are not met).

Anna Freud's work constituted an elaboration of these findings and a plea to analysts to realize that the alleviation of neurotic symptoms and character dispositions had to proceed from changes in the ego's tolerance of and responses to danger situations. The effort of psychoanalysis, increasingly, became the delineation and alteration of the characterologic maladaptive defenses as these became manifest in the resistance and transference of the treatment situation. Hartmann extended this view by emphasizing the effort of the ego at every moment to achieve the best adaptation available given and its particular repertoire of capacities and defenses. Hartmann contradicted earlier views in which the instincts were seen as all-powerful forces dominating a puny ego attempting to operate with borrowed energies of the id. Instead, in Hartmann's conception, the ego has its own line of development, beginning as a body ego, and many of its functions (*i.e.,* anticipation, affect) are not resultants of conflict but were the ego's integral apparatus for achieving adaptedness to the environment. He labeled these the autonomous ego functions.

The superego, a specially developed self-critical agency of the ego, also became the object of scrutiny under the ego-psychological point of view. Two portions of the superego are distinguished: (1) the ego ideal, the internalized set of standards against which all behavior is measured, and (2) the unconscious conscience, which demands punishment in the form of guilt and suffering if ego-ideal standards are not met. It is a characteristic of the superego that it tends to be far more harsh than the parents, whose standards presumably were internalized, perhaps because the child's defiant rage at having to give up his own hedonic regulation in favor of that of his parents is added to the punitiveness of the actual parents. Furthermore, the uncon-

sciously operating conscience does not distinguish thoughts from acts—a murderous thought is the equivalent of a murderous deed, and the demand for guilt is as great as if the act had occurred.

The observation of ego and superego functioning constituted an important advance in analytic theory and technique, possibly saving psychoanalysis from a sterile emphasis on primitive functioning of drives. This would have neglected the all-important mediating processes that distinguish each individual and encode the individual's history, which he has internalized. Ego psychology also has the merit of retaining Freud's basic concepts of development, psychic structure, neurosogenesis, and the central role of the Oedipus complex.

There have been many variants and modifications of ego psychology, but only the work of Erikson is discussed here.[18] Erikson emphasized that the psychosexual stages of development expressed not only a biological need but also cultural and interpersonal needs of the developing individual. He described a "life cycle" of stages, each of which presented the organism with tasks to be achieved and a developmental "crisis" during its attempted achievement. Where Freud centered development around the psycho*sexual* stages of the infant and child, Erikson was interested in the psycho*social* stages throughout the life cycle. His famous chart of the life cycle demonstrates his effort (Fig. 1).

The infant in the psychosexual oral-sensory stage (his bodily zone for contacting the outside world is the mouth and his mode of contact is sensation) has the psychosocial task of establishing "basic trust" in his tending mother (against tendencies to mistrust because of failures of parental care). The infant who establishes a firm sense of basic trust (the ability to see the world as both gratifying and predictable with an accompanying growth of self confidence) will be better equipped to negotiate the next phase in which he is confronted with the task of establishing a sense of autonomy. Failure to achieve a sense of growing autonomy, either because of already damaged adaptive capacities or because of the failure of adequate support from the environment, will leave the young child with excessive shame and doubt, further handicapping his ability to surmount the "crisis" of the next developmental stage. Erikson viewed development as proceeding through phases of epigenesis (*i.e.,* the changes of maturation were not gradual and smooth, but proceeded by leaps from one form of organization to another, the later phase not necessarily prefigured in the earlier one.

	1.	2.	3.	4.	5.	6.	7.	8.
I. INFANCY	Trust vs. Mistrust				Unipolarity vs. Premature Self-Differentation			
II. EARLY CHILDHOOD		Autonomy vs. Shame, Doubt			Bipolarity vs. Autism			
III. PLAY AGE			Initiative vs. Guilt		Play Identification vs. (oedipal) Fantasy Identities			
IV. SCHOOL AGE				Industry vs. Inferiority	Work Identification vs. Identity Foreclosure			
V. ADOLESCENCE	Time Perspective vs. Time Diffusion	Self-Certainty vs. Identity Consciousness	Role Experimentation vs. Negative Identity	Anticipation of Achievement vs. Work Paralysis	Identity vs. Identity Diffusion	Sexual Identity vs. Bisexual Diffusion	Leadership Polarization vs. Authority Diffusion	Ideological Polarization vs. Diffusion of Ideals
VI. YOUNG ADULT					Solidarity vs. Social Isolation	Intimacy vs. Isolation		
VII. ADULTHOOD							Generativity vs. Self-Absorption	
VIII. MATURE AGE								Integrity vs. Disgust, Despair

FIG. 1. Erikson's life cycle of stages. (Erikson E: Childhood and Society. New York, WW Norton, 1950).

One cannot predict the butterfly from the morphology of the chrysalis).

Erikson's work provided an important corrective to a tendency to view behavior simply as the result of sexual and aggressive drives and their modulation. He provided for the role of culture in shaping the special human meanings that these drive derivatives acquire, and he showed how complex culturally based "virtues" evolve from biologically determined somatic origins. In some respects Erikson's work has been a bridge between ego psychology and object relations theory; his views of identification, introjection, and ego identity as core processes for building the personality provide mechanisms for understanding the ways in which the environment of child rearing is internalized.

OBJECT RELATIONS THEORY

Klein was one of the originators of child psychoanalysis, perhaps the inventor of play therapy, and she developed her theories of object relations on the basis of her direct experience with children.[19–21] It was her view that the capacity for fantasy is one of the earliest, primitive psychological abilities and that these fantasies follow a regular sequence of patterning reflecting the infant's experience of interaction with the mother. In contrast to Freud's original psychosexual schema, which described development as a set of internal pressures leading to action in the outside world, Klein focused on the changing landscape of the internal world as development proceeded. She assumed the infant to be involved with the mother from the start of life, both in external reality and in internal fantasy. Originally, the infant is prone to experience himself as the omnipotent source of all gratifications and to perceive the outside world—mother—as a source of frustration. Klein described this as the *paranoid position,* believing that in this early stage (perhaps birth to 6 months) the infant views himself as the hostile target of the giant mother's evil manipulations and projects into the mother all of his own angry feelings. In the normal course of events, the infant also begins to internalize the mother's loving ministrations and increasingly has a sense of his dependence on and need for the loved and loving mother. Although providing feelings of comfort and safety, this new realization also, however, leads to what Klein termed the *depressive position,* as the infant becomes guiltily aware of his murderous rage toward the loved mother and fears the loss of that mother. Klein believed that these internalized object relations to the mother, initially paranoid, later depressed, are part of the psychic core of all humans, and are points of regression in later life.

Klein's views have been modified in many respects, but the term *object relations theory* applies to the many derivatives of her work. The term emphasizes the view that the mind is, from the start, made up of internal representations of the relationship of the infant to its objects. This is in contrast to Freud's view that the mind begins with instinctual urges that are object seeking, with the objects only secondarily becoming part of the mental contents. Klein gave great emphasis to complex, apparently "pre-wired" fantasies in the very early infant, implying an unlearned knowledge of sexuality, the Oedipus complex, and the experiences of envy and gratitude and paranoia and depression. Many others have objected to the degree of psychological organization hypothesized for a relatively unformed nervous system. Analysts who found merit in Klein's views constructed numerous variants of her theory, emphasizing the central role of early internalized infant–object interaction in shaping the development of psychic structure. Among these should be mentioned Fairbairn,[22] Bion,[23] Winnicott,[24] Guntrip,[25] and Kernberg.[26]

Although these workers have different views on many aspects of psychoanalytic theory and technique, they agree that the drives are amalgams of id wishes, internalized objects, and accompanying affect states, differing from the traditional Freudian view of drives. The object relations theorists also give central importance to processes of "splitting"; the capacity of the infant to divide a single object—mother—into separate good and bad mothers depending on the infant's experience of gratification or frustration. The successful integration of these split images, the achievement of "object constancy" some time around age 2 1/2, enables the child to retain a single mental representation of an object that is both frustrating and gratifying, a whole person, and is an essential step in development. Regression to, or fixation on, splitting mechanisms is common in more severe pathologic states particularly the borderline personality.

SELF THEORY

Kohut developed a powerful and influential variant of psychoanalysis that held the structure and vicissitudes of the self to be the central organizer of psychic development.[27,28] In his view, self-psychology was the logical next step following id-psychology and ego-psychology. Its primary focus is on the maturation of the sense of self from its infantile state of fragility and fragmentation into the cohesive and stable structure of adulthood. Concern with the self or identity is to be found in earlier analytic writings, but Kohut placed it in a central position.

Kohut postulated that the infant psyche is endowed with the germs of a bipolar self-organization characterized by two major trends. At one pole are the tendencies toward grandiosity and exhibitionism—the beginnings of assertiveness and ambition—and at the other pole are the tendencies toward idealization of the parents—the beginnings of ideals and values. Both the exhibitionist wish for an audience and the idealizing admiration of the parents contribute to the strong self-object ties between infant and parent, which are the basis for the achievement of a healthy self. These two poles are connected by a tension arc of talents and skills that develops over time and provides the means for connecting grandiose ambitions with internalized idealized goals. One aspect of appropriate maternal care is the way in which the empathically resonant mother provides the mirroring approval of the child's exhibitionisms and also allows herself to be idealized by the adoring child. This empathic mothering is an essential ingredient for the development of a healthy self.

The sexual and aggressive drives so emphasized by Freud and central to his theory of development are viewed by self psychology as "disintegration products" that appear when self-development is disturbed; they are not the movers of psychic development. That role is played by the self, which is an independent center of initiative. Kohut uses the term *selfobject* to refer to the infant's failure entirely to distinguish inside and outside in its earliest relationships; the selfobject is a significant object in the environment perceived as a part of oneself, without which one feels incomplete. Although all humans require relationships to objects to maintain a firm sense of self, there are great variations in the *extent* to which the object is perceived as either separate and having its own needs, or as an integral part of the self. Patients who present with narcissistic personality disorder are characterized by their failure to separate adequately from the selfobject and are thus unable to perceive or respond to the individuality of these valued persons.

Kohut maintained that the major pathology of most patients seeking psychoanalytic help was not conflictual (the conflicts were secondary phenomena) but was a deficit in the structure of the self. Due to failure of early empathic mothering, aspects of the self, in one or both its poles, had become enfeebled. It was this lack of firm self structure that led to the conflicts on which classical psychoanalysis had focused its attention. Humans engaged in these conflicts of what Kohut termed Freud's "Guilty

Man," the effort to achieve relief from inner inhibition and punishment, contrasted to the plight of "Tragic Man," who attempted to realize his inherent inner program of self-fulfillment in the world. The emphasis on deficit, rather than conflict, leads to different prescriptions for the role of the analyst in the psychoanalytic situation. Rather than attempting to be a neutral screen, the analyst needs to be aware of the damage done by a previously unempathic environment and to be alert to the ways in which the psychoanalytic situation reproduces or alters that earlier experience. Change occurs through the effect of "transmuting internalizations" of the new experience with the analyst—the same process by which development originally occurs. The building of new structure is given precedence over conflict resolution, and the process requires that the patient be permitted to regress to early stages of self-development so that the resumption of new healthy growth may begin at the point of its disruption during development. Kohut emphasized the need for empathic responsiveness on the part of the analyst, recognizing the individual needs of each patient, rather than adopting a standard analytic rule to be applied to all patients. Some patients require muted responsiveness on the analyst's part, while others require a more vivid presence, depending on the nature of the earlier failures of empathic response.

Kohut's work began as an attempt to replace the abstruseness of Freud's metapsychology with an experience-near description of the developmental process as it was revealed in the analysis of severe narcissistic personality disorders. He placed great weight on the importance of empathy as both the investigative mode of psychoanalytic investigation and as the essential ingredient of the mother–infant tie. As Kohut's theory grew, it became highly abstract in its own right and claims were made that it serves as a replacement of Freud's theoretic structure rather than as correction of it. Kohut's work bears marked similarities to aspects of the works of Sullivan, Winnicott, and Rogers. Winnicott emphasized the core structure of the "True Self" in the healthy psyche, a structure that could develop only in the presence of what he called "good-enough mothering." Winnicott, like Kohut, also viewed the patient's transference responses as reflecting both the patient's previous experiences and the actual behavior of the analyst in precipitating a recurrence of the patient's response. Transference is an interactive process, rather than one that the patient alone brings to a neutral situation.

Self-psychology has generated a heated debate in American psychoanalysis, with charges that it represents a return to a shallow therapy of corrective emotional experience, rather than depth psychology, an avoidance of sex and aggression, and a loss of the conflict-based theory of traditional analysis in favor of a holistic and less penetrating theory and technique. Many claim that it is "nothing new." The verdict is certainly not in, but the dispute has so far led to a useful scrutiny of traditional propositions and subtle changes in analysts' acknowledgement of the mutuality of the psychoanalytic situation. It has also led to an as yet inconclusive debate of the question of whether psychoanalysis deals only with psychic reality (the constructed reality of the adult patient who presents his past through the filter of his needs and defenses) or whether the psychoanalytic situation provides a reasonably accurate picture of the actual environment of development. Kohut firmly believed the latter; patients fall ill because of real failures of empathy, not because of isolated drive and superego predispositions. This view has much in common with the interpersonal theory.

INTERPERSONAL PSYCHOANALYSIS

Sullivan, an American working in New York and Washington, developed what he termed *interpersonal psychoanalysis*.[29] At the core of Sullivan's system is the view that there is no possibility of conceiving of a human in isolation: we are only human as a part of a human environment. Rather than theorizing about the infant as an autonomous unit housing its instinctual innate program of development, he conceived the mother–infant dyad as the original unit out of which the infant self will take on the particular features of its individuality. The idea of the "individual" is a philosophic fiction, since we assume our human attributes only in interpersonal interactions, whether internal or external. Sullivan attempted to replace the 19th century mechanistic, scientific base of psychoanalysis with a more modern relativistic stance. He also tried to construct an operational language that would replace the traditional language of metapsychology.

In Sullivan's view the basic motivators of behavior are the satisfaction of bodily needs (*e.g.*, hunger, sex, attachment) and security needs (*e.g.*, love, approval). The empathic relationship of mother and child is crucial for the child's development. Core affects such as anxiety are learned by the child through their transmission by the mother. It is assumed that the child is an accurate registrar of the mother's emotional state, which is communicated subtly. The child's need to avoid the intolerable affect of anxiety and to feel a sense of control over its environment leads to the construction of defenses and psychic structures.

Central importance is given to what Sullivan termed the *self-dynamism*, a dynamic regulatory structure that includes the self-representation and the state of self-esteem. The self-dynamism arises through the reflected appraisals of others, basically approving or disapproving. Basic good and bad feeling states lead to internalized constructs of good and bad self and good and bad nipple (mother). Under optimal conditions, the child receives a preponderance of positive reinforcements, has a predominant sense of good experience, and condenses the two selves and mothers into a single satisfying representation. Neurosis is the consequence of bad experience with an unsatisfying mother, leading to maladaptive defenses and defective self-dynamism.

Interpersonal theory proposes that the psychoanalyst is always a "participant observer" in his interaction with the patient and must acknowledge his full role as a person, being changed by the patient as he helps the patient to change. The therapeutic task is to help the patient, under conditions of a new experience, to change his self-esteem patterns, to reduce perceptual distortions, and to devise new and more adaptive patterns of defense and coping. Like a good mother, the good analyst depends on empathy to guide him in recognizing and helping the patient to reduce his anxieties.

For many decades, Sullivan was accorded little recognition within mainstream psychoanalysis. In recent years, with increasing attention to the self, and the enhanced role accorded the environment in shaping inner development, there has been renewed recognition of the importance of Sullivan's work.

ADDITIONAL SOURCES OF MODERN PSYCHOANALYSIS

At least three major nonanalytic sources have played an important role in shaping the current psychoanalytic model. These sources are ethology, infant observation and experimentation, and hermeneutic philosophy. Others, such as linguistics and systems theory have had significant influence but not to the extent of these three. It is likely that each of these fields will continue to nourish psychoanalytic thinking, and a few of the influences already apparent are mentioned here.

Bowlby, in his major work on separation, attachment, and loss[30] drew heavily on the observations of the major ethologists (particularly Tin-bergen, Lorenz, and Harlow) to outline a different model of the instinctual endowment of the child. His own work with children served as the laboratory to confirm the utility of the views he put forward. Bowlby asserted that the infant's instinctual apparatus is primarily designed to ensure its proximity to and continuing emotional interaction with its mother. The relation to the mother is not a phenomenon secondary to the infant's need for food or warmth but is a primary array of instinctual behaviors that release caring and attachment responses from the mother, who in turn elicits new stimuli from the infant. Bowlby described a regular sequence of protest, despair, and detachment occurring when a child is separated from its mother and produced data indicating irreparable emotional damage if the mother–child tie is disrupted during the second year of life. Spitz had already demonstrated that children who lack a reliable tie to a mothering, loving tender person during earliest infancy will not thrive. Bowlby's work, shedding new light on the sources of anxiety and depression, has demonstrated that the development of the child's instinctual endowment is embedded in the relationship with the mother and continuously shaped by interactions between the two. He also demonstrated the value of incorporating observations from animal studies into psychoanalytic theory and research.

Infant researchers, including Piaget,[31] Mahler,[32] Stern,[33] and Emde[34] have revealed a surprisingly sophisticated array of endowments with which the infant confronts his universe. Abilities for recognition, memory, and classification of simple and complex states (*e.g.*, colors and affective states) develop far earlier than had been previously been assumed. In many instances, these were a part of the process of maturation and do not require learning. The realization of the infant's complex capacities at a few months of age has led to reconsideration of the phasing of many of the crucial psychological events of development.

Mahler has played a very important role in current psychoanalytic thought with her and her colleagues' focused researches on the processes by which the child moves from an originally symbiotic attachment in order to achieve separation from his mother and gradually to develop a sense of his own individual self. Clinicians have given increasing attention to the vicissitudes of separation-individuation in attempting to understand some of the more severe personality disorders, and the subtleties of the mother–infant interaction in negotiating the infant's increasing capacity for separateness and the accompanying fears and angers.

There has been considerable disagreement in recent years concerning the value of Freud's higher-level theoretic formulations—his metapsychology. Although Freud was deeply concerned to ensure that psychoanalysis would remain rooted in biology, other psychoanalysts, including Klein,[35] Schafer,[36] and Gill and Holt,[37] have asserted that the valuable propositions of psychoanalysis are the clinical ones and that these are entirely psychological, deriving their power from their capacity to give meaning to otherwise incomprehensible human experiences. Ricouer, a philosopher of religion, in his book *Freud and Philosophy*,[38] emphasized that psychoanalysis was essentially a hermeneutic (*i.e.,* interpretive) activity. It sought for meanings in human creations, particularly the meanings in the communications to the analyst, treating these as a special text. The biological roots of the communication are not relevant, since what is sought is not the cause but the ways in which symbols are endowed with meaning. Schafer has emphasized the narrative aspects of the patient's analytic history—the tale that unfolds during analysis—and the ways in which that narrative changes during the multiple retellings of the story during the course of the analysis, as both teller and listener progressively change. For Schafer, the issue is not to discover the "true" version of the history but to help the patient to come to as complete and coherent a version of his history as he can at that time. The hermeneutic point of view is currently productive and persuasive to many psychoanalysts.

Validation

In recent years, there has been increasing pressure both from within and outside the psychoanalytic community for validation studies testing psychoanalytic hypotheses and clinical results. Many studies have been conducted testing specific and usually peripheral hypotheses, but little research has been done concerning major clinical findings and treatment outcome. There has also been continuing controversy whether psychoanalytic propositions are cast in a form that is amenable to scientific investigation.

The difficulties of testing psychodynamics hypotheses include the following:

Many propositions are difficult to operationalize.
It is difficult to construct reliable instruments to measure subtle, inferred, unconscious mental processes.
Each behavior involves multiple interacting determinants so that it is difficult to isolate the influence of single variables.
Variables of interest are often by their nature difficult or impossible to control.
Psychoanalysis extends over long periods of time and research designs often require great patience.
Psychoanalytic education is conducted outside academic institutions, and psychoanalysis has not evolved a research tradition and method.

Psychoanalysis developed its scientific base through naturalistic data collection and inductive reasoning. Many of Freud's hypotheses were closely derived from clinical observation and validated with further observations. Validation through the weight of evidence is a legitimate scientific technique and, despite the epistemologic weaknesses of this approach, is often the only one available in complex fields. Medicine has advanced through the combination of systematic, clinical observation and controlled experimentation.

The scientific maturation of psychoanalysis and political and social forces are creating new opportunities and demands for high quality research in psychoanalysis. The availability of increasingly powerful, multivariate statistical methods and number-crunching computers make more complex and interesting questions amenable to study. There are many signs that the psychoanalytic profession has begun to apply itself to do the research the field requires. The relatively recent emergence of brief forms of psychodynamic (*i.e.,* focal) therapy provides a convenient arena for psychodynamic process and outcome research and for comparisons of psychodynamic with other types of psychotherapy to determine if specific interventions have specific effects. Malan's naturalistic studies[39] indicate that transference/parent linking interpretations have a significant correlation with psychodynamic change. Psychodynamic therapies remain the most prevalent in psychiatric practice and deserve to be studied extensively. The availability of focal therapy and instruments that measure psychodynamic process and outcome make this increasingly technically feasible.

There have been numerous psychodynamic studies relating anxiety to oral, anal, and genital levels of psychosexual development and their associated personality types. Specific mothering styles have been associated with the development of individuals with the oral personality traits of anxiety and separation difficulties.[40–42]

In a longitudinal study, Kagan and Moses[43] demonstrated that oral traits (dependency, passivity, and separation anxiety) correlate with one another and persist from birth to adulthood, especially in females. In attempts to distinguish oral and anal anxiety, Rapaport[44] and Sarnoff and Zimbardo[45] found that oral characters chose to affiliate when faced with an oral stress and that anal characters chose to be alone when faced with a situation stressful to an anal character. Rosenwald[46] found that the degree to which individuals expressed anxiety about anal matters predicted their obstinacy and need to arrange piles of magazines. Many other studies have confirmed intercorrelations of aspects of the oral and anal personality and that predictions about behavior can be made based on this level of diagnosis.[47]

Castration anxiety has been investigated in a number of studies measuring whether men are more fearful of bodily injury than are women.[48–50] Findings have been consistently in the expected direction in studies of different age-groups and using different methods of measurement (including projective test, manifest content of dreams, and verbal samples). Moreover, several other studies[51] indicate that castration anxiety in males is increased in response to sexually exciting stimulation. Other studies have confirmed Freud's view that anxiety about loss of love is more common in females.[52–54] There is also evidence that castration anxiety is especially prominent in homosexual males.[55,56]

The literature on psychoanalytic research has been reviewed most thoroughly by Fisher and Greenberg.[57] Although they found that many of Freud's hypotheses have yet to be tested adequately, and that some results contradict his view of the oedipal situation, most of the available experimental and observational evidence confirms Freud's observations about psychosexual stages of development and their associated fears and demonstrates the internal consistency of the model. Obviously, much more needs to be done and it seems that the tools are now available for testing both psychodynamic hypotheses and treatment methods.

Conclusion

For many years, psychoanalysis was riven by splits among different schools and was handicapped by a failure to pursue scientific aims of achieving reliable observation and scientific validation. During the past decade, this situation has begun to change. Analysts have become less interested in discovering ways in which their propositions do or do not mesh with Freud's. Instead, there are efforts toward finding the most useful and parsimonious integrations of the new data derived from infant research and neurobiology with the growing yield of psychoanalytic investigation. It is likely that the psychoanalytic model will change more rapidly in the future than it has in the past and will continue to be an extraordinarily rich and interesting way to understand normal and pathologic behaviors and to treat selected patients with personality disorders and neuroses.

REFERENCES

1. Holt RR: Manifest and latent meanings of metapsychology. Annu Psychoanal 10:247, 1982

2. Marcus S: The Other Victorians. New York, Basic Books, 1964

3. Gay P: The Bourgeois Experience. New York, Oxford University Press, 1984

4. Jones E: The Life and Work of Sigmund Freud, vols 1–3. New York, Basic Books, 1957

5. Clark RW: Freud: The Man and the Cause. New York, Random House, 1980

6. Freud S: Studies on hysteria. In Strachey J (ed): The Standard Edition of the Complete Works of Sigmund Freud, vol 2. London, Hogarth Press, 1961

7. Freud S: Project. In Strachey J (ed): The Standard Edition of the Complete Works of Sigmund Freud, vol 1, pp 283–357. London, Hogarth Press, 1961

8. Freud S: The interpretation of dreams. In Strachey J (ed): The Standard Edition of the Complete Works of Sigmund Freud, vol 4. London, Hogarth Press, 1961

9. Freud S: Three essays on sexuality. In Strachey J (ed): The Standard Edition of the Complete Works of Sigmund Freud, vol 7. London, Hogarth Press, 1961

10. Freud S: Inhibitions, symptoms and anxiety. In Strachey J (ed): The Standard Edition of the Complete Works of Sigmund Freud, vols 20 and 22. London, Hogarth Press, 1961

11. Ellenberger HF: The Discovery of the Unconscious. New York, Basic Books, 1970

12. Havens LL: Approaches to the Mind. Boston, Little Brown, & Co, 1973

13. Wyss D: Psychoanalytic Schools From the Beginning to the Present. New York, Jason Aronson, 1973

14. Munroe RL: Schools of Psychoanalytic Thought. New York, Dryden Press, 1955

15. Freud S: The ego and the id. In Strachey J (ed): The Standard Edition of the Complete Works of Sigmund Freud, vol 19, pp 3–68. London, Hogarth Press, 1961

16. Freud A: The Ego and the Mechanisms of Defense. New York, International Universities Press, 1946

17. Hartmann H: Ego Psychology and the Problem of Adaptation. New York, International Universities Press, 1958

18. Erikson E: Childhood and Society, p 273. New York, WW Norton, 1950

19. Klein M: Contributions to Psycho-analysis. London, Hogarth Press, 1948

20. Klein M, Riviere J: Love, Hate and Reparation. London, Hogarth Press, 1967

21. Klein M, Heimann P, Money-Kyrle R (eds): New Directions in Psychoanalysis. New York, Basic Books, 1955

22. Fairbairn WRD: An Object-Relations Theory of the Personality. New York, Basic Books, 1952

23. Bion WR: Seven Servants. New York, Jason Aronson, 1977

24. Winnicott DW: The Maturational Processes and the Facilitating Environment. New York, International Universities Press, 1965

25. Guntrip HJS: Personality Structure and Human Interaction: The Developing Synthesis of Psycho-dynamic Theory. New York, International Universities Press, 1961

26. Kernberg O: Object Relations Theory and Clinical Psychoanalysis. New York, Jason Aronson, 1976

27. Kohut H: The Analysis of the Self. New York, International Universities Press, 1971

28. Kohut H: The Restoration of the Self. New York, International Universities Press, 1977

29. Swick-Perry H, Ladd M, Gibbon G et al (eds): The Collective Works of Harry Stack Sullivan, M.D. New York, WW Norton, 1956

30. Bowlby J: Attachment and Loss, vols 1–3. New York, Basic Books, 1969, 1973, 1980

31. Piaget J: The Origins of Intelligence in Children. New York, International Universities Press, 1952

32. Mahler MS, Pine F, Bergman A: Psychological Birth of the Infant. New York, Basic Books, 1975

33. Stern D: The Course of Life: Psychoanalytic Contributions Toward Understanding Personality Development. Washington, DC, Mental Health Administration, 1980

34. Emde R: The Development of Attachment and Affiliative Systems. New York, Plenum Press, 1982

35. Klein G: Psychology vs. Metapsychology. New York, International Universities Press, 1976

36. Schafer R: A New Language for Psychoanalysis. New Haven, Yale University Press, 1976

37. Gill MM, Holt RR: The Primary Process: Motives and Thought. New York, International Universities Press, 1967

38. Ricouer P: Freud and Philosophy. New Haven, CT, Yale University Press, 1970

39. Malan DH: Toward the Validation of Dynamic Psychotherapy. New York, Plenum Press, 1976

40. Finney JC: Some maternal influences on children's personality and character. Genet Psychol Monogr 63:199–278, 1961

41. Goldman-Eisler F: The problem of ''orality'' and of its origins in early childhood. J Ment Sci 97:765–782, 1951

42. Whiting JW, Child IL: Child Training and Personality: A Cross-cultural Study. New Haven, CT, Yale University Press, 1953

43. Kagan J, Moses HA: The stability of passive and dependent behavior from childhood through adulthood. Child Dev 31:577–591, 1960

44. Rapaport C: Character, Anxiety and Social Affiliation, unpublished Ph.D. dissertation, New York University, 1963

45. Sarnoff I, Zimbardo PG: Anxiety, fear and social affiliation. J Abnorm Soc Psychol 62:356–363, 1961

46. Rosenwald GC: Effectiveness of defenses against anal impulse arousal. J Consult Clin Psychiatry 39:292–298, 1972

47. Lazare A, Klerman GL, Amor DJ: Oral, obsessive and hysterical personality patterns. Arch Gen Psychiatry 14:624–630, 1966

48. Blum GS: A study of the psychoanalytic theory of psychosexual development. Genet Psychol Monogr 39:3–99, 1949

49. Gottschalk LA, Glesar GC, Springer KJ: Three hostility scales applicable to verbal samples. Arch Gen Psychiatry 9:254–279, 1963

50. Pitcher EG, Prelinger E: Children Tell Stories: An Analysis of Fantasy. New York, International Universities Press, 1963

51. Sarnoff I, Corwin SM: Castration anxiety and the fear of death. J Personality 27:374–385, 1959

52. Bradford JL: Sex Differences in Anxiety, unpublished Ph.D. dissertation, University of Minnesota, 1968

53. Gleser GC, Gottschalk LA, Springer KJ: An anxiety scale applicable to verbal samples. Arch Gen Psychiatry 5:593–605, 1961

54. Manosevitz M, Lanyon RI: Fear survey schedule: A normative study. Psychol Rep 17:699–703, 1965

55. Bieber L, Dain HJ, Dince PR et al: Homosexuality: A Psychoanalytic Study of Male Homosexuals. New York, Basic Books, 1962

56. Schwarz BJ: The measurement of castration anxiety and anxiety over loss of love. J Personality 24:204–219, 1955

57. Fisher S, Greenberg RP (eds): The Scientific Evaluation of Freud's Theories and Therapy. New York, Basic Books, 1978

Social Learning Models

Any cursory review of the field of psychopathology cannot help but leave us with an uncomfortable feeling. Matters are, at best, in disarray. And, from the viewpoint of logic and structure, the field may best be characterized by that all-too-familiar diagnosis (epithet?) "borderline organization." Except for colleagues of more doctrinaire and insular persuasions, we suffer from an "uncertainty about several issues relating to identity" and by "marked shifts of attitude, idealization, devaluation," and so on.

It may be of little comfort to know that this discouraging state of affairs is not unique to psychopathology; it is endemic in all fields of science. We, of course, know our science best and, without the blinders that some of us place on our usual keen observations, cannot be other than acutely aware of the controversies, inconsistencies, and unknowns that beset our own field. The fact is that any review, other than a cursory one, will show us to be in no more a borderline state than luminous fields such as molecular biology and nuclear physics. Our status is the natural state in which to be when a science seeks to move beyond its established frontiers; it is a state shared with all sciences that are open to new concepts and knowledge.

It is inevitable that a subject as broad as psychopathology would exhibit a diversity of viewpoints. Complex clinical problems lend themselves to many approaches, and divisions in research and theory become not only a matter of choice but also one of necessity. Fortunately, this diversification has resulted in a broad spectrum of knowledge about pathologic phenomena. Unfortunately, random evolutions in science have marked disadvantages as well. Scientists guided by only one approach or segment of the field often have little knowledge of the work of others. Intent on a narrow theoretic model, they lose sight of perspective. Potentially complementary contributions become scattered and disconnected. What is needed then is a synthesis in which divergent perspectives and elements of knowledge are brought together to be seen as parts of an integrated whole. Until a psychological Newton or Einstein comes along, however, the serious clinician must do the next best thing: develop an attitude by which the various branches and levels of psychopathology are viewed as an interrelated, if not an integrated unit. He should become acquainted with the language and orientation of each of the major approaches as if they were part of an indivisible piece. Until such time as a bridge is created to coordinate each theory and level of approach to the others, no one theory or approach should be viewed as all-embracing or accepted to the exclusion of the others. A multiplicity of viewpoints must prevail. It is in this open-minded spirit that the reader should approach the subject of this chapter.

Principles, Sources, and Continuity of Social Learning

The use of learning concepts to explain psychopathology is based on the assumption that principles demonstrated in controlled research settings may be generalized to more complex behavior. Accordingly, psychopathology is considered by social learning theorists to be complicated patterns of learned, maladaptive responses, and nothing else; all response patterns—normal or abnormal—are conceived, understood, and derived from a few basic principles of learning.

Several alternative models have been proposed to represent the rubric of "social learning" theory; despite their differences they do share one basic and integral assumption: social experiences, especially those occurring during the early formative years, are the main determinants of behavior and personality. Moreover, differences observed among individuals, whether judged normal or abnormal, directly reflect the particular conditions under which social learning occurred. Any effort to explicate individual behaviors, cognitions, and affects will be best achieved with direct reference not to genetic factors, maturational processes, or unconscious conflicts but to the specific social experiences that led to their acquisition.

It would not be surprising if readers are wondering how this social learning formulation differs from what theorists of other orientations have to say. The answer is the central role given the learning process as contrasted to its content. To learning theorists, social or otherwise, attention is directed to the task of carefully specifying the conditions that determine how behaviors are both learned and unlearned. Not only do social learning theorists contend that psychopathology is deficiently or maladaptively learned behaviors, but also they assert that most therapies unwittingly apply learning principles in their treatment procedures. Therapists of other orientations are seen as formulating their methods in elaborate conceptual systems and engaging in circuitous maneuvers, such as providing interpretations or promoting the release of repressed emotions. The crucial element in their technique, according to social learning theorists, is the indirect and largely inadvertent manner in which they teach the patient to strengthen adaptive behaviors and to unlearn those that are maladaptive. They contend, further, that the benefits of psychological treatment will be maximized when therapists knowingly apply learning principles in a planned and systematic fashion.

LEARNING PRINCIPLES

What are the basic principles of social learning? Several of the major concepts employed to explicate the acquisition and elimination of learned behaviors will be briefly described in the following paragraphs.

Contiguity Learning

The simplest formulation proposed to account for the acquisition of new behaviors and perceptions has been referred to as contiguity. In essence this principle states that any set of environmental elements that occurs either simultaneously or in close temporal order will become associated with each other. If one of these elements recurs in the future, the other elements with which it had previously been associated will be elicited. Some years ago, for example, I had the unpleasant experience of running out of gas as my car was crossing a heavily trafficked bridge. For several months thereafter, I sensed an uncomfortable feeling whenever I drove over this particular bridge and found myself anxiously checking the gas gauge.

The principle of contiguity may be applied to the progressive development of both *response learning* and *expectancy learning*. Response learning refers to associative bonds established between stimulus events and responses. Using the contiguity concept as a model, we can formulate this type of learning as follows: any stimulus pattern accompanying or immediately preceding a response will tend, if it recurs, to elicit that response. Expectancy learning refers to associative bonds established among stimulus events. It does not relate to the learning of responses to stimuli but to the learning of relationships among stimuli. Described in contiguity terms, it states: any environmental stimulus that previously has occurred in temporal or spatial contiguity with other stimuli will, if it recurs, elicit the expectation (*i.e.*, perception, cognition, or prediction) that the other stimuli will follow.

Instrumental Learning

In time, the organism learns to discriminate between those stimuli that result in pain and those that promise pleasure. This stage of learning takes the form of an expectancy in which it avoids stimuli that led to discomfort and exposes itself to those that provide rewards. With these cognitions in mind it is able to circumvent future negative reinforcements and invite future positive reinforcements. Moreover, it begins to engage intentionally in a series of acts designed to obtain the reinforcements it seeks. It anticipates and actively manipulates the events of its environment to suit its needs since it has learned that reinforcements are contingent on the performance of certain prior acts.

The process of acquiring these anticipations and manipulative behaviors is known as *instrumental learning* or operant conditioning. Either through direct tuition or chance events, the person learns which of his acts ultimately "produces" the desired result of obtaining a positive reinforcement or escaping a negative one. For example, a fussy and cranky child is offered candy or ice cream as a means of pacifying him. Although the child has been subdued for the time being, the parent, in effect, has given the child a positive reinforcement consequent to his misbehavior. On subsequent occasions, when the child wants candy or other similar reinforcements, he will engage in cranky and fussy behavior again since it "succeeded" previously in producing a reward for him.

If these "successful" manipulative acts prove effective in a variety of similar subsequent situations, they may take the form of an ingrained and widely generalized behavior pattern. These learned sequences of instrumental responses serve as the basis for the development of coping strategies, that is, a complex series of manipulative acts, employed in relation to events or persons, in which the individual avoids negative reinforcements and obtains positive ones.

Vicarious Learning

Human patterns of behavior are extraordinarily complex. For each child to learn the intricacies of civilized behavior by trial and error or reinforcement methods alone would be no less possible than it would be for an isolated primitive culture to advance, in one generation, to a full-fledged industrial and scientific society. Rather than struggling to acquire and integrate each of the many components of human behavior piece by piece, the child learns by adopting whole sequences of behaviors provided for him through the incidental actions of older members of his social group. These learnings are acquired *in toto* merely by observing, vicariously learning, and then imitating what others do and think. It is an efficient and necessary means by which the child becomes a "civilized human" in an amazingly short period of time.

This form of vicarious learning may be acquired quite incidentally by simple contiguity (*e.g.*, being exposed to established associations among stimuli such as are found in social belief systems or observing exemplary forms of behavior) or by complex instrumental strategies (*e.g.*, identifying with and adopting patterns of behavior manifested by parents as a means of obtaining their approval). Thus, intricate sequences of model-matching behaviors and attitudes are learned by incidental exposure to social models, by deliberate parental guidance and reinforcement, or by the child's own instrumental maneuvers.

Implicit Learning

Much of what is learned, especially after the early years of childhood, occurs implicitly, that is, without being a direct consequence of external environmental effects. Clearly, the "thinking" organism is capable of arranging memories of experiences into new patterns of association. As the child develops an extensive symbolic repertoire of words and images, he no longer is dependent on "real" environmental experience to form and strengthen new learnings. By manipulating his storehouse of symbols and images, he can reinforce himself by fantasy attainments and can concoct new instrumental strategies for dealing with his environment. By reorganizing his internal symbolic world, then, he supplements the objective world with novel thoughts that provide him with new learnings and self-administered reinforcements.

SOURCES OF ABNORMAL LEARNING

Attitudes and behaviors may be learned as a consequence of instruction on the part of parents, but most of what is learned arises from a haphazard series of casual and incidental events to which the child is exposed. Not only are rewards and punishments meted out most often in a spontaneous and erratic fashion, but the everyday activities of parents also provide the child with "unintended" models to imitate. Without their awareness or intention, parents suggest, through incidental aspects of their behavior, how "persons" think, talk, fear, love, solve problems, and relate to others. Aversions, irritabilities, attitudes, anxieties, and styles of interpersonal communication are adopted and duplicated by children as they observe the everyday reactions of their parents and older siblings. Children mirror these complex behaviors without understanding their significance and without parental intentions of transmitting them. The old saying, "practice what you preach," conveys the essence of this thesis. Thus, a parent who castigates the child harshly for failing to be kind to others may create an intrinsically ambivalent learning experience; the contrast between parental manner and verbalized statement teaches the child simultaneously to think "kindly" but to "behave" harshly.

The belief that early interpersonal experiences within the family play a decisive role in the development of psychopathology is well accepted among professionals, but reliable data supporting this conviction are difficult to find. The deficits in these data are not due to a shortage of research efforts. Rather, they reflect the operation of numerous methodologic and theoretic difficulties that stymies progress. For example, most of the data depend on retrospective accounts of early experience. These data are notoriously unreliable. Patients interviewed during their illness are prone to give a warped and selective accounting of their relationships with others. Information obtained from relatives often is distorted by feelings of guilt or by a desire to uncover some simple event to which the disorder can be attributed. In general, then, attempts to reconstruct the complex sequence of events of previous years that may have contributed to pathologic learning are fraught with almost insurmountable methodologic difficulties. Nevertheless, in the following sections I will attempt to outline some of the more reliable findings of recent research.

Parental Feelings and Attitudes

The most overriding aspect of learned experience, yet the most difficult to appraise, is the extent to which the child develops a feeling of acceptance or rejection by his parents. With the exception of cases of blatant abuse, investigators have extreme difficulty in specifying, no less measuring, the signs of parental disaffection. Despite the methodologic difficulties that researchers encounter, the child who is the recipient of rejecting cues has no doubt but that he is unappreciated, scorned, or deceived.

To be exposed throughout one's early years to parents who view one as unwanted and troublesome can only establish a deep and pervasive feeling of isolation in a hostile world. Deprived of the supports and security of home, the child may be ill disposed to venture forth with confidence to face struggles in the outer world. Rejected by his parents, he may anticipate equal devaluation by others. As a defense against further pain, he may learn the strategy of avoiding others. He may use apathy and indifference as a protective cloak to minimize the rejection he now expects from others. Different strategies may evolve, of course. Children may imitate parental scorn and ridicule and learn to handle their disturbed feelings by acting in a hostile and vindictive fashion.

Rejection is not the only parental attitude that may result in insidious damage to the child's personality. Attitudes represented by terms such as seduction, exploitation, and deception contribute their share of damage as well. However, it is usually the sense of being unwanted and unloved that proves to have the most pervasive and shattering of effects. A child can tolerate substantial punishment

and buffeting from his environment if he senses a basic feeling of love and support from his parents. Without them, his resistance, even to minor stress, is tenuous.

Methods of Behavior Control

What training procedures are used to regulate the child's behavior and to control what he learns? As noted earlier, incidental methods used by parents may have a more profound effect than what the parent intended; that is, the child acquires a model of interpersonal behavior by example and imitation as well as by verbal precept.

What are some of the pathogenic methods of control?

First among these are *punitive methods*. Parents disposed to intimidate their offspring, using punitive and repressive measures to control their behavior and thought, may set the stage for a variety of maladaptive patterns. If the child submits to pressure and succeeds in fulfilling parental expectations (*i.e.*, learns instrumentally to avoid the negative reinforcement of punishment), he is apt to become an overly obedient and circumspect person. Quite typically, these individuals learn not only to keep their impulses and contrary thoughts in check but, by vicarious observation and imitation, to adopt the parental behavior model and begin to be punitive of deviant behavior on the part of others. Thus, an otherwise timid and very tense 16-year-old-boy, whose every spark of youthful zest had been squelched by harshly punitive parents, was observed to be "extremely mean" and punitive when given the responsibility of teaching a Sunday school class for 7-year olds.

Should these youngsters fail to satisfy excessive parental demands, and be subject to continued harassment and punishment, they may develop a pervasive anticipatory anxiety about personal relationships, leading to feelings of hopelessness and discouragement, and resulting in such instrumental strategies as social avoidance and withdrawal. Others, faced with similar experiences, may learn to imitate parental harshness and develop hostile and aggressively rebellious behavior. Which of these reactions or strategies evolves will depend on the larger configuration of factors involved.

A second approach to control behavior may be termed *contingent reward methods*. Some parents rarely are punitive but expect certain behaviors to be performed prior to giving encouragement or doling out rewards. In other words, positive reinforcements are contingent on approved performance. Youngsters reared under these conditions tend to be socially pleasant and, by imitative learning, tend to be rewarding to others. But, quite often, we observe that they seem to have acquired an insatiable and indiscriminate need for social approval. For example, a 15-year-old girl experienced brief periods of marked depression if people failed to comment favorably on her dress or appearance. In early childhood she had learned that parental approval and affection were elicited only when she was "dressed up and looked pretty." To her, failure on the part of others to note her attractiveness signified rejection and disapproval. It would appear then that contingent reward methods condition children to develop an excessive need for approval. They manifest not only a healthy social affability but also a dependency on social reinforcement.

A third approach, usually unintended, are the more-or-less *inconsistent methods*. Parental methods of control often are irregular, contradictory, and capricious. Some degree of variability is inevitable in the course of every child's life, but there are parents who display an extreme inconsistency in their standards and expectations and an extreme unpredictability in their application of rewards and punishments. Youngsters exposed to such a chaotic and capricious environment cannot learn consistently and cannot devise nonconflictive strategies for adaptive behavior.

To avoid the suspense and anxiety of unpredictable reactions, the child may protectively become immobile and noncommittal. Others, imitatively adopting what they have been exposed to, may come to be characterized by their own ambivalence and their own tendency to vacillate from one action or feeling to another. Irregular reinforcements build behavior patterns that are difficult to extinguish. Thus, the immobility or ambivalence of these youngsters may persist long after their environment has become uniform and predictable.

A fourth approach is best labeled *protective methods*. Some parents so narrowly restrict the experiences to which their children are exposed that these youngsters fail to learn even the basic rudiments of autonomous behaviors. Overprotective mothers, worried that their children are too frail or are unable to care for themselves or make sensible judgments on their own, not only succeed in forestalling the growth of normal competencies but, indirectly, give the child a feeling that he is inferior and frail. The child, observing his actual inadequacies, has verification of the fact that he is weak, inept, and dependent on others. Thus, not only is this youngster trained to be deficient in adaptive and self-reliant behaviors but he also learns to view himself as inferior and becomes progressively fearful of leaving the protective "womb."

Fifth among the techniques of parental control are what can be described as *indulgent methods*. Overly permissive, lax, or undisciplined parents allow children full rein to explore and assert their every whim. These parents fail to control their children and, by their own lack of discipline, provide a model to be imitated that further strengthens the child's irresponsibility. Unconstrained by parental control, and not guided by selective rewards, these youngsters grow up displaying the inconsiderate and often tyrannical characteristics of undisciplined children. Having had their way for so long, they tend to be exploitive, demanding, uncooperative, and antisocially aggressive. Unless rebuffed by external disciplinary forces, these youngsters may persist in their habits and become irresponsible members of society.

Family Styles of Communication

Each family constructs its own style of communication, its own pattern of listening, attending, and conveying thoughts to others. The styles of interpersonal communication to which the child is exposed serve as a model for reacting to the expressions of others. Unless this framework for learning interpersonal communication is rational and reciprocal, the child will be ill equipped to function in an effective way with others. Thus, the very symbolic capacities that enable humans to transcend their environment so successfully may lend themselves to serious misdirections and confusions.

The effects of confusing patterns of family communication have been explored by numerous investigators. Not only are messages attended to in certain families in an erratic or incidental fashion, with a consequent loss of focus, but when they are attended to, they frequently convey contradictory meanings. The transmission of ambivalent meanings produces what has been referred to as a *double-bind*. For example, a seriously disturbed 10-year-old boy was repeatedly implored in a distinctly hostile tone by his equally ill mother as follows: "Come here to your mother; mommy loves you and wants to hug and squeeze you, hug and squeeze you." The contradictory nature of these double-bind messages precludes satisfactory reactions; the recipient cannot respond without running into conflict with one aspect of the message (*i.e.*, he is "damned if he does and damned if he doesn't"). Exposed to such contradictions in communication, the youngster's foundation in reality becomes increasingly precarious.

PERSISTENCE OF EARLY LEARNINGS

Childhood experiences are crucially involved in shaping lifelong patterns of behavior. To support this view several conditions of early upbringing and their learned consequences are noted. In this section I will concentrate on the notion of continuity in behavior, since social learning theorists believe that the significance of early experience lies not only in its impact but also in its durability and persistence. Experiences in early life are not only ingrained more pervasively and forcefully, but their effects also tend to persist and are more difficult to modify than later experiences.

Acquired behaviors and attitudes usually are not fixed or permanent. What has been learned can be modified or eliminated under appropriate conditions, a process referred to as *extinction*. Extinction usually entails exposure to experiences that are similar to the conditions of original learning but that provide opportunities for new learning to occur. Essentially, old habits of behavior change when new learning interferes with and replaces what previously had been learned. Failure to provide opportunities for interfering with old habits means that they will remain unmodified and persist over time. In other words, learnings associated with events that are difficult to reproduce are resistant to extinction.

Are the events of early life experienced in such a manner as to make them difficult to reproduce and, therefore, resistant to extinction? An examination of the conditions of childhood suggests that the answer is yes! The reasons for this assertion may be formulated with reference to three features that distinguish early learning.

Presymbolic Learning

Biologically, the young child is a primitive organism. His nervous system is incomplete, he perceives the world from momentary vantage points, and he is unable to discriminate many of the elements of his experience. What he sees and learns about his environment through his infantile perceptual systems will never again be experienced in the same manner in later life.

The infant's presymbolic world of impressions recedes gradually as he acquires the ability to discriminate and symbolize experience. By the time he is 4 or 5 years of age, he views the world in a way quite different from that of infancy. He can no longer duplicate the amorphous experiences of his earlier years. Unable to reproduce early experiences in later life, he will not be able to extinguish what he learned in response to them. No longer perceiving events as initially sensed, he cannot supplant his early reactions with new ones.

Random Learning

The young child lacks not only the ability to form a precise image of his environment but also the equipment to discern logical relationships among its elements. His world of objects, persons, and events is connected in an unclear and random fashion. He learns to associate events that have no relationship. Thus, when he experiences fear in response to his father's harsh voice, he may learn to fear not only that voice but the setting, the atmosphere, the pictures, the furniture, and any incidental objects that by chance were present at that time. Unable to discriminate the precise source in his environment that "caused" his fear, he connects his discomfort randomly to all associated stimuli. Now each stimulus can become a precipitant for these feelings.

Random associations of early life cannot be duplicated as the child develops the capacity for logical thinking. By the time he is 4 or 5 years of age he can discriminate cause-and-effect relationships with considerable accuracy. Early random associations do not "make sense" to him. When he reacts to one of the precipitants derived from early learning, he is unable to identify what it is in the environment to which he is reacting. He cannot locate the source of his difficulty, since he now thinks more logically than before. To advise him that he is reacting to a picture or piece of furniture simply will be rejected. He cannot fathom the true features that evoke his feelings since these sources are so foreign to his new, more rational mode of thought.

Generalized Learning

The young child's discriminations of his environment are crude and gross. As he begins to differentiate the elements of his world, he groups and labels them into broad and unrefined categories. All men become "daddy"; all four-legged animals are called "doggie"; all foods are "yum-yum." When the child learns to fear a particular dog, for example, he will learn to fear not only that dog but all strange, mobile four-legged creatures. To his primitive perception, all of these animals are one of a kind.

As the mass of early experiences becomes more finely discriminated, learning gets to be more focused, specific, and precise. A 10-year old will learn to fear bulldogs as a result of an unfortunate experience with one, but he will not necessarily generalize this fear to collies or poodles, since he knows and can discern differences among these animals.

Generalized learning is difficult to extinguish. The young child's learned reactions are attached to a broader class of objects than called for by his specific experiences. To extinguish these broadly generalized reactions in later life, when his discriminative capacities are much more precise, will require that he be exposed to many and diverse experiences. This may be an elusive point to convey, and an illustration may be useful to clarify it.

Let us assume that a two-year-old child was frightened by a cocker spaniel. Given his gross discriminative capacity at this age, this single experience may have conditioned him to fear dogs, cats, and other small animals. Let us assume further that in later life he is exposed repeatedly to a friendly cocker spaniel. As a consequence of this experience, we find that he has extinguished his fear, but only of cocker spaniels, not of dogs in general or cats or other small animals. His later experience, seen through the discriminative eye of an older child, was that spaniels but not dogs in general are friendly. The extinction experience applied then to only one part of the original widely generalized complex of fears he acquired. His original learning experience incorporated a much broader range of stimuli than his later experience, even though the objective stimulus conditions were essentially the same. Because of his more precise discriminative capacity, he now must have his fear extinguished in a variety of situations to compensate for the single but widely generalized early experience.

These three interlocking conditions—presymbolic, random, and generalized learning—account in large measure for the unusual difficulty of reexperiencing the events of early life, and the consequent difficulty of unlearning the feelings, behaviors, and attitudes generated by these events.

SOCIAL REINFORCEMENT OF LEARNED BEHAVIORS

Of the many factors that contribute to the continuity of early behavior patterns, none plays a more significant role, according to social learning theorists, than relationships with significant others. As pointed out in an earlier section, ingrained learned patterns of behavior develop as a consequence of enduring experiences generated in intimate and subtle relationships. The attention of social learning theorists is not on the content of what is learned as much as on those aspects of relationships that strengthen what has been learned and

that lead to their perpetuation. Three such influences will be described: repetitive experiences, reciprocal reinforcement, and social stereotyping.

Repetitive Experiences

The typical daily activities in which the young child participates are restricted and repetitive. There is not much variety in the routine experience to which the child is exposed. Day in and day out he eats the same kind of food, plays with the same toys, remains essentially in the same physical environment, and relates to the same persons. This constricted environment, this repeated exposure to a narrow range of family attitudes and training methods, not only builds in deeply etched habits but prevents the child from new experiences that are essential to change. Early behaviors fail to change, therefore, not because they may have gelled permanently but because the same slender band of experiences that helped form them initially continues and persists as influences for many years.

Reciprocal Reinforcement

Whatever the initial roots may be—constitutional or learned—certain forms of behavior provoke, or "pull" from others, reactions that result in the repetition of these behaviors. For example, a suspicious, child who is defiant and has a chip on his shoulder eventually will force others, no matter how tolerant they may have been initially, to counter with exasperation and anger. An ever-widening gulf of defiance may develop as parents of such children "throw up their hands in disgust." Affections that might have narrowed the gulf of suspicion and hostility break down. Each participant, in feedback fashion, contributes his share, and the original level of hostile behavior is aggravated and intensified.

Social Stereotypes

The dominant features of a child's early behavior form a distinct impression on others. Once this early impression is established, persons expect that the child will continue to behave in his distinctive manner. In time, they develop a fixed and simplified image of "what kind of person the child is." The term *stereotype*, borrowed from social psychology, represents this tendency to simplify and categorize the attributes of others.

Persons no longer view a child objectively once they have formed a stereotype of him. They now are sensitized to those distinctive features they have learned to expect. The stereotype operates as a screen through which the childs behaviors are selectively perceived so as to fit the characteristics attributed to him. Once cast in this mold, the child will experience a consistency in the way in which others react to him. No matter what he does, he finds that his behavior is interpreted in the same fixed and rigid manner. Exposed time and time again to the same reactions and attitudes of others, he may give up efforts to convince them that he can change. For example, if a "defiant" child displays the slightest degree of resentment to unfair treatment, he will be jumped on as hopelessly recalcitrant. Should he do nothing objectionable, questions will be raised as to the sincerity of his motives.

SELF-PERPETUATION OF LEARNINGS

The residual of the past does more than passively contribute its share to the present. By temporal precedence, if nothing else, memory traces of the past guide, shape, or distort the character of current events. Not only are they ever present, but also they transform new stimulus experiences in line with past ones. Two of these processes of perpetuation, perceptual and cognitive distortion and behavior generalization, will be elaborated on here.

Perceptual and Cognitive Distortion

As noted previously, certain psychological processes not only preserve the past but also transform the present in line with the past. Once a person acquires a system of threat expectancies, he responds with increasing alertness to similar threatening elements in his life situation. Thus, a person who has learned to believe that "everyone hates him" will tend to interpret the incidental and entirely innocuous comments of others in line with this premise.

The role of habits of language as factors shaping a person's perceptions are of particular interest. The words persons use transform experiences in line with the meaning of these words. For example, a child who has been exposed to parents who respond to every minor mishap as "a shattering experience" will tend to use these terms himself in the future. As a consequence, he will begin to feel that every setback he experiences is shattering because he has labeled it as such. Instead of interpreting events as they objectively exist, the individual selectively distorts them to "fit" his expectancies and habits of thought.

This distortion process has a cumulative and spiraling effect. By misconstruing reality in such ways as to make it corroborate his learned expectancies, the individual, in effect, intensifies his misery. Thus, ordinary, even rewarding events may be perceived as threatening. As a result of this distortion, the patient subjectively experiences neutral events "as if" they were, in fact, threatening. In this process, he both creates and accumulates painful experiences for himself when none exists in reality.

Behavior Generalization

A number of factors that lead individuals to perceive new experiences in a subjective and frequently warped fashion have just been described. Perceptual and cognitive distortions may be viewed as the defective side of a normal process in which new stimulus conditions are seen as similar to those experienced in the past. This process, although usually described in simpler types of conditions, commonly is referred to as *stimulus generalization*. In the present section, another closely related form of generalization, the tendency to react to new stimuli in a manner similar to the way that one reacted in the past is discussed. This process is referred to as *behavior generalization*.

Stimulus generalization and behavior generalization often are two sides of the same coin. Thus, if an individual distorts an objective event so as to perceive it as identical to a past event, it would be reasonable to expect that his response to it would be similar to that made previously. For example, let us assume that a child learned to cower and withdraw from a harshly punitive mother. Should the child come into contact with a somewhat firm teacher, possessing physical features similar to those of the mother, the child may distort his perception of the teacher, making her a duplicate of the mother, and then react to her as he had learned to react to his mother.

This tendency to perceive and to react to present events as if they were duplicates of the past is the same as the well-known psychoanalytic concept of *transference*, signifying the observation that patients in treatment magnify minor similarities between their parents and therapist and then transfer to the therapist responses learned within the family setting.

The tendency to generalize inappropriate behaviors has especially far-reaching consequences since it often elicits reactions from others that not only perpetuate these behaviors but also aggravate the conditions that gave rise to them. A person whose past experiences led him to anticipate punitive reactions from his parents may be hyperalert to signs of rejection from others. As a consequence of his suspiciousness he may distort neutral comments, seeing them as indications of hostility. In preparing himself to counter the hostility he expects, he freezes his posture, stares coldly and rigidly, and passes a few aggressive comments himself. These actions communicate a message that quickly is sensed by others as unfriendly and antagonistic. Before long, others express open feelings of disaffection, begin to withdraw, and display real, rather than imagined, hostility. The person's suspicious behavior has evoked the punitive responses he expected. He now has experienced an objective form of rejection similar to what he received in childhood. This leads him to be more suspicious and arrogant, beginning the vicious circle all over again.

Major Social Learning Models

Nature was not made to suit our need for a tidy and well-ordered universe. The complexity and intricacy of the natural world make it difficult not only to establish clear-cut relationships among observed phenomena but also to find simple ways in which these phenomena can be classified or grouped. In our desire to discover the essential order of nature we are forced to select only a few of the infinite number of elements that could be chosen; in this selection we narrow our choice only to those aspects of nature that we believe best enable us to answer the questions we pose. The elements we have chosen may be labeled, transformed, and reassembled in a variety of ways. However, we must keep in mind that these transformations are not "realities." The definitions, concepts, and theories scientists create are only optional tools to guide their observation and interpretation of the natural world; it is necessary to recognize, therefore, that different concepts and theories may coexist as alternative approaches to the same basic problem. A major source of confusion for both scientists and clinicians stems from their difficulty in recognizing the existence of these different levels of observation and conceptualization.

With this perspective in mind, let us narrow our field of interest and inquiry to the question, what is psychopathology?

Mental disorders are expressed in a variety of ways. Clearly, psychopathology is a complex phenomenon that can be approached at different levels and can be viewed from many angles. On a behavioral level, for example, mental disorders may be

conceived of as a complicated pattern of responses to environmental stress. Cognitively, they may be seen as expressions of personal discomfort and anguish. Approached from a biological viewpoint, they may be interpreted as sequences of complex neural and chemical activity. Psychodynamically, they may be organized into unconscious processes that defend against anxiety and conflict.

Given these diverse possibilities, it should readily be understood why mental disorders may be approached and defined in terms of any of several levels that we may wish to focus on and any of a variety of functions or processes that we may wish to explain. Beyond this, each level of approach lends itself to a number of different theories and concepts, the usefulness of which must be gauged by their ability to help classify the particular problems and purposes for which they were created. For example, within the framework of psychodynamic thinking clear distinctions are drawn among those following an orthodox Freudian approach, those stemming from ego-analytic viewpoints, orientations that reflect self- and object-relations theories, as well as a host of other less known, yet intrapsychically based formulations.

Similarly, social learning can be studied from many vantage points; it can be observed and conceptualized in legitimately different ways by behaviorists, cognitivists, psychodynamicists, and biologists. No point of observation or conceptualization alone is sufficient to encompass all of the complex and multidimensional features that comprise social learning. Processes may be described in terms of conditioned habits, reaction formations, cognitive expectancies, or genetic dispositions. These levels of conceptualizing the processes and determinants of social learning cannot be arranged in a hierarchy, with one level viewed as reducible to another, nor can they be compared in terms of some "objective truth value." These alternative levels of approach merely are different; they make possible the observation and conceptualization of different types of data and lead, therefore, to the enhancement of different realms of knowledge.

There are many ways in which the subject matter of social learning can be differentiated according to "data levels." What classification will represent the current state of thinking best?"

The major historical traditions in psychopathology suggest a particularly useful basis to follow and one that corresponds closely to significant orientations in social learning theory today. These contemporary orientations not only reflect relatively distinct historical traditions but, perhaps more importantly, also differ in the kinds of data they elect to conceptualize. For example, those who favor formulations based on a mind–body synthesis have focused on the *biological* substrate of social learning; those who follow psychoanalytic traditions are likely to deal with unconscious *psychodynamic* processes; theorists who work within a phenomenological-existential framework will most probably be concerned with conscious *cognitive* experience; and those holding to the academic traditions of psychology will attend primarily to overt *behavioral* data. These levels—biological, psychodynamic, cognitive, and behavioral—reflect, therefore, both different sources of data and the major theoretic orientations in social learning.

BEHAVIORALLY ORIENTED SOCIAL LEARNING THEORIES

Taken in its strictest form, behaviorally oriented learning theories require that all concepts and propositions be anchored exclusively and precisely to measurable properties in the observable world. Empirically unanchored speculation is anathema to behaviorists; hypothetical constructs, which abound in psychoanalytic and cognitive theories, are presumably not to be found in behavioral theories.

Behaviorism originated with the view that subjective introspection was "unscientific" and that it should be replaced by the use of objectively observable behaviors. Furthermore, all environmental influences on behavior were likewise to be defined objectively. If unobservable processes were thought to exist within the individual, they were to be defined strictly in terms of observables that indicate their existence. Bindra[1] states this position strongly:

> Research on the problems of causation, diagnosis and treatment of behavior disorders should concentrate, not on "psychodynamics" or other hypothetical processes, but on observed behavior. Descriptions of subjective states, not being subject to publicly observable or objective reliability checks, should not be considered as statements about crucial psychopathological events.

Behaviorally oriented theorists limit themselves to concepts generated in experimental learning research. They are not simple translations of developmental or psychoanalytic concepts into behavioral terms but are based on the ostensible "empirical" laws of learning. Theorists using these concepts lay claim to the virtues of science since their heritage lies with objective research and not with what they conceive to be the dubious methods of clinical observation and speculation.

Who are the social learning theorists who have expounded this view? A short discussion of an historical nature will provide a context and orientation to contemporary behavioristic thinking.

Pavlov and Watson

The origin of modern learning theory may be traced back to the seminal "law of effect" idea formulated by Edward Lee Thorndike[2] at the turn of the 20th century. Thorndike stressed the signal importance of reward and punishment in learning, formulating his concept succinctly as follows:

> Any act which in a given situation produces satisfaction becomes associated with that situation, so that when the situation recurs the act is more likely than before to recur also. Conversely, any act which in a given situation produces discomfort . . . (subsequently) when the situation recurs the act is less likely than before to recur.

Despite the clarity of Thorndike's statement, it remained for the great Russian physiologist Ivan Petrovitch Pavlov[3] to demonstrate experimentally that behavior is modified as a function of learning. Pavlov's discoveries resulted from an unanticipated observation made in 1902 during studies of digestive reflexes. While measuring saliva secreted by dogs in response to food, he noticed that dogs salivated either at the sight of the food dish or on hearing the footsteps of the attendant who brought it in. Pavlov realized that the stimulus of the dish or the footsteps had become, through experience, a substitute or signal for the stimulus of food. He soon concluded that this signaling or learning process must play a central part in the adaptive capacity of animals. Because of his physiologic orientation, however, he conceived these observations as processes of the brain. Initially, he referred to them as "psychic secretions." Later, he coined the term *conditioned reflex* for the learned response and labeled the learned signal as a *conditioned stimulus*. As his work progressed, Pavlov noted that conditioned reflexes persisted over long periods of disuse. They could be inhibited briefly by various distractions and completely extinguished by repeated failure to follow the signal or conditioned stimulus with the usual reinforcement.

Despite his lifelong predilection for conceptualizing these conditioning processes as physiologic activities of the "higher nervous system," his experiments served more directly to replace the focus on subjective introspection that characterized learning research at the turn of the century. In his substitution of measurable and objective reactions to stimuli, he laid the groundwork, not only for the next three fourths of a century of Russian research but also for American "behaviorism" and modern learning theory, as well.

Pavlov came to realize in his later studies that words could replace physical stimuli as signals for conditioned learning. He divided human thought into two signal systems, stating the following:

Direct impressions of the surrounding world are primary signals of reality. Words are secondary signals. They represent themselves as abstractions of reality. The human brain is composed of the animal brain, the first signaling system, and the purely human part related to speech, the second signaling system.

Pavlov noted that under emotional distress behavior shifts from the symbols of the second signal system to the bodily expression of the first signal system. Not only did he recognize this "regression" as a part of mental disorders, but he also used the concept of the second signal to show how verbal therapy can influence the underlying first signal system it represents. Thus, words could alter malfunctioning "brain processes" in the neurotic individual by way of persuasion and suggestion.

In 1913 the American psychologist John Broadus Watson[4] formally espoused a point of view called *behaviorism* that was intended as an antidote to the preoccupation with consciousness and introspection among his contemporaries. To him, consciousness was a subjectively private experience; as such, it failed to meet a major tenet of science that data should be objective or publicly verifiable. Watson became acquainted with the conditioned reflex studies of Pavlov and his Russian contemporary V. M. Bechterev in 1915, and he saw quickly that this method could be used to circumvent introspective reports and give him the overt and objective data he sought. From that point, and with each succeeding publication, Wat-

son made the conditioned reflex a central concept in behaviorism. He rejected the physiologic orientation of Pavlov, however. He had no interest in the inner structure or processes of the animal, stating that concepts defined at the level of behavior were sufficient to account for all learning processes.

Watson was perhaps the first psychologist to apply learning principles to induce a "neurotic fear" response, as well as to provide a method for its extinction. In collaboration with his associate Rosalie Rayner, Watson[5] set out to produce a learned fear of white rats in an 11-month-old child named Albert. Prior research showed that sudden loud noises would naturally elicit trembling and crying reactions in the youngster, whereas the sight of a white rat had no such effect. They arranged to place Albert and the white rat in close proximity; when Albert extended his hand to touch the furry animal they immediately sounded the loud noise. After seven such pairings over two separate sessions, they recorded that the mere presence nearby of the white rat produced the fear response in Albert. The once neutral stimulus of the rat now evoked a "neurotic" reaction comprising both avoidant behavior and tearfulness. In addition, Albert gave evidence of what is termed *stimulus generalization*, that is, his learned fear response extended to a sealskin coat, a rabbit, and a dog, objects with which he had no prior experiences of a frightening nature.

Subsequent to the Albert study, Watson guided the work of another research associate, Mary Cover Jones,[6] who tried two ways of extinguishing a child's fear of white furry animals. The child, a 2½-year old dubbed Little Peter, was seen to exhibit less fear when he observed other children calmly handling a white rat. By introducing several such "fearless" children as models for Peter to observe, Jones was the first to demonstrate empirically the contemporary behavior modification technique of "model imitation." In another study with Peter, Jones progressively exposed the child to a formerly feared white rabbit by a series of graduated steps that brought him into closer and closer contact with the animal; in due course, Peter was able to fondle the rabbit calmly. By following a course of progressive "toleration" of what previously produced anxiety, Jones' technique was the forerunner of the now well-established behavioral procedure termed *desensitization*.

Skinner

The first modern theory of social learning to restrict its concepts entirely to objective behavioral processes, eschewing all reference to internal phenomena such as the unconscious, innate anxiety dispositions or self-reinforcing thoughts, was formulated by B. F. Skinner.[7,8] According to Skinner, it is misleading and unnecessary to posit the existence of unobservable emotional states or cognitive expectancies to account for behavior pathology. Skinner explicitly disavows the notion of disease entities, arguing that individuals are not disordered or sick but rather have failed to learn adaptive responses to the normal stimulus conditions of social life.

Skinnerians prefer to view maladaptive responses as a simple product of environmentally based reinforcing experiences. They dismiss the attention that other social learning theorists give to internal mediating processes such as expectancies and self-reinforcing thoughts. Hypothetic inner states are discarded, and explanations are formulated solely in terms of external sources of stimulation and reinforcement.

Environmental reinforcements shape the behavioral repertoire of the individual, and differences between adaptive and maladaptive behaviors can be traced entirely to differences in the reinforcement pattern to which individuals were exposed. To Skinner, the so-called neuroses and psychoses are merely the upshot of defective or peculiar reinforcement histories. Some pathologies stem from deficits in the behavior repertoire of the individual, owing to inadequacies in his reinforcement history; an example here might be a dependent personality who failed to acquire the competencies requisite to mature and independent functioning.

Other cases may represent a mismatch between an individual's response repertoire and the reinforcers available in his environment. Thus, even in persons with a broad range of adaptive responses, the inability to find or elicit positive reinforcers (*e.g.*, attention, approval) may result in a marked decrement in motoric, cognitive, and affective behaviors or what is usually labeled depression. In another maladaptive case a person may be observed who is "out of touch" with the available reinforcers that usually elicit adaptive responses; this individual might properly be diagnosed as schizophrenic. A case such as this may reflect a history in which the individual was positively reinforced when attending unusual or "superstitious" stimulus cues. As a consequence, he now responds to socially deviant or idiosyncratic elements in his environment, portraying a clinical picture in which behaviors are bizarre and thinking is peculiar.

Wolpe

Following the classical conditioning paradigm originated in Pavlov's research, Joseph Wolpe[9] conceived neurotic behaviors to be simple conditioned fear responses. Although Wolpe recognizes that situations that elicit intense and opposing responses may give rise to anxiety, he contends that conflict is neither necessary to such neurotic responses nor does he find it to be the most common reason for its development. To Wolpe, anxiety stems most frequently from the unfortunate conjunction of a neutral stimulus with a painful psychological or physical event. Once a concurrence of this nature occurs, the conditioned anxiety may be further conditioned to an ever-widening array of events that are either similar to or happen by mere coincidence to be present during the original situation. Anxiety reactions may spread, therefore, both to stimuli that are alike, as well as to those that bear little resemblance to the conditions in the initial event. He notes further that the neurotic response itself is often a mere repetition of the complex of behaviors, including anxiety, the person happened to be experiencing and doing at the time of the original conditioning. Subsequently, other symptoms may become attached to the syndromal picture of anxiety by virtue of their often entirely coincidental concurrence at times of anxiety reduction.

Wolpe has formulated a variety of methods for extinguishing learned neurotic responses such as these by adopting a procedure originally developed by Mary Cover Jones. In Jones' early study, children were given attractive foods in the distant presence of a previously conditioned feared object. Over time the feared object was brought progressively closer to the child while it ate the desired food, until such time as the object no longer evoked the fear response but rather became conditioned to the positive feelings associated with food. Terming this process *reciprocal inhibition*, Wolpe described the technique as follows:

> If a response antagonistic to anxiety can be made to occur in the presence of anxiety-evoking stimuli so that it is accompanied by a complete or partial suppression of the anxiety response, the bond between these stimuli and the anxiety response will be weakened.

The most highly developed of Wolpe's therapeutic techniques for fashioning conditions that are antagonistic to anxiety is known as *systematic desensitization*, a method of presenting imagined events on an anxiety hierarchy while the patient maintains a learned relaxation response. However, in drawing on cognitive processes such as imagination, Wolpe deviated in an important way from the radical behaviorism espoused by Watson and Skinner.

PSYCHODYNAMICALLY ORIENTED SOCIAL LEARNING THEORISTS

Numerous learning theorists and researchers developed ideas at variance with the views of Watson and Skinner. According to this group, there was an inner world of events and processes somewhere between observable stimuli and responses that could be fruitfully investigated within the tenets of scientific respectability. Not only did this group disagree with Skinner's adherence to an orthodox behaviorism, which asserted that internal processes were not a proper subject for scientific inquiry, but many were intrigued by, if not active adherents of, psychoanalytic thought. They not only claimed that learned behaviors involved inner motivations, drives, and conflicts, as well as mechanisms for their acquisition and resolution, but also that higher intrapsychic processes were integral to the task of understanding all normal or abnormal behaviors. To them, behavior was invariably the result of a complex network of internal sequences that could never be adequately represented, no less explicated, by a reflexive stimulus–response paradigm.

These psychodynamically oriented social learning theorists differed, however, from those whose views derived from classical psychoanalytic roots. Their attentions were directed to the mechanisms and principles by which maladaptive behaviors were acquired, rather than the content of experience that gave rise to them. Also noteworthy was their philosophic allegiance to the values of scientific empiricism. Despite their willingness not only to accept but also to study internal processes that transpire ''unobservably'' between stimuli and responses, they insisted that ''intervening variables'' such as these be defined objectively and be measured quantitatively, albeit in indirect form.

Investigators of Experimental Neuroses

Interestingly, while one branch of learning theory, the disciples of Watson and Skinner, actively disavowed psychodynamic concepts, another branch were just as active in embracing them. As early as 1914, several of Pavlov's students undertook a series of conditioning studies in which dogs were taught to discriminate between a circle and an ellipse; the dogs were always fed when the circle was displayed on a screen but never when the ellipse was shown. As expected, the dogs learned to salivate whenever the circle was flashed but reacted indifferently to the ellipse. Once the discrimination was clearly established, the experimenters contin-

ued to present both stimuli in random sequence, but they altered the shape of the ellipse so as to progressively transform it to look more and more like a circle. Faced repeatedly with this increasingly difficult discrimination task, the dogs became confused, began to squeal in their stand, bit at their harnesses, and tore through the tubes connecting the recording apparatus. Furthermore, when they were led either to or from the experimental room, they wailed or barked violently, signs of troubled emotions that were distinctly different than their prior tranquil behaviors.

Sequences similar to these prompted Pavlov to term this phenomenon an *experimental neurosis*, a descriptive label that was adopted in later years by other investigators. These researchers sought to find a laboratory setting that would enable them to manipulate antecedent conditions that they judged critical to the ''learning'' of abnormal behaviors. Among American investigators who adopted Pavlov's experimental paradigm in the 1930s were W. Horsely Gantt, who traveled to Russia to work with Pavlov; N. R. F. Maier, who did extensive laboratory research with rats; and H. S. Liddell, who carried out comparable experiments with sheep. All confirmed the findings that Pavlov and his associates had earlier reported. In essence, animals faced with circumstances that frustrate learned responses or with conflict-producing demands or treated in random rather than expectable ways almost invariably developed manifest disturbances that strongly resembled those seen in humans.

Of special note in this research area were the studies of Jules Masserman,[10] who sought to connect the findings of experimentally induced neuroses explicitly to psychoanalytic concepts. Arranging conditions that produced severe ''conflicts'' in cats, he was able to record not only their consequent and extreme startle reactions to incidental stimuli but also their physiologic disturbances, notably tachycardia, irregular breathing, and profuse perspiration. Masserman took a major step in attempting to ''treat'' his animals. For example, by increasing a cat's desire to achieve one of a pair of competing drives, he was able to overcome its state of immobility. Similarly, he introduced cat ''models'' who demonstrated normal behaviors and served as exemplars to be emulated by disturbed animals. Most successful among his ''therapeutic'' techniques were procedures that enabled cats to achieve mastery over a feared situation, such as being able in a conflict setting to have full control over when it would receive a desired reinforcement. Ultimately, these animals showed a marked reduction of ''neurotic'' behaviors, such that they could not be distinguished from their counterparts who had not been disturbed.

Dollard and Miller

There are a number of assumptions that social learning and psychodynamic theorists share, notably those that assert that clinical behaviors are, first, traceable to the impact of historical events in the background of the individual and, second, reflect the operation of drives and reinforcements. It should not be surprising, therefore, that an increasing number of learning researchers began to turn to psychoanalytic theory as a source of ideas and inspirations. Most central to building this bridge was the role played by Clark Hull in the 1930s and 1940s. While serving as professor of psychology at the Institute of Human Relations of Yale University, perhaps the first think tank designed to bring together perspectives from all of the behavioral sciences, Hull established an ongoing seminar and initiated a series of research studies designed to translate psychoanalytic concepts into formal and testable hypotheses that could be investigated in controlled laboratory settings. Among Hull's younger research associates were several who had undergone formal psychoanalyses and were sufficiently versed in dynamic theory, learning concepts, and experimental methodology to provide a basis for implementing Hull's aspirations. On the institute's junior faculty possessing backgrounds such as these were John Dollard, Neal Miller, and O. Hobart Mowrer.

Dollard and Miller[11] proposed, as did Freud, that intense emotional conflicts are the basis of psychopathology. By conflict they meant the existence of two or more mutually incompatible drives; thus, conflicts could occur between innate physiologic needs, such as hunger or sex, or socially acquired emotional responses, such as fear, anger, or anxiety. The components of these conflicts were categorized as *approach* or *avoidant*. For example, a college student who wished to marry his girl friend (approach) but feared parental disapproval of this desire (avoidant) would experience conflict.

Disorders, according to Dollard and Miller, will not arise unless the individual represses or is otherwise unaware of his conflict; the problem takes on serious proportions because unconscious conflicts are not accessible to realistic thought and intelligent resolution. The consequence of this repression is far reaching. To stop thinking about the conflict, the individual tends also to inhibit thinking about other problem areas, as well; as a consequence, the person's overall capacity to reason and plan is impaired. Symptoms of disorder are seen by Dollard

and Miller as efforts to deny painful conflicts. For example, a phobia of crowded places may cover up conflicting feelings toward others; similarly, antagonisms to women may arise in "moralistic" men as a cloak for disturbing sexual desires. To Dollard and Miller then, pathology consists of unconscious conflicts that cannot be resolved since they are not available to conscious reasoning. As a result, the individual engages in shortsighted partial resolutions, many of which may invite more serious conflicts and complications.

Dollard and Miller limited themselves to translating the therapeutic processes of psychoanalysis into the language of learning theory. Although these writings suggested a new way of conceptualizing and explaining traditional forms of therapy, they suggested no new techniques as to how therapy might be executed. In later years, instead of merely restating psychodynamic forms of treatment in the vernacular of learning concepts, clinicians began to use principles that were derived first in social learning research to create entirely new forms of therapy.

As is evident from the foregoing, the social learning theory proposed by Dollard and Miller is not substantially different than that formulated by psychodynamic theorists. As noted, they translated the concepts of traditional Freudian psychoanalysis into the language of Pavlovian conditioning and Hullian learning theory. Some critics have noted that a proper application of learning principles should have led them to a new conception of psychopathology. However, their work did make the study of abnormal processes more palatable to research psychologists; if nothing else then, Dollard and Miller built an important bridge between previously incompatible fields of interest.

Mowrer

An important distinction, insofar as the elements that comprise learning are concerned, was proposed by O. Hobart Mowrer,[12] another student of Carl Hull. In accord with his "two factor" model, Mowrer set out to differentiate *solution* from *sign* learning. In solution learning a person acquires response habits by finding a solution to some problem, perhaps the reduction of a primary drive. In sign learning the individual does not acquire a response habit but instead an expectation, belief, or set.

Mowrer employed his two-factor learning model to explicate both neuroses and psychotherapy. Neuroses are considered the product of solution learning since neurotics use their problem-solving capacities defensively. They engage in actions that protect themselves against new learnings that, in the long run, might be useful. It is at this point that psychological abnormalities begin. To Mowrer, neuroses are seen as problem-solving situations in which the person represses impulses he ought to acknowledge. Repression, therefore, is conceived of as learning not to learn. Therapy, to him, should consist of a combination of fear extinction and the reinforcement of being "realistic" and expressing drives that have been denied.

Related to Mowrer's theory of abnormal behavior is a concept he terms the *neurotic paradox.* Mowrer points out that the behavior of neurotics is self-perpetuating as well as self-defeating. For example, a compulsive handwasher will continue to clean and rub his fingers endlessly even though much time is wasted and nothing is achieved other than getting sores and irritations. Mowrer explains the paradox by stating that neurotics suffer from a learning deficit. At some point in the developmental process, they have become fixated or bogged down, rather than overcoming their fruitless habits. To go forward, however, is to give up their successfully learned response situations. On the other hand, however, not to give them up is to prevent themselves from acquiring new, more adaptive competencies. Their "successful" learning has proved, therefore, to be self-defeating.

Mowrer's own theoretic views did not become fixated, however. In later writings he gave greater weight to the role that sign rather than solution learning played in psychopathology. In this work, he anticipated many of the ideas of the "cognitive" theorists. In these writings, Mowrer asserted that social learning is less a matter of acquiring methods of solving problems than it is the acquisition of appropriate attitudes, meanings, and expectations.

COGNITIVELY ORIENTED SOCIAL LEARNING THEORISTS

According to phenomenologic theory, each individual reacts to the world in terms of his unique perception of it. No matter how transformed or unconsciously distorted this perception may be, it is the person's way of construing events that determines his behavior. Concepts and propositions must be formulated, therefore, not in terms of objective realities, as stressed by the behaviorists, or of unconscious processes, as done by psychodynamic theorists, but in accordance with how events actually are cognitively perceived by the individual. Concepts must not disassemble these experiences

into depersonalized or abstract categories but rather represent these phenomenologic processes directly. Cognitive theorists have taken this philosophy seriously. This is most clearly seen in their introduction of terms such as *cognitive expectancies, vicarious learning,* and *self-reinforcing thoughts.* Although sharing with phenomenologic philosophers their concern with cognitive factors and subjective experiences, cognitive learning theorists are much more explicit in spelling out and articulating their concepts, as well as in strongly endorsing the need to employ precise assessment and systematic therapeutic methods.

Cognitive social learning theorists have moved from their origins in behavioral psychology to the psychodynamic focus on internal mediating events. They emphasize the importance of thoughts, perceptions, and beliefs; recognize the role of internal mediations in learning; and attend to the unique relationship between each individual and his environment. Since people interpret and respond differently to situations, they conclude that each individual's distinctive cognitive appraisal of environmental events is extremely important.

Cognitive theorists have not given up the basics of classical and reinforcement conditioning models. However, they insist that neither environmental nor personal variables alone can explain human behavior; both are necessary, and they invariably interact. Cognitive theorists do not accept the psychodynamic assertion that behaviors can be fully understood by evaluating the individual's personality dispositions and structures. On the other hand, they reject the behavioristic view that behavior can be adequately grasped with reference solely to environmental conditions. They contend that both internal and external forces are necessary elements. Most pertinent to their model is how each individual's distinctive cognitions and expectations shape his special interpretation of objective situations.

Rotter

In line with the major tenets of the cognitive social learning model, Julian B. Rotter[13] has emphasized the importance of subjective expectancies and of a person's perceived judgment of the reinforcement consequences of his behavior. Rotter proposed two concepts as basic to his theory: (1) *behavior potential* and (2) *expectancy.* The first refers to the thesis that behaviors that have most frequently led to positive reinforcements (rewarding experiences) in the past have the greatest potential for occurring again. The second concept is defined as "the probability held by the individual that a particular reinforcement will occur as a function of a specific behavior in his part''; in other words, this refers to the likelihood, as the person sees it, that what he does will prove rewarding. For a particular behavior potential to remain high, the individual must continue to expect that it will lead to positive reinforcement. The continuation of any behavior indicates that the individual's expectancy for reward remains higher than his expectancy for punishment. A problem in understanding abnormal behavior is to explain why a person subjectively expects to gain satisfaction for behaviors that appear to be judged by others as undesirable and that experience should show him leads to negative consequences. On closer analysis, however, it may be found that the individual's environment does, in fact, encourage it. Sometimes the encouragement is rather open and direct, as in the case of a dependent and anxiety-ridden child whose fears are continually reinforced by the fact that his parents respond to them with protectiveness, attention, and a hesitation about allowing him to experience even a modicum of danger. Sometimes the encouragement of abnormal behaviors is very subtle, involving the needs and reactions of others who, without realizing it, are more comfortable if the problem behavior occurs than they would be if it did not occur. Other forms of disturbed and deviant behavior also are positively reinforced by the concern and special privileges they evoke, as would be the case in a nurturant hospital setting.

Rotter recognized that expectancies differ in terms of the range of conditions or settings to which they apply. Most individuals acquire a number of *generalized expectancies* that operate across a wide variety of situations. For example, neurotics often have a generalized expectancy of disapproval from others if they act assertively in any situation; they may have encountered disapproval so consistently in the past that they now expect it in all situations. A fundamental type of generalized expectancy, according to Rotter, concerns people's beliefs about whether they, or the environment, control their reinforcements. Rotter refers to this as the internal versus external *locus of control* of reinforcement. The impact of reinforcements on behavior will depend, according to Rotter, on whether individuals perceive events to be contingent on their behavior or as independent of it, that is, whether or not they believe they have control over their environment. At one end of this dimension are those who are internal locus-of-control types, that is, who perceive rewards as contingent on their own behavior. At the opposite pole are external locus-of-control types, those who perceive rewards as determined by persons or forces beyond their control.

Therapy is viewed by Rotter as a specially arranged process of unlearning and relearning that is no different in its fundamental character and principles than that of other learning settings. In fact, as Rotter notes, formal therapy, despite its concentrated and focused nature, is often a less efficient vehicle for change than repetitive everyday experiences, since it is limited to a few hours a week at most and takes place in a setting that is appreciably different than that to which its effects must be generalized.

Therapeutic processes are designed to change maladjustive reinforcement expectancies. Hence the task is lowering the expectancy that a particular behavior will lead to gratifications or increasing the expectancy that alternate behaviors would lead to greater gratification in the same situation. In general learning terms, the therapist has the choice of either weakening the inadequate response, strengthening the correct or adequate response, or doing both.

Of utmost importance as a therapeutic goal is strengthening the expectancy that problems can be resolved. As Rotter notes, it is the purpose of therapy not to solve all of the patient's problems but rather to increase the patient's ability to solve his own problems. From a cognitive social learning point of view, one of the most important goals of treatment is to reinforce in the patient the expectancy that problems are solvable.

Bandura

In addition to Rotter's expectancy-reinforcement thesis and the other more traditional notions of how learning occurs, Albert Bandura[14,15] proposes such concepts as *vicarious conditioning* and *self-reinforcement systems*. The first pertains to the fact that persons can learn their pathologic attitudes simply by observing the experiences and feelings of others; for example, if a youngster happened to be glancing out the window when he saw a neighborhood dog chasing another child, the observing youngster may learn to fear that dog even though he had no frightening experience with it himself. The second concept refers to the fact that persons reinforce their attitudes and emotions simply by thinking about them; moreover, repetitive self-reinforcements often supplant the objective reinforcements of reality. Bandura notes that until recently, self-reinforcing behavior was virtually ignored in learning theory, perhaps because of a preoccupation with animal research. Unlike human subjects, who engage in self-evaluative behavior, animals are disinclined to pat themselves on the back for commendable performances or to berate themselves for getting into difficulties. By contrast, humans typically make self-reinforcement contingent on their performing in ways they have come to value as an index of personal merit. They often set relatively explicit standards, and a failure to meet them may not only be considered undeserving of reward but may also elicit self-denial or even self-punishment. Conversely, most people usually reward themselves well when they attain their self-determined standards. Self-administered positive and negative stimuli may serve, according to Bandura, both as powerful incentives for learning and as effective reinforcers in maintaining behaviors. Moreover, behavior may become completely controlled by fictional contingencies and fantasized consequences that are powerful enough to override the influence of real social reinforcements.

Bandura's conception of psychopathology emphasizes the acquisition of maladaptive behaviors and expectancies as a consequence largely of direct observational learning. Particularly important are learned expectancies of harm and a parallel sense of inefficiency in the ability to cope with perceived threat. Such fear expectancies and lowered self-evaluations lead to defensive behaviors that are difficult to unlearn because they appear to be subjectively confirmed as efficacious when harm does not occur. Maladaptive behaviors are often learned as a result of exposure to inadequate or maladaptive models. Bandura suggests that the degree to which parents themselves exhibit forms of abnormal behavior is a significant factor in the development of parallel deviant behaviors in their children. There is no need, according to Bandura, to look for traumatic early incidents or for psychodynamic conflicts. Once the behaviors have been learned through observational learning, it is likely that they will become manifest and be maintained by direct and vicarious reinforcement.

Although the acquisition of overt maladaptive behaviors remains important to an understanding of psychopathology, increasingly the cognitive approach to social learning theory has placed greater emphasis on the role of *dysfunctional expectancies* and *self-conceptions*. Persons may have erroneously learned to expect painful events to follow certain life situations. As a result they may act to avoid these events or to act in a way that creates the very situation they sought to avoid. An example would be a person who anticipates that closeness will result in pain, leading him to act in a defensively brusque way, which then results in social rejection,

as well as confirmation of his expectancy that closeness leads to rejection.

Learned cognitive processes not only lead to dysfunctional expectancies but also to *dysfunctional self-evaluations*. An example here would be a person who fails to value himself as a source of reward and thus experiences boredom when alone and an almost complete dependency on others for esteem and pleasure. Also common are problems associated with the acquisition of severe standards. Such learnings may present in excessive self-criticism, which gives rise, in turn, to depressive reactions, chronic discouragement, feelings of worthlessness, and a lack of purposefulness.

The cognitive learning approach to psychopathology can be contrasted to the psychoanalytic view of anxiety and defense. In cognitive social learning, anxiety results from a perceived inefficacy in coping with aversive events rather than being the result of unconscious impulses. Moreover, anxiety is not seen as leading to defensive behaviors; rather both anxiety and defensive behaviors are conceived to result from the expectancy of pain. According to Bandura, it is this expectation and the perceived inability to cope that results in both anxiety and defensive behaviors. Bandura notes further that defensive behaviors are difficult to unlearn because they often succeed in removing the person from troubling circumstances. Avoidance behavior prevents the individual from learning that life circumstances may have changed. Since the anticipated difficulty fails to materialize, this reinforces the assumption that the defensive behavior succeeded in turning it away. With this confirmation in hand, the neurotic's defensive behavior is reinforced erroneously and, hence, likely to be repeated again and again.

Perhaps cognitive social learning theorists should be called phenomenologic humanists since they have taken over the major features of these philosophic traditions. By including in their model processes such as self-reflection, personally established standards, reasoning, and other cognitive functions, as well as strategies to gain control over oneself, they have certainly introduced features to traditional learning formulations that are totally at variance with the originating philosophy of behaviorism.

Ellis

When emotions are highly aroused, cognitive functions are greatly impaired, according to Albert Ellis.[16,17] In what he speaks of as "emotional behavior," Ellis states that emotions are in control rather than cognitions, with the consequence that behaviors are frequently unrealistic and neurotic. During emotional episodes, efforts to act rationally are likely to fail. To Ellis, the time to control emotions is when reason can have the upper hand. Ellis believes we can learn and rehearse strategies for cognitive control. Like other cognitive theorists, he maintains that persons can learn a variety of effective cognitive strategies. These can be worked out on one's own by profiting from past mistakes or by anticipating problems and preventing them. One can learn both from direct experience and vicariously, that is, by observing how others handle difficult situations. Most important is that we can rehearse self-instructions, or what Ellis terms *self-verbalizations.*

Ellis has taken a powerful cognitive principle and developed its therapeutic implications extensively. Thus, if faulty behavior and emotions stem from faulty thinking and reasoning, then it is necessary to trace and modify the sources of faulty thinking itself. Ellis asserts that a major problem are false beliefs (cognitions) that are unrecognized among middle-class Americans because they are quite common. Among these fallacious beliefs, according to Ellis, are (1) we should be loved by almost everyone we know because to be disliked means we are flawed; (2) we should be competent and successful in all possible things if we are to think well of ourselves; (3) we have a right to expect that our friends will meet our perfectionistic ideals; (4) we are justified in believing that we are victims of circumstances that we cannot do much about; (5) because we cannot be successful at everything, we should avoid life's difficulties; (6) whatever strongly affected our lives will forever be a problem since we cannot get over things from the past; and (7) if we do not solve our problems, we are to blame.

BIOLOGICALLY ORIENTED SOCIAL LEARNING THEORISTS

A major theme of biologically-oriented social learning theorists is that psychopathology develops as a result of an intimate interplay of intraorganismic and environmental forces; such interactions start at the time of conception and continue throughout life. Individuals with similar biological potentials emerge with different personalities and clinical syndromes depending on the environmental conditions to which they are exposed.

According to these theorists there are a number of ways in which biological factors can shape, facil-

itate, or limit the nature of the individual's experiences and learning. For example, the same objective environment will be perceived as different by individuals who possess different biological sensibilities; people register different stimuli at varying intensities in accord with their unique pattern of alertness and sensory acuity. From this fact they assert that significant differences in experience itself is shaped at the outset by the biological equipment of the person.

Most biologically oriented learning theorists recognize further that the interaction between biological and psychological factors is not unidirectional such that biological determinants always precede and influence the course of learning and experience; the order of effects can be reversed, especially in the early stages of development. These theorists refer to research that shows that biological maturation is largely dependent on favorable environmental experience. The development of the biological substrate itself can be disrupted, even completely arrested, by depriving the maturing organism of stimulation at sensitive periods of rapid neurologic growth.

Beyond the crucial role of these early experiences, these theorists argue further that there is a circularity of interaction in which initial biological dispositions in young children evoke counterreactions from others that accentuate their disposition. They claim that the child plays an active role in creating environmental conditions, which, in turn, serve as a basis for reinforcing his biological tendencies.

Most learning and psychodynamic theorists of psychopathology have viewed disorders to be the result of detrimental experiences that the individual has had no part in producing himself. This is seen as a gross simplification by biosocial theorists. Each person possesses a biologically based pattern of sensitivities and behavioral dispositions that shapes the nature of his experiences and may contribute directly to the creation of environmental difficulties. Two facets of the interactive biological social learning system might be noted because of their special pertinence to the development of pathology.

First, the biological dispositions of the maturing individual are important because they strengthen the probability that certain kinds of behavior will be learned. For example, highly active and responsive children relate to and learn about their environment quickly. Their liveliness, zest, and power may lead them to a high measure of personal gratification. However, their energy and exploratory behavior may result in excess frustration if they over-aspire or run into insuperable barriers; unable to gratify their activity needs effectively, they may grope and strike out in erratic and maladaptive ways. Adaptive learning in constitutionally passive youngsters also is shaped by their biological equipment. Ill disposed to deal with their environment assertively and little inclined to discharge their tensions physically, they may learn to avoid conflicts and step aside when difficulties arise. They are less likely to develop guilt feelings about misbehavior than active youngsters, who more frequently get into trouble, receive more punishment, and are therefore inclined to develop aggressive feelings toward others.

Second, it appears to biosocial learning theorists that early temperamental dispositions evoke counterreactions from others that accentuate these initial tendencies; that is, a child's biological endowment shapes not only his behavior but that of his parents as well. For example, if a youngster's disposition is cheerful and adaptable and has made his upbringing easy, his parents will tend to display positive reciprocal attitudes. Conversely, if the child is tense and wound up, or if his upbringing is difficult and stressful, parents will react with dismay, fatigue, or hostility. Through his own behavioral disposition, then, the child elicits a series of parental behaviors that reinforce his initial temperament.

The reciprocal interplay of temperamental dispositions and parental reactions has been explored primarily by this group of theorists. It may be one of the most fruitful spheres of research concerning the etiology of psychopathology. The biosocial learning approach that characterizes the following theorists stems largely from the thesis that the child's genetic and constitutional endowment shapes and interacts with his social reinforcement experiences.

Eysenck

Hans Jurgen Eysenck[18,19] has proposed three major dimensions underlying all dispositions to psychopathology: extraversion, neuroticism, and psychoticism.

Neuroticism, at times referred to as stability-neuroticism, has several components. The most important is high emotionality, that is, a tendency to become physiologically aroused easily. Eysenck asserts that the tendency of the autonomic nervous system to be easily aroused is both an inherited characteristic and a major determinant of neurosis. The *introversion–extraversion* dimension refers primarily to sociability. It corresponds to the dichotomy between those who are less sociable, more solitary, and more contemplative (introverts) and those who are more gregarious, less inhibited, and more impulsive (extraverts). To Eysenck, extraverts acquire conditioned responses more slowly than introverts. Lastly, the *psychoticism* factor refers to the individual's contact with reality, that is, whether one's thought processes are impaired sufficiently to exhibit delusions or hallucinations. Eysenck notes that psychoticism is not a true dimension with opposite poles but an ingredient present in varying and inheritable degrees in all individual personalities. Eleven characteristics of those high on psychoticism are specified, including items such as being solitary and not caring for people, behaving in a troublesome manner and not fitting in, showing a lack of feeling, liking odd and unusual things, and engaging in little personal interaction.

An active laboratory researcher, Eysenck found direct empirical evidence on a variety of performance, metabolic, and personality measures that the dimension of extroversion–introversion could help distinguish two groups of neurotic illnesses. To represent the first group of neuroses, Eysenck labeled them as exhibiting *dysthymia.* Eysenck employed the label *hysteric* for the second group.

To Eysenck, *neurotic introverts* show a tendency to develop anxiety and depressive symptoms. They are characterized by obsessional tendencies, irritability, and apathy and suffer from a lability of the autonomic nervous system. According to their own statements, their feelings are easily hurt, they are self-conscious, nervous, given to feelings of inferiority, and moody; daydream easily; keep in the background on social occasions; and suffer from sleeplessness. In contrast, *neurotic extraverts* show a tendency to develop hysterical conversion symptoms and a hysterical attitude to their symptoms. Furthermore, they show little energy, narrow interests, have a bad work history, and are hypochondriacal. According to their own statements, they are troubled by stammering, are accident prone, are frequently absent from work owing to illness, are disgruntled, and troubled by aches and pains.

To Eysenck, dysthymic disorders are biologically grounded *learned* fears. Introverts who become dysthymic do so, because their high cortical and high emotional arousal facilitates rapid and strong anxiety conditioning. Dysthymic neurotic symptoms, such as phobias and anxiety attacks, are interpreted by Eysenck as conditioned maladaptive responses that are acquired by neurotic introverts. By contrast, hysterical disorders reflect failures to learn anxiety-based responses that are normally acquired during socialization. Extraverts who become hysterics or antisocial personalities do so because their cortical and emotional underarousal impedes the learning of anxiety-based self-restraints and moral inhibitions.

Eysenck suggests that extraverts may also be divided into two types. In the first, an outgoing sociability and stimulus-seeking behavior predominates. In the second extravert type, impulsivity and an inability to restrain antisocial urges predominate. The first type resembles the normal personality, whereas criminal behavior is more characteristic of the second. This second type contrasts most sharply to the dysthymic. The criminal or antisocial individual has failed to acquire by conditioning the normal socialization restraints that in the dysthymic have been exaggerated into chronic anxiety symptoms.

According to Eysenck, a simple learning model cannot explain satisfactorily why some neurotic symptoms persist unmodified despite severe negative consequences. Furthermore, some neurotic behaviors appear to be founded on irrational fears that are so removed from reality that the dreaded outcome never occurs. Nevertheless, despite the failure of the fear to be reinforced, the symptom is never extinguished as it should be according to standard learning theory. As a consequence of these observations, Eysenck believes that learning models of neuroses must recognize the possibility that some anxieties and fears are based on a biologically anchored and innate sensitivity to certain noxious objects. He suggests the probable development of an evolutionary mechanism by which organisms have been biologically ''prepared'' to react to certain stimuli with fear. For example, there would be survival value in a disposition to fear darkness, poisonous snakes, certain insects, and high places. Conditioned neurotic fears that were based on these evolved survival phobias might not obey the ordinary principles of learning for their extinction. Evolutionary preparedness might also explain why certain phobias tend to be restricted to a small class of events when conditioning theory would predict that *any* stimulus should be able to be made fearsome by learned associations. To Eysenck, biological preparedness suggests that only neurologically ''wired in'' response tendencies will display this difficult-to-extinguish form of neurotic anxiety.

Meehl

Although Paul Meehl's[20] biologically oriented social learning model is limited to one major syndrome, that of schizophrenia, it is notable both for its elegance and specificity. He hypothesized that only a certain class of people, those with a particular genetic constitution, have any liability to schizophrenia. Meehl suggests that the varied emotional and perceptual-cognitive dysfunctions displayed by schizophrenics are difficult to explain in terms of single region disorders. The widespread nature of these dysfunctions suggests the operation of a more diffuse ''integrative neural defect.'' Although a combination of different neurologic disturbances can account for this defect, Meehl opts for an explanation in terms of deficits in synaptic control. More specifically, he believes that the major problem in schizophrenia lies in a malfunctioning of the two-way mutual control system between perceptual-cognitive regions and the limbic motivation center.

Meehl's proposal is that integrative neural defects are the only direct phenotypic consequences produced by the genetic disorders; given the label *schizotaxia*, it is all that can properly be spoken of as inherited. The imposition of certain social learning histories on schizotaxic individuals results in a personality organization that Meehl, following Rado,[21] calls the *schizotype*. Four core behavior traits, namely anhedonia, cognitive slippage, interpersonal aversiveness, and ambivalence, are not innate. However, Meehl postulates that they are universally learned by schizotaxic individuals, given any existing social learning regimen, from the best to the worst. If the social environment is favorable and the schizotaxic person has the good fortune of inheriting a low anxiety readiness, possesses physical vigor, and a general resistance to stress, he will remain a well-compensated schizotype and may never manifest symptoms of clinical ''schizophrenia.'' He will be like the gout-prone male, according to Meehl, whose genes determine him to have an elevated blood uric acid titer but who never develops clinical gout.

Meehl considers the most important causal influence pushing the schizotype toward schizophrenic decompensation to be the schizophrenogenic mother. If this interaction were free of maternal ambivalence and aversive inputs to the schizotaxic child, even compensated schizotypy might be avoided. At worst there might be faint signs of cognitive slippage, minimal neurologic aberrations, including body image deviations, but not the interpersonal aversiveness that Meehl considers central to the clinical picture.

The relation between schizotaxia, schizotypy, and schizophrenia is class inclusion: all schizotaxics become, on all social learning regimens, schizotypic in personality organization; most, however, remain compensated. A minority, disadvantaged by other, largely polygenically determined constitutional weaknesses and exposed to ambivalent learning regimens by schizophrenogenic mothers, are potentiated into clinical schizophrenia. What makes schizotaxia etiologically specific is that it is a *necessary* condition. Meehl postulates that a nonschizotaxic individual, whatever his other genetic makeup and whatever his social learning history, would at most develop a nonschizotypal personality disorder or a psychoneurosis.

Millon

In what I have termed a *biosocial* learning theory, I have stressed the fact that there are manifold biogenic and psychogenic determinants of psychopathology, the relative weights of each varying widely as a function of time and circumstance.[22,23] These determinants are seen to operate conjointly to shape the pattern of an illness. Furthermore, interaction effects operate across time; that is, the course of later events are related in a determinant way to earlier events. I view the etiology of psychopathology as a developmental process in which intraorganismic and environmental forces display not only a reciprocity and circularity of influence but also an orderly and sequential continuity throughout the life of the individual.

The maturation of biological substrates for psychological capacities are anchored initially to genetic processes, but their development is substantially dependent on environmental stimulation. I use the concept of *stimulus nutriment* to represent the belief that environmental experience activates chemical processes requisite to the maturation of neural collaterals. Stimulus "impoverishment" is seen to lead to irrevocable deficiencies in neural development and their associated psychological functions; stimulus "enrichment" may prove equally deleterious by producing pathologic over-developments or imbalances among these functions.

Numerous theorists have proposed, either by intention or inadvertently, schemas based on a concept of sensitive developmental periods. None has formulated this notion in terms of neurologic growth stages. Freud's theory of stages of psychosexual development, in which particular early experiences at specified times in development have deeply etched and lasting effects, may be viewed as the first major psychopathologic theory based on a concept of sensitive periods. Despite Freud's early training as a neurologist, I believe that his schema was founded *not* in terms of internal neurologic maturation but in terms of a peripheral sphere of maturation, that of sexual development. His concern lay with variations in external sensory erogenous zones (*e.g.,* oral, anal, and genital), not with the more central neurologic structures that underlie and are basic to them.

A more profitable basis for organizing a system of developmental periods would be in terms of internal neurologic growth potentials. Relationships certainly exist between these inner variables and other less centrally involved variables, such as Freud's concept of erogenous zones. However, to focus on peripheral spheres of maturation, as did Freud, is, in my view, to put the proverbial "cart before the horse."

I propose three neuropsychological stages of development, representing peak periods in neurologic maturation. Each developmental stage reflects transactions between constitutional and experiential influences that combine to set a foundation for subsequent stages; if the interactions at one stage are deficient or distorted, all subsequent stages will be affected since they rest on a defective base.

The first stage, termed *sensory attachment*, is seen to predominate from birth to approximately 18 months of age. This period is characterized by a rapid maturation of neurologic substrates for sensory processes and by the infant's attachment and dependency on others. The second stage, referred to as *sensorimotor autonomy*, begins at about age 12 months and extends in its peak development through the sixth year. It is characterized by a rapid differentiation of motor capacities that coordinate with established sensory functions; this coalescence enables the young child to locomote, manipulate, and verbalize in increasingly skillful ways. The third stage, called the period of *intracortical initiative*, is considered primary from about the fourth year through adolescence. There is rapid neurologic growth during this stage, enabling the child to reflect, plan, and act independent of parental supervision. Integrations developed during earlier phases of this period undergo substantial reorganization as a product of the biological and social effects of puberty.

Maladaptive consequences arise as a result of either stimulus impoverishment or stimulus enrichment at each of the three stages. Thus, marked stimulus impoverishment during the sensory-attachment period will produce deficiencies in sensory capacities and a marked diminution of interpersonal sensitivity and behavior. There is little evidence available with regard to the effects of stimulus enrichment during this stage; I propose, however, that excessive stimulation may result in hypersensitivities, stimulus-seeking behaviors, and abnormal interpersonal dependencies. Next, children deprived of adequate stimulation during the sensorimotor stage will be deficient in skills for behavioral autonomy, will display a lack of exploratory and competitive activity, and will be characterized by timidity and submissiveness. In contrast, excessive enrichment and indulgence of these sensorimotor capacities may result in uncontrolled self-expression, narcissism, and social irresponsibility. Among the consequences of understimulation during the intracortical-initiative stage is an identity diffusion, an inability to fashion an integrated and consistent purpose for one's existence and an inefficiency in channeling and directing one's energies, capacities, and impulses. Excessive stimulation in the form of overtraining and overguidance was seen to result in the loss of several functions, notably spontaneity, flexibility, and creativity.

Trust of others is the central attitude learned during the sensory-attachment stage. Feelings of self-competence are acquired first during the stage of sensorimotor autonomy. Attitudes concerning one's personal identity are formed primarily during the intracortical-initiative period.

Personality strategies and disorders are complex forms of instrumental learning, that is, ways of achieving positive reinforcements (pleasure) and avoiding negative reinforcements (pain). These strategies reflect what reinforcements the individual has learned to seek or avoid, where he looks to obtain these reinforcements, and how he performs in order to elicit or escape them. I proposed a 4×2 classificatory scheme, which is briefly touched upon in another chapter of this text,[24] as a theoretic foundation for the personality disorders of Axis II in the *Diagnostic and Statistical Manual of Mental Disorders*. This scheme is based on three dimensions: (1) the relative role played by positive (pleasure) and negative (pain) reinforcements as determinants of behavior; (2) the tendency to obtain reinforcements either from other persons or from oneself; and (3) the proclivity either to seek these reinforcements actively or to wait passively for their occurrence.

Eleven personality disorders are derived from the theoretic model. A product of both biogenic and psychogenic factors, and developed as an instrumental means of coping with one's environment, the personality disorders frequently prove self-defeating in that they exhibit an adaptive inflexibility and a tendency to perpetuate and foster, rather than resolve new problems.

CONCLUSIONS

The vast number of figures, the conflicting theories, and the divergent interests that have shaped the historical course of social learning theory can all but stagger the reader who is first becoming acquainted with this model. Although sketchy in detail, this review has outlined the major concepts that have led to present theories and directions in social learning. It is hoped that it will serve as a perspective through which future readings may be evaluated and integrated.

That psychopathology should incorporate a variety of different approaches is not an invitation to ill-conceived notions and random speculations; tolerance of diversity is not license for scientific incompetence.

None of the theories discussed in this chapter, nor I suspect in any other, approaches the ideal of a complete scientific system for psychopathology. Hence, what I have written in this section is likely to apply to models discussed elsewhere.

The formal structure of most theories is haphazard and unsystematic; concepts often are vague, and procedures by which empiric consequences may be derived are tenuous. Many theories are written in a hortatory and persuasive fashion. Facts are mixed with speculations, and literary allusions and colorful descriptions are offered as substitutes for testable hypotheses. In short, instead of presenting an orderly arrangement of concepts and propositions by which hypotheses may be clearly derived, most theories present a loosely formulated pastiche of opinions, analogies, and speculations. Brilliant as many of these speculations may be, they often leave the reader dazzled rather than illuminated.

Confusion stems further from the interweaving of concepts based on different and occasionally quite distinct sources of data. Thus, concepts generated in learning research are adopted by some theorists and used as if they were synonymous with neurophysiologic processes on the one hand and clinical behavior on the other. Terms are interchanged because of some vague similarity in meaning. Further difficulties arise because of the excessive use of hypothetic constructs; even worse, these constructs often are reified into entities. Thus, concepts are presented as if they represented tangible clinical phenomena and then assigned powers of the most illusory nature.

Ambiguous concepts in structurally weak theories make it impossible to derive systematic and logical hypotheses; this results in conflicting derivations and circular reasoning. Most theories of psychopathology have generated brilliant deductions and insights, but few of these ideas can be attributed to their structure, the precision of their concepts, or their formal procedures for hypothesis derivation.

REFERENCES

1. Bindra D: Experimental psychology and the problem of behavior disorders. Canad J Psychol 13:135–150, 1959

2. Thorndike EL: The Elements of Psychology. New York, Seiler, 1905

3. Pavlov ID: Lectures on Conditioned Reflexes, vol 1. New York, International Publishers, 1928

4. Watson JB: Psychology from the Standpoint of a Behaviorist. Philadelphia, JB Lippincott, 1919

5. Watson JB, Rayner R: Conditioned emotional reactions. J Exp Psychol 3:1–14, 1920

6. Jones MC: The elimination of children's fears. J Exp Psychol 7:382–390, 1924

7. Skinner BF: What is psychotic behavior? In Theory and Treatment of the Psychoses. St. Louis, Washington University Press, 1956

8. Skinner BF: Cumulative Record. New York, Appleton-Century-Crofts, 1959

9. Wolpe J: Psychotherapy by Reciprocal Inhibition. Stanford, CA, Stanford University Press, 1958

10. Masserman JH: Behavior and Neurosis. Chicago, University of Chicago Press, 1943

11. Dollard J, Miller N: Personality and Psychotherapy. New York, McGraw-Hill, 1950

12. Mowrer OH: Learning theory and behavior therapy. In Wolman B (ed): Handbook of Clinical Psychology. New York, McGraw-Hill, 1965

13. Rotter JB: Social Learning and Clinical Psychology. Englewood Cliffs, NJ, Prentice-Hall, 1954

14. Bandura A: Principles of Behavior Modification. New York, Holt, Rinehart & Winston, 1969

15. Bandura, A: Social Learning Theory. Englewood Cliffs, NJ, Prentice-Hall, 1977

16. Ellis A: Reason and Emotion in Psychotherapy. Secaucus, NJ, Lyle Stuart, 1962

17. Ellis A: Theoretical and Empirical Foundations of Rational-Emotive Therapy. Monterey, CA, Wadsworth, 1979

18. Eysenck HJ: The Biological Basis of Personality. Springfield, IL, Charles C Thomas, 1967

19. Eysenck, HJ: A genetic model of anxiety. In Sarason IG, Speilberger CD (eds): Stress and Anxiety, vol 2. New York, John Wiley & Sons, 1975

20. Meehl P: Schizotaxia, schizotypy, schizophrenia. Am Psychol 17:827–838, 1962

21. Rado S: Psychoanalysis of Behavior. New York, Grune & Stratton, 1962

22. Millon T: Modern Psychopathology. Philadelphia, WB Saunders, 1969

23. Millon T: Disorders of Personality: DSM-III, Axis II. New York, John Wiley & Sons, 1981

24. Millon T: The avoidant personality. In Cavenar JO Jr (ed): Psychiatry. Philadelphia, JB Lippincott, 1985

Richard I. Shader, Edward L. Scharfman, and Daniel A. Dreyfuss

A Biological Model for Selected Personality Disorders

Despite the emphasis that was at times placed by Freud on the consequences of conflict and early infantile wishes and experiences, much of his theory of personality was based on notions of energy distributions within the mind, motive forces, energies present even in the absence of neurotic inhibition, and the need to maintain psychophysiologic homeostasis. He spoke directly about the mistaken impression that he did not acknowledge the importance of innate factors.[1-3] Federn was among the few of his contemporaries who also concerned himself with possible constitutional determinants of personality.[4] The unfortunate neglect of the biological determinants of personality by some of the most experienced and articulate shapers of concepts of personality has left us without adequately tested, workable, and accepted concepts in this basic aspect of human functioning and psychology.

Traits such as gregariousness or shyness with strangers, impulsivity, explosivity, dependency, and passivity are easy to notice as enduring characteristics in ourselves and others, and yet even some of the more popularized traits such as schizoid, introversion, and extraversion remain controversial, ill defined, and without adequate research and documentation about their fundamental existence, basic biology, and genetics.

In the absence of such clear lines of research, what we offer in this chapter are observations that we believe argue for the need for a new, broader, more pluralistic, more fluid model of personality. Although there are several widely used concepts and definitions of personality, most share the idea that personality, once formed, is constant and immutable. Descriptive adjectives of personality include "pervasive," "deeply ingrained," and "con-

stant over time." The determinants of personality have too often been understood in simplistic, reductionistic terms, with the assumptions of a cause-and-effect relationship between the adult personality, the final outcome, and early developmental and experiential events.

During the past several decades, the use of psychopharmacologic probes has facilitated the preliminary dissection and identification of possible subpopulations of patients from among the broad, poorly defined macropopulations conceptualized as having personality disorders. The potential validity of these subpopulations as discrete entities with reliable diagnostic criteria is currently gaining support from psychogenetic family studies, prospective longitudinal studies of patients with personality disorders, experimental procedures such as rapid eye movement (REM) latency measurements and dexamethasone suppression testing, and the "response" of patients in these newly defined subpopulations to specific psychopharmacologic treatments. By "response" we refer to the modifications of maladaptive emotions, affects, behavior patterns, and cognitions that have been causing the patient dysfunction and/or dysphoria. These ideas will be described more fully below.

We do not believe that palliation of target symptoms alone causes symptom substitution, and experiences with behavioral therapy, hypnotherapy, cognitive therapy, and pharmacotherapy lend support to this impression. Nor do we believe that diminution or palliation of target symptoms decreases a patient's motivation for continued hard work in the psychotherapeutic process. On the contrary, a patient, less overwhelmed by anxiety or intolerable painful affects, can invest a psychotherapy with more focused attention, concentration, and communication. The ability to tolerate anxiety and painful affects can even lessen resistance and facilitate exploration and uncovering in areas that had previously been too threatening.[5-7] Because we view personality as a final common pathway with multiple determinants, we advocate a treatment plan with a multimodal approach—never pharmacotherapy alone, but pharmacotherapy (if indicated) in combination with some form of psychotherapy (*e.g.,* therapeutic listening and communication, clarification, support for mastery and self-esteem, education, and increased tolerance for ambiguity and uncertainty).

The idea that constitution and environment act together to bring out pathology is well known in medicine. A patient with genetically determined sickle cell trait, for example, may remain asymptomatic until a stressor such as sepsis or dehydration, acting on the patient's constitutional diathesis, leads to a medical emergency—the sickle cell crisis. Freud believed that infantile sexuality had a "polymorphous perverse" quality (*i.e.,* an innate diathesis that could be expressed through a variety of different channels leading to a perverse or normal outcome depending on the environmental conditions that acted jointly on this predisposition).[8] Thomas and Chess,[9,10] in some of the rare longitudinal research in this area, observed neonates, following them into early adulthood. They suggest the presence of a number of innate temperaments, extant and identifiable from the very beginning of life. These include level of activity, adaptability, attention span, persistence, distractability, intensity of reaction, stimulus threshold, and approach–withdrawal.

Our concept of personality as being interactive or fluid rather than fixed derives from some of the observations and evidence that we will develop in this chapter (*i.e.,* on the interdependency of personality and one's internal and external environments). Not only can personality predispose to and shape psychopathology, but psychopathology can reshape and remodel personality, causing marked alterations that did not exist in the premorbid state. This idea of fluidity in a construct conceptualized as constant and immutable is analogous to theories and observations about bone. On the surface, bone appears hard, rigid, and fixed in shape, size, and form. Its shape as a tibia or scapula, its length, and its size are all genetically determined; yet bone requires growth hormone and sex hormones for this to be accomplished. There is a constant influx and efflux of calcium salts, governed by diet, kidney function, levels of vitamin D, and the hormones calcitonin and parathormone. There is continual reshaping of structure and architecture, with reabsorption here and redeposition there. Bone functions to provide form, structure, and protection and to bear weight and stress. It serves a creative function as an endless reservoir of blood and in times of stress, such as infection, it pours out an abundance of white blood cells. The analogies to personality are endless. However, bone can also demineralize, become brittle, and fracture. The nature of this complex interdependency of all of the above systems would require a thorough multimodal approach to the diagnosis and appropriate treatment in case of fracture. It is precisely this that we advocate with respect to the approach to personality and personality disorders, (*i.e.,* a holistic, pluralistic overview, that considers fluidity, interdependency, and multiplicity of determinants in the diagnosis and treatment of such disorders).

What follows is a discussion of five broad, ill-defined categories of personality disorder from which we will further develop our thesis. These groups are not meant to be a representative sample but rather illustrations. We posit that for subpopulations in each of these heterogeneous groups the primary underlying disorder is biologically mediated and the character pathology is often secondary. Having identified such subgroups, we propose that psychopharmacologic treatment is necessary, although not sufficient, to effect the best possible outcome and response. Many patients, particularly those who invoke negative countertransference in the therapist, and who make little progress in psychotherapy, are often "condemned" with the pejorative and hopeless diagnosis of having "character pathology." We hope to offer convincing evidence that pharmacotherapy and psychotherapy in specific cases will alleviate much dysfunction and dysphoria in these patients.

Disorders of Affect

It is commonly held in psychiatric lore that the major affective disorders are characterized by a discrete onset, a finite course, and a return to baseline premorbid functioning following the termination of the core episode. On the other hand, patients with chronic protracted milder depressions have been conceptualized as suffering from neurosis or character pathology. A continuum between the two groups was not believed to exist, until recently.

We will describe and review evidence supporting the idea that major affective disorders can have chronic, protracted, subclinical courses and that many patients who have been subsumed under the umbrella of neurosis or character disorder in reality suffer from primary, subsyndromal affective disorders that are muted and attenuated and on a continuum with major affective disorder. A brief digression to review the psychophysiologic, psychometric, and psychopharmacologic techniques used to accumulate this evidence will now be presented.

Kupfer[11,12] has demonstrated that in patients with primary depression there are characteristic changes in sleep architecture. Frequently, the time between sleep onset and the beginning of the first REM cycle, known as REM latency, is significantly shortened in this group, and REM activity is increased.

Neuroendocrine studies have revealed a disrupted circadian cortisol pattern and an abnormally high secretion of cortisol in patients with primary depression. Carroll[13,14] found that a large portion of inpatients with primary major depression who have anhedonia and autonomy of mood will have high serum cortisol levels on the day following the administration of the potent exogenous steroid dexamethasone. This group escapes the normal physiologic suppression of cortisol that one would expect and is said to have a positive dexamethasone suppression test.

Psychogenetic studies examine the prevalence of illness in the first-degree relatives of an identified patient proband group, studying whether the illness under study is more prevalent in such relatives as compared with relatives of controls. Positive results imply probable genetic determinants in the transmission of the illness. To control for environmental input, studies have been made of children of parents with known illnesses who are adopted into so-called normal families. Finally, concordance rates for illness in monozygotic twins are contrasted to concordance rates for dizygotic twins. Primary affective disorders have been shown by these methods to have important genetic underpinnings.

Prospective longitudinal studies of an illness over time allow one to follow the vicissitudes of such an illness. Frequently, the diagnosis, prognosis, and treatment plan will change. We will now review studies indicating how neuroses and personality disorders may shift into primary affective disorders over time.

Pharmacotherapy can serve as a diagnostic tool in addition to being a curative or palliative treatment. The response of syndromes to drug treatment, particularly syndromes thought to have pre-dominantly developmental or psychological causes clearly raises questions about the existence of multiple causes and, moreover, questions about which of these multiple causes is primary and which is secondary. Furthermore, treating a depressed patient with a previously unknown bipolar affective disorder diathesis with antidepressants may often precipitate a hypomanic episode, allowing a more accurate diagnosis of bipolar disorder and a more effective treatment with lithium. These examples form some of the basis for the concept of the pharmacologic diagnostic probe.

None of the above tools is meant to substitute for careful clinical evaluation and experience-derived judgment. None alone is foolproof. However, when used together, and in combination with clinical judgment, the result should be a more accurate definition of more homogeneous patient subgroups, amenable to specific pharmacotherapies. Many such patients have until now been lost in the seemingly heterogeneous haystack referred to as character or personality disorders.

Akiskal and his colleagues have been among the major proponents of the idea that primary major affective disorders can follow chronic, protracted, subclinical courses, that these subclinical entities are on a continuum with full-blown clinical affective disorders, and that patients who suffer from these chronic "subaffective" disorders are often misunderstood, misdiagnosed, and inadequately treated.[15-21] They studied patients with "neurotic depression" in a 3-year longitudinal, prospective study. These patients were characterized by mildly depressed mood (without incapacitation); no psychosis; no vegetative signs; the presence of a psychosocial stressor (usually a loss); a dependent, object-hungry style; and a pattern of reaction to stress with depression. During the course of the study, 18% became manic or hypomanic and 22% developed a primary major depressive episode. Given that 40% of this group developed a major affective disorder, he concluded that the diagnostic concept of "neurotic depression" was heterogeneous and imprecise and that these 40% represented either a precursor, or an interepisode state of major affective disorder. What is clear is that although characterologic depressions are typically chronic, "not all chronic depressions are characterological!"[19] In another group, they studied 50 patients diagnosed as having characterologic depressions: 40% responded to antidepressants, 35% became hypomanic on antidepressants, and many who responded to antidepressants had a shortened REM latency. All these findings are typical of patients with primary affective disorder. Akiskal and co-workers[19] infer that "some characterological depressions represent a subsyndromic and lifelong version of primary affective illness." Finally, in discussing the concept of dysthymic disorder, they describe 65 patients with chronic characterologic depression.[17] One third responded to antidepressants, had shortened REM latencies, and had family histories positive for major affective illness.

An interepisode or post-depressive personality has also been described.[16] Reintegration into the family and vocational and social rehabilitation were disturbed in a fourth of these cases following remission of the core major depression. After 2 years, these patients displayed helplessness, dependency, irritability, obsessional brooding, clinging, phobias, and a decrease in emotional ties. It is stressed that these changes in personality did not exist as premorbid traits but arose secondary to the insult of the primary major depression. "The clinician is admonished not to equate their interepisodic manifestations of affective illness with primary characterologic pathology,"[16] and the authors advocate the use of adjunctive pharmacotherapy when it can be demonstrated that there is a subaffective disorder presenting as a personality disorder.

Cyclothymia is another personality disorder with a subaffective determinant. In addition to short, irregular fluctuations in affect, these patients may display explosive outbursts, irritability, lability, marital failure, unstable employment, impulsivity, wanderlust, substance abuse, promiscuity, chaotic interpersonal relationships, and injudicious, self-destructive behavior. Such patients have been diagnosed as hysterical, narcissistic, antisocial, and borderline character disorders. The Akiskal group studied 50 such patients over time and found that 36% became manic, 44% became hypomanic on antidepressants, and 30% had first-degree relatives with bipolar illness.[20] Moreover, 60% responded to lithium with a reduction in impulsivity, explosivity, promiscuity, chaotic employment records, and substance abuse. Their conclusion is that cyclothymic personalities represent a genetically mediated, subclinical affective disorder, on a continuum with bipolar illness. "Unpredictability in mood was a major source of distress . . . as they could not know from moment to moment how they would feel. It undermined their 'sense of self' . . . after lithium, their 'sense or self' had finally acquired the stability which came from significant control of unpredictable mood swings." For this group of patients, lithium had to be added to psychotherapy to achieve a more complete ego re-

construction in the sphere of "sense of self." The results were quite rewarding!

Rifkin and the Klein group described a group of patients similar to cyclothymics but with more prominent antisocial behavior.[22] Usually adolescent girls, these patients are truant, have poor tolerance of authority, and are manipulative, seductive, promiscuous, and prone to malingering. In addition, they experience mood swings lasting hours to days that are not preceded by a psychosocial precipitant and are nonreactive to environmental stimuli. This behavior is not attention seeking. Called emotionally unstable character disorders, 14 of 21 of this subgroup when treated with lithium (in a double-blind crossover study with placebo) showed improvement in mood, aggression, and sociability. What appeared to be a personality disorder with antisocial, histrionic, narcissistic, and borderline features is postulated to be a secondary manifestation or epiphenomenon of an underlying primary disturbance in affect.

Klein and colleagues[23,24] have identified still another subgroup of patients (usually diagnosed as having avoidant, narcissistic, histrionic, or borderline personality disorder) by virtue of their preferential response to monoamine oxidase inhibitors (MAOIs). They are referred to as hysteroid or rejection-sensitive dysphorics and display a marked vulnerability to rejection, with a crushlike depression, and feelings of hopelessness, low self-esteem, anergy and lethargy, suicidal gestures, and "reversed" vegetative signs such as hypersomnia and hyperphagia. They frequently binge on sweets and abuse cocaine, amphetamine, and alcohol. Their depression, although severe, may remit with attention, admiration, and applause, after which these patients may become elated and energetic until the next rejection. In the interepisode phase they are flamboyant, ebullient, histrionic, seductive, impulsive, indiscrete, and possessive. Their attachments are intense, idealized, and short-lived. Job changes and romances at work are typical. By middle age, they tend to avoid close contact for fear of rejection. In a double-blind, crossover study of psychotherapy plus MAOI versus psychotherapy plus placebo, the patients on the drug showed a more stabilized mood, a more stabilized work record, more stabilized interpersonal relationships, palliation of vegetative signs, a decrease in substance abuse, and less promiscuity.[25] This response to MAOIs and the similarity of this subgroup to patients described as having atypical depression[26] led Klein and Shader[24] to conclude that, in such patients, the pharmacologically responsive underlying affective disorder is primary. When the rejection-induced depression is tempered by medication, these patients feel less desperate and engage in fewer "reparative," maladaptive behavior patterns, which, prior to medication, were in the service of modulating their affective vulnerability to social approval or rejection. Without pharmacotherapy for the underlying dysregulated affect, the secondary character pathology is less amenable to modification in psychotherapy.

In this section we have presented information about subpopulations of patients whose personality disorders we view as epiphenomenal, while the affective, subaffective, or interepisodic affective determinants are the underlying prime mover. These "chronic low grade depressions are . . . conditions where the trait and the state are so closely interwoven that it is hard to separate . . . lifestyles from illness."[21] We have reviewed the methodology currently available to help make these separations. The results have been gratifying and rewarding for both patients and clinicians.

Borderline Personality Disorders

Patients with borderline personality disorders are a heterogeneous group that has been in the forefront of psychiatric literature for about 2 decades, and although there are a number of noncongruent theories about etiology, there is good general agreement about how these patients appear phenomenologically. They are not psychotic yet are prone to brief periods of psychosis, or psychosis-like experiences; they are not neurotic yet certainly have neurotic symptoms. Disturbances in mood and affect are common, but such patients are not conceptualized as having major affective disorders. Some consider these patients unanalyzable, while others advocate that modification of classic analytic techniques can yield good results. In the past these patients were believed to be on the "borderline" of psychosis and were diagnosed as having latent schizophrenia, preschizophrenia, or pseudoneurotic schizophrenia. Gunderson and colleagues[26,27] have collated a constellation of eight traits typical of these patients:

1. Low achievement and diminished work capacity, despite talent
2. Impulsivity, low frustration tolerance, and polysubstance abuse
3. Manipulativeness, with suicide threats and gestures
4. Intense affect, with rage and depression
5. Chaotic, disturbed interpersonal relationships with dependence, devaluation, idealization, and intrusiveness
6. Difficulty tolerating being alone
7. Brief periods of psychosis and regression usually precipitated by psychosocial stress
8. The emergence of primitive material in unstructured psychological testing.

Kernberg complements these ideas with the perspective that these patients have intact reality but an impaired integration in their sense of self.[28,29] Chronic and intolerable feelings of emptiness are part of the description in the *Diagnostic and Statistical Manual of Mental Disorders (DSM-III)*.[30]

In attempting to understand the causes of these conditions, Stone[31] and the Klein group[32] were both impressed with instability of affect as the primary disorder, which, when coupled with certain developmental and experiential vicissitudes, could forge the borderline personality as a final common pathway. The Klein group postulates that the "peculiar behavior might be an attempt to express or cope with recurrent intolerable affective states and reactions" and that "with the development of pharmacological agents whose mode of actions seems to be the direct amelioration of disordered affects . . . or the reduction of specific affective vulnerabilities, that character and ego defect may be seen as more secondary then primary."[32]

In our discussion of characterologic depressions in the first section, we implicated this theory and presented evidence that subgroups of such patients could respond dramatically to antidepressants or lithium. In addition to the disturbance in affect and the response to affect-regulating medication, most of the patients described in the prior section also meet the descriptions for borderline personality disorder by Gunderson, Kernberg, and the *DSM-III*. Cole reviewed a study of 62 patients who met Gunderson's criteria for borderline personality disorder.[32] Of these, 15 also met *DSM-III* criteria for major depression and 16 met *DSM-III* criteria for dysthymic disorder. We agree with Cole's conclusions that borderline personality disorder and major affective disorder (or subsyndromal affective disorders) can co-exist and are not mutually exclusive. However, we go a step farther and agree with the Klein group that for some patients with co-existing affective disorder and borderline personality disorder, the so-called borderline behavior and organization are secondary, "reparative" attempts to modulate an overwhelming dysregulation in affect that developed and expressed itself early in life, particularly when object-constancy, self-object differentiation, and separation anxiety were important.

Returning to methodology to support our thesis, it is useful to examine a review by Stone[31] of two psychogenetic studies of patients diagnosed as having borderline personality organization by Kernberg's criteria. Thirty percent of the first-degree relatives of 23 borderline probands studied at the New York State Psychiatric Institute had psychiatric illness, mostly primary affective disorder. In addition, the 23 probands themselves had several symptoms of primary affective disorder and two had frank bipolar illness. The second psychogenetic study supported the first, with findings that there was a significantly higher prevalence of primary affective disorder in the first-degree relatives of 34 patients who met Kernberg's criteria for borderline personality organization when compared with first-degree relatives of neurotic controls.

As commentary on these issues, Akiskal and Lemmi[15] state, "There is converging evidence from phenomenologic, familial, longitudinal, neuroendocrine, and sleep EEG findings to suggest that as many as two-thirds of patients labeled borderline . . . represent *formes frustes* of recurrent affective disorders . . . the unstable 'sense of self' characteristic of these conditions may, in a substantial number of cases, be epiphenomenal to unpredictable mood swings that prevent optimum ego development." In another paper, Akiskal[17] adds, "the affective component is often overlooked because borderline patients present with complicated biographies and give histories of affective instability in a setting of tempestuous interpersonal relationships." We would argue that under the rubric of borderline personality disorder, subpopulations of patients are subsumed who have a dysregulation of affect. Once identified, these patients should benefit from affect-regulating medication, in addition to psychotherapy.

For those patients whose borderline personality disorder is in part determined by a predisposition to psychotic disorganization, the pharmacotherapy may need to include antipsychotic or neuroleptic medication. Spitzer[33] has discussed the difficulty in defining this subgroup, many of whom we would classify as schizoid and/or schizotypal. Although these patients seldom require hospitalization, many can benefit from antipsychotic medication. "Soft" elements of formal thought disorders, ideas of reference, and other target symptoms that "bor-

der" on frank psychosis are common. The relationship of this group of patients to those patients with schizophrenia is as yet unclear.

Bellak[34] has described a group of patients with adult attention deficit disorder who have a behavior disorder characterized by impulsivity, minipsychotic episodes, tremendous irritability, difficulty in their object relations, and polysubstance abuse. These patients also meet *DSM-III* criteria for borderline personality disorder. Such patients may respond to psychostimulants, especially if there is a positive childhood history of inattention, impulsivity, easy distractability, and hyperactivity and a generally normal level of intelligence.

We fully support the importance and possible role of separation-individuation, introjects, and object-relations theory, but we propose that such experiences impact on patients with a certain genetic diathesis to produce the borderline personality disorder. In some patients the diathesis has more subaffective determinants, while in others, more subpsychotic determinants. These multifactorial determinants should be approached with a multidimensional treatment plan.

Panic Anxiety and Agoraphobia

Anxiety has been a central subject in psychiatry from the beginning. Freud proposed and revised theories of anxiety as did his successors. However, it is the Klein group, using medication as a diagnostic probe, who draws our attention to the need to dissect panic anxiety away from anticipatory, generalized, and signal anxiety and to identify the spontaneous panic attack as a potentially discrete entity.[32,35] The Klein group postulates a relationship between panic anxiety and the secondary development of anticipatory anxiety and agoraphobia, in which acute spontaneous panic attacks induce agoraphobia, and not vice versa. They describe a group of patients seen as dependent, needy, clinging, regressed, demanding, and manipulative, who are also chronically anxious, depressed, fearful, helpless, and agoraphobic. Such patients have severe disturbances of impairment in social and vocational function. Most consult a variety of medical and/or mental health professionals over the years and carry diagnoses such as "obsessional, hysterical, depressive, borderline, pseudoneurotic-schizophrenic, passive-aggressive and/or addictive personality disorders, or hysterical conversions."[32] None demonstrated hallucinations, delusions, or thought disorder. Sheehan[36] describes a patient who had consulted 30 physicians including six psychiatrists over a 12-year span. She was in psychoanalysis for 5 days per week over the course of 2 years, had 3 years of psychotherapy, 1 year of behavior therapy, ECT, and minor tranquilizers, all to no avail. The patients described by Klein did not respond to anxiolytics, antipsychotics, or either supportive or intensive insight-oriented psychotherapy. However, after their patients responded to the antidepressant imipramine, they realized that these patients constituted a specific, perhaps homogeneous, subgroup, distinct from patients with generalized anxiety who do respond to psychotherapy and/or anxiolytics. Their concept of panic attacks as the primary event, with secondary anticipatory anxiety and subsequent agoraphobia was constructed after careful review of the evolution of patients' symptoms. For each, a spontaneous, unexpected paroxysm of profound anxiety, without any warning or precipitant, was an initial event. Although attending to normal routine daily functions, such patients become overwhelmed with terror, fears of dying, of going insane, or having a "breakdown," and an impulse to flee. Somatic and autonomic experiences accompanying these feelings including palpitations, dyspnea, diaphoresis, numbness, nausea, weak legs, hot or cold flashes, dizziness, a churning stomach, choking and/or derealization—the entire episode lasting minutes to hours. Following several similar episodes, such patients begin to develop an interepisode anxiety in anticipation of the next attack, since by now they know that by nature the attacks are sudden, unexpected, and unpredictable. The anticipatory anxiety becomes chronic and continual, not episodic, and is less intense than the panic attacks. In attempts to master or even prevent the attacks, patients begin associating the occurrence of these attacks with certain events or places, as a cause-and-effect relationship. They hope that by avoiding these events and places, the attack can be forestalled. In extreme cases some patients become housebound, fearing (via the process of stimulus generalization) that going anywhere could promote panic. When questioned carefully, it can be discovered that the "phobia" is not of the crowd, the tunnel, the subway, or the theater, but rather a fear that if a panic attack occurs in such a setting, there will be no help readily at hand, the patient will not be able to, or may find it impossible, to flee. A further confirmation that the panic attack is a discrete event derives from the finding that imipramine blocks the panic attacks but does little to ameliorate the anticipatory anxiety or the phobic avoidance behavior. However, when the panic attacks are interrupted by the imipramine, patients are then able to make considerable gains with the anticipatory anxiety and the phobic-avoidance behavior through treatment via psychotherapy, behavior therapy, and/or anxiolytics. (The converse has not been found: psychotherapy, behavior therapy and anxiolytics do not block the panic attack). Major symptom remission is usually not achieved until or unless the panic attacks are first alleviated with imipramine, monoamine oxidase inhibitors, or, more recently, the benzodiazepine alprazolam.

Recently both psychogenetic and biochemical evidence has supported the concept that "panic disorders are a discrete metabolic disease to which there may be a genetic vulnerability."[37] It has been shown that infusions of sodium lactate and inhalation of 5% carbon dioxide can precipitate panic attacks more frequently in patients who experience spontaneous panic attacks than will occur in controls. Moreover, when such patients are pretreated with imipramine, monoamine oxidase inhibitors, or alprazolam, these induced panic attacks are prevented.[38,39] Pretreatment with more customary anxiolytics does not prevent induced attacks. Genetic studies reveal concordance for panic attacks in monozygotic, but not dizygotic, twins,[35] and family studies suggest that a fourth of the first-degree relatives of patients with panic attacks have an increased incidence of panic attacks but not of generalized anxiety.[37]

We propose that in this disorder a primary underlying biophysiologic disorder exists in certain people with a genetic predisposition and that in turn there are secondary maladaptive changes in the personality as described above, including regression, helplessness, depression, and dependency. Treatment that has focused on these character traits as the primary pathology has been notoriously unhelpful, but it has been most effective when combined with appropriate medications.

The Klein group's theory of panic anxiety deserves brief mention. They formulate that panic anxiety in adults is analogous to severe separation anxiety in children and liken the panic response to the protest response described in children by Bowlby[40,41] following infant–mother separation in humans. Clinical support for this comes from the observation that children with "school phobia" respond better to play therapy or family therapy *plus* imipramine than to play therapy alone.[35] As with the adult suffering from panic-induced agoraphobia, the child with school phobia avoids going to school out of separation anxiety rather than a true fear of school. If there is a central regulatory biophysiologic mechanism that modulates response to separation, some individuals with one type of low threshold may experience panic, while others without this threshold change may experience only manageable levels of anxiety. Effective agents may act by raising the threshold of such an impaired central mechanism in these patients. As of now, this theory is heuristic and challenging and its presentation here is meant to stimulate thoughts and ideas. Much of the data has been corroborated and replicated in trials and clinical experience, and we conclude that it is the primary vulnerability to panic disorder that produces the secondary personality changes seen in this subgroup of patients.[42–45]

The Lithium-Responsive Labile or Explosive Personality

Lithium is of course best known and most directly used for patients with affective and subaffective disorders. It is fascinating to note that during the past 12 or so years, lithium has been used with impressive results in the treatment of patients characterized by impulsivity, unpremeditated aggression, violence, assaultiveness, destructiveness, and antisocial personality traits. These patients do not have affective or subaffective illness, are not psychotic, and for the most part do not have established seizure disorders. They generally have a clear sensorium at the time of their actions, with an accurate recall for the details of the acts they committed and the affects they felt.

Sheard[46] describes a double-blind study of 66 prisoners with "short fuses" as a descriptor of their anger control, who had records of being chronically impulsive and aggressive. They had been convicted of crimes such as murder, rape, manslaughter, antisocial behavior, and assault and were thought of as "extremely manipulative, hostile and aggressive . . . highly impulsive and action oriented." Many had chaotic developmental histories including adoption, foster homes, divorced parents, death of a parent before age 16, and antisocial behavior by age 12. Eighty percent had spent at least 1 year in prison by age 18. Of these 66, half were treated with lithium and half with placebo for 3 months. A significant decrease in the total number of rule infractions, particularly those reflecting violent behavior infractions, was recorded for the lithium group. Minor, nonviolent infractions were unchanged in frequency. Sheard concluded that lithium worked in some way to decrease and inhibit aggressive and impulsive actions. Since the number of minor infractions was not affected, it seems unlikely that lithium exerted a global inhibitory affect on behavior but rather a more specific effect for aggression, violence, and impulsivity in these patients.

This study is consistent with the results of a nonblind study conducted by Tupin.[47] He describes 27 male convicts whose behavior was characterized by recurrent, angry, rapid, and often violent reactions to even the smallest of provocations. These subjects were treated with lithium for up to 1½ years, and they were evaluated by self-report, their guards, and the research team. Both violent and nonviolent sociopathic behavior was reduced in the lithium group, although nonviolent behavior was reduced less. There was a significant decrease in the number of disciplinary actions for violent infractions, and a significant decrease as well in the number of inmates who received maximum security classifications. Subjects rated themselves as having a greater degree of control. One said "now I can *think* about whether to hit or not." The psychiatric staff noted "an increase in the capacity to reflect on the consequences of actions . . . to control angry feelings when provoked . . . a more reflective mood." Of note is that phenothiazines did not produce this improvement, making it unlikely that sedation or tranquilization alone brought about this observed and welcome change.

Shader and colleagues[48] described a case of a 34-year-old woman who demonstrated antisocial behavior from age 14, including running away from home, assault, car theft, drug abuse, and multiple suicide attempts. She spent the 16 years between ages 14 and 30 in either a prison or a psychiatric hospital. She carried a diagnosis of "personality disorder, antisocial . . . characterized by aggressiveness, assaultiveness and destructiveness." She frequently broke windows, cut herself, and assaulted staff members. She was never psychotic. Her full-scale IQ was 117. Phenothiazines and minor tranquilizers had no meaningful influence on her violent, impulsive behavior. One week after being treated with lithium she was improved. She was calm, more reflective, less impulsive, and less explosive. "For the first time she was able to *talk* about her affective responses to her environment . . . she did not seem on the verge of acting." This response continued at a 1-year follow-up. We concluded, "it is as if a delay factor is added as a way-station in patients who previously went automatically from stimulus to response."

All these clinical reports indicate that lithium may have facilitated certain functions in these subjects such as thinking, judging, reflecting, and weighing the consequences of actions *before* acting. The reflex arc of stimulus-response was broken and rerouted, such that the circuit now included the cortex and, metapsychologically speaking, the psychic apparatus. Thought, judgment, reflection, control of impulsivity, increased frustration tolerance, and modulation of raw aggression are basic ego functions. Lithium is postulated to facilitate the appropriate recruitment of these ego functions that are masked and unavailable before the lithium trial.

Is there some central regulatory center for impulsive aggression that can be modulated either directly or indirectly by lithium (exclusive of lithium's effect on mania, depression, and cyclothymia) with a resulting change in personality from pharmacotherapeutic intervention? The inference for us is that here, too, there is good reason to assume that personality has multiple determinants, some of which are organic and chemically modifiable. We encourage the reader to consider the potential role for lithium in their treatment evaluations of nonpsychotic, nonaffective, impulsive, violent, aggressive antisocial patients.

Personality Disorders with Neuroanatomical Determinants

It is well known that personality changes accompany states in which the patient suffers from an underlying toxic and/or metabolic derangement. These changes have specific features. They frequently interfere with social, interpersonal, and vocational function and are often accompanied by cognitive and intellectual impairment. They tend to follow the course of the underlying insult, and usually the personality reverts back to the premorbid state soon after the underlying toxic-metabolic imbalance remits. Finally, the personality "changes" are often exaggerations of premorbid traits: a suspicious person becomes paranoid; a neurasthenic

person becomes listless and apathetic. The social disinhibition caused by alcohol, the paranoia induced by cocaine or amphetamine, and the apathy induced by hepatic encephalopathy are common examples.

In this section we will describe personality changes with strikingly different features. They result from a neuroanatomical focus and not a toxic-metabolic derangement. There is no impairment in cognitive or intellectual function. Social, vocational, and interpersonal activities are usually preserved and intact. The changes do not parallel the episodic course of the illness but rather interestingly appear *between* the acute episodes and begin to emerge up to years after the illness is originally diagnosed. Moreover, these personality changes may become permanent and autonomous of the acute episodes and are not prevented from occurring despite control of the acute episodes with medication. Lastly, these changes are *not* exaggerations of premorbid traits but are distinct from them. We are referring to the interictal personality changes observed in patients with temporal lobe epilepsy (TLE).

The interictal personality changes have been described by several investigators.[49–55] Such patients are characterized by the following traits:

Hypereligiosity, or an intense preoccupation with religious, divine, or demonic themes. Patients have been known to undergo multiple religious conversions over the years. They are at times grandiose; a patient described by Waxman and Geschwind said, "I am the cosmic minister to the world."[51,54]

Hypergraphia, or the tendency for the patient to produce copious volumes of writing. These patients write prayers, novels, poetry, prose, and diaries. The writing typically includes frequent use of parentheses, quotations, underlining, italics, and commentary in the margins; a page of such writing appears quite meticulous with each line directly below the one above.[52]

Hypermorality, or the preoccupation of the patient with global, moral and philosophical issues. The patient may brood incessantly about "life, love, God, and 'why'?" There is often a rigid sense of crime, sin and wrong.

Viscosity, or the feeling of the observer who feels he can never be rid of the long-winded circumstantial patient.

Hyperemotionality, which describes the intense investment by the patient of neutral, minute stimuli with a subsequent deepened affect. Their affect is frequently labile, with mood swings of depression or elation; anger, paranoia, anxiety, and humorlessness are also common.

Behavior changes, with the emergence of obsessional or dependent traits. Sexual activity varies and includes hypersexuality, hyposexuality, fetishism, and transvestism.

Details of two studies are particularly interesting. Slater and Beard[53] described 69 patients who developed interictal personality changes up to 14 years after the onset of temporal lobe seizures. Several developed a schizophreniclike state, with formal thought disorder, hallucinations, and delusions. However, their affect remained full, supple, and appropriate, and there was no downhill deteriorating course. The premorbid personalities of these patients do not reveal schizoid or schizotypal traits.

Bear and Fedio[51] noticed that interictal personality traits differed depending on whether the primary epileptic focus was in the right or the left temporal lobe. Fifteen patients with right-sided TLE displayed what were described as "emotive traits," including elation, sadness, hyperemotionality, hypermoralism, viscosity, and decreased libido. Twelve patients with left-sided TLE were described as "ideative" and displayed traits such as anger, paranoia, humorlessness, dependence, hyperreligiosity, and a sense of cosmic personal destiny. Recent studies of "split brain" subjects support these findings, that is, that hemispheric asymmetry can influence the preferential emergence of specific personality and affective states.

The theoretic understanding proposed by these researchers is somewhat vague but involves a temporal lobe–limbic modification causing previously neutral stimuli to become more affectively cathected. What is clear is that the personality changes occur as a result of the temporal lobe focus yet are autonomous. These personality traits are generally not observed in other seizure disorders. Although personality changes are common in neurologic disorders such as Parkinson's disease and Huntington's disease, these illnesses are associated with degeneration of brain tissue, which does not occur in TLE. It seems probable that such personality changes do become independent of the seizure disorder; they evolve despite control of seizures with anticonvulsants, and they may begin years following the onset of the seizure disorder. These observations, we believe, lend further support to our theme that personality is fluid, interdependent, and influenced by multiple determinants, many of which are often organic.

Conclusion

It has been our stance throughout to present research that supports the concept of a broad, interdependent, fluid model of personality—a model comprising multiple determinants. We advocate the identification of those subgroups of patients who may have organic and constitutional determinants to their character pathology, not in lieu of, but in addition to, experiential and developmental determinants. We propose that for such patients the most effective treatment should include a combination of appropriate pharmacotherapy and psychotherapy.

Current clinical research is being conducted in the use and benefits of pharmacotherapy in disorders such as bulimia, anorexia nervosa, and obsessive-compulsive disorders. Preliminary results are promising. Finally, it has been our goal and hope that the ideas we have presented will stimulate interest, thought, and speculation.

REFERENCES

1. Freud S: New introductory lectures. In Strachey J (ed): The Standard Edition of the Complete Works of Sigmund Freud, vol 22, p 154. London, Hogarth Press, 1963
2. Freud S: An outline of psychoanalysis. In Strachey J (ed): The Standard Edition of the Complete Works of Sigmund Freud, vol 23, p 182. London, Hogarth Press, 1963
3. Freud S: The dynamics of transference. In Strachey J (ed): The Standard Edition of the Complete Works of Sigmund Freud, vol 12, p 99. London, Hogarth Press, 1963
4. Federn P: Psychoanalysis of the psychoses. Psychiatr Q 17:246, 1943
5. Marmor J: The adjunctive use of drugs in psychotherapy. J Clin Psychopharmacol 1:312–315, 1981
6. Marmor J: Systems thinking in psychiatry: Some theoretical and clinical implications. Am J Psychiatry 140:833–838, 1983
7. Rainer JD: Heredity and Character Disorders. Am J Psychol. 33:6–15, 1979
8. Freud S: Three essays on sexuality. In Strachey J (ed): The Standard Edition of the Complete Works of Sigmund Freud, vol 8, pp 191–242, London, Hogarth Press, 1963
9. Thomas A, Chess S: Temperament and Development. New York, Brunner/Mazel, 1977
10. Thomas A, Chess S: Genesis and evolution of behavioral disorders: From infancy to early adult life. Am J Psychiatry 141:1–9, 1984
11. Kupfer DJ, Foster G, Coble P et al: The application of EEG sleep for the differential diagnosis of affective disorders. Am J Psychiatry 135:69–74, 1978
12. Kupfer D: Interaction of EEG sleep, antidepressants, and affective disease. J Clin Psychiatry 43:30–36, 1982
13. Carroll BJ, Feinber M, Greden JF et al: A specific laboratory test for the diagnosis of melancholia. Standardization, vali-

dation, and clinical unity. Arch Gen Psychiatry 38:15–22, 1981

14. Carroll BJ: Use of the dexamethasone test in depression. J Clin Psychiatry 43:44–50, 1982

15. Akiskal HS, Lemmi H: Clinical, neuroendocrine and sleep EEG diagnosis of "unusual" affective presentations: A practical review. Psychiatr Clin North Am 6:69–83, 1983

16. Cassano GB, Maggini C, Akiskal HS: Short term, subchronic and chronic sequelae of affective disorders. Psychiatr Clin North Am 6:55–67, 1983

17. Akiskal HS: Dysthymic disorder: Psychopathology of proposed chronic subtypes. Am J Psychiatry 140:11–20, 1983

18. Akiskal HS, Hirschfeld RMA, Yerevanian B: The relationship of personality to affective disorders. Arch Gen Psychiatry 40:801, 1983

19. Akiskal HS, Rosentho T, Haykel R et al : Characterological depressions: Clinical and sleep EEG findings separating "subaffective dysthmymias" from character spectrum disorders. Arch Gen Psychiatry 37:777–783, 1980

20. Akiskal HS, Khani M, Scott-Strauss A: Cyclothymic temperamental disorders. Psychiatr Clin North Am 2:527–554, 1979

21. Yerevanian BI, Akiskal HS: Neurotic characterological and dysthymic depressions. Psychiatr Clin North Am 2:595–617, 1979

22. Klein DF, Gittelman R, Quitkin F et al: Diagnosis and Drug Treatment of Psychiatric Disorders: Adults and Children, 2nd ed. Baltimore, Williams & Wilkins, 1980

23. Liebowitz MR, Klein DF: Hysteroid dysphoria. Psychiatr Clin North Am 2:555–575, 1979

24. Klein DF, Shader RI: Psychopharmacologic treatment approaches to an undiagnosed case. In Shader RI (ed): Manual of Psychiatric Therapeutics, pp 281–293. Boston, Little, Brown & Co, 1975

25. Davidson JR, Miller RD, Turnbull CD et al: Atypical depression. Arch Gen Psychiatry 39:527–534, 1982

26. Gunderson JG, Singer MT: Defining borderline patients, an overview. Am J Psychiatry 132:1–13, 1975

27. Gunderson JG, Kolb JE: Discriminating features of borderline patients. Am J Psychiatry 135:792–796, 1978

28. Kernberg O: Borderline personality organization. J Am Psychoanal Assoc 15:641–685, 1967

29. Kernberg O: Borderline Conditions and Pathological Narcissism. New York, Jason Aronson, 1975

30. Diagnostic and Statistical Manual of Mental Disorders, 3rd ed, pp 321–323. Washington, DC, American Psychiatric Association, 1980

31. Stone MH: Contemporary shift of the borderline concept from a schizophrenic disorder to a subaffective disorder. Psychiatr Clin North Am 2:577–594, 1979

32. Cole JO: Drug therapy of borderline patients. McLean Hosp J 2:110–125, 1980

33. Spitzer R et al: Crossing the border into borderline personality and borderline schizophrenia. Arch Gen Psychiatry 36:17, 1979

34. Bellak LP (ed): Psychiatric Aspects of Minimal Brain Dysfunction in Adults. New York, Grune & Stratton, 1979

35. Klein DF: Anxiety reconceptualized. Compr Psychiatry 21:411–427, 1980

36. Sheehan DV: Panic attacks and phobias. N Engl J Med 307:156–158, 1982

37. Shader RI, Goodman M, Gever J: Panic disorders: Current perspectives. J Clin Psychopharmacol 2:25–105, 1982

38. Pitts FN, McClure JN: Lactate metabolism in anxiety neurosis. N Engl J Med 227:1329–1336, 1967

39. Kelly D, Mitchell-Heggs N, Sherman D: Anxiety and the effects of sodium lactate assessed clinically and physiologically. Br J Psychiatry 119:129–141, 1971

40. Bowlby J: Attachment and Loss, vol 1. New York, Basic Books, 1969

41. Bowlby J: Attachment and Loss, vol 2. New York, Basic Books, 1973

42. Sheehan DV: Current perspectives in the treatment of panic and phobic disorders. Drug Ther 179–190, 1982

43. Muskin PR, Fyer AJ: The treatment of panic disorder. J Clin Psychopharmacol 1:81–90, 1981

44. Sheehan DV, Sheehan KH: The classification of anxiety and hysterical states: I. Historical review and empirical delineation. J Clin Psychopharmacol 2:235–344, 1982

45. Sheehan DV, Sheehan KH: The classification of anxiety and hysterical states: II. Toward a more heuristic classification. J Clin Psychopharmacol 2:386–393, 1982

46. Sheard MH, Marini JL, Bridges CI: The effect of lithium on impulsive aggressive behavior in man. Am J Psychiatry 133:1409–1413, 1976

47. Tupin JP, Smith DB, Clanon TL et al: The long term use of lithium in aggressive prisoners. Compr Psychiatry 14:311–317, 1973

48. Shader RI, Jackson AH, Dodes LM: The antiaggressive effects of lithium in man. Psychopharmacologia 40:17–24, 1974

49. Waxman SG, Geschwind N: The interictal behavior syndrome of temporal lobe epilepsy. Arch Gen Psychiatry 32:1580–1586, 1975

50. Bear DM, Arana G: Neurologic syndromes affecting emotions and behavior. Weekly Psychiatry Update Series, vol 3, lesson 39, 1980

51. Bear DM, Fedio P: Quantitative analysis of interictal behavior in temporal lobe epilepsy. Arch Neurol 34:454–467, 1977

52. Waxman S, Geschwind N: Hypergraphia in temporal lobe epilepsy. Neurology 24:629–636, 1974

53. Slater E, Beard AW: The schizophrenia-like psychoses of epilepsy. Br J Psychiatry 109:95, 150, 1963

54. Dewhurst K, Beard AW: Sudden religious conversion in temporal lobe epilepsy. Br J Psychiatry 117:497–507, 1970

55. Geschwind N, Shader RI, Beard AW et al: Behavior changes with temporal lobe epilepsy. J Clin Psychiatry 41:89–95, 1980

Interpersonal Methods of Diagnosis and Treatment

Overview

In the world of nature, onlookers regularly neglect the gigantic but buried tap-root as they stand engrossed in the grandeur of a tree's jutting branches and limbs. Analogously, many prominent therapeutic offshoots in present-day psychiatry and psychology derive their existence and sustenance from Sullivan's seminal ideas,[1-6] yet few proponents demonstrate much appreciation of their ontogenetic source.

Sullivan's pivotal contribution was to reject boldly psychiatry's and psychology's prevailing investigative focus on the conceptually isolated individual. Instead, he arrogantly insisted that a person's actions can be understood only as they derive *conjoint* meaning from the historical and present interpersonal transactions in which they are embedded. A patient's actions, then, need to be understood as communicative "force fields" that influence, and simultaneously are influenced by, other "force fields" from present-day interactants in important lawfully reciprocal ways.

A personality can be comprehended only as "the relatively enduring pattern of recurrent interpersonal situations which characterize a human life."[2] Hence, to be fully cognizant of oneself or of another requires an observational stance offering a clear view of the sequence of events played out tenaciously and recurrently by a person or patient in encounters with significant others.

From this new *systems* perspective, transferences (parataxic distortions) and countertransferences— although admittedly expressed and evoked rigidly and extremely by psychotherapy patients—are phenomena not at all unique to the therapy situation. Rather, their more or less rigid and extreme expressions by all persons constitute the essence of human living—the "stuff" of human relationships. Perhaps the most distinctive aspect of interpersonal therapy, in regard to both diagnosis and intervention, is its unswerving emphasis on these transference–countertransference sequences as they unfold between patient and therapist. A patient's central problems in living are played out "live" in the therapist's office and as they emerge must be counteracted by the therapist through use of multifaceted interventions.

Appropriately, then, interpersonal diagnosis requires that therapists continually monitor the inner experiences and overt reactions evoked from them by their patients within the sessions. The important purpose of this monitoring process is to pinpoint the patient's maladaptively rigid "bids" for self-confirmation. Likewise, interpersonal intervention requires therapists to provide metacommunicative feedback that labels the interpersonal impacts they experience, as a springboard to collaborative exploration with the patient of their self-defeating and "self-fulfilling prophecy" meanings.

In sum, an interpersonal approach to psychotherapy assumes that a patient's central problems in living reside in maladaptive transaction cycles with significant others, including the therapist. The therapist's overriding diagnostic task is to identify the specific components of the self-defeating maladaptive pattern. The therapist's major interventive task is to disrupt the identified transaction cycle by various interpersonal moves that refuse to reinforce, that insist on exposing, and that push to alter the patient's self-defeating pattern both within and outside the therapy sessions.

This chapter details the principles and methods of interpersonal diagnosis and intervention currently available in the literature. It can provide only an overview and is heavily shaped by my own integrations. The reader can find much greater detail and other emphases both in Sullivan's writings and in other more recent interpersonal volumes.[7-12]

Several cautionary comments need to be made before proceeding. First, with the exception of Sullivan's writings, no systematic and comprehensive interpersonal theory of psychotherapy has as yet appeared that might guide current practice or research. What is available are several initial but incomplete systematic attempts.[8,10,13-15] Second, historically interpersonal theorists have resisted attempts to establish an interpersonal "school" of psychotherapy. Instead, they most often insist that basic aspects of interpersonal theory offer a framework comprehensive enough to subsume and integrate concepts and findings from other therapy approaches. Third, these theorists caution that we have little reliable information regarding the limits of applicability of interpersonal theory to abnormal behavior. Interpersonal theorists have concentrated their efforts on what currently are referred to as *DSM-III* Axis II personality disorders. However, the extent to which interpersonal therapy needs to be modified or expanded to address the multiple interactive factors operative among major or minor Axis I disorders is unknown and can be determined only through future theoretical and empirical efforts.

Interpersonal Diagnosis

Basic to understanding of both interpersonal diagnosis and intervention are two conceptual models that provide structure and guidance to the interpersonal therapist. The first, the *interpersonal circle*,[8,10,14,16] is a model that specifies the range of individual differences in normal and abnormal interpersonal behavior. Through use of one or more inventories one can assess a patient's interpersonal behavior and precisely locate that behavior on the surface of the interpersonal circle. This placement, in turn, permits both exact specification of the patient's maladaptive pattern of living as well as precise prediction of various components of the opti-

mal treatment program for that patient. The second model, Kiesler's *maladaptive transaction cycle*,[17] provides a framework for depicting the specific transactional pattern present in any patient's self-defeating interpersonal relationships. It also pinpoints cognitive and behavioral components that need to be targeted for intervention in order to disrupt the patient's pattern of maladaptive transactions.

THE INTERPERSONAL CIRCLE

The latest version of the interpersonal circle[14] is shown in Figure 1. The original[10] and all subsequent circles are constructed on the assumption that human interpersonal behavior represents blends of two basic motivations: the need for control (power, dominance) and the need for affiliation (love, friendliness). That is, persons interacting with each other (including patient and therapist) continually are negotiating two major relationship issues: how friendly or hostile they will be with each other, and how much in charge or in control each will be in their encounters. The interpersonal circle directly incorporates this assumption by placing control (dominance–submission) and affiliation (friendliness–hostility) along its vertical and horizontal axes respectively.

Any interpersonal action represents a composite or blend of relative components of these two factors—so many units of control, so many units of affiliation. The 16 segments found on the circumference in Figure 1 define the range of possible blends of the two underlying dimensions. For example, exhibitionistic actions fall at segment O and represent approximately two units of dominance and two units of friendliness. In contrast, inhibited actions (segment G) represent the polar opposite to O and represent approximately two units of submission and two units of hostility.

The sixteen circle radii represent continua of normal (near the midpoint) to abnormal (near the circumference) versions of each segment's interpersonal acts. In other words, component actions subsumed by each segment vary in terms of their intensity or extremeness. The more extreme the act, the more maladjusted it is, and the more aversive its effects on interactants. For example, along the range of segment O, exhibitionistic acts, $level_2$ histrionic actions (loquacious/divulging, histrionic, impulsive, and hypersuggestible) are more maladaptive than milder segment O versions at $level_1$ (talkative/disclosing, demonstrative, casual/spontaneous, and suggestive). Note that Figure 1 provides $level_1$ (mild–moderate) and $level_2$ (extreme)

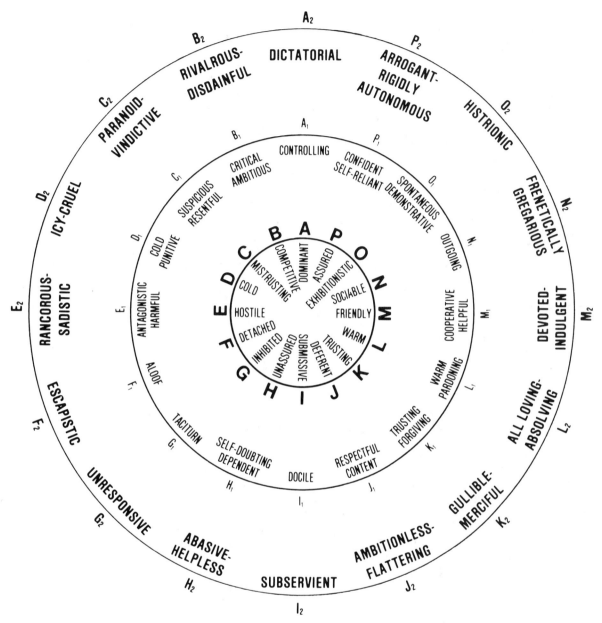

FIG. 1. The 1982 interpersonal circle.

labels for each of the 16 segments of interpersonal behavior.

Besides being intense or extreme, the interpersonal acts of a maladjusted individual are characterized by their rigidity. That is, the person's acts are constricted to expressions of only a few segments of circle behaviors. For example, a patient diagnosed *DSM-III* histrionic personality tends to

enact extreme behaviors exclusively from segments O and N. He does not seem to be able to respond to others with actions from the 14 other segments.

In sum, the maladjusted person is one who lacks the flexibility to use the broad range of interpersonal behaviors (depicted around the circle circumference) that different interpersonal situations may warrant. Instead, the person continually enacts the same rigid and extreme interpersonal behaviors with virtually all significant persons. As Leary observed, the maladjusted individual

> tends to overdevelop a narrow range of one or two interpersonal responses. These are expressed intensely and often, whether appropriate to the situation or not . . . [Further,] the more extreme and rigid the person, the greater his interpersonal "pull"—the stronger his ability to shape the relationship with others.[10]

In contrast, the more normal individual enacts varied sets of interpersonal acts appropriately tuned to the persons with whom he is interacting. In each new case he negotiates a mutually agreed upon and satisfying definition of self and other, in response to the unique aspects of the particular interaction.

An important implication of these notions regarding abnormal behavior is that in the therapy context the patient's interpersonal actions of necessity will override the actions of the hopefully more normal therapist. Especially during their earlier sessions, the patient will exhibit greater interpersonal "pull" than the therapist—will demonstrate a stronger ability to shape the therapy relationship. It follows from this that it is crucial for the therapist to form a clear notion of the overriding impacts or pulls the patient evokes from him in their sessions.

Fortunately, once the patient's interpersonal behavior has been assessed as falling at specific segments of the circle, the therapist can make precise predictions regarding the objective countertransference reactions he will experience (also locatable on the circle). These predictions derive from Sullivan's "theorem of reciprocal emotion" and assume the form of *complementary* interpersonal reactions.[8,10,14] Figure 2 depicts the predicted complementary response for each quadrant and segment of the interpersonal circle.

Laws of complementarity are based on the assumption that a patient's interpersonal actions tend to initiate, invite, or evoke from interactants reactions that lead to a repetition of the patient's original actions. In a relatively unaware, automatic, and unintended fashion, interpersonal behaviors tend to pull, draw, or entice from interactants restricted classes of reactions that are reinforcing of, consistent with, and confirming of a person's proffered self-definition. If complementary reactions are not forthcoming from interactants, the relationship will either not endure or will be altered in such a manner that complementarity is established.

On the interpersonal circle, *complementarity* oc-

curs on the basis of "reciprocity" in respect to the control dimension or axis (dominance pulls submission, submission pulls dominance), and "correspondence" in respect to the affiliation axis (hostility pulls hostility, friendliness pulls friendliness). In the therapy context a complementary encounter exists when the therapist reacts to the patient with interpersonal acts reciprocal in terms of control and corresponding in terms of affiliation. By this reaction, the therapist accepts and confirms the patient's self-presentation on both the control and affiliation dimensions. *Anticomplementarity* exists when the therapist responds to the patient with behavior both nonreciprocal in terms of control and noncorresponding in terms of affiliation. In the anticomplementary situation, the therapist rejects the patient's "bids" or "claims" for self-definition on both the control and affiliation dimensions. *Acomplementarity* exists when the therapist reacts to the patient with actions either reciprocal in control or corresponding in affiliation, but not both. In this case the therapist accepts the patient's bid on one dimension but rejects it on the other.

Of the three transactional possibilities, the one most comfortable for the patient occurs when the therapist provides the complementary response. The most aversive and uncomfortable situation for the patient is that in which the therapist insists on providing the anticomplementary reaction. The middle level of discomfort for the patient occurs when the therapist reacts with acomplementary responses. However, since the patient's interpersonal behavior is more extreme and rigid than the therapist's, the patient has considerably more power to determine the nature of their relationship by overriding the therapist's preferred style of interpersonal transaction. In early therapy sessions, therefore, the therapist cannot avoid being pulled into the complementary response with a patient, cannot avoid experiencing objective countertransference.

Circle Inventories of Interpersonal Behavior

In interpersonal therapy, the circle is a key conceptual map that guides interpersonal diagnosis and therapy of psychiatric patients. A repertoire of interpersonal measures is available for use to obtain empirical scores that profile a given patient's interpersonal behavior at specific segments of the circle. It includes the Interpersonal Check List (ICL),[18,19] the Interpersonal Behavior Inventory (IBI),[20,21] the Interpersonal Adjective Scales (IAS),[22,23] the Impact Message Inventory (IMI),[24,25] the Check List for Psychotherapy Transactions (CLOPT), the Check List for Interpersonal Transactions

FIG. 2. Complementary quadrants and segments of the 1982 interpersonal circle.

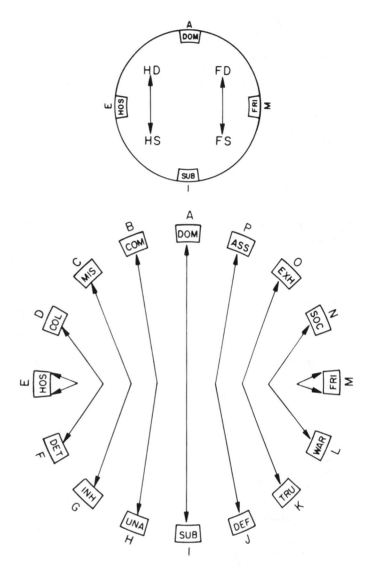

(CLOIT),[26] and various questionnaires that constitute the Structural Analysis of Social Behavior (SASB).[27,28] For the reader interested in more detail, Wiggins provides an excellent summary and critique of these measures.[16]

By use of these measures, a therapist can assess the interpersonal behavior of a particular patient in one or all of several distinct ways. First, one can administer to the patient directly the self-report versions of these circle inventories (ICL, IAS). Second, significant others in the patient's life can be asked (with the patient's permission) to rate the patient's interpersonal behavior at various points over the course of therapy. Alternatively, groups of observers can be shown videotaped samples of therapy sessions and asked to rate the patient's be-

havior from these transcriptions. Either of these rating tasks can be accomplished through use of the ICL, IAS, IBI, CLOPT, or CLOIT measures. Third, significant others, observers of videotaped sessions, and the therapist, through use of the IMI, can also be asked to report the internal, covert emotional, and other experiences they observe in themselves when interacting with the patient. The IMI measures the covert complementary response (the objective countertransference) experienced by the therapist and other persons who have interactions with the patient. Further, application of any or all of these measures at sequential points of the treatment process permits direct measures of outcome or improvement in the patient's interpersonal problem behaviors.

Although these measures are at various stages of psychometric development, work in progress is likely to provide increasingly reliable and valid versions. Administration of any one of these instruments permits assessment of the patient's pattern of interpersonal actions. This assessment, in turn, produces an exact profile of that patient's interpersonal behavior on the interpersonal circle, which permits precise prediction of reactions that are complementary, anticomplementary, or acomplementary to the patient's actions and of interventions that are optimal for facilitating change in the patient's maladaptive pattern.

Diagnosis of DSM-III Personality Disorders

At present, interpersonal diagnosis is most clearly relevant to the *DSM-III* personality disorders. Future theory and research will determine the extent to which the circle might be useful for diagnosis of DSM Axis I disorders.

Kiesler has detailed the principles that guide interpersonal diagnosis using the circle as a conceptual framework.[29] He also offers Translations of *DSM-III* personality disorders in regard to their respective profiles on the circle. Table 1 presents a summary of these translations. Several conclusions can be drawn from the circle descriptions provided in this table.

First, the structural pattern of interpersonal behavior found for patients with various personality disorders is not the same. Five of the eleven disorders are located at a particular circle octant (two adjacent segments), two are defined at one segment only, two are characterized by a triad of adjacent segments, and two are represented by segments from different quadrants. Clearly, circle diagnosis of the personality disorders reveals no patterns that directly support the three "clusters" described by *DSM-III:* odd or eccentric; dramatic, emotional, or erratic; and anxious or fearful.

Second, it also is apparent from Table 1 that the *DSM-III* personality disorders are classified predominantly in the hostile left half of the 1982 circle. Two exceptions, narcissistic and histrionic, are found in the top right (friendly–dominant) quadrant. Further, for various reasons,[29] persons exhibiting abnormal behavior patterns not represented in *DSM-III* and falling in the bottom right (friendly–submissive) or extreme top left of the circle seldom appear voluntarily in psychiatric treatment settings.

TABLE 1.   Placement of *DSM-III* Personality Disorders on the 1982 Circle

DSM-III Disorder	1982 Circle Segment	
"Octant" prototypes		
Histrionic	N_2O_2:	Frenetically gregarious–histrionic
Narcissistic	O_2P_2:	Histrionic–arrogant/rigidly autonomous
Dependent	HI:	Unassured–submissive (levels unspecified)
Compulsive	F_1G:	Aloof–inhibited (G level unspecified)
Passive–aggressive	E_1F_1:	Antagonistic/harmful–aloof
"Triad" prototypes		
Paranoid	$C_2D_1E_1$:	Rivalrous/disdainful–cold/punitive–antagonistic/harmful
Avoidant	$F_1G_1H_1$:	Aloof–taciturn–self-doubting/dependent
"Segment" prototypes		
Antisocial	E:	Hostile (level unspecified)
Schizoid	F_2:	Escapistic (without F_{2c}): autistic/eccentric
"Mixed quadrant" prototypes		
Schizotypal	C_1F:	Suspicious/resentful–detached (F level unspecified)
Borderline	$B_2 \leftrightarrow J_2$:	Rivalrous/disdainful ↔ ambitionless/flattering
	$E_2 \leftrightarrow M_2$:	Rancorous/sadistic ↔ devoted/indulgent

A–P, segments; subscripts 1 and 2, segment levels.

Kiesler also discusses at length the principles that govern interpersonal diagnosis based on circle measures. He argues that interpersonal diagnosis combines both dimensional and typological assessment toward the goal of Roschian "prototype" classifications of psychiatric disorders.[29]

In sum, as various writers have argued,[14,16,29,30] the interpersonal circle offers considerable advantages to psychiatric classification and should be considered seriously as a theoretical and empirical base for future revisions of *DSM-III*. Regardless, the interpersonal circle provides the first essential conceptual model for diagnosis in interpersonal psychotherapy.

THE MALADAPTIVE TRANSACTION CYCLE

What the circle does not provide, however, is a conceptual model that might guide understanding of the sequence of transactions—the evolving momentary actions and reactions, moves and countermoves—that occur over a session between patient and therapist and, outside the sessions, between the patient and significant others.

The circle offers a static characterization at a frozen moment in time of the transactional behaviors exhibited by one or the other interactants. If measures of the behavior of both interactants are taken at intervals over an evolving relationship, the circle can provide some "macro" description of the emerging trends in the transaction. What it does not offer, however, is a conceptual guide that predicts the specific components of the recurrent pattern of actions and reactions that define the patient's self-defeating maladaptive transactions with others. With a conceptual map describing the key steps in the patient's maladaptive sequence with others, the therapist would be able to discover the specific content for each key component. The key components would include the covert and overt aspects of the patient's behavior that are chained circularly to the covert and overt aspects of the interactant's (or therapist's) reactions.

Figure 3 depicts Kiesler's maladaptive transaction cycle, which defines the essential components in the maladaptive action–reaction sequence.[17] The squares to the far left of the figure represent person A (in our case, the psychotherapy patient) in a transaction. The squares to the far right represent interactant B (in our case, the therapist as well as other persons significant to the patient). The arrows depict the direction of overriding influence between A and B, indicating the flow of action and reaction and their causal interrelatedness. What is evident from the flow is that a major effect of B's reactions is to confirm or validate the cognitive, emotional, and other inner experience of patient A and, in turn, to escalate A's repetition of the extreme and rigid actions originally enacted. Overall what is depicted is the "vicious cycle" that characterizes maladaptive interpersonal behavior in which, mostly without awareness, the patient produces and maintains his own maladaptive predicament.

In the figure, stage one describes the earlier sequence in patient A's transactions with a particular interactant (B). In line with the principle of complementarity, B will be pulled to experience constricted covert reactions producing complementary overt actions that confirm A's expectancies, cognitions, emotions, and other inner experience. This confirmation leads to A's continued production of his original maladaptive interpersonal behaviors. In this earlier stage of A's and B's relationship, the complementary fit makes their transactions somewhat mutually satisfying and confirming.

The difficulty develops over time as the relationship continues. As they continue to replay the cycle, interactant B increasingly experiences the aversive impacts that result from being "pushed around" by patient A's superior and rigid power. Patient A cannot alter his behavior toward enactment of behaviors from other segments of the circle because of chronic vulnerability but also now because B continues to confirm his expectancies and cognitions through enactment of complementary responses. On the other hand, B now begins to experience more hostile and rejecting impacts and, if possible, will escape from or avoid further encounters. But if, for a variety of reasons, escape is not possible, B will continue to enact complementary responses, yet simultaneously will "leak" subtle messages of hostility and rejection. These rejecting cues will be picked up by patient A's selectively attuned perceptual system and trigger anxiety in response to this threat to his self-system. Now more desperate, patient A escalates enactment of the same interpersonal behaviors that form the constricted core of his maladaptive self-presentation. In stage two, then, the transaction between A and B is at "impasse"—is locked into recurrent enactment of the cycle of maladaptive self-fulfilling prophecy and behavior.

The therapist and other significant persons in patient A's life initially cannot *not* be pulled into the patient's specific version of the maladaptive

STAGE 1

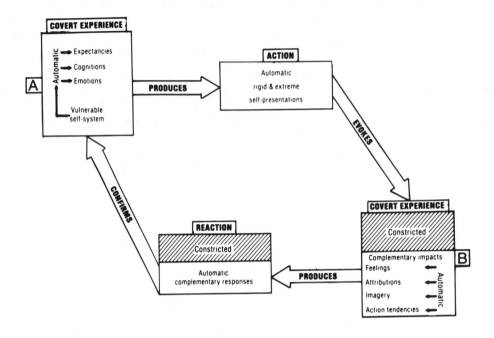

STAGE 2

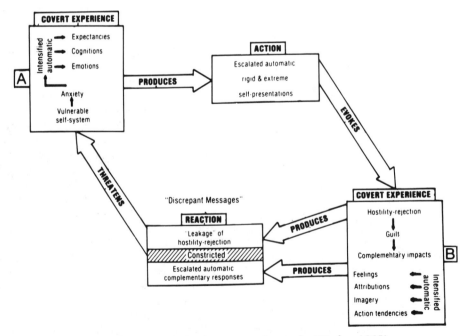

FIG. 3. The maladaptive transaction cycle (Kiesler, 1985)

transaction cycle. Unless they cease to be significant, others cannot avoid experiencing over time aversive feelings and reactions when transacting with the patient. The therapist also cannot avoid this aversive consequence unless the therapist first detects the pattern of the cycle and, then, makes interventive moves to begin to disrupt patient A's maladaptive pattern.

The second crucial step in interpersonal diagnosis, then, consists of the therapist's identification for a particular patient of the specific components of the maladaptive transaction cycle. Without this specification the therapist easily can get lost in the maladaptive drift of the relationship. With clear specification the therapist has available a conceptual blueprint that defines the sequential covert and overt steps of the maladaptive cycle toward which interventions can be aimed. The essential goal of these interventions is to disrupt the patient's maladaptive cycle and, then, to test out with him more flexible and less extreme cognitive hypotheses and overt behaviors with others, including the therapist.

A TRANSACTIONAL CONCEPTUALIZATION OF DEPRESSION

Figure 4 depicts application of the maladaptive transaction cycle to the depressed patient. Some of the contents found in Figure 4 are adapted from Coyne's interpersonal analysis of depression.[31]

Coyne conceptualizes depressive symptoms and behavior as messages that solicit and pull reassurance and support from others—as communications that probe and test for acceptance. As Figure 4 shows, the depressive's inner experiences consist of cognitions, memories, fantasies, emotions, and so forth characterized by low self-worth, sadness, self-effacing automatic thoughts, hopeless expectations, and the like. This phenomenologic experience (reflecting a vulnerable self-system) leads the depressive to enact unassured, submissive, and deferent behaviors (circle segments H, I, J).

Application of the principle of complementarity reveals that significant others will be pulled to experience covert reactions of sympathy, concern, and responsibility which lead the others to enact behaviors of reassurance, support, advice giving, and taking charge (the complementary circle segments of B, competitive; A, dominant; and P, assured). In the earlier stage of their relationship, the friendlier components (A, dominant; P, assured)

will predominate in B's reaction, and both parties, to some extent, will find their transactions satisfying and confirming.

The difficulty develops as the relationship continues. The bottom half of Figure 4 depicts this later stage. The basic problem is that the depressive's actions do not change or improve. Interactant B now begins to experience more hostile and rejecting impacts. The portion of B's reaction that "leaks" rejection intensifies the depressive's negative cognitions, irrational expectancies, and other experience. As patient A becomes increasingly vulnerable, he is anxiously driven to evoke supportive and accepting reactions and desperately escalates the depressive maladaptive behavior pattern. J, deference now becomes less evident in patient A's actions toward B, while G, inhibited becomes more prominent. In correspondence to A's shift, interactant B's response now includes a new C, mistrusting element (in complementary response to A's new G, inhibited), while the P, assured components begin to subside.

Their interaction now is in a clear state of conflict for both participants. Patient A is increasingly vulnerable to B's potential rejection but perceives no options that might replace escalation of inhibited, dependent, and submissive behaviors. Interactant B now vacillates between anger and guilt. Direct expression of anger is inhibited by B's perception of the depressive's abject suffering and profound helplessness, and these same perceptions intensify B's guilt for having hostile and rejecting thoughts in the first place. Interactant B is now trapped into expression of discrepant or incongruous messages that simultaneously are supportive and reassuring yet subtly hostile and rejecting. Because of the depressive's low perceptual thresholds for cues of hostility, patient A takes in primarily the messages of rejection and interprets B's reassurance and support as nongenuine. Thereby the depressive finds further confirmation of his maladaptive beliefs and expectancies. The depressive's unique maladaptive transaction cycle is now complete, with A and B remaining at an impasse.

The maladaptive transaction cycle needs to be applied concretely to other *DSM-III* disorders. Other seminal interpersonal conceptualizations are appearing for the histrionic personality,[32] the paranoid personality,[33] the alcoholic,[34] and for the general personality disorders.[29] Yet none has been articulated with the specificity required for translation into the form shown for the depressive in Figure 4. Obviously much work remains for interpersonal therapists.

STAGE 1

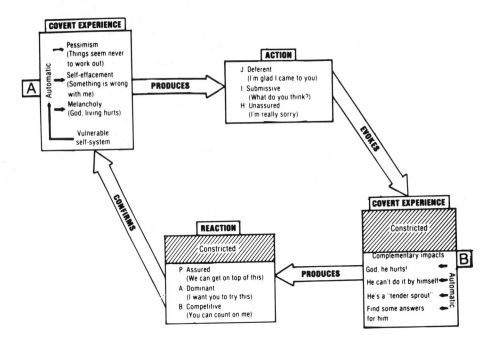

STAGE 2

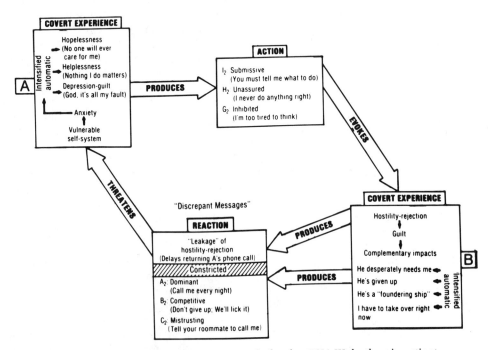

FIG. 4. The maladaptive transaction cycle for the *DSM-III* dysthymic patient.

OTHER INTERPERSONAL DIAGNOSTIC PROCEDURES

An Inventory of Interpersonal Problems

Horowitz and colleagues set out to investigate the relationships among three classes of complaints that bring patients into psychotherapy: symptoms, specific behavioral difficulties, and self-defeating thoughts.[35] In the process they examined complaints in the form of interpersonal problems (e.g., I can't seem to make friends, I find it hard to say "no" to my friends) gathered from samples of patients about to begin therapy. Observers viewed videotaped intake interviews and recorded each problem that began with the phrase "I find it hard to . . ." or with a synonym such as "I can't . . .," as well as statements that began "I find it hard NOT to . . ." or with a synonym such as "I can't STOP . . ." Nearly 200 problems were identified and over three quarters were judged to be interpersonal in nature.

By various sorting and scaling procedures, three major problem dimensions were identified among the 200 problem statements: control, degree of psychological involvement, and nature of the involvement. A clustering procedure grouped the problems further into five thematic clusters concerning intimacy, aggression, compliance, independence, and socializing. A final analysis yielded a list of 87 problem statements scored under one of these five clusters. These 87 items represent the present version of the Inventory of Interpersonal Problems.[35]

The inventory has been used in two formats. A group administration requires that patients indicate which statements they find self-descriptive. After first circling all problem statements "that are like you," the patient then identifies his "top five most familiar problems," and the "next five most familiar problems." The second format involves a more individualized testing that requires patients to use the Q-sort procedure to assign problem statements (printed on cards) to category piles that range from "most familiar as a problem" to "least familiar as a problem."

Research provides evidence for both good internal consistency and stability reliability for the inventory. Initial validity studies are also encouraging. Readers interested in more detail and in the complete version of the inventory can consult the work of Horowitz and colleagues.[35]

Comprehensive interpersonal assessment requires some form of inventory of interpersonal problems. Its application can determine the correspondence of patient-presenting problems to clusters of overt interpersonal behaviors defined by the 16 segments of the interpersonal circle and to various *DSM-III* disorders. The Inventory of Interpersonal Problems shows considerable promise for serving that function in an eventual standardized battery of interpersonal measures.

Assessment of Patients' Relationships

Within interpersonal theory, the preeminent situational determinants of a patient's maladaptive actions are other persons, especially those whom the patient considers "significant." Significant persons are those whose opinions about the patient "as a person" matter, with whom the patient spends considerable time in either imaginary or real transactions, and who serve as potential sources of intimacy and regard in the patient's life. Until recently, however, no systematic procedures have been available to the clinician or researcher to help chart the scope and nature of these past and present relationships.

Klerman and associates, as part of their interpersonal approach to depression, emphasize an assessment procedure called the "interpersonal inventory," which is completed through the process of the therapist's questions in early therapy sessions.[36] The questioning has as its goal a review of key persons and issues in the patient's life, past and present. The therapist has the option of pursuing this exploration by asking the patient to write an autobiographical statement containing interpersonal information.

Either exploration seeks to gather the following information about each person who is important in the patient's life:

> (1) interactions with the patient including frequency of contact, activities shared, etc.; (2) the expectations of each party in the relationship, including some assessment of whether the expectations were or are fulfilled; (3) a review of the satisfactory and unsatisfactory aspects of the relationship with specific, detailed examples of both kinds of interactions; and (4) the ways the patient would like to change the relationships, whether through changing his or her own behavior or bringing about changes in the other person.[36]

Chewning constructed a Significant Other Survey for standardized use in interpersonal research and therapy[37] and presently is collecting reliability and validity data. Her survey asks the patient to "list the names of all the persons who you consider to be highly significant in your life." For each person listed the patient then supplies the following information: a rating of the importance of the person's opinion of the patient as a person; a rating of how much imaginary and real time is devoted by the patient to that person; a list of three positive and three negative "traits, characteristics, or behavior patterns" characteristic of himself; a list of three positive and three negative traits that characterize each significant person listed; a rating of the extent to which the patient has actually discussed each of his traits in actual conversations with each significant other; and, finally, a rating of the extent to which each significant other has actually discussed his traits in actual conversations with the patient.

In interpersonal therapy it is crucial that the therapist be able to identify the significant relationships in a patient's life in order to explore, define, and alter the patient's maladaptive transaction pattern. Perhaps the assessment procedures of both Chewning[37] and Klerman and associates[36] will develop toward an integrated measure that also can become part of an eventual standardized interpersonal assessment battery.

Sequential Analysis of Transactions

The potentially most useful procedures for identifying specific components of the maladaptive transaction cycle for patient disorders are various possibilities of *sequential* or *stochastic* analysis of the evolving patterns of action–reaction between patients and significant others. Stochastic statistical procedures have been developed but remain in a relatively primitive state.

Peterson has developed several sequential analysis methods that can be applied by clinicians and researchers alike.[38] So far he has applied his assessment procedures primarily to marital therapy. He argues that the flow of actions and reactions that occurs as spouses meet, deal with one another, and then part must first be described at a very specific and concrete level. Only subsequently should the therapist attempt to understand this flow in terms of deeper relationship meanings.

One of Peterson's methods is called an "interaction record." On separate forms each spouse describes the most important interaction they had on a given day. In their own words, and from their respective viewpoints, each independently describes in specific detail the conditions under which the exchange took place, how the interaction started, and what happened then. The third point is especially crucial in that the spouse is asked to write a fairly detailed account of the exchange from start to finish, including: Who did and said what to whom? What were you thinking and feeling as the action went on? What ideas and emotions did your partner seem to have? How did it all come out?

In interpreting interaction records, Peterson first identifies the major acts or moves that each person has made in the course of the exchange. Then an interpersonal meaning or message is inferred for each act. Each message contains three kinds of meaning: a report of the emotion the person is feeling at the time, a report of the way the person construes the situation, and an expectation about the response of the other. Peterson reports that, despite the rather high level of inference required for these interpretations, clinicians agree fairly closely about them. He finds interesting differences between normal and disturbed couples regarding the kinds of affect, construal, and expectation they report with this procedure.

Peterson also advocates use of videotaped samples of "analogue interactions" between spouses in which they are directed to discuss conflicts, plan vacations, and so on. Descriptions of recurrent interaction patterns can be derived from these videotapes by clinicians or other observers. Once obtained, the causal governing regularities in interpersonal behavior between marriage partners or other dyads can be inferred provisionally. Peterson uses the phrase, "functional analysis of interpersonal behavior," to designate this "cyclical process of describing interaction patterns, formulating ideas about the conditions that maintain the patterns, testing the propositions by planned interventions, and describing the interaction patterns that follow" to determine whether changes have or have not occurred. Changes "in predicted directions confirm hypotheses about the causes of the disorder. Persistence of the problem tends to disconfirm the hypothesis and requires conceptual reformulation."[38]

Peterson's modifications of behavioral procedures for study of interpersonal disorders have much to offer interpersonal assessment, especially in regard to discovery of specific components of maladaptive transaction cycles prototypical of distinct psychiatric disorders.

Interpersonal Intervention

In interpersonal therapy the therapist's essential task is to disrupt the patient's vicious circle of self-defeating actions depicted in the maladaptive transaction cycle. In attempting to accomplish this task, the therapist has available important components of intervention that are derivable from the interpersonal circle. Although interpersonal therapists have yet to articulate comprehensive treatment packages applying these principles to specific disorders, some important first steps have been taken.

This part of the chapter first summarizes five general principles of interpersonal intervention derivable from the interpersonal circle. It then reviews some creative "stage models" constructed by their authors as guides to the process of interpersonal therapy. Finally, it discusses several recent attempts to provide comprehensive treatment programs for specific patient disorders.

GENERAL PRINCIPLES

Available as guides to interpersonal intervention are five basic principles, each of which is derivable and specifiable from the interpersonal circle.[14] Underlying them all is the assumption that in order for a patient's maladaptive transaction cycle to be disrupted, the therapist must respond to the patient in a manner markedly different from others in the patient's life. That is, the therapist must respond to the patient with something other than complementary responses. If the patient is permitted to continue to restrict the therapist's reactions to only complementary responses, the therapist simply continues to confirm or reinforce (as do others) the patient's maladaptive cognitions and behaviors.

Another embarrassing possibility is evident at the point of impasse, which occurs in the later stage of the maladaptive transaction cycle. During impasse the therapist sends incongruent messages (enacts discrepant behaviors) expressing the unrecognized conflict that the patient's maladaptive pattern evokes. The general form of the therapist's conflict consists of hostile–rejecting feelings and cognitions toward the patient. The therapist then experiences guilt about these feelings and cognitions that are so much at variance with himself and his role definitions as an accepting and nurturant caregiver. The extreme of these hostile–rejecting feelings and their concomitant threat to the therapist have been vividly described by object-relations theorists characterizing the treatment process with borderline and narcissistic personalities. In interpersonal therapy the preeminent objective is to avoid this impasse, which represents the extreme of unhelpful "treatment" by a therapist.

Principle One. The goal of therapy is to facilitate an increased frequency and intensity of interpersonal actions with significant others from segments OPPOSITE on the circle to the segments that define the patient's pattern of maladaptive interpersonal behavior. The direct effects of attainment of this goal are reductions of (1) the extremeness of the patient's maladaptive behaviors with others by pulling him toward the center of the circle, and (2) the rigidity of the patient's behavior by increasing the range of acts available to the patient in transactions with others. Both reductions make the patient more "normal"—better able to adjust his actions more appropriately to different interpersonal situations. These new options provide the patient a much better probability for attaining the intimacy with others that is essential for genuine self-esteem and for satisfaction of basic interpersonal needs.

To illustrate, if a patient is diagnosed as *DSM-III* compulsive personality, interpersonal measures will profile the patient at the FG octant of the 1982 circle (see Table 1). The therapeutic goal, then, is to facilitate an increased frequency and intensity of patient actions from octant NO, which is directly opposite to FG on the circle. Improvement for the compulsive patient results from helping him interact with others in a manner more like that of a normal histrionic individual. Specifically, where F, detachment, and G, inhibition, prevail, more N, sociable, and O, exhibitionistic behavioral possibilities with others need to be introduced. The hopeful outcome is that by facilitating greater occurrence and egosyntonicity of sociable and exhibitionistic behaviors, the compulsive patient will enjoy greater options of being detached or not, inhibited or not, based on real characteristics of an interactant and his significance to the patient.

In sum, once a patient's interpersonal behavior is precisely diagnosed on the circle, the goal of therapy for that patient is specifically determined.

Principle Two. In early therapy sessions especially, the patient will evoke or pull covert and overt responses from the therapist that are precisely characterized at segments of the circle that are COMPLEMENTARY to those that define the patient's maladaptive interpersonal style. In the case of the FG compulsive patient, this means that the therapist inevitably will be hooked or pulled to enact behaviors from the DC, cold–mistrusting, octant of the circle. The therapist quickly will begin to experience an objective countertransference manifested by actions that are cold, stern, and strict/punitive (segment D) as well as vigilant, suspicious/jealous, cunning, resentful, and covetous/stingy (segment C).

By his statements and nonverbal behaviors, the

patient sends evoking messages that shape the therapist to respond from a narrow portion of his inner experience and behavioral repertoire. The therapist inevitably is pulled to provide the complementary response because the patient is more adept, more expert in his distinctive, rigid, and extreme game of interpersonal encounter. The position the patient pushes the therapist to adopt is one that is least threatening to and most confirming of roles central to the patient's self-definition. By eliciting the complementary role from the therapist, the patient continues to validate his crippled self-definition and hangs on to the self-in-world view that maladaptively organizes his experience and behavior.

As the therapist becomes hooked, he experiences greater or lesser intensities of the various classes of "impact messages": feelings, action tendencies, cognitive attributions, and fantasies.[24,25,39] If the therapist does not disengage from these impacts, he in effect unwittingly reinforces the maladaptive behavior of the patient. As their sessions continue the therapist will increasingly feel more negative feelings such as boredom, anxiety, frustration, irritation, and depression. The maladaptive transaction cycle shows that as the therapist continues to be unaware of the hooking, his experience of these feelings is inevitably communicated to the patient through a package of the therapist's own discrepant acts. These events not only compound the transactional impasse but, by his own incongruent communications, the therapist is placed in the embarrassing position of modeling maladaptive communication for the patient.

The therapist cannot *not* be hooked temporarily into providing the complementary response to the patient. Indeed, getting hooked probably is necessary for establishment of a working therapeutic alliance. It also permits the therapist to experience first-hand the aversive interpersonal consequences of the patient's maladaptive transactions.

Principle Three. The first therapeutic priority is for the therapist to DISENGAGE from the complementary covert and overt responses being pulled from him by the patient. Since relationship messages typically are automatic and outside the direct awareness of both participants, the therapist of necessity experiences feelings and other internal engagements before he can notice or label them.

Accordingly the first task in the disengagement process is for the therapist to detect, attend to, and label the engagements being evoked in him by a given patient. From the first session the therapist must ask these essential questions about his internal reactions: What is this patient trying to do to me? What am I feeling when I'm with this patient? What do I want to do or not to do with this patient? The Impact Message Inventory provides a useful format for this self-exploratory process.[24,25]

A second disengagement maneuver available to the therapist is to discontinue the complementary response. When the therapist realizes that he has been enticed to provide answers and advice, he must withhold these responses. When he has been pulled to be entertained, the therapist must cease enjoyment of the entertainment. When pushed into feeling cautious and constricted, he must find a way to be more spontaneous. When trapped into protecting the patient from more intense emotion, he must begin to help the patient face the feared feelings.

A third disengagement option involves use by the therapist of various techniques to help the patient interrupt his distinctive pattern of interpersonal behavior. When the compulsive patient uses abstractions and qualifications to describe his problems, the therapist can push for concrete elaborations through pinpointing and situational analysis procedures. When the histrionic patient entertains the therapist with anecdotes and dramatic displays, the therapist can reflect the patient's feelings of fragility and encourage him to attend to and elaborate the feelings being avoided.

Through the process of disengagement, the therapist prevents the relationship from ending in alienation. Unlike most others with whom the patient interacts, the therapist hangs in in a supportive fashion to help the patient face tuned-out aspects of his experience. The patient avoids these aspects in order to keep his self-definition and esteem from being devastated—to keep himself from emerging naked and vulnerable in a totally unpredictable new world. Finally, through disengagement the therapist regains his options to act therapeutically toward the patient and to use a more varied repertoire of interventions.

Principle Four. The therapist can produce cognitive ambiguity and uncertainty for the patient, as the first step toward disrupting the patient's maladaptive style, by shifting from complementary responses to therapeutic ASOCIAL[40] responses. The therapist responds to the patient in an asocial or disengaged way whenever he withholds the customary, preferred, or expected complementary response. As a direct first result, the patient experiences a sense of "beneficial uncertainty,"[40] since the patient's preferred style does not produce the expected and familiar interpersonal consequences.

In the case of the compulsive patient, asocial therapist responses would require that (1) the therapist in no way provide the DC, cold–mistrusting complementary response bid for so vigorously by the FG, detached–inhibited compulsive patient, and (2) that any therapist response have ambiguous meaning in the sense that the compulsive patient cannot pinpoint a position on the circle from which the therapist is responding. As examples of therapeutic asocial responses, Young and Beier list delay responses such as long therapist silences, reflection of content and feeling, labeling the patient's interaction style, and use of therapeutic paradox.[41]

Kiesler emphasizes that the asocial response of "metacommunicative feedback" has interventive priority throughout the course of therapy.[13,15,39] Metacommunication means that the therapist talks directly to the patient about the transactional engagements transpiring between them and refers directly to the evoking or impact messages he experiences. Since it is far from the norm that persons talk directly to each other about their subtle relationship messages, metacommunication is very much an asocial response. With maladjusted individuals who have problems, others most frequently take the easiest way out by simply leaving the scene. Even those who do not flee usually stay with the implicit agreement that talking about what they might be doing to each other is forbidden. Generally metacommunication remains a remote option in everyday affairs because of the threat that it can eventuate in rejection, withdrawal of affection, various forms of punishment, or social isolation—that it might lead to dramatic disconfirmation of one's identity. The advantages of metacommunication as well as principles that guide its use in therapy are discussed in detail elsewhere.[39]

In the case of the compulsive patient, the therapist might find himself feeding back to the patient the following kinds of internal engagements: "I'm trying to figure out why it is that I feel so emotionally distant from you—feel that you have to do all this by yourself without any help from me." "You know, often when you talk, it's difficult for me to follow your train of thought—you start off in one direction, shift to another, then another; and all the time I'm wondering where you're going and whether you're going to bring it back to the original topic." "Often I find myself being cautious and careful about what I'm going to say to you—as if, if I'm not careful, you will disapprove of what I say and lose respect for me."

By addressing the patient–therapist relationship directly, the therapist not only disrupts the patient's maneuvers with a surprising asocial response, but importantly provides the patient with new information about the undesirable effects the patient has on others. Open feedback brings the attention of both patient and therapist to the relationship issues occurring between them and interfering with the self-exploratory task and permits pinpointing of the distinctive patterns these maneuvers have taken. Through collaborative exploration of each participant's contribution to the transactional effects experienced by the therapist, they begin to clarify the patient's central maladaptive patterns with others—to detail the content of the patient's particular maladaptive transaction cycle. And the therapist, by his willingness to address the patient–therapist relationship openly, models a powerful technique for the patient to use with significant others outside his sessions.

The success of metacommunication depends crucially on the commitment of the therapist to open, direct, unambiguous communication to the patient about the therapist's feelings, fantasies, and pulls as well as on the skill with which the therapist can provide feedback in a manner that is simultaneously confrontative and protective of the patient's self-esteem. To be assimilated by the patient, feedback first must be heard. Hence, in using impact messages the therapist must always consider, in addition to his own possible subjective countertransference, the potential threat to the patient's shaky conception of self.

Principle Five. In later sessions the therapist can exert the greatest pressure for change in the patient's interpersonal behavior (for increasing the frequency and intensity of actions from opposite segments of the circle) by initiating responses that are ANTICOMPLEMENTARY on the circle to the patient's maladaptive interpersonal profile. Recall that if the therapist enacts an anticomplementary response, he is rejecting both components (control and affiliation) of the patient's self-presentation. That is, the therapist's response is both nonreciprocal on the control axis and noncorresponding on the affiliation axis. Anticomplementary responses come from the opposite vertically divided half of the circle and from the same horizontally divided half. The anticomplement to friendly–dominant behavior is hostile–dominant action, to friendly–submissive behavior is hostile–submissive action, and vice versa. More detailed specification of the anticomplementary segments on the circle can be found elsewhere.[14]

Since use of the anticomplementary response involves total rejection of the patient's self-presentation, its application early in therapy would likely result in the patient's rejection of treatment and/or premature termination. These patient reactions would represent very sensible responses to a threatening and aversive situation. It seems probable, then, that effective use by the therapist of anticomplementary responses can occur only in later stages of the therapy transaction. The therapist must first "hook" the patient—establish a working therapeutic alliance—by reacting with some components of the complementary response, so that later injections of the anticomplementary response do not elicit the strong and disruptive patient anxiety probable in earlier sessions.

In the case of the compulsive patient, the therapist would provide responses anticomplementary to the patient's maladaptive FG, detached–inhibited behaviors whenever the therapist responds from the KL, trusting–warm octant. By these actions the therapist offers a stance characterized as unguarded, trusting, innocent, forgiving, and generous (segment K) as well as warm, gentle, and lenient/pardoning (segment L). These acts are bipolar opposites to the complementary responses the compulsive is working so hard to pull from the therapist, that is, reactions that are vigilant, suspicious/jealous, cunning, resentful, and covetous/stingy (segment C) and cold, stern, and strict/punitive (segment D). To provide the anticomplementary response, then, the therapist must struggle to find a way to enact behaviors diametrically opposite to the complementary acts being pulled from him so relentlessly by a patient.

In sum, the most powerful response available to the interpersonal therapist requires use of actions from circle segments anticomplementary to those that define the patient's rigid and extreme maladaptive style. Effective use of these responses probably occurs only after a working therapeutic alliance has been established.

INTERPERSONAL STAGE MODELS OF PSYCHOTHERAPY

The basic therapeutic principles just described need to be further elaborated into treatment packages, consisting of distinct stages, which are tailored for specific psychiatric disorders. This section summarizes attempts by therapists to articulate the distinct stages within the process of interpersonal therapy. The final section reviews the few comprehensive treatment programs offered by interpersonal therapists for specific psychiatric disorders.

Cashdan's notions provide a useful framework for organizing these stage model attempts. According to him a psychotherapy process is "essentially a miniature theory that specifies how therapist operations are sequenced [and that] predicts what changes can be expected in the patient as therapy progresses."[42] Process, thus, represents a series of "stages," each of which is composed of a set of "rules" for the therapist to follow, as well as specified corresponding behavioral shifts for the patient. Rules for a given stage are principles that guide the therapist's "technique" (the concrete responses of the therapist).

Most of the following process conceptualizations offer models that articulate the sequential stages of intervention occurring over the course of interpersonal therapy. As will be evident, however, the extent to which these models provide the precise detail advocated by Cashdan varies considerably.

Interactional Psychotherapy

Cashdan's interactional therapy dictates five stages of transaction between therapist and client.[42,43] In the first stage, *hooking*, the therapist establishes the conditions that enable him to be viewed by the patient as a significant other. This is accomplished primarily through use of "emotional coupling" techniques. A major function of hooking is to prevent the patient from bolting in later stages when the going gets rough.

In stage two, *maladaptive strategies*, the patient's self-defeating patterns of relating start to emerge full-blown in the patient–therapist relationship. Through use of techniques of "direct confrontation" and "dare ploys," the therapist attempts to elicit clear and direct expressions of the patient's maladaptive patterns within the therapy sessions.

In stage three, *stripping*, the therapist confronts, challenges, and ultimately refutes the appropriateness of the patient's basic maladaptive strategy. This is accomplished by use of "refutation–affirmation" techniques in which the therapist refuses to respond to the patient in strategic ways, but at the same time expresses a continuing commitment to the patient and the patient's welfare.

In stage four, *adaptive strategies*, the therapist helps the patient to fill the void by finding new options for relating to others in more meaningful ways. To accomplish this goal the therapist uses "transactional feedback" and maintains a supportive, affirming manner.

In the fifth and last stage, *unhooking* or *termination*, the therapist and patient apply their transactional learnings to the patient's relationships outside therapy. As diminishing returns begin to set in, the therapist openly discusses the experience of separation and loss with the patient, and the therapy comes to a close.

Interpersonal Behavior Therapy

DeVogue and Beck offer a four-stage process model in which interpersonal and behavior therapy strategies are integrated.[44] In stage one the therapist tries to avoid any interpersonal actions that would be classified as intense or extreme on any of the circle segments. As a result of this tactic the patient will begin to use his preferred interpersonal tactic to initiate a comfortable form of intimacy with the therapist.

In stage two the therapist invites the patient directly into a conversation about their "here-and-now" relationship. In stage three the therapist refuses to enact any behavior that is complementary to the patient's preferred interpersonal stance. Instead, he launches an unemotional and logical attack against the patient's position, while providing the patient with a clear message of the therapist's desire to continue the relationship.

Finally, at stage four, various behavioral techniques such as social skills and assertiveness training are instituted.

Interpersonal–Cognitive Therapy

Carson has written convincingly about the cognitive components of interpersonal therapy.[8,45] He notes that "by far the most important cause of persistently maladaptive behavior is the tendency of the interpersonal environment to confirm the expectancies mediating its enactment."[45] In Carson's view, and as depicted in the maladaptive transaction cycle, an unbroken causal loop exists among the patient's social perceptions or cognitions, behavioral enactments, and reactions of interactants that confirm the patient's maladaptive cognitions or expectancies. This loop reflects another interpersonal assumption: that a patient's rigid and extreme interpersonal actions tend to evoke complementary responses that confirm the maladaptive perceptions, expectations, or constructions that organize the patient's phenomenal world.

From Carson's interpersonal–cognitive viewpoint, "a major task of the psychotherapist is that of explicit identification of the client's habitual, disorder-related, parataxic distortions of social cognition, an examination of their sources, and a comprehensive analysis of the manner in which they affect the client's behavior, particularly in its maladaptive aspects."[45] Further, the therapy relationship itself is the major arena in which corrective experiences occur. In addressing specific parataxic distortions projected by the patient onto the therapist, the therapist encourages a nondefensive and participatory exploration of the patient's more problematic "person–schematas" by undertaking a "thorough examination of the evidential basis of the characteristics assigned to him, and repeatedly asserts[s] his willingness to be put to *fair* tests, having *explicit* criteria, concerning his personal attitudes and commitments."[45]

Safran amplifies Carson's notions regarding the cognitive components of interpersonal therapy and argues convincingly for a rapprochement between cognitive–behavioral and interpersonal therapies.[46,47] His first paper details a number of ways in which Sullivan's concepts are compatible with the contemporary cognitive behavioral tradition. He also details specific ways in which incorporation of interpersonal principles can broaden and enrich its theoretical and practical scope. Namely, interpersonal theory provides a systematic framework for understanding and dealing with problems in therapeutic compliance and for understanding what variables can lead to problems in therapeutic maintenance, and at the same time allows cognitive behavior therapists to broaden their conceptualization of the role of emotions in psychotherapy.

In his second paper, Safran, like Carson, argues that "cognitive activities, interpersonal behaviors, and repetitive interactional or *me-you patterns* are linked together and maintain one another in an unbroken causal loop."[47] Expanding on the metacommunicative principles described above,[39] Safran emphasizes that "in addition to pinpointing and providing feedback to the patient about the interpersonal impact of dysfunctional behavior, the process of pinpointing dysfunctional interpersonal behaviors can provide the cognitive therapist with markers indicating the need for cognitive exploration."[47] This process involves the therapist-led exploration of the automatic thoughts accompanying or preceding the behaviors. Once some of the automatic thoughts and beliefs have been identified, the therapist can assign a variety of homework tasks described in detail by Safran.

Safran concludes that "a full assessment in the context of a *cognitive-interpersonal* therapy requires that the therapist conduct a comprehensive exploration of both the specific interpersonal behaviors and *me-you patterns* that impair the client's interpersonal relations, and the particular cognitive activities that are linked to them."[47]

Relational Psychotherapy

McLemore and Hart describe a "relational psychotherapy" that consists of five process stages.[48] In their first stage, *inquiry*, the therapist gathers information about the patient and the presenting problems. He accomplishes this primarily through use of open-ended questions.

In stage two, *stabilization,* the therapist and client establish the transactional rhythm into which they both settle for purpose of joint exploration of the patient's life. During this stage the patient is encouraged to take the lead, with the goal being "emotional immersion," which the therapist encourages through use of "triadic reflection" responses.

Stage three, *assimilation,* involves the therapist's use of free-association technique to explore the patient's mental representations of significant others. Jointly they clarify the patient's powerful introjects or personifications, and the therapist helps the patient to accept aspects of an introject that the patient deems desirable and to reject the rest.

In the fourth stage, *confrontation,* the therapist directly helps the patient to extend learnings about introjects to ongoing relationships in the patient's life. As a major means of accomplishing this goal, McLemore and Hart use an intervention they call "the disclosure," which consists of bringing into the therapy session at the same time the patient and one or more significant others. This focal intervention has the purpose of assisting the patient "at the appropriate time, and in the appropriate manner, to inform his or her significant other(s) of what the patient thinks and feels about some private 'something.' This is done with the therapist present to ensure clear communication, to encourage benevolence, and to prevent the patient from getting stuck or diverted."

Their fifth and final stage, *transition,* leads to a discontinuance of regular therapy sessions, but with the clear understanding that patients may consult the therapist later at any point in their lives. A careful analysis is also conducted of the degree to which the patient's goals have been reached as the patient's visits gradually decrease in frequency.

A Brief Strategic Therapy

Coyne and Segal extend and systematize the brief strategic therapy developed by Watzlawick and colleagues at the Palo Alto Mental Research Institute.[49] They offer detailed descriptions and examples of five basic maladaptive "metapatterns of interpersonal solutions." These metapatterns include attempts to be spontaneous deliberately; attempts to have others behave in a desired fashion even while requiring that they do so spontaneously; seeking a nonrisk method where some risk is inevitable; attempting to reach accord through argument; and attracting attention by attempting to be left alone.

Coyne and Segal detail five stages of their version of brief strategic therapy. In the first stage, *pretreatment,* a concerted effort is made to identify the members of an interpersonal problem situation who are most committed to change. If the person calling for an appointment fails to meet this criterion, they use a number of strategies either to increase that person's motivation for therapy or to identify a more appropriate point of intervention in the system.

In stage two, *obtaining a problem description,* the therapist takes pains to gather clear and concrete information that provides a comprehensive description of the ongoing interactions that characterize a problem in the interpersonal system.

In stage three, *describing attempted solutions,* the emphasis is on obtaining behaviorally relevant descriptions of specific interactions that characterize the patient's attempts to handle or resolve the identified problem. In this stage the therapist looks for commonalities in what the patient is trying to accomplish and how he goes about doing this.

In stage four, *eliciting a goal statement,* the therapist seeks from the patient a clear behavioral description of the kind of interaction that could signify that the problem has been resolved. Attempts are made to have the goal stated in terms of the occurrence of a positive event that involves a small but strategic change.

The fifth and final stage, *strategic planning,* involves the therapist's attempts to influence the patient "to take a new tack that is not a variation of the basic solution so that the behaviors perpetuating the problem are abandoned." This is accomplished through use of reframing interventions that change "the meaning attributed to the [problem] situation, and therefore its consequences, but not the concrete facts."[49] The particular reframing that is chosen is carefully constructed to reflect the patient's values, beliefs, and attitudes.

Interpersonal Communication Psychotherapy

The distinctiveness of my "interpersonal communication psychotherapy" derives from its integration of three conceptual traditions: Sullivan's interpersonal therapy and its derivatives, interactional psychiatry, and research in nonverbal communication.

My initial formulation was made in the context of construction of a differential treatment for the obsessive (*DSM-III* compulsive) personality.[50] This was subsequently updated in another unpublished paper.[51] Seventeen propositions of interpersonal communication and psychotherapy were systematically offered and used to critique the behavior therapies of that period.[15] A comprehensive interpersonal communication analysis of relationship in psychotherapy appeared that specified six measurable indices, which together constitute a valid assessment of therapy relationship factors.[13] Twelve propositions that constitute the basic assumptions of interpersonal approaches to personality and psychotherapy were outlined.[52]

I presented a taxonomy of interpersonal behavior in the form of the 1982 interpersonal circle designed to integrate findings from previous circle inventories and also defined 11 propositions of complementarity as they apply to personality, psychopathology, and psychotherapy.[14] I provided an interpersonal analysis of *DSM-III* personality disorders and outlined six principles that can guide interpersonal diagnosis conducted within the framework of the interpersonal circle.[29] I offered a model of interpersonal supervision of therapy that emphasizes both the therapy and supervisory transactions and that describes various interventions a supervisor can use to help the supervisee learn to disengage from transactional impasses with patients.[53] Finally, I provided a detailed analysis of impact messages registered by therapists during their transactions with patients and offered eight principles that govern the therapist's use of metacommunicative feedback with patients.[39]

The latter report also offers a two-stage process model detailing the optimal sequence that objective countertransference events should take over the course of therapy. In the *engaged* or *hooked* stage, the therapist invariably is pulled into enactment of covert and overt complementary reactions to the patient. A side-effect of this engagement is that it permits the therapist to experience live the interpersonal consequences of the patient's maladaptive behavior and also to "hook" the patient into a working therapeutic alliance wherein the therapist attains "significant-other" status.

The second, *disengaged*, stage requires that the therapist prevent his objective countertransference responses from building to intense levels. As the therapist experiences intense covert reactions to the patient, it is easy for subjective, irrational countertransferences to emerge full-blown, blocking any possibility of therapeutic intervention. Further, by becoming intensely trapped in the patient's maladaptive style, the therapist's reactions dramatically reconfirm and reinforce the patient's maladaptive cognitions and behavior. I have detailed methods of disengagement the therapist can use to avoid transactional impasses with patients.[39] These procedures were described briefly in an earlier section of this chapter.

DIFFERENTIAL INTERPERSONAL TREATMENTS

The interpersonal stage models reviewed above offer guides for a therapist's efforts with any psychotherapy patient. None has much, if anything, to offer in regard to the types of patients with whom a given stage model is more or less effective. Likewise, none describes any principles that might guide differential applications to the various psychiatric disorders.

As emphasized above, the distinctive power of interpersonal therapy derives from its potential for concrete specification of distinctive maladaptive cognitions and behaviors corresponding both to the maladaptive transaction cycle and to distinctive profiles on the interpersonal circle. This power can be realized only as differential treatment programs are constructed for patients prototypical of various *DSM-III* disorders or for patients exhibiting prototypical profiles of circle interpersonal behaviors. At present, attempts at systematic differential interpersonal treatments of this sort are few and far between.

Interpersonal Psychotherapy of Depression

Klerman and associates provide a detailed description of a comprehensive interpersonal treatment program for depressed patients.[36] Interpersonal psychotherapy (IPT) of depression is a time-limited treatment that focuses on interpersonal behavior rather than on intrapsychic phenomena. It concentrates on the patient's current life situations and is directed toward alleviation of one or two problem areas by changing the way the patient thinks, feels, and acts in current problematic relationships. In IPT the therapist first identifies one of four problem areas that depressed patients commonly encounter: grief reactions, interpersonal disputes with a significant other, role transitions, and interpersonal deficits resulting in isolation and loneliness.

The strategies of IPT are applied in three stages of the treatment process. During *phase one*, the depression is diagnosed within a medical model and the disorder is explained in some detail to the patient. Initial sessions are devoted to identification of the major problem areas associated with the onset of depression and to establishment of a treatment contract. Also, a primary problem area is defined in order to identify and clarify the most recent stress with which the patient is trying to cope. The defined problem area then becomes the focus of the therapy sessions.

In the second or *intermediate* phase, the therapist and patient begin the hard work on the defined major current interpersonal problem area. The therapist's main tasks are to help the patient discuss topics pertinent to the problem while constantly attending to the patient's affective state and to the therapeutic relationship. These tasks are necessary in order to maximize the patient's intimate self-disclosure and to prevent the patient from sabotaging the treatment. Exploration of the problem area entails general exploration of the problem, a focus on the patient's expectations and perceptions, an analysis of possible alternative ways to handle the problem, and attempts at new behavior.

In the third phase, *termination*, two to four sessions are devoted to discussing the patient's feelings about termination, to reviewing progress, and to outlining the work remaining to be done. Areas of potential difficulty are discussed, the therapist guides the patient through an exploration of how various contingencies might be handled, and he emphasizes the importance of the patient's ability to judge when help needs to be sought again.

The work of Klerman and associates serves as an IPT training manual that standardizes the strategies and techniques to be followed by therapists treating depressed patients.[36] It provides detailed instructions and guidelines for the actual conduct of the treatment, a list of operationalized techniques from which the therapist can choose, detailed outlines of strategies for approaching the patient's interpersonal problem depending on which of the four problem areas is presented, a set of guidelines for handling specific issues that usually arise in the sessions, instructions about the sequence of events to be followed in the various stages of therapy, and descriptions of the defining features of the relationship the IPT therapist attempts to form with the patient.

Interpersonal Psychotherapy of the Histrionic Personality

Andrews provides a conceptualization of the hysteric (*DSM-III* histrionic) personality and a plan of differential interpersonal treatment.[32] His interpersonal analysis of the hysteric's personality centers on a self-presentational style characterized by excessive use of agreeable, affiliative, and overconventional behavior (the NO segments of the 1982 interpersonal circle). He describes a transactional cycle in which the hysteric sends conflicting and indirect messages to others. The messages combine both symbolic sexual overtones (to gain interest and attention) and simultaneous but subtle hostile messages (to keep the other person at a distance).

No matter which part of the hysteric's message an interactant responds to—the interactant who shows disinterest is regarded as rejecting and mean; the interactant who reciprocates the advances is regarded as guilty of sexual exploitation—the effect is the same: namely, confirmation and strengthening of the hysteric's overconventional self-image. In addition, the hysteric's cognitive experience is distinguished by his tendency to perceive in global, diffuse, and impressionistic ways (field dependence) and to exhibit a weak differentiation of self from the environment. He is oversensitive to external stimuli and confused as to what is external and internal.

The therapy package Andrews advocates for the hysteric patient consists of strategies and techniques designed to counteract the above stylistic components. They are designed to attain the following objectives: symptom reduction, development of a clear sense of identity, acceptance of negative feelings, greater assertiveness, and enhanced cognitive differentiation.

The most important relationship issue posed for the therapist stems from the patient's eagerness for approval, which leads the hysteric to try to discover the therapist's attitudes, which are then used as an external guide for being a "good" patient. The aim is to gain the therapist's confirmation of the patient's self-image as an agreeable, nonhostile person. The therapist counters this ploy by using the ambiguity inherent in the free-association rule of psychoanalysis, insisting that the patient share all thoughts, feelings, and associations no matter how bizarre or unacceptable they may seem. What this ambiguous stance accomplishes is a paradoxical attack on the patient's facade of overconventionality. For if the hysteric religiously follows the rule (as might be expected from one who conforms to conventions, rules, and expectations), he inevitably will come up with censored hostile, sexual, and other troublesome feelings that contradict his self-presentation. On the other hand, for the hysteric to openly resist or deliberately censor his thoughts introduces conflict or deceit that is equally incompatible with the agreeable self-image. Change will occur no matter what the patient does, since the only way to please the therapist is to bring up that which is unpleasant and conflictual about oneself.

To accomplish this paradoxical attack, the therapist must establish and maintain a realistic middle ground between pleasing and disappointing the hysteric patient. Thus, the therapist maintains a neutral, steady, but flexible attitude in which he is willing to accept some of the hysteric's demands for dependency.

To enhance development of more discriminating cognitive skills, the therapist continually provides reflective comments to the patient's spontaneous associations and self-disclosures. This labeling provides cognitive structure for the hysteric's inner experiences, facilitates conceptual clarity, and reinforces early steps toward cognitive control of emotionally laden internal experiences.

Finally, the hysteric is helped to learn new communication skills, including how to express his needs effectively even in the face of conflict, and how to be a more effective and less manipulative elicitor of attention.

In sum, Andrews' interpersonal therapy directs the therapist to create a setting in which the hysteric's repeated efforts to elicit attention from the therapist by symptomatic and other manipulative maneuvers are not reinforced. Once this has been accomplished, new ways of living with himself and with others are fostered.[32]

Conclusion

Despite the facts that the earlier works of Sullivan and Leary were remarkably innovative and provocative and that interpersonal theory had pervasive subterranean influence on psychology and psychiatry, until recently few sustained or systematic theoretical or empirical follow-ups appeared. This chapter demonstrates that this era of sporadic and abortive interpersonal startups has come to an end. Sustained momentum is now established, and exciting theoretical and empirical work is proliferating.

Systematic interpersonal diagnosis is an increasingly viable and practicable option. A battery of psychometrically sophisticated interpersonal inventories, all tied closely to the interpersonal circle, is a real probability for the near future. Even now Benjamin's SASB system, although conceptually divergent from the mainstream of circle inventories, demonstrates vividly the clinical utility and power of such comprehensive and sophisticated interpersonal assessment. In addition, new procedures for measuring both the interpersonal problems and significant interpersonal relationships of the patient will, over time, provide additional range to this psychometric arsenal. Most importantly, as we gain increased sophistication in sequential analysis procedures, we will evolve perhaps the most powerful methods for assessing the crucial maladaptive transaction cycles that are at the heart of various interpersonal psychopathologies.

The most potent feature of interpersonal therapy resides in the close theoretical and empirical hookup it offers between psychodiagnosis and intervention. Its central models of individual differences in psychopathology, the interpersonal circle and the maladaptive transaction cycle, offer conceptual and empirical guides to the design of distinct treatment programs for various psychiatric disorders. Although as yet differential process-stage models have not been articulated either systematically or in detail, clearly the potential is there and creative first attempts are emerging.

Finally, what interpersonal theory also provides is a conceptual structure for explanations of psychopathology and psychotherapy that is sufficiently comprehensive to subsume and integrate concepts and methodologies from other treatment approaches. In turn, other orientations can offer much toward filling in gaps found in current interpersonal approaches. For one, interpersonal therapy needs a systematic developmental theory, and developmental conceptualizations from ego psychology, cognitive psychology, and object relations have much to offer. Likewise, current interpersonal therapy lacks any systematic or comprehensive theory explaining the cognitive, affective, and other covert events associated with, or isomorphic in structure to, overt interpersonal actions depicted on the interpersonal circle. In this regard, exciting developments in experimental cognitive psychology and from experimental studies of emotion provide the possibility for these badly needed integrations. Still other gaps exist and need to be filled in by integrative efforts with other disciplines.

Much remains to be done. Nonetheless the unifying possibilities of the interpersonal paradigm for the fields of personality, psychopathology, and psychotherapy seem staggering indeed and warrant serious contributory efforts by all concerned at this unusually propitious point in the field's scientific and clinical development.

REFERENCES

1. Sullivan HS: Conceptions of Modern Psychiatry. New York, Norton, 1953
2. Sullivan HS: The Interpersonal Theory of Psychiatry, pp 110, 111. New York, Norton, 1953
3. Sullivan HS: The Psychiatric Interview. New York, Norton, 1954
4. Sullivan HS: Clinical Studies in Psychiatry. New York, Norton, 1956

5. Sullivan HS: Schizophrenia As a Human Process. New York, Norton, 1962

6. Sullivan HS: The Fusion of Psychiatry and Social Science. New York, Norton, 1964

7. Anchin JC, Kiesler DJ: Handbook of Interpersonal Psychotherapy. New York, Pergamon, 1982

8. Carson RC: Interaction Concepts of Personality. Chicago, Aldine, 1969

9. Chrzanowski G: Interpersonal Approach to Psychoanalysis: A Contemporary View of Harry Stack Sullivan. New York, Gardner, 1977

10. Leary T: Interpersonal Diagnosis of Personality. New York, Ronald, 1957

11. Wachtel PL: Psychoanalysis and Behavior Therapy: Toward an Integration. New York, Basic Books, 1977

12. Witenberg E (ed): Interpersonal Psychoanalysis. New York, Gardner, 1978

13. Kiesler DJ: An interpersonal communication analysis of relationship in psychotherapy. Psychiatry 42:299, 1979

14. Kiesler DJ: The 1982 interpersonal circle: A taxonomy for complementarity in human transactions. Psychol Rev 90:185, 1983

15. Kiesler DJ, Bernstein AB, Anchin JC: Interpersonal Communication, Relationship and the Behavior Therapies. Richmond, Virginia Commonwealth University, 1976

16. Wiggins JS: Circumplex models of interpersonal behavior in clinical psychology. In Kendall PC, Butcher JK (eds): Handbook of Research Methods in Clinical Psychology. New York, John Wiley & Sons, 1982

17. Kiesler DJ: The Maladaptive Transaction Cycle. Richmond, Virginia Commonwealth University, 1985

18. LaForge R: Using the ICL: 1976. Unpublished manuscript, 1977

19. LaForge R, Suczek RF: The interpersonal dimension of personality: III. An interpersonal check list. Personality 24:94, 1955

20. Lorr M, McNair DM: Expansion of the interpersonal behavior circle. Pers Soc Psychol 2:823, 1965

21. Lorr M, McNair DM: The Interpersonal Behavior Inventory, Form 4. Washington, DC, Catholic University of America, 1967

22. Wiggins JS: A psychological taxonomy of trait-descriptive terms: The interpersonal domain. J Pers Soc Psychol 37:395, 1979

23. Wiggins JS: Revised Interpersonal Adjective Scales. Vancouver, University of British Columbia, 1981

24. Kiesler DJ: Research Manual for the Impact Message Inventory. Palo Alto, Consulting Psychologists Press, 1985

25. Kiesler DJ, Anchin JC, Perkins MJ et al: The Impact Message Inventory. Richmond, Virginia Commonwealth University, 1976

26. Kiesler DJ: Check List of Psychotherapy Transactions and Check List of Interpersonal Transactions. Richmond, Virginia Commonwealth University, 1984

27. Benjamin LS: Structural analysis of social behavior. Psychol Rev 81:392, 1974

28. Benjamin LS: Validation of structural analysis of social behavior (SASB). Madison, Wisconsin Psychiatric Institute, 1980

29. Kiesler DJ: The 1982 interpersonal circle: An analysis of DSM-III personality disorders. In Millon T, Klerman G

(eds): Contemporary Issues in Psychopathology. New York, Guilford, 1986

30. McLemore CW, Benjamin LS: What ever happened to interpersonal diagnosis? A psychosocial alternative to DSM-III. Am Psychologist 34:17, 1979

31. Coyne JC: Toward an interactional description of depression. Psychiatry 39:28, 1976

32. Andrews JDW: Psychotherapy with the hysterical personality. Psychiatry 47:211, 1984

33. Lemert EM: Paranoia and the dynamics of exclusion. Sociometry 25:2, 1962

34. Gorad SL, McCourt WF, Cobb JC: A communications approach to alcoholism. Q J Studies Alcoholism 32:651, 1971

35. Horowitz LM, Weckler DA, Doren R: Interpersonal problems and symptoms: A cognitive approach. In Kendall PC (ed): Advances in Cognitive-Behavioral Research and Therapy, vol 2. New York, Academic Press, 1983

36. Klerman GL, Weissman MM, Rounsaville BJ et al: Interpersonal Psychotherapy of Depression, pp 86, 87. New York, Basic Books, 1984

37. Chewning MC: Significant Other Survey. Richmond, Virginia Commonwealth University, 1984

38. Peterson DR: Functional analysis of interpersonal behavior. In Anchin JC, Kiesler DJ: Handbook of Interpersonal Psychotherapy, p 164. New York, Pergamon Press, 1982

39. Kiesler DJ: Confronting the client–therapist relationship in psychotherapy. In Anchin JC, Kiesler DJ (eds): Handbook of Interpersonal Psychotherapy. New York, Pergamon Press, 1982

40. Beier EG: The silent language of psychotherapy. Chicago, Aldine, 1966

41. Young DM, Beier EG: Being asocial in social places: Giving the client a new experience. In Anchin JC, Kiesler DJ (eds): Handbook of Interpersonal Psychotherapy. New York, Pergamon Press, 1982

42. Cashdan S: Interactional psychotherapy: Stages and Strategies in Behavioral Change, pp 3, 4. New York, Grune & Stratton, 1973

43. Cashdan S: Interactional psychotherapy: Using the relationship. In Anchin JC, Kiesler DJ (eds): Handbook of Interpersonal Psychotherapy. New York, Pergamon Press, 1982

44. DeVogue JT, Beck S: The therapist–client relationship in behavior therapy. In Hersen M, Eisler RM, Miller PM (eds): Progress in Behavior Modification, vol 6. New York, Academic Press, 1978

45. Carson RC: Self-fulfilling prophecy, maladaptive behavior, and psychotherapy. In Anchin JC, Kiesler DJ (eds): Handbook of Interpersonal Psychotherapy, pp 64, 67. New York, Pergamon Press, 1982

46. Safran JD: Some implications of Sullivan's interpersonal theory for cognitive therapy. In Reda MA, Mahoney MJ (eds): Cognitive Psychotherapies: Recent Developments in Theory, Research and Practice. Cambridge, Ballinger, 1984

47. Safran JD: Assessing the cognitive–interpersonal cycle. Cog Ther Res 8:333, 1984

48. McLemore CW, Hart PP: Relational psychotherapy: The clinical facilitation of intimacy. In Anchin JC, Kiesler DJ (eds): Handbook of Interpersonal Psychotherapy. New York, Pergamon Press, 1982

49. Coyne JC, Segal L: A brief, strategic interactional approach to psychotherapy. In Anchin JC, Kiesler DJ (eds): Hand-

book of Interpersonal Psychotherapy, p 257. New York, Pergamon Press, 1982

50. Kiesler DJ: A communications approach to modification of the obsessive personality: An initial formulation. Atlanta, Emory University, 1973

51. Kiesler DJ: Communications assessment of interview behavior of the obsessive personality. Richmond, Virginia Commonwealth University, 1977

52. Kiesler DJ: Interpersonal theory for personality and psychotherapy. In Anchin JC, Kiesler DJ (eds): Handbook of Interpersonal Psychotherapy. New York, Pergamon Press, 1982

53. Kiesler DJ: Supervision in interpersonal communication psychotherapy. Richmond, Virginia Commonwealth University, 1982

5

Aaron Lazare, Sherman Eisenthal, and Anne Alonso

Clinical Evaluation: A Multidimensional, Hypothesis Testing, Negotiated Approach

The clinical evaluation consists not only of the clinician's perspective as to what is wrong and what should be done but also of the patient's perspective and the ways in which the inevitable differences between clinician and patient are negotiated.[1] This approach rests on six assumptions regarding the nature of the data base, the manner in which the data are acquired, and the nature of the interaction between patient and clinician:

1. An essential, but commonly overlooked, aspect of the evaluation includes an assessment of the patient's perspective as to his definition of the problem, goals of treatment, methods of treatment, conditions of treatment, and desired treatment relationship.[2,3]
2. The clinician's perspective is based on categorical diagnosis and on an individualistic perspective, which includes biomedical, psychodynamic, sociocultural, and behavioral/conceptual frameworks.[4]
3. Data for the clinician's perspective are elicited by an hypothesis testing approach.[5]
4. Special techniques of observations, referred to as the psychodynamic mental status examination, are required for the confirmation and refutation of psychodynamic hypotheses.[6]

This chapter is adapted in part from Lazare A, Eisenthal S, Wasserman L: The customer approach to patienthood: Attending to patient requests in a walk-in clinic. Arch Gen Psychiatry 32:553–558, 1975, Copyright 1975, American Medical Association; Lazare A, Eisenthal S: Patient requests in a walk-in clinic: Replication of factor analysis in an independent sample. A Nerv Ment Dis 165:300–340, 1977; Lazare A: The psychiatric examination in the walk-in clinic: Hypothesis generation and hypothesis testing. Arch Gen Psychiatry 33:96–102, 1976, Copyright 1976, American Medical Association.

5. Differences or conflicts between the patient's perspective and the clinician's perspective are inevitable in the vast majority of clinical encounters, particularly in the initial evaluation.[3]
6. Differences or conflicts between the patient's perspective and the clinician's perspective are best resolved through the process of negotiation. The clinical evaluation is therefore a negotiated outcome.[3]

In this chapter we will attempt to elaborate these six assumptions. More specific aspects of evaluation for the individual neuroses and personality disorders are detailed in subsequent chapters.

The Patient's Perspective

The patient's perspective of his problem is a critical but commonly overlooked aspect of the clinical evaluation. We will attempt to provide in this section a clinically and pedagogically useful categorization of the patient's perspective with a specific listing of patient requests. We will then attempt to illustrate the clinical value of eliciting such a perspective. It is our experience that patient dissatisfaction, poor compliance, and failure to develop a therapeutic alliance can be traced to differences between clinician and patient on one or more of the aspects of the patient's perspective that are discussed in the following sections.

CLASSIFICATION OF THE PATIENT'S PERSPECTIVE

The *definition of the problem* refers to what the patient thinks is wrong. This is embodied in the "chief complaint" and its elaboration. The definition of the problem also includes the illness attribution or the patient's theory as to the cause and pathogenesis of what he thinks is wrong. Attributes vary widely, ranging from life events and social problems outside the patient ("I lost my farm"; "My wife is threatening to leave.") to more patient-centered causes ("I have a weak nervous system"; "I am being neurotic again"; "I am not coping well"). With multiple problems, the definition includes a statement of priorities ("My biggest problem is my marriage—after that it is my drinking").

The *goals of treatment* refer to the patient's wish for the ultimate outcome of the encounter or treatment ("I want to be able to leave my house without fear"; "I want to be able to have relationships with people that are not so stormy and frustrating"; "I want this crisis to be behind me"; "I want to stop washing my hands so frequently").

Methods or requests for treatment refer to what the patient wants the clinician to do in order to achieve his goals. Knowledge of the definition of the problem and the goals in no way predicts the request or methods. For instance, a patient whose problem is anxiety and whose goal is symptom relief may request medication, psychodynamic psychotherapy, or a family meeting. Methods or requests must be distinguished from expectations. The request is what the patient wants. The expectation refers to what the patient anticipates will happen. For example, a patient who expects to be treated with medication might request psychotherapy.

Conditions of treatment include issues such as by whom (psychiatrists, psychologists, social workers, nurses), where (in the clinic, private office, home), how frequently, and for how much.

The patient's perspective of the *desired relationship* includes wishes for the type of expertise, empathy, caring, activity, and authoritarianism on the part of the therapist.

PATIENT REQUESTS OR DESIRED METHODS FOR TREATMENT

One aspect of the patient's perspective that has been the subject of considerable study is the request or method the patient makes of the clinician. In a series of studies, Lazare and Eisenthal have developed a list of 15 discrete requests on samples of patients presenting to a psychiatric walk-in clinic.[7,8] This listing has been replicated in college student health services and psychiatric outpatient clinics. The requests include administrative request, advice, clarification, community triage, confession, control, medical, nothing, psychological expertise, psychodynamic insight, reality contact, set limits, social intervention, succorance, and ventilation and are elaborated on below:

Administrative request. The patient is seeking administrative or legal assistance from the clinic to help him with his current dilemma. The specific request may be to provide a disability evaluation, a draft deferment, a medical excuse to leave work, medical permission to return to work, permission to drive, admission to a hospital, or testimony in court. These powers are delegated by society to particular professionals or institutions. The power may be subsequently rescinded or, as in the case of therapeutic abortions, may no longer be necessary.

Advice. The patient wants guidance about what to do in personal or social matters. He may already have formed an opinion but now wants professional advice. He wants to know the "right" thing, the "best" thing, or the "wisest" thing to do. He may want the advice in order to have the clinician share the responsibility for a decision he is about to make.

Clarification. The patient wants help to put his feelings, thoughts, or behavior in some perspective. He does not want to be told what to do but would rather take an active role in the therapeutic process. Often the patient wants the help to be able to make a decision. He wants to understand; he wants to see his choices. The patient usually sees his problem as being acute and not a part of an ongoing neurotic pattern.

Community triage. The patient is requesting information as to where in his community he can get the help he needs. He sees the clinic as an available resource that has the necessary information.

Confession. The patient feels guilty about what he has said, thought, or done and hopes that by talking to the therapist he will feel better. Specifically, the patient wants to be forgiven. He hopes the clinician (authority figure) will see the misdeed as medical or psychological in origin and therefore not bad.

Control. The patient is feeling overwhelmed and out of control. He may fear hurting himself or someone else, or going crazy. He is saying: "Please take over. I can no longer manage."

Medical. The patient sees his problem as being physical in origin, like any other medical condition, as opposed to psychological or situational in origin. He often refers to his problem as "nerves," or as a "nervous condition." The patient, accordingly, hopes for a medical kind of treatment such as pills, electroconvulsive treatment (ECT), hospitalization, or medical advice. He expects to take a passive role in the treatment.

Nothing. Patients who make no request are a heterogeneous group. They may have been referred without proper preparation; they may be psychotic; they may have problems but are not seeking help at this time; they may want help but are reluctant to state the problem; they may not need help; they may be in the wrong clinic.

Psychological expertise. The patient believes that the source of his problem is psychological rather than physical or situational. He is asking the professional to provide an explanation as to why he thinks, feels, or acts the way he does. The patient anticipates playing a passive role in the interaction, contributing only that information which the expert requires.

Psychodynamic insight. The patient perceives his problem as psychological in origin, as evolving from his early development, and as having a repetitive quality. As a result, he is left feeling unhappy, unfulfilled, but not overwhelmed or out of control. He expects to take an active, collaborative role in talking about the roots of his problem and hopes that a better understanding of his problem will enable him to change.

Reality contact. The patient feels that he is losing hold of reality. He wants to talk to someone who is psychologically stable and "safe." The request is for the clinician to help him "check out" or "keep in touch with" reality so that he will feel he is thinking straight and not losing his mind.

Set limits. The patient believes he is behaving in a way that is harmful to himself. He would like the clinician to help by setting firm and consistent limits. The patient is aware that he has final control over the responsibility for what he does.

Social intervention. The patient sees the problem as residing primarily in the people or situations around him. Because he feels that he does not possess the resources to effect the necessary change, he is asking the clinic to intervene on his behalf. He is asking not for the legal powers of the clinic but for its social influence.

Succorance. The patient is feeling empty, alone, not cared for, deprived, or drained. He wants the clinician to care, to be involved, to be comforting, and to be warm and giving so that he can feel replenished and warm inside. It is not so much the content of the interchange that is requested as its affective quality of warmth and caring.

Ventilation. The patient would like to tell the clinician about various feelings and affect-laden experiences. The patient anticipates that "getting it out" or getting it off his chest will be therapeutic. He feels like he is carrying around a burden that he would like to leave with the clinician. In contrast to confession, the patient does not feel guilty and does not need or want forgiveness.

CLINICAL VALUE OF ELICITING PATIENT REQUESTS

Diagnostic Issues

The patient's response to the clinician's elicitation of the request provides information that is diagnostic in the broadest sense. Indeed, some diagnostic data may not become apparent, or will be delayed, until the request is elicited.

When the patient's request is clinically appropriate, making a careful diagnosis of the request can be important in determining the precise clinical response. Take for example, the requests for ventilation, confession, and reality contact in three separate patients and assume that these requests represent valid clinical needs. An accurate diagnosis of the request or need will lead to three distinct clinical responses. For the patient who needs ventilation, the clinician can best help by taking the role of the interested listener. If he interrupts to make interpretive comments, the patient is likely to tolerate the interruption, ignore the clinician's words, and go on with his story. For the patient who needs confession, the clinician can best help by an attitude and verbal response that (when the guilt is neurotic) puts the deed in a medical or psychological perspective or that (when the guilt is real) communicates compassion and empathy necessary to help the patient bear his pain and search for his own forgiveness. If the clinician were to assume the role of the passive listener (as for ventilation), the patient would take this response as confirmation of his guilt. For the patient who needs reality contact, it may be important for the clinician to share his thoughts about what is real. Again, the role of the passive listener might aggravate the condition.

The patient's response to the clinician's elicitation of the request may also have special diagnostic meaning when the patient is reluctant or refuses to state what he wants. If the clinician pursues the matter, he will often learn important psychologic data about the patient. Patients have told us, for instance, that they are not worthy enough to ask for anything, that they are unwilling to commit themselves to a request, or that they will be obligated to give the clinician something in return. Without these responses, exploration of important psychological issues may be delayed.

Process Issues

There is likely to be a great deal of wasted time and energy during an interview in which the patient request is verbalized either late in the interview or not at all. Instead of speaking freely about his problem, the patient may be preoccupied, wondering whether or not the clinician is kind enough, respectful enough, wise enough, understanding enough, and flexible enough to hear the request: "When will the clinician be ready to hear?" "When will I have the courage to come right out with it?" The clinician, meanwhile, often unaware of these concerns, goes about the business of establishing diagnoses and making treatment recommendations. He does not understand why the patient participates only reluctantly during the interview. On the other hand, when the patient has stated the request early in the interview and believes it has been supportively heard, he is likely to participate more freely and feel more satisfied at the end.

Sometimes the clinician unwittingly discourages the patient from stating his request. One may observe in this situation a sparring between the clinician and the patient. For example, the patient offers a hint about the request: "I think I may need to be watched over for a time" (alluding to a request for hospitalization). The clinician then changes the subject without acknowledging the request. "Have you had any physical illness recently?" The patient responds with hostility: "I'm just fed up with everything!"

Sometimes the patient, believing there is no opening, waits until the end of the interview before stating the request: "By the way, would you . . . ." The clinician now has new and essential data but not enough time to evaluate or act on them. For example, a patient comes to a clinic allegedly for a problem with his nerves. As he is about to leave the office after the examination, he states the real request: "Doctor, you don't think I need to be watched, do you?" (expressing suicidal concerns). Had the patient made the request earlier and had the clinician perceived the request as legitimate and important, the clinician could have explored the depth of depression and related issues not verbalized throughout the interview.

In many clinical situations, acknowledging the request or giving the patient what he asks for satisfies needs that must be met before a healthier request can be made. For instance, patients who first request control, reality contact, or succorance cannot be expected to progress to requests requiring their active collaboration, such as clarification or psychodynamic insight, until the more basic requests are dealt with. We refer to this process of shifting requests from "sicker" to "healthier" as progressive. Contrariwise, patients whose initial requests are rejected or not acknowledged may sub-

sequently present with a sicker or regressive request. For example, if a request for social intervention is denied, the patient may request control or reality contact.

The elicitation of the patient request has, in many situations, an important impact on the clinician that, in turn, affects the entire course of the interview. For instance, the clinician's feelings may change from anger to compassion as he learns he is not helpless and that there is something to do.

It is not uncommon for overworked clinicians, often dealing with patient populations culturally different from their own, to believe that the patient wants radical changes in character and symptomatology that are hard to fulfill. The clinician also believes that the patient will expect him to effect these changes and then becomes angry at the patient for having such unreasonable demands. Having the patient state his request undercuts this series of projections, since what the patient wants is usually more modest than what the clinician had anticipated. Patients do not want to be different human beings. They want to feel better.

EXPRESSION OF PATIENT REQUESTS

Eliciting Requests

Since the patient's statement of the request during the initial interview is a critical beginning of the negotiated approach, how the clinician elicits the request deserves special attention.

Sometimes the patient will state his request spontaneously at the beginning of the interview. When this does not occur, the patient request is best elicited after the clinician learns the patient's complaint and a meaningful part of the present illness. This preliminary interaction establishes the rapport necessary for the elicitation of the patient request. Eliciting the request at the very start of the interview before the patient has stated his problem increases the chances of placing the patient in the position of adversary rather than collaborator in the diagnostic and therapeutic process. "You asked me what I want. You do not even know what is wrong with me." Eliciting the request at the end of the interview deprives the clinician of the opportunity to negotiate or work with the request.

We have been most successful in eliciting the patient request by asking, "How do you hope (or wish) I (or the clinic) can help?" The questions "What do you want?" or "What do you expect?" should be avoided because they are likely to be perceived as a confrontation. The words "wish" or "hope," in contrast, give the patient permission to state requests he does not necessarily expect will be granted. Even when the clinician finally asks the patient what he hopes for, the response is commonly, "I don't know. You are the therapist," or "I just want to feel better." In this kind of situation, the patient frequently has a specific request in mind that he is reluctant to state for reasons we will describe later. The elicitation of the request then requires persistence, persuasion, and compassion. "You must have had some idea when you decided to come," or "It may be important for me to know what your wishes are even though I may not be able to fulfill them."

The initial statement of the request may be incomplete or stated in such general terms that it requires elaboration to achieve the specificity necessary for clinical use. "You said you want me to help you understand things better. What in particular do you want to understand?" or "You thought you would feel better if I would fix up your family situation. How do you hope I can fix it up?" When the request has finally been stated and elaborated, it is important that the clinician acknowledge that he has heard and understood the request. Otherwise, the patient may wonder whether the clinician heard the request, was offended by it, or did not believe it worthy of a response.

The elicitation of the request undoubtedly depends on more than timing and phraseology. Certainly, the clinician's attitude of interest and receptivity is crucial. We have observed, for instance, that the patient frequently hints at or alludes to the request, apparently waiting for some response from the clinician that will indicate that it is acceptable to continue or to become more specific.

As the interview proceeds, the clinician should listen for elaborations of or changes in the request resulting from the developing relationship between clinician and patient. The patient thinks to himself, "Now that I have more trust in you, let me tell you what I really want," or "Now that you have responded to my initial request, it occurs to me that there is something more important that I need."

Resistance to Expressing Requests

We have observed an extraordinary amount of resistance (not used in the psychoanalytic sense) on the part of the clinicians and patients in the elicitation and expression of patient requests. It is as if there were a conspiracy between both parties in which the patient agrees not to say what he wants and the clinician agrees not to ask.

Clinicians describe several reasons why they neither elicit nor respond to patient requests. Some believe that from hearing the target complaint and the goal, they know the patient's requests, even though it has not been made explicit. In other words, the clinician is likely to assume that a bright, intelligent, insightful person who describes some personality inadequacy or conflict wants psychotherapy. Other clinicians believe either that patients cannot verbalize what they want or that the verbalizations are conscious distortions of unconscious processes. For some, the issue of professional norms is at stake. It is feared that the patient will regard the clinician who elicits the patient's request as not professionally responsible: "You should know; you are the therapist." Another important issue has to do with authority. In these circumstances, the clinician may believe that asking the patient what he wants is tantamount to turning over the authority for treatment to the patient. However, perhaps the most important issues that keep the clinician from finding out how the patient would like him to intervene are those of feared impotence and helplessness. There is the concern in many of us that eliciting the request will open up a Pandora's box of unending, overwhelming, and depleting demands that the clinician would rather avoid.

We have observed three major reasons why patients find it difficult to tell the clinician what they want. The first has to do with the patient's belief that it is his role to state the problem but not his evaluation of how the help should be provided. The patient, nevertheless, reserves the right to take his business elsewhere if he is not satisfied. The second reason has to do with the patient's perception of the clinician as the adversary who has the power to say no. As a result, the patient must hint at his request or present it in an indirect way that may maximize his chances of "winning." The third reason has to do with a wide range of personality variables that are reflected in feelings of aggression, guilt, humiliation, or uncomfortable intimacy when patients ask for something of value.

The Clinician's Perspective

The clinician's perspective in the clinical evaluation is no less complicated than that of the patient. His definition of what is wrong as well as the desired goals, methods, conditions of treatment, and treatment relationship are determined in practice by many factors. Two major conceptual issues involved in the clinician's understanding of human behavior and psychopathology are (1) the use of categorical versus individualistic approaches and (2) the use of one or a combination of conceptual models.

CATEGORICAL VERSUS INDIVIDUALISTIC PERSPECTIVES

Throughout the history of medicine, psychiatry, and psychology, there has been an ongoing debate over whether individualistic or categorical approaches best explain the nature of human suffering.[4] The individualistic approach (also referred to as biographical or historical) has as its main interest the meticulous study of various manifestations of illness and disease in individual patients. Diseases are regarded as states of disequilibrium or deviations from the normal, rather than discrete, independent, or "ontologic" entities. Physicians representing this approach include Hippocrates, Galen, Virchow (in his early years), and Wunderlich. Representative psychiatrists include Benjamin Rush, Sigmund Freud, Adolph Meyer, and Karl Menninger. The categorical approach regards diseases as distinct entities with characteristic natural histories. A disease is generally considered to be qualitatively different from normality and from other diseases. Physicians representing this approach include Paracelsus, Sydenham, deSauvages, and Laennec. Representative psychiatrists include Kahlbaum, Kraeplin, Guze, and Spitzer. The intellectual evolution of this controversy is more than a debate. It is better understood as a dialectic with both sides clashing, interacting, and affecting each other before again going their separate ways.

Contemporary psychodynamic clinicians with their interest in a developmental approach tend to think in an individualistic mode, while contemporary biological clinicians with their interest in target symptoms and syndromes tend to think in a categorical mode. These psychological-individualistic and biological-categorical relationships, however, are not fixed and have not stood the tests of history. Biologists have been and are individualistic, and psychologists have been and are categorical.

The categorical approach has become for some the essential defining characteristics of the medical model.[9,10] This is a mistake. The categorical approach has not been a consistent feature of medicine's concept of disease. Both Hippocratic physicians as well as the 19th century German physiologists were advocates of individualistic approaches to disease.

What is the relevance of these issues for the clinical evaluation of neuroses and personality disorders? Even after acknowledging the considerable contributions of the *Diagnostic and Statistical Manual of Mental Disorders,* 3rd ed (*DSM-III*), including its individualistic multiaxial approach, it is clear that its categories have varying degrees of validity and provide us with limited amounts of information about each patient's suffering. Undue reliance on the *DSM-III,* a common mistake of beginners, results in an oversimplification of the patient's pathology. *We advocate an assessment of each patient by both categorical and individualistic approaches.* Although the clearest statement of categories are found in the *DSM-III,* we must be open to other syndromal diagnoses based on psychodynamic or other theoretical frameworks. We must also consider the possibility that the multicausal nature of some psychopathology leads to such complex pathogeneses that the behavioral manifestations of much of human distress do not form clear and predictable syndromes. The questions we must ask, therefore, in any evaluation include the following:

What known syndromes can we observe?
What other "unofficial" syndromes can be observed using psychodynamic and other theoretic frameworks?
What other nonsyndromal aspects of human suffering can we observe using biomedical, psychodynamic, sociocultural, and behavioral perspectives?

A MULTIDIMENSIONAL APPROACH

Although "human beings are simultaneously biological organisms, psychological selves, behaving animals, and members of social systems," we lack a theory of human behavior that satisfactorily integrates these four dimensions.[11] Attempts by psychoanalysts, behaviorists, or general system theorists to describe a comprehensive theory of human behavior are either too cumbersome or not adequately inclusive. Clinicians, in the absence of such a comprehensive theory, implicitly use one or a combination of models that include the biomedical, psychodynamic, sociocultural, and behavioral. These models may be thought of as different lenses through which one can observe a single object. Each lens has its own value, and each has its own limitations.

The choice of conceptual approach in clinical

practice has serious implications, since it may determine the method by which one collects data, the data that are considered relevant, and the treatment that is most appropriate. For example, a clinician using a psychodynamic approach to examine a depressed patient may elicit a history of unresolved grief or may explore the psychological meaning of the precipitating event in order to understand the issues that have led to the depression. A clinician using a social approach to examine the same patient may determine how the disruption of the social matrix led to the patient's becoming depressed. It is hoped that there will be some way of reestablishing some social equilibrium. Using a biomedical approach, the clinician will inquire into the signs and symptoms of a unipolar or bipolar depression, previous episodes of depression, and family history of depressive illness in the hopes of diagnosing a syndrome for which there is a somatic treatment. Using a behavioral approach, the clinician will elicit the undesired behaviors together with their antecedent and reinforcing conditions in the hopes of positively reinforcing normal behavior or extinguishing depressive behavior.

In clinical practice, the use of one or a combination of the four conceptual models is implicitly determined by many variables. These include the ideology of the therapist, the diagnosis, the responsiveness of the symptoms to somatic treatment, the treatment resources, the social class of the patient, and other personal attributes such as verbal intelligence, psychological mindedness, young adult age, psychological strengths, likeability, and attractiveness.

Clinicians are sometimes unaware of how these variables influence their clinical judgment. When this happens, they run the risk of dealing with diffuse and incomplete data, an approach that may be inappropriately termed *eclectic.*

In the examination of patients in a variety of clinical settings for whom various conceptual frameworks may be relevant, the pitfalls described above can be minimized by simultaneously formulating the problem from biomedical, psychodynamic, sociocultural, and behavioral perspectives. This means that hypotheses from all four theoretic frameworks are considered. In this way, the chances of making the appropriate clinical mix to yield the optimal gain will be enhanced.

THE INTERVIEW AS HYPOTHESIS TESTING

A clinician brings to the interview partial formulations based on his previous experience. A formulation is defined here as a concept that organizes, explains, or makes clinical sense out of large amounts of data and influences the treatment decision.[5] These concepts include clinical syndromes, such as anxiety disorders; personality styles, such as the hysterical personality; social conditions, such as social isolation; and even symptoms such as suicidal behavior. These concepts may be "apples and oranges," but they do represent clusters of information that clinicians find useful in understanding patients. "This is the nature of communication between people—to operate on many levels at once with different words, different objects, and different meanings."[5] These concepts are partial formulations because any one alone is insufficient to provide adequate understanding of any given patient. In the process of bringing these partial formulations to the interview for consideration, they become hypotheses to be tested.

The clinician by thinking in terms of hypotheses keeps himself from being bombarded or overloaded with large amounts of unstructured data. Each new observation can now be considered in terms of its relevance to a limited number of hypotheses under consideration instead of being one of thousands of possible facts.

Two problems immediately arise in applying this approach to the psychiatric evaluation. The first is that in considering a new hypothesis usually generated early in the interview, the clinician may come to premature closure, thereby ignoring more relevant hypotheses. The second is that, given the rich and varied data of clinical psychiatry, there must be thousands of possible hypotheses or ways of organizing data. A solution to both problems would be the development of a manageable list of hypothesized partial formulations based on current psychiatric knowledge that would organize most of the observations that might relate to decision making. The entire range of hypotheses could then be considered, at least briefly, during each interview. The composition of such a list might vary with the clinical setting and would undoubtedly change with advances in the field.

In this chapter we will propose 18 hypotheses that we have found useful in evaluating and treating patients in various outpatient settings. They are organized under four major headings: (1) biomedical, (2) psychodynamic, (3) sociocultural, and (4) behavioral (according to the conceptual approach whose theory and methods generate, confirm, or refute the hypothesis). These hypothesized partial formulations are intended to become neither decision trees nor a complete list of diagnoses. Rather, they are intended to assist in the clinical understanding of individual patients so that decisions can more effectively be made and to provide a basis for important theoretic discussion as to which hypotheses belong in such a list. These partial formulations are intended to supplement not replace official diagnostic categories.

There is some overlap between various partial formulations since they may explain similar observations from different perspectives. For instance, calling a patient "schizoid" or "socially isolated" may be describing some of the same phenomena from different perspectives.

For any given patient, several partial formulations will be necessary to approach a more comprehensive understanding; for example, knowing that a patient is suffering from unresolved grief tells us a great deal. Add to this partial formulation the knowledge of an obsessional personality style, the ego's incapacity to bear painful affective states, relative social isolation, and a behavioral system that punishes grieving behavior. These additional partial formulations provide the clinician with considerably more power to understand and treat the patient.

BIOMEDICAL HYPOTHESES

The five biomedical hypotheses address psychopathology characterized by organic etiology, biological markers, responsiveness to somatic treatment, and functional conditions that simulate physical conditions. Considerations of these hypotheses, therefore, requires specific biomedical expertise.

The patient's problem can be understood in part as resulting from a known medical disorder. Organic mental disorders, according to the *DSM-III,*[12] include the dementias, substance-induced disorders, delirium, amnestic symdrome, organic delusional syndrome, organic hallucinations, organic affective syndrome, organic personality syndrome, and atypical or mixed organic syndrome. Patients with these conditions invariably present with a history or signs characteristic of organic conditions. They may also present with psychiatric symptoms such as anxiety, mania, depression, disturbance in thinking, perceptual disturbance, motor disturbances, disturbance in sleeping, sexual dysfunction, and alterations in personality that may be explained by known medical disorders. These patients may have clear sensorium and normal intellectual functioning.

The patient's problem can be understood in part as being related to a concomitant physical condition. Many patients with psychiatric disorders have concomitant physical conditions that may be important in psychological and biological management. These conditions are often undiagnosed in psychiatric patients. The physical condition is listed in Axis III of the *DSM-III.*

The patient's problem can be understood in part as a physical condition affected by psychological factors. This hypothesis derives from the *DSM-III* category "Psychological Factors Affecting Physical Conditions" for which the diagnostic criteria include the following: psychologically meaningful environmental stimuli are temporally related to the initiation or exacerbation of a physical condition; the physical condition has either demonstrable organic pathology or a known pathophysiologic process; or the condition is not due to a "somatoform" disorder.

The patient's problem can be understood in part as a "somatoform" disorder. The somatoform disorders are characterized by "physical symptoms suggesting physical disorder for which there are no demonstrable organic findings or known physiological mechanisms and for which there is positive evidence, or a strong presumption, that symptoms are linked to psychological factors or conflicts."[12] Somatoform disorders include somatization disorder, conversion disorder, psychogenic pain disorder, hypochondriasis, and atypical somatoform disorder.

The patient's problem can be understood in part as a "functional" symptom or syndrome characterized by genetic transmission, biological markers, and/or responsiveness to somatic treatment. This hypothesis applies to a wide variety of psychiatric syndromes including some affective disorders, schizophrenic disorders, and anxiety disorders.

PSYCHODYNAMIC HYPOTHESES

The four psychodynamic hypotheses deal with the choice of psychodynamic model, the meaning of the precipitating event, the meaning of the developmental crisis, and the nature of personality.

The patient's problem can be understood in part in the context of one of three major psychodynamic models. There are three major psychodynamic models of the mind that the clinician can use to understand a patient's problems. These are the structural model, the object relational model, and the self-psychology model.[13] These models have in common an historical, developmental orientation but focus on different lines of personality development and place a different emphasis on the importance of certain historical events and attitudes. Although each model may be applied to certain historical events, clinicians find a particular model most helpful for particular types of patients.

The structural model, or classic Freudian model, places emphasis on the intrapsychic development of structures, namely, the id, ego, and superego. It postulates two primary instincts, libido and aggression, as the drives that lead to the development of these structures. The expression of these drives ultimately lead to conflict.

The object relational model is primarily focused on the individual's relationships with important people in the environment (both historical and current). Attachment is the primary drive. Difficulties in the early maturational environment are seen as impediments to personal and interpersonal integrations.

The self-psychology model focuses on the earliest experiences in the development of the individual and on the deficits in personality that are the residual of failures in this early development. It is a model frequently used in the assessment of severely impaired patients, especially those with borderline or narcissistic character pathology.

The patient's problem can be understood in part by knowledge of the precipitating event and its dynamic meaning. It is essential to learn the stress or precipitating event (when present) that precedes the onset of symptoms. At least as important is the psychological meaning of this event. Does the event mean to the patient that he is now hopeless, weak, powerless, out-of-control, destructive, bad, a failure, unreal, unloved, alone, or void of self-esteem? Does it mean to him that he is attacked, penetrated, violated, damaged, overwhelmed, smothered, ridiculed, humiliated, insulted, cheated, or abandoned? Is the precipitating event evidence of a recurrent neurotic theme? Knowing the psychological meaning of the event improves rapport because the patient now believes the clinician appreciates what is happening. At least as important, the clinician may know with considerable specificity the psychological work that needs to be done. The meaning of the precipitating event may depend on the choice of psychodynamic model the clinician applies to the patient and the situation.

The patient's problem can be understood in part as a developmental crisis. When it is difficult to understand the patient's presentation as a reaction to a discrete event, the problem may be better understood as part of a developmental crisis. Using this approach, the clinician considers what series of issues the patient at his stage of development is apt to be suffering from. For instance, a 50-year-old woman may well be struggling simultaneously with menopause, children leaving home, strains in the marital relationship, and the death of a parent. With the developmental crisis hypothesis in mind, the clinician can elicit specific historical data that may clarify the clinical problem. Here, too, the meaning of the developmental crisis may depend on the choice of the psychodynamic model the clinician applies to the patient and the situation.

The patient's problem can be understood in part by knowledge of the patient's personality style. Knowledge of the personality style may be important in understanding the patient's psychological vulnerabilities and, therefore, the meaning of the precipitating event or developmental crisis. It may also predict the defensive posture that the patient will employ to keep the clinician from getting to the important psychological issues surrounding the current problem. Armed with this knowledge, the clinician can avoid the patient's diversionary tactics and more effectively get to the issues. Again, personality constructs differ according to which psychodynamic model is applied to the patient.

SOCIOCULTURAL HYPOTHESES

The patient's problems can be understood in part by cultural factors. It is important to consider to what degree cultural factors influence perceptions, beliefs, values, behavioral norms, and expectations that give clues as to the choice, expression, and seriousness of symptomatology. Cultural factors also influence the choice of an attitude toward treatment and even the basic communicative processes between clinician and patient.

The patient's problem can be understood in part in terms of the nature and social impact of stressful life events. The clinician investigates the content, intensity, amount, temporal onset, and duration of stress, noting whether the change is desirable or undesirable, predicted or unpredicted, and whether there is an entrance or exit from the social field. This analysis helps provide a cognitive map of the patient's social field, thereby helping the patient see his reactions as meaningful and somewhat within control.

The patient's problem can be understood in terms of the extent, nature, and accessibility of social support. The clinician should review members of the patient's social support system, including friends, relatives, working relations, and religious affiliations. The assessment should include the nature of the available social support as well as recent changes in membership or access of the social support system.

The patient's problem can be understood in part as a social communication. The symptom or even the clinic visit can be understood as an attempt to influence or to communicate something to some person, social group, or institution. This hypothesis, like the previous one, can be determined by reviewing the persons or groups in the patient's life space. The questions are as follows: Who wants what from whom, and who is doing what to whom? Sometimes the communication can be discerned by watching the patient with a relative in the waiting room or at a family conference. The communication may or may not be conscious.

BEHAVIORAL HYPOTHESES

The patient's problem can be understood in part as disordered thinking, feeling, or acting causally related to antecedent events. The clinician, in considering this hypothesis, studies the varying situations in the patient's daily life that appear to be causally related to the occurrence of the disordered behavior from the time the symptoms first appeared until the patient presents to the clinician.

The patient's problem can be understood as disordered thinking, feeling, or acting resulting from reinforcing consequences of the behavior. The clinician determines, for this hypothesis, the events that maintain or reinforce the disordered behavior. The reinforcing events may be the changes produced in the behaviors of those with whom the patient is interacting. They may also be avoidance of anxiety or discomfort by escaping from adversive conditions.

The patient's problem can be understood as disordered thinking, feeling, or acting in response to sociocultural and biological events. The clinician explores to what degree cultural, social, and biological conditions determine the immediate stimulus condition activating the disordered behavior, the experiences a patient is subject to in the present, and how the individual expects to behave in a given situation in the future.

The patient's problem can be understood in part as a deficit of behavior in the areas of thinking, acting, and feeling. The clinician considers for this hypothesis that the individual never acquired the necessary repertoire for functioning effectively in his environment. The deficits may include areas of cognition, emotional responsiveness, and motor skills. Anxiety is conceptualized here as a secondary reaction to the lack of skills rather than a primary causative factor.

The patient's problem can be understood in part by an analysis of areas of effective functioning. The clinician focuses on effective functioning to reinforce verbally patients who might otherwise feel demoralized and to devise an overall treatment strategy to revise the pathological process.

A PSYCHODYNAMIC MENTAL STATUS EXAMINATION

The mental status examination (MSE), a time-honored part of the clinical evaluation, named and described in 1918 by Adolph Meyer, is an invaluable tool for the diagnosis of various psychiatric syndromes. Binstock and Lazare have suggested that the observations of the MSE have limited value for the testing of psychodynamic hypotheses and need to be supplemented by a new set of observations referred to as the psychodynamic MSE.[6] These are observations that are used in everyday psychodynamic practice (but not recorded as such) to make inferences for concepts such as intrapsychic conflict, ego strength, personality style, defensive strategies, self-concept, ego ideal, and object relations. So that these observations can be incorporated into the traditional MSE, we follow Binstock and Lazare's method of using the usual organizational headings: general appearance, associations, affect and mood, context, and intellectual functions.

General Appearance. The observer notes dress and grooming, posture and movement, entry and exit, blemishes and handicaps, and how the patient develops a relationship with the interviewer to provide data about autonomy, basic trust or mistrust, capacity for a therapeutic alliance, management of aggression, strategies for dealing with shame and guilt, overall functions of superego and ego ideal, management of self-esteem, fear of separation, and tolerance for frustration.

Associations. The observer notes the general development of themes in the interview, the spontaneity of associations, specific associative connections, the relationship of the patient's responses to the clinician's words, and the balance of primary process and secondary process organization. From these observations, inferences can be made about major conflictual themes, relative psychological health, psychological mindedness, disorganization, compliance, defensiveness, fragility of self-esteem, and other dimensions of personality.

Affect and Mood. The observer notes the general range, expression, and appropriateness of affect; the general level of anxiety and capacity to bear it; the general level of depression and capacity to bear it; the ability to express anger; the management of ambivalence; sadomasochism; the capacity for enjoyment; the ability to tolerate affective interchange. These observations have bearing on estimation of ego strength and assessment of personality style.

Content. The observer notes general content and recurrent themes; style of content; omissions, evasions, specific amnesia; slips of speech or hearing; words, phrases, or metaphors with loaded meaning; content highlighted with associated change in affect, posture, stuttering, or rhythm of speech or speech that is inappropriately intimate or of primary process content. These observations are useful in assessing personality, ego functioning, and areas of conflict.

Intellectual Functioning. The observer notes behavior that suggest inferences about cognitive style, defensive strategy, psychological mindedness, concept of self, and conflict-free areas.

SUBJECTIVE RESPONSE OF THE CLINICIAN

An overlooked kind of diagnostic information available to the clinician is his subjective reactions to the patient. The clinician's reactions may be similar to those of other clinicians or idiosyncratic reactions based on his own personal experience. Whether universal or idiosyncratic, the reactions tend to be diagnostically reliable. The same kinds of patients will reliably elicit feelings of warmth; caring; sexual excitement; anger, suspiciousness, or disgust; and desires to help, rescue, or reject.

This kind of data is included in the rich psychoanalytic literature on countertransference and in the writing of Messner under the rubric of "autognosis" by which he means diagnosis by the use of the self.[14]

The Clinical Evaluation as a Negotiation

It is commonly assumed that the clinician's perspective is all that matters. According to this view, the disagreeing by the patient with this perspective or his refusal to participate in the treatment plan is a manifestation of resistance (in psychodynamic terms) or deviant behavior (in social psychologic terms). Based on a large body of literature, an analysis of the patient's perspective presented earlier, and our clinical experience, we believe that conflict is present in the vast majority of clinical encounters. It is particularly evident in the initial evaluation when the clinical interaction between patient and clinician is just beginning. Taking the argument one step further, for the best results conflict should be regarded as normative behavior, inherent in the clinical encounter. Every clinical evaluation, therefore, must note the areas of conflict and the attempts at resolution during the evaluation process.

A classification of conflict follows the classification of the patient's perspective described earlier. There may be conflicts over the definition of the problem, the goals of treatment, the methods of treatment, the conditions of treatment, and the desired relationship.

The diagnosis and expression of conflict in the clinical evaluation is complicated by the expression of and awareness of conflict on the part of the clinician and patient. Conflicts may be explicit versus implicit, displaced versus direct, and conscious versus unconscious.

A conflict is explicit when clinician and patient verbalize divergent viewpoints, and it is implicit when at least one party fails to make explicit a divergent position. Often after the patient or clinician makes his position clear, the other party will not openly disagree and cause a confrontation. Rather he will wait for an opportunity subtly to persuade or reeducate the other. For instance, when a patient says his anxiety has its cause in everyone but himself, the clinician, rather than confront the patient, will take a careful history in the context of an empathic relationship to help the patient own to at least some of the problem.

Conflicts are often displaced from their original target. The most common displacement is from the relationship to the conditions or methods of treatment. For example, when the patient feels unloved, uncared for, or not trusting of the clinician, he is apt to request more medications or more frequent visits.

Some conflicts, such as those over the relationship, may be out of the awareness of the patient and/or clinician. What two people want from each other, particularly when they are based on neurotic aspects of past relationships, is often outside awareness.

Conflicts between individuals and groups may be resolved by a wide variety of methods, including force, chance methods such as flipping a coin, or binding arbitration. In psychiatric practice, the most common and effective method of resolving conflict is negotiation.

This method was clearly described and prescribed by Meyer as recollected by Muncie: "The patient comes with his own view of the trouble; the physician has another view . . . Treatment is a matter of negotiation of viewpoints and attributes."[15] Balint, a British psychoanalyst commenting on medical practice, described the "chronic haggling" in a relationship that was "always and invariably the result of a compromise between the patient's offer and demands and the doctor's response to them."[16] Scheff, a social psychologist, describes the interview as a process of "negotiating reality."[17] Levinson, a social psychologist, describes the psychiatric evaluation as a process of developing a negotiated consensus between patient and clinician.[18]

The point of the negotiation is not to convince the patient that the clinician is correct. The goal of negotiation is mutual influence so that the intellectual scope of both parties is enhanced. The patient's perspective, although not a professional one, is often an uncommon source of wisdom. Furthermore, what we recommend under the guise of professional expertise is often negotiable: individual versus group therapy, a tricyclic antidepressant or a monoamine oxidase inhibitor, twice weekly psychotherapy versus psychoanalysis. Even what we name a disorder is negotiable. A patient might prefer the diagnosis of chronic loneliness to schizoid character disorder. Similarly, in medicine, there is much that is negotiable, such as the route of medication, the timing of a diagnostic procedure, whether to have preoperative medicine, and whether to have a general versus local anesthetic. As Meyer stated, "Treatment consists of the joint effort to bring about that approximation of those views (the patient's view and the physician's view) which will be the most effective and the most satisfying in the situation."[15]

A series of negotiating strategies can be developed based on observations of expert clinicians and an extensive literature in the field of social psychology. They can be organized around developing and sustaining an atmosphere for negotiation, establishing the nature of the conflict, and specific negotiating strategies. Lazare and Eisenthal have described the dynamics of negotiating in psychiatric settings.[3]

Suggestions for the Clinical Record

To the degree that the clinical evaluation described above is found to be useful, it should be incorporated in the clinical record. Here it will not only serve as a source of important information but will capture essentials of the clinical process, thereby serving as an aid for clinical care, teaching, and supervision. We recommend four changes from the traditional record:

PATIENT'S PERSPECTIVE

The section of the record traditionally labeled "Chief Complaint" should be renamed "Patient's Perspective" to include the following data when available and relevant: a brief statement of the patient's description of the problem including the complaint, the attributions, and the fears; the patient's priority of problems if there is more than one; the patient's goal of treatment; the patient's desired method of treatment; the patient's desired conditions of treatment; and the patient's desired treatment relationship. For instance, the patient may state that his major problem is anxiety. The secondary problem is his relationship to his wife. He fears he will "lose my mind" and "lose control." He wants a doctor to "check me out physically" and "prescribe tranquilizers."

MENTAL STATUS EXAMINATION

The section of the record labeled "Mental Status Examination" should include the data described earlier in this chapter. This will encourage the observation and recording of data necessary for psychodynamic inferences.

CASE FORMULATION

Following a *DSM-III* diagnosis, the record should include a section entitled "Case Formulation," which would discuss the process by which the *DSM-III* categorical and individualistic diagnostic dimensions were reached based on biomedical, psychodynamic, sociocultural, and behavioral hypotheses.

NEGOTIATED TREATMENT PLAN

The section labeled "Treatment Plan" should be renamed "Negotiated Treatment Plan." It should describe how the clinician has responded to various aspects of the "Patient Perspective," which conflicts have been negotiated, which conflicts remain, and future plans for conflict resolution. For instance, this section may read, "The patient felt less anxious by the end of the evaluation. He seemed to accept the idea that there was some connection between his rage at his wife and his anxiety attacks. He agreed not to take any medications until after our next visit but insisted on a physical examination.

Plan: **1.** Return in one week for continued negotiation over individual or couples therapy.
2. Continue assessment for panic disorder.
3. Refer for medical consultation and physical examination."

REFERENCES

1. Lazare A, Eisenthal S, Wasserman L: The customer approach to patienthood: Attending to patient requests in a walk-in clinic. Arch Gen Psychiatry 32:553–558, 1975
2. Lazare A, Eisenthal S: A negotiated approach to the clinical encounter: I. Attending to the patient's perspective. In Lazare A (ed): Outpatient Psychiatry: Diagnosis and Treatment, pp 141–156. Baltimore, Williams & Wilkins, 1975
3. Lazare A, Eisenthal S, Frank A: A negotiated approach to the clinical encounter: II. Conflict and negotiation. In Lazare A (ed): Outpatient Psychiatry: Diagnosis and Treatment, pp 157–170. Baltimore, Williams & Wilkins, 1975
4. Lazare A: Psychiatric diagnosis: A perspective from the history and philosophy of medicine (unpublished manuscript)
5. Lazare A: The psychiatric examination in the walk-in clinic: Hypothesis generation and hypothesis testing. Arch Gen Psychiatry 33:96–102, 1976
6. Binstock WA, Lazare A: A psychodynamic mental status examination. In Lazare A (ed): Outpatient Psychiatry: Diagnosis and Treatment. pp 215–229. Baltimore, Williams & Wilkins, 1975
7. Lazare A, Eisenthal S, Wasserman L et al: Patient requests in a walk-in clinic. Compr Psychiatry 16:467, 1975
8. Lazare A, Eisenthal S: Patient requests in a walk-in clinic: Replication of factor analysis in an independent sample. J Nerv Ment Dis 165:330–340, 1977
9. Spitzer RL, Sheehy M, Endicott J: DSM-III: Guiding principles. In Rakoff VM, Stancer HC, Kedward HB (eds): Psychiatric Diagnosis. New York, Brunner/Mazel, 1976
10. Guze SB: The validity and significance of the clinical diagnosis of hysteria (Briquet's syndrome). Am J Psychiatry 132:2, 1975
11. Lazare A: Hidden conceptual models in clinical psychiatry. N Engl J Med 288:345–351, 1973
12. Diagnostic and Statistical Manual of Mental Disorders, 3rd ed. Washington, DC, American Psychiatric Association, 1980
13. Gedo JE, Goldberg A: Models of the Mind: A Psychoanalytic Theory. Chicago, University of Chicago Press, 1973
14. Messner E: Autognosis: Diagnosis by the use of the self. In Lazare A (ed): Outpatient Psychiatry: Diagnosis and Treatment, pp 230–237. Baltimore, Williams & Wilkins, 1975
15. Muncie WS: The psychological approach, In Arieti S (ed): American Handbook of Psychiatry, 2nd ed. New York, Basic Books, 1974
16. Balint M: The Doctor, His Patient, and the Illness. New York, International Universities Press, 1957
17. Scheff TJ: Negotiating reality: Notes on power in the assessment of responsibility. Soc Problems 16:3–17, 1968
18. Levinson DJ, Merrifield J, Berg K: Becoming a patient. Arch Gen Psychiatry 17:385–406, 1967

6

John F. Clarkin and John A. Sweeney

Psychological Assessment

Clinical interviewing is a time-honored assessment technique for arriving at diagnoses and planning treatment interventions. Psychological assessment instruments provide additional information for making such decisions. The use of these instruments reflects an attempt to use the empiric and theoretic potential of the science of psychology in the clinical setting. As an adjunct to the clinical evaluation, testing provides an alternative source of data such as quantitative assessment of symptom severity and change, assessment of cognitive functioning useful for localizing cerebral impairment, and inferences about personality dynamics. By virtue of their relative degrees of standardization and normative data, assessment instruments provide the advantages of *quantified* and easily communicated information, and allow comparison of the patient with others.

Definition and Nature of Psychological Tests

A psychological test is a standardized method of sampling behaviors (defined broadly to include feelings, thoughts, overt behavior, and intellectual functioning) in a reliable and valid way.[1] The immediate goals of testing are to extrapolate from representative samples of behavior in order to predict behaviors other than those being directly sampled by the tests and to measure change over time.

Tests are administered and scored in a standardized manner to ensure reliability and to allow meaningful comparisons and generalizations. There are several forms of reliability. *Test–retest reliability* is the correlation between scores on the same test by the same subject at two different points in time. For most tests, it is desirable to have high test–retest reliability at least over a short period of time. When a longer period of time is under question, trait measures will remain stable while state measures vary because of changes in subjective experience and accumulation of life experience. *Alternate form reliability* measures the correlation between scores obtained by the same person on different forms or versions of the same test. A third form of reliability is *split-half reliability,* which is used to evaluate the internal consistency of a test by correlating an individual's performance on one half of the test with that on the other half.

The ultimate criterion of any assessment instrument is its validity—does it really tap what is is intended to measure? Reliability and validity are interrelated because reliability determines the upper limit for validity indices—only a reliable test can be valid. Validity is determined by the relationship between test scores and external criteria of what the test is designed to measure. For example, a valid test of intelligence might have a positive relationship with school performance as a criterion; a valid test of depression might have a high correlation with a clinician's assessment of depression or with response to treatments. There are three major categories of validity: (1) content, (2) criterion-related, and (3) construct validity.

Content validity refers to whether the test content adequately samples the dimension of interest (*e.g.,* an intelligence test should cover various content areas of intellectual functioning, such as vocabulary knowledge, arithmetic skills, and abstracting abilities). A test of depression can be examined to see if the items adequately sample the manifestations of depression (*e.g.,* cognitive, vegetative, and behavioral).

Criterion-related validity involves the relationship between test scores and outside criteria. *Concurrent validity* is the correlation of a measure with outside criteria in the present and *predictive validity* is the correlation with future behavior. A valid test of depression would correlate with the clinician's assessment of depression (concurrent) and might predict future episodes of depression or treatment response (predictive).

Construct validity refers to the ability of a test to measure a specific theoretic construct, such as intelligence or depression.

The specific instruments to be discussed in this chapter vary considerably in their scientific standards[2] and technical attributes. For detailed, specific information on these and other tests excellent test reviews are available.[3]

Goals of Assessment

The goals of clinical assessment have changed considerably with modification in treatment aims and methods over the past 40 years. During and shortly after World War II, Rapaport and associates[4] developed what became in various modified forms the "standard battery" of tests. All patients were given the same battery of tests (typically, the Wechsler Adult Intelligence Scale, Rorschach Inkblot Test, and Thematic Apperception Test), with various examiners regularly including other tests such as the Bender Gestalt, Human Figure Drawings, and/or a sentence completion test. The rationale was that the same structured cognitive tests and unstructured projective tests would be given to each patient, allowing an assessment of the organization of thinking and of psychodynamic conflicts. A battery of tests provided potential for overlapping confirmatory clues from different sources of information. In this way, the severity of regression and the idiographic features of an individual's personality could be specified. Because of a limited availability of differential therapeutic interventions (with emphasis on psychotherapy as the primary treatment), assessment of ego functions and of person-

ality conflicts that could be addressed in psychotherapy became the appropriate aim of psychological testing. Emphasis was placed on constructing an individualized description of what was unique about patients rather than what characteristics they might share with patients of different diagnostic categories. Research relating test findings to clinical diagnoses has not been convincing with regard to the diagnostic utility of the standard test battery, and there have been few attempts to relate test findings with current diagnostic criteria.

Over the past 2 decades there have been major shifts in diagnostic and treatment practice. These changes include significant concern with the development and use of reliable diagnostic criteria and increasing knowledge about the differential utility of various psychotherapeutic and psychopharmacologic treatments. Also, there has been a dramatic change in the philosophy of inpatient psychiatric treatment, the setting in which the full battery of tests was developed. The typical aim of care has become the stabilizing of severely disturbed patients rather than the use of psychodynamically oriented psychotherapy to significantly alter personality organization. These developments have led to changes in psychological assessment strategies and techniques, including the following:

1. A shift from qualitative description of personality traits to more quantitative assessments of symptom severity
2. A shift away from the use of a standard battery of tests to a more focal approach where tests are selected and administered to evaluate particular dimensions of interest
3. A wider use of objective tests of current state and history, such as self-report instruments and structured interviews, with a concomitant decline in the use of projective tests
4. The development of measures of social adjustment and recent life stress that may begin to broaden the evaluation of these dimensions as assessed on Axes IV and V of the *Diagnostic and Statistical Manual of Mental Disorders* (*DSM-III*)
5. An increased role of neuropsychological evaluation in the assessment practice of clinical psychologists resulting from the growing understanding of brain–behavior relationships
6. The wider use of screening instruments administered to evaluate new admissions, particularly with the aid of microcomputers
7. The emergence of "behavioral assessment" that emphasizes clearly defined patient/environmental interactions by self-report, direct observation, and psychophysiologic measurement.

Indications for Assessment

The most frequent indications for testing in the clinical psychiatric setting are uncertainty about categorization (diagnosis) and the severity of salient dimensions, such as depression, suicide intent, or thought disorder.[5] In contrast to the unstructured interview situation, which generates clinical impressions, test materials yield scores that facilitate comparisons of one patient with others. Such comparison is often helpful in solving otherwise puzzling diagnostic problems. Tests also can be used to focus more clearly and specifically on issues that will be addressed within the context of the general treatment plan (*e.g.*, to provide a particular focus for a brief dynamic therapy, for pharmacotherapy, or for behavioral intervention). Moreover, psychological testing is very useful in allowing the consultant or therapist to compare symptoms or dynamic conflicts before, during, and after treatment to assess progress and the need for further intervention.

Psychological assessment also serves as a valuable aid in "role-inducing" the patient into a therapeutic mode. By taking time for reflection about specific ideas, attitudes, feelings, and behaviors, the patient is encouraged to become a self-observer. This facet of the testing situation is important not only because it prepares a patient for treatment in a goal-directed and self-reflective fashion but also because the examiner is given the opportunity to evaluate ability and willingness of patients to reflect about and evaluate themselves.

In a survey of inpatient units at 101 hospitals maintaining clinical psychology internship training programs,[5] it was found that questions about *DSM-III* Axis I diagnosis were most frequently the primary referral questions (69%), followed by questions of Axis II disorders (15%) and questions concerning treatment planning, including requests about specific recommendations for psychotherapy. In contrast, referral questions for testing in day hospital settings often emphasize the assessment of specific cognitive and vocational assets that will enable an adequately diagnosed patient to function. Behavior therapists working in a phobia clinic may want assessment to measure the severity of fears and to list each environmental situation in which the fears arise. A psychoanalyst in private practice is likely to ask quite different questions of psychological testing, such as impressions about the nature of internal conflicts, defensive patterns, ego strengths necessary for long-term insight-oriented treatment and potential transference paradigms. Questions about neuropsychological functioning, including the nature, degree, and localization of impairment, are often a major focus of concern with children and elderly patients and in neurology clinics.

Categorical and Dimensional Assessment

A central issue in assessment is the tension between categorical (diagnostic) and dimensional approaches to evaluating psychopathology. The categorical approach is exemplified in the work of Kraepelin, who attempted to define distinct syndromes of psychopathology. The dimensional approach is reflected in traditional psychological tests, in which an effort is made to assess and quantify functioning on dimensions of importance such as personality variables, symptom severity (*e.g.*, anxiety or depression), or assets (*e.g.*, intelligence).

Kendell[6] has described the advantages and disadvantages of categorical versus dimensional systems. He points out that while most natural objects are categorized in everyday thinking and language (*e.g.*, cow, star, apple), there are everyday situations that are dimensionalized (*e.g.*, height, intelligence), in part because appropriate measuring instruments are available. Diseases, like real or empirical classes, are polythetic rather than monothetic; that is, they are defined not by a single necessary attribute but by the presence or some or most of a number of attributes, none of which is mandatory for class membership. In addition, the defining characteristics of empirical classes have quantitative variation rather than being only present or absent, which reduces confidence about the decision of membership or nonmembership. Although totally convincing empirical data are not available, Kendell[6] argues that the advantages outweigh disadvantages for a categorical system in the realm of psychotic illness, while in the area of neurotic and personality disorders, arguments for a dimensional system are more convincing.

Theoretic and technical advances in psychiatric diagnosis have significantly changed the practice of clinical assessment. At the theoretic level, clarification of the differences between classic and prototypic models of categorization have added conceptual flexibility to recent attempts to define syndromes. In comparison with classic models, prototypic models of classification do not require the presence of necessary and sufficient signs or symptoms to allow the assignment of a diagnosis. Rather, the prototypic model allows categorization on the basis of a sufficient degree of shared characteristics. For many diagnoses, *DSM-III* is implicitly prototypic in orientation in that it describes diagnostic categories with sets of correlated features rather than criterial ones and recognizes the heterogeneity of patients who reach the same diagnosis by fulfilling different sets of criteria. There are 93 potentially different ways, for example, to meet at least five of the specified eight criteria for borderline personality disorder.

Tests that Yield Classic/Prototypic Classification

In the past psychologists typically used tests to construct a full, integrated description of a patient's personality organization, however, some of the more recently developed assessment instruments have attempted to survey behavioral and phenomenologic symptoms that would allow prototypic or classic categorization in terms of *DSM-III* criteria. Typically these instruments are in the form of structured interviews, where an examiner systematically determines the presence or absence of specific symptomatic features.

The clinical interviewer has the advantage of probing selectively and emphasizing specific areas that seem most important. In contrast, a semi-structured interview ensures the comprehensive coverage of all relevant areas so that a broad range of questions (that could be missed inadvertantly in even a brilliant clinical interview) are asked in a standard way to generate a score or categorization. Because of the different advantages of structured and unstructured interviews, in practice the approaches are usually combined, allowing an evaluator to ask questions in a structured way from rating scales while pursuing other topics that seem relevant in a clinically informed fashion.

The most widely used of these instruments has been the Schedule for Affective Disorders and Schizophrenia (SADS), which was developed by Endicott and Spitzer.[7] The SADS is a semi-structured interview guide that enables the clinician to assess the presence and severity of symptoms and impairment in patient functioning. The content of the interview covers symptoms related to affective and thinking disturbances and is most useful when the differential diagnosis between affective and schizophrenic disorders is crucial. The data obtained from the semi-structured interview enable the clinician to arrive at a Research Diagnostic Criteria (RDC) categorization. Although it is too long and detailed for routine clinical assessment, sections of the SADS can, at times, be administered to evaluate specific symptom areas of clinical importance for a given patient. The use of instruments such as the SADS by trainees can help teach a thoroughness in the evaluation of phenomenology. Structured interviews such as the SADS, Current and Past Psychopathology Scales (CAPPS),[8] and Present State Examination (PSE)[9] review a sufficiently broad range of symptoms to determine the presence or absence of criteria defining most Axis I disorders. Other structured interviews focus on different groups of disorders, such as those used to evaluate patients for the presence of personality disorders (*DSM-III*, Axis II). Examples of such tests are the Diagnostic Interview for Borderlines (DIB)[10] and the Structured Interview for the *DSM-III* Personality Disorders (SIDP).[11]

An alternative approach to reviewing a broad range of possible symptoms in a structured interview is the use of self-report instruments. Self-report instruments systematically ask the patient about the symptoms as he experiences them. Instruments such as the Millon Multiaxial Clinical Inventory (MMCI)[12] and the Personality Disorders Questionnaire (PDQ)[13] use self-report data to generate Axis II diagnoses. These instruments have the advantages of economy and of direct standardized measurement of the patient's perception of his difficulties and assets. At the same time, of course, the validity of the information obtained by self-report rests on the patient's accurate self-perception and willingness to report with candor. This does not mean that self-report is invalid or useless but that it should usually not be used alone, especially with very ill patients who most probably have less accurate self-perception or with individuals having any obvious reason to bias their self-description. In some situations an individual may feel more comfortable completing a test in privacy than when confronted by an inquisitive examiner, in which case self-report data may provide more valid information than those gathered in an interview. The various methods of data collection supplement one another by providing different types of information.

Tests that Yield Dimensional Scores

MULTIDIMENSIONAL ASSESSMENT INSTRUMENTS

The tests described previously are used with the intent of determining the presence or absence of specific symptomatic or personality syndromes. In contrast, the dimensional approach is rarely used with categorization as the primary goal. Issues of symptom severity and the relative importance of different features of a patient's presentation are better addressed with dimensional tests. Some of these tests are multidimensional self-report inventories of symptomatology, which are particularly useful for screening purposes, while others focus on specific dimensions of functioning. One multidimensional test is the SCL-90-R,[14] which evaluates dimensions including depression, anxiety, psychoticism, hostility, and interpersonal sensitivity. This brief self-report instrument is useful in tracking the response of patients to treatment intervention.

By far the most widely used multidimensional self-report instrument is the Minnesota Multiphasic Personality Inventory (MMPI).[15] Although labeled a personality test, the MMPI was constructed to assess what are now considered Axis I syndromes as well as to assess a limited number of dimensions of personality. Despite the original intent, the MMPI now may find its greater usefulness in characterizing dimensions of personality rather than categorizing it.

Devised in the 1940s by McKinley and Hathaway, the MMPI is a self-report inventory with items taken from lists of psychiatric symptoms and complaints compiled from textbooks of psychiatry and previously constructed personality inventories. With a large sample of such items, they used the method of contrasting criterion groups to arrive at final scale construction. This empiric approach consisted of giving the item pool to criterion groups, such as diagnosed hypochondriacs and a group of "normals" and then constructing a scale that would best differentiate these groups. For scale 1, hypochondriasis was defined as a neurotic concern over bodily health, and 50 patients with hypochondriasis uncomplicated with psychosis or other psychiatric features were selected. Their responses to the MMPI items were contrasted to those of "normals," who consisted of 724 friends or relatives seen at the University Hospitals in Minneapolis. Using this method of criterion-keyed scoring, nine clinical scales were constructed: scale 1 (hypochondriasis), scale 2 (depression), scale 3 (hysteria), scale 4 (psychopathy), scale 5 (masculinity–femininity), scale 6 (paranoia), scale 7 (psychasthenia), scale 8 (schizophrenia), and scale 9 (hypomania).

In addition to the clinical scales, validity scales assess the test-taking attitudes of the patient. Meehl and Hathaway focused on the necessity of assessing two test-taking attitudes of defensiveness or minimizing symptoms and problems ("faking good") and of maximizing problems ("faking bad"). Validity scales were constructed to evaluate these dimensions, which are helpful in interpreting the severity of symptomatic complaints on the clinical scales.

The increased availability of small computers at low cost has led many hospitals to purchase systems allowing patients to respond to questions presented on a video display terminal. These systems are interactive, so that after a patient responds to a question, the computer stores the response and presents the next question. Future questions can be presented depending on the nature of prior answers. These systems can store data over time to generate base rates of symptoms in specific hospital settings. Computers can also be used to monitor and sample psychophysiologic data on dimensions related to psychopathology such as the electroencephalogram (EEG), galvanic skin response (GSR), and eye tracking. The patient's responses on the MMPI and other self-report instruments can be scored by the computer, which then generates a profile of scores. Although the results of computer-assisted assessment need to be reviewed by an experienced psychologist familiar with the base rates of different presentations to evaluate the validity and specificity of conclusions, the cost–benefit ratio in terms of professional time required to review a broad range of symptoms is very advantageous.

INTELLIGENCE

Alfred Binet[16] constructed the first widely used instrument to assess intelligence. The test was designed for use with schoolaged children and was found to be useful in predicting the future academic performance of young children. It was used to place children in academic tracts of varying degrees of difficulty. The Stanford-Binet, which is the English translation of Binet's test, has normative American data and is still widely used to assess intelligence of children. Although a large number of tests have been developed to assess intelligence in both children and adults, the most commonly used tests today are those developed by David Wechsler, including the Wechsler Intelligence Scale for Pre-School Children (WPPSI), the Wechsler Intelligence Scale for Children–Revised (WISC-R), and the Wechsler Adult Intelligence Scale–Revised (WAIS-R). The WAIS-R[17] consists of 11 subtests, 6 of which (information, comprehension, arithmetic, similarities, digit span, and vocabulary) are grouped into a verbal scale and five of which (digit symbol, picture completion, block design, picture arrangement and object assembly) are grouped into a performance scale. Raw scores on each of the subtests are transformed into standard scores, which are used to generate verbal, performance, and full-scale intelligence quotients. The test is normed so that the average individual achieves a score of 100, and the standard deviation is equal to 15 points. The norms are constructed for different age ranges, so an individual's IQ reflects the comparison of his score with an age-matched comparison group.

Intelligence is a crucial asset needed for daily functioning as well as for different forms of therapeutic intervention. For these reasons, assessment of intellectual functioning traditionally has been considered an important part of patient assessment. By using a test such as the WAIS-R, which evaluates several types of cognitive activity, performance on different subtests can be compared to determine relative areas of strength and weakness in a patient's current functioning. For example, the presence of specific areas of deficit such as problems of concentration, attention, new learning, and abstract reasoning can be determined. Greater variability on the different subtests usually indicates more severe problems of cognitive organization.

Qualitative aspects of performance on these different intellectual tests also has importance in clarifying diagnostic issues. For example, hypervigilance to detail in performing tests can indicate an overideational obsessional or paranoid disorder. Poor practical and social judgment and an impulsive problem-solving style can indicate psychopathic character features. On a more general level, idiosyncratic approaches to tests, peculiar verbalizations, and episodic inabilities to solve simple tasks raises questions about reality relatedness and psychosis.

The evaluation of intelligence also has important implications for treatment planning. This is particularly true when insight-oriented psychotherapy is being planned. A higher level of abstract thinking is necessary to grasp symbolic meanings and relationships between the past and current behavior. In a review by Luborsky and co-workers,[18] 10 of 13 studies showed a positive correlation (.24 to .46) between intelligence and outcome in psychotherapy.

Intelligence tests currently in use, such as the WAIS-R, were not constructed on the basis of any clear empiric or theoretic model of human cognition. Rather, they comprised reasonably well-correlated subtests that measure what the test constructor believed intelligence to be. At the present time, several research laboratories are attempting to construct intelligence tests based on information processing models of cognition. Relatively discrete components of cognition are assessed, such as exchanges of information between sensory input, working memory, and long-term memory; speed of manipulation and efficiency of different strategies used in rearranging information in working memory; and storage of information in long-term memory.[19] This approach may allow a more careful analysis of the elements of everyday mental competence and, in time, lead to the development and wide clinical use of a new "generation" of intelligence assessment procedures. These procedures may be especially useful in evaluating the specific impairments of cognitive processing that characterize different psychopathologic groups.

NEUROPSYCHOLOGY

There has been great interest in recent years in the application of cognitive and motor performance tests to evaluate patients with known or suspected neurologic disorders. The aim of neuropsychological testing is typically to identify the nature and severity of different forms of cognitive impairment known to be associated with specific neurologic disorders. In practical terms, this involves administering a series of tests with the intent of specifying the areas of deficit manifest in a patient's current cognitive functioning. This information is useful in terms of localizing a focus of *cerebral impairment,* since different areas of the brain are primary substrates for different higher cortical functions. The tests are also used to clarify the nature and severity of *functional impairment* associated with known or suspected neurologic impairment.

Examining patients for the presence of neurologically based cognitive impairment has been for many years an aim of psychologists who administer tests. In the past, these evaluations were often done by administering a test of visual spatial relations and constructional ability (*e.g.*, the Bender Gestalt Test). With growing sophistication in the field of neuropsychology, it became clear that such tests did not evaluate the wide range of cognitive functions that could become compromised following focal cerebral impairment and that only a broad-ranging battery of tests or a thorough neuropsychologically informed mental status examination could appropriately rule out all the deficits of cognitive function that can result from cerebral impairment.

A battery of such tests developed by Halstead[20] and revised by Reitan[21] is commonly referred to today as the Halstead-Reitan battery. A more recently developed battery of tests constructed by Golden is the Luria-Nebraska battery.[22] This latter battery was constructed in an attempt to measure the types of cognitive functioning thought to be mediated by discrete areas of the cortex on the basis of Luria's model of higher cortical functions.[23] Research comparing the Halstead-Reitan and the Luria-Nebraska batteries is active and ongoing; however, the Halstead-Reitan battery remains more widely used,[5] which in part reflects the lack of sufficient validity studies evaluating the more recently developed Luria-Nebraska battery.

These test batteries evaluate a number of cognitive and psychomotor skills, including the dexterity, speed, and strength of motor functioning; the ability to enact sequential hand movements; computational skills, constructional skills; tactile sensitivity; visual and verbal memory; and receptive and expressive speech. Research demonstrating an association between specific cognitive impairments and focal neurologic impairment generally supports the use of these tests in the localization of neurologic impairment clinically.[24]

To a large degree, neuropsychological tests attempt to quantify dimensions that have traditionally been evaluated in a neurologic mental status examination. In contrast to clinical behavioral neurology, the psychometric testing approach has the advantage of quantitative measurement and therefore the degree of functional impairment as well as the behavioral response to pharmacologic, surgical, or rehabilitation treatment can be more readily evaluated and communicated. Although it is certainly wise to obtain multiple sources of information about possible cerebral impairment (*e.g.*, computed tomographic scans and electroencephalograms), neuropsychological testing is particularly useful in settings where access to sophisticated neurologic evaluations is limited or when a functional evaluation is desired rather than knowledge of cerebral localization of a disorder.

THOUGHT DISORDER

A prominent traditional use of psychological tests has been the assessment of the organization and goal directedness of thinking. The degree of thought disorder is widely used as an index of the severity of psychotic regression. The most widely used test to examine patients for thinking disorders is the Rorschach Inkblot Test,[25] which was developed by the Swiss psychiatrist Hermann Rorschach.

In this test, patients are shown a relatively ambiguous stimulus (a colored or achromatic inkblot) and asked to state what the blot looks like. Responses are scored as to the location (the area of the card that elicits a response), the determinants of the response (form, movement, color, and shading), form quality (the degree to which percepts match to the inkblot area responded to), and content. Scoring systems were developed by Rapaport and co-workers,[4] Beck,[26] and Klopfer and Kelley.[27] More recently, Exner[28] has developed a scoring system that attempts to integrate the best aspects of the older systems.

Johnson and Holzman[29] have developed a quantitative scoring system for the assessment of the severity of thought disorder manifest in Rorschach responses. Responses are scored for the presence of different indices of thought disorder such as peculiar word usage, autistic logic, incongruous combinations (*e.g.*, "a bear sitting on a butterfly"), and loss of distance (*e.g.*, "my blood on the card"). Initial validation studies[30] suggest that this quantified approach to the assessment of disorder in the formal organization of thought and perceptual processes may have considerable clinical use. This is true not only in the assessment of more disorganized patients but also for patients in the borderline range of pathology where a therapist suspects that more disorganized thinking may be concealed by a patient's bland, guarded, or histrionic manner.

Another approach to the assessment of thought disorder is exemplified in the work of Chapman,[31] who has developed tests of mild psychotic symptoms or "psychotic proneness." These instruments, which allow an examiner to rate several phenomenologic symptoms on severity continua, include measures of physical anhedonia and perceptual aberration. The Object Sorting Test, developed by Goldstein,[32] presents patients with a group of common objects. The patient is instructed to select an object and then categorize with that object any of the rest that should be grouped with the selected object. The results are useful in evaluating the overinclusiveness or concreteness of a patient's conceptual organization. Jung,[33] in his early studies of dementia praecox, developed the procedure of testing a patient's free association to common words to assess the typicality or looseness of verbal associations.

DEPRESSION AND ANXIETY

Dimensional tests have frequently been employed in evaluating the severity of depression and the response of depressed patients to treatment. The two most widely used self-report depression inventories are those developed by Beck[34] and Zung.[35] In these tests, patients rate themselves regarding the severity of depressive symptoms. These self-report instruments are frequently used in conjunction with the Hamilton Rating Scale for Depression,[36] on which a clinician rates the severity of depressive symptoms following a semi-structured interview with the patient. Although dimensional, these various tests of depression place variable emphasis on the diverse symptoms of depression (cognitive, motoric, affective, vegetative). For example, the Beck test emphasizes cognitive symptoms, while the Hamilton test is more systematic in evaluating neurovegetative signs.

The suicide potential of patients has obvious treatment planning implications. Review of recent literature indicates that suicide threats, suicide planning and/or preparation, suicidal ideation, and recent parasuicidal behavior are direct indicators of current risk.[37] These factors should be assessed in detail in a clinical interview. Self-report instruments, which focus specific and detailed attention on known predictors of suicidality are often clinically useful. Such scales include the Suicide Intent Scale (SIS) and the Index of Potential Suicide, developed by Beck and Zung[38,39] An especially troublesome and difficult clinical situation is assessment of suicide potential with a patient who denies suspected depression and/or suicidal ideation. In such instances, projective tests such as the Rorschach Inkblot Test or Thematic Apperception Test are sometmes used in hope that the patient's responses will indicate such ideation without his conscious intent or awareness.

The assessment of anxiety can be done in the context of the total personality or in isolation as a specific dimension. As one factor in the larger context of personality, anxiety can be assessed with the 16-Personality Factor Inventory (16-PF),[40] the Eysenck Personality Inventory (EPI),[41] and the Taylor Manifest Anxiety Scale (TMAS).[42]

Other instruments assess only anxiety or other forms of fearfulness, and these instruments may be more clinically useful as dimensional measures of the severity of anxiety or when anxiety will most probably become a target for therapeutic intervention. Zung[43] has constructed two instruments to measure anxiety: the Anxiety Status Inventory (ASI), which is a rating of anxiety by a clinician following an interview guide, and the Self-Rating Anxiety Scale (SAS), which is a self-report by the patient of various symptoms of anxiety. Both scales use a full range of anxiety symptoms to assess anxiety, fear, panic, physical symptoms of fear, nightmares, and cognitive effects. These anxiety scales are recommended for the serial measurement of the effects of therapy on anxiety states.

Spielberger[44] has constructed an extensively used measurement of anxiety called the State Trait Anxiety Inventory (STAI). In self-report format the items ask patients to describe how they feel in general (trait) and how they feel at a particular point in time (state). Endler[45] has criticized the STAI for measuring only interpersonal anxiety and, in contrast, has developed a person-by-situation interaction model for anxiety. The Endler S-R Inventory of Anxiousness[46] measures by self-report the interaction between the individuals and interpersonal, physically dangerous, and ambiguous anxiety situations. This instrument has been widely used as a therapy outcome measure[47] and is recommended as an instrument that may be helpful in tailoring the treatment to the individual nature of the patient's anxiety.

PERSONALITY

The dimensional assessment of personality has traditionally been a major focus of psychological testing. Two approaches have characterized work in this area. The first is the nomothetic psychometric approach, which evaluates specific personality dimensions such as introversion or the need for dominance. Tests of this sort typically evaluate many predetermined dimensions. Examples of such tests include Cattell's 16-Personality Factor Inventory, the Maudsley Personality Inventory,[48] the California Psychological Inventory,[49] and the Personality Research Form.[50] These tests have the advantages of normative data to which patient's performance can be compared as well as a relatively high degree of reliability.

Foulds[51] has proposed the distinction that personality differences among people should be viewed as either personality attributes that typically vary among people (*e.g.*, introversion/extraversion) or as psychiatric syndromes of psychopathologic personality types (*e.g.*, psychopathy). Tests such as the 16-Personality Factor Inventory were constructed to assess stable personality traits that are relatively independent and universal among people, such as emotional stability and need for dominance. Tests of this sort emphasize continuities among people, while tests of personality disorder syndromes such as the SIDP and MMCI tend to evaluate personality types defined as syndromes on the basis of their discontinuity from "normal" people. The distinction initially appears to be a fine one, but closer inspection reveals that some implications are quite important. First, tests that assess personality types are not likely to evaluate personality dimensions that are not useful in identifying and differentiating personality disorder syndromes, even if they are important for understanding a patient's basic personality organization. Second, because measures of personality disorder syndromes tend to be more symptom oriented, they may be less appropriate for assessing the ongoing personality traits of patients who do not have a gross Axis II disorder. This point is particularly relevant for the assessment of healthier patients who are to be treated with a more unstructured psychotherapy, since the focus of such treatment is personality organization as a whole rather than only a focused problem area. This point is also relevant when a more or less normal group of patients is to be evaluated, such as in personnel evaluations, where the 16-Personality Factor Inventory is widely used. Third, change measurement is complicated when initial assessment focuses on the presence of a syndrome because information about the degree of change is lost. Fourth, assessment of personality assets may be lost when only the presence or severity of syndromal features is evaluated.

The second approach to the assessment of personality is the ideographic and typically psychodynamic model of projective testing, which uses such tests as the Rorschach Inkblot Test, the Thematic Apperception Test, human figure drawings, and sentence completion tests. The rationale of these tests is that given a relatively standardized but unstructured situation, the unique features of a patient's personality dynamics and structure will emerge in a way that is, for the patient, less obvious and less consciously monitored. In contrast to the psychometric approach, projective testing has a lower reliability of interpretation because the evaluation of test responses is more qualitative and intuitive. The advantage of the approach is that the evaluation is not limited to specific predetermined dimensions, so that the more unique and conflicted areas of personality can emerge and be evaluated.

INTERPERSONAL AND ENVIRONMENTAL ASSESSMENT

Because of increasing awareness that the interaction of the patient with their environment has profound impact on behavior and psychiatric symptomatology, tests of recent stress and social adjustment have gained wide clinical and research acceptance.

Horowitz[52] has pointed out that 76% of applicants for outpatient treatment reported problems that were interpersonal in nature, suggesting that in assessing psychotherapy outcome, social adjustment should be measured to assess change in interpersonal behavior in addition to change in symptoms. Self-report instruments that assess interpersonal behavior include the Interpersonal Checklist,[53] the Interpersonal Behavior Inventory (IBI),[54] the Structural Analysis of Social Behavior Questionnaires,[55] and the KDS-15[56] for marital functioning/dysfunctioning.

Stress is now acknowledged in the standard psychiatric diagnostic system (*DSM-III*) by a rating on Axis IV. In assessing stress and coping, one can measure the stress stimuli, the response to the stress, or the interaction of the person and the stress. Stimulus-oriented measures of stress would include the Recent Life Changes Questionnaire (RLCQ),[57] the Social Readjustment Rating Scale (SRRS),[58] and the Life Experiences Survey (LES).[59] To capture the subjective reaction to the life events, Horowitz and colleagues have developed another life events scale.[60] The Jenkins Activity Survey (JAS)[61] is the prototype of an interaction measure of stress, since it focuses on the cognitive and perceptual characteristics of the individual that mediate responses to stress. This instrument has shown predictive validity in studies of reactions to coronary heart disease. Obviously, measures using an interactional approach are needed for general areas of psychiatry. The Derogatis Stress Profile (DSP),[62] which measures stimuli from job, home, and health, as well as characteristic attitudes and coping mechanisms, may be helpful in this area, but further validation studies are needed with this instrument.

Conclusions

There are a number of reasons why there has been a steady decline in the amount of testing done by psychologists—from 44% of their time in 1959, to 28% in 1969, to 10% in 1976.[63] In a review of clinical testing, Korchin and Schuldberg[64] argued that the main aim of traditional psychodiagnostic testing has been to make characterologic (rather than psychiatric) diagnoses in order to describe the individual in as full and multifaceted manner as possible. As long as the major or sole aim of testing remained to describe the person in full multifaceted detail, psychological testing had a low cost–benefit ratio (cost was high due to expensive professional time, and benefit was low when the yield was broad-based statements about personality dynamics from projective tests). Shifts in emphasis in the clinical practice of psychological assessment have been toward focal assessment of specific problem areas. This "problem oriented" approach uses tests appropriate for a selective evaluation of limited problem areas, which is quite different from the "test oriented" full battery approach that considers problems after a battery of tests has been administered.

Beyond the change to more focused assessments, other developments include a wide use of screening tests (often in a computer-assisted fashion) and greatly increased emphasis on neuropsychology. Psychological testing also is practiced more at the interface of categorical and dimensional approaches to assessment, as psychologists flexibly select tests and focus consultations simultaneously on categorical diagnostic classifications and on careful quantitative measurement of psychological dimensions of interest. In practice, this frequently involves an integration of concerns with careful diagnostic classification and interest in the social and intrapsychic forces affecting an individual's behavior.

Psychological consultations need to be tailored to the individual case in order to assist in making specific treatment planning decisions. This is particularly true in settings where the majority of referral questions request a clarification of psychiatric diagnosis or an evaluation of neuropsychological functioning. With the emergence of more focal pharmacologic and psychosocial treatments, and with advances in neuropsychology and psychiatric diagnostic practice, a flexible selective use of categorical and dimensional assessment approaches depending on patient problems and the treatment setting offers the most promising future for psychological assessment.

REFERENCES

1. Anastasi A: Psychological testing, 5th ed. New York, Macmillan, 1982
2. Standards for Educational and Psychological Tests. Washington, DC, American Psychological Association, 1966
3. Buros OK (ed): The Eighth Mental Measurements Yearbook. Highland Park, NJ, Gryphon Press, 1978
4. Rapaport D, Gill M, Schafer R: Diagnostic Psychological Testing. Chicago, Yearbook Medical Publishers, 1945–1946
5. Sweeney JA, Clarkin JF: Survey of utilization of psychological assessments in psychiatric teaching centers (unpublished manuscript)
6. Kendell RE: The Role of Diagnosis in Psychiatry. London, Blackwell Scientific Publications, 1975
7. Endicott J, Spitzer RL: A diagnostic interview: The Schedule of Affective Disorders and Schizophrenia. Arch Gen Psychiatry 35:837–844, 1978
8. Endicott J, Spitzer RL: Current and Past Psychopathology Scales (CAPPS): Rationale, reliability and validity. Arch Gen Psychiatry 27:678–687, 1972
9. Wing JK, Nixon JM, Mann SA et al: Reliability of the PSE (9th edition) used in a population study. Psychol Med 7:505–516, 1977
10. Gunderson JG, Kolb JE, Austin V: The diagnostic interview for borderline patients. Am J Psychiatry 138:896–903, 1981
11. Pfohl B, Stangl D, Zimmerman M: Structured interview for the DSM-III personality disorders (SIDP). Iowa City, University of Iowa, Department of Psychiatry, 1983
12. Millon T: Millon Multiaxial Clinical Inventory Manual. Minneapolis, National Computer Systems, 1977
13. Hurt, SW, Hyler S, Frances A et al: Methods of assessing borderline personality disorder: Self-report versus clinical interview versus semistructured interview. Am J Psychiatry (in press)
14. Derogatis LR: The SCL-90R. Baltimore, Clinical Psychometric Research
15. Hathaway SR, McKinley JC: Minnesota Multiphasic Personality Inventory Manual (revised). New York, Psychological Corporation, 1967
16. Binet A, Simon T: Méthodes nouvelles pour le diagnostic du niveau intellectuel des anormaux. Annee Psychol 11:191–244, 1905
17. Wechsler D: Wechsler Adult Intelligence Scale (revised). New York, Psychological Corporation, 1981
18. Luborsky L, Chandler M, Auerbach AH et al: Factors influencing the outcome of psychotherapy: A review of quantitative research. Psychol Bull 75:145–185, 1971
19. Hunt E: On the nature of intelligence. Science 219:141–146, 1983
20. Halstead WC: Brain and Intelligence. Chicago, University of Chicago Press, 1947
21. Reitan RM: Investigation of the validity of Halstead's measures of biological intelligence. Arch Neurol Psychiatry 48:474–477, 1955

22. Golden CJ, Hammeke TA, Purisch AD: Diagnostic validity of a standardized neuropsychological battery derived from Luria's neuropsychological tests. J Consult Clin Psychol 46:1258–1265, 1978

23. Luria AR: Higher Cortical Functions of Man. New York, Basic Books, 1966

24. Golden CJ, MacInnes WD, Ariel RN, et al: Cross-validation of the ability of the Luria-Nebraska neuropsychological battery to differentiate chronic schizophrenics with and without ventricular enlargement. J Consult Clin Psychol 50:87–95, 1982

25. Rorschach H: Psychodiagnostics. New York, Grune & Stratton, 1949

26. Beck SJ: Introduction to the Rorschach Method. New York, American Orthopsychiatric Association, 1937

27. Klopfer B, Kelley DM: The Rorschach Technique. Yonkers, NY, World Book, 1942

28. Exner JE Jr: The Rorschach: A Comprehensive System. New York, John Wiley & Sons, 1974, 1978

29. Johnston MH, Holzman PS: Assessing Schizophrenic Thinking. San Francisco, Jossey-Bass, 1979

30. Hurt SW, Holzman PS, Davis JM: Neuroleptic treatment affects schizophrenic thought disorder. Arch Gen Psychiatry 40:1281–1285, 1983

31. Chapman LJ, Edell WS, Chapman JP: Physical anhedonia, perceptual aberration, and psychosis proneness. Schizophr Bull 6:639–653, 1980

32. Goldstein K, Scheerer M: Abstract and concrete behavior: An experimental study with special tests. Psychol Mono 53 (2, whole No. 239): 1–151, 1941

33. Jung CG: The Psychology of Dementia Praecox. Brill AA (trans). New York, Nervous and Mental Disease Publishing, 1936

34. Beck AT, Ward CH, Mendelson M et al: An inventory for measuring depression. Arch Gen Psychiatry 4:561–571, 1961

35. Zung WWK: A self-rating depression scale. Arch Gen Psychiatry 13:508–516, 1965

36. Hamilton M: A rating scale for depression. J Neurol Neurosurg Psychiatry 23:56–61, 1960

37. Linehan MM: A social-behavioral assessment of suicide and parasuicide: Implications for clinical assessment and treatment. In Clarkin JF, Glazer HI (eds): Depression: Behavioral and directive intervention strategies. New York, Garland Press, 1981

38. Beck AT, Schuyler D, Herman I: Development of suicidal intent scales. In Beck AT, Resnik HLP, Lettieri DJ (eds): The Prediction of Suicide. Bowie, MD, Charles Press, 1974

39. Zung WWK: Index of Potential Suicide (IPS): A rating scale for suicide prevention. In Beck AT, Resnik HLP, Lettieri DJ (eds): The Prediction of Suicide. Bowie, MD, Charles Press, 1974

40. Cattell RB, Stice G: The sixteen personality factor questionnaire. Champaign, IL, Institute for Personality and Ability Testing, 1949–1950.

41. Eysenck HJ, Eysenck SB: The Structure and Measurement of Personality. San Diego, CA, RR Knapp, 1969

42. Taylor-Spence JA, Spence KW: The motivational components of manifest anxiety: Drive and drive stimuli. In Spielberger CD (ed): Anxiety and Behavior. New York, Academic Press, 1966

43. Zung WK: A rating instrument for anxiety disorders. Psychosomatics 12:371–379, 1971

44. Spielberger CD, Gorsuch RL, Luchene RE: Manual for the Stait-Trait Anxiety Inventory. Palo Alto, CA, Consulting Psychologists Press, 1976

45. Endler NS: A person-situation interaction model for anxiety. In Spielberger CD, Sarason IG (eds): Stress and Anxiety. New York, Hemisphere, 1975

46. Endler NS, Hunt J McV, Rosenstein AJ: An S-R inventory of anxiousness. Psychol Mono: Gen Applied 76(17, whole no 536):1–31, 1962

47. Lambert MJ: Introduction to assessment of psychotherapy outcome: Historical perspective and current issues. In Lambert MJ, Christensen ER, DeJulio SS (eds): The Assessment of Psychotherapy Outcome. New York, John Wiley & Sons, 1983

48. Eysenck HJ: Manual of the Maudsley Personality Inventory. London, University of London Press, 1959

49. Gough HG: California Psychological Inventory. Palo Alto, CA, Consulting Psychologist Press, 1956–1957

50. Jackson DN: Personality Research Form Manual. Goshen, NY, Research Psychologists Press, 1967

51. Foulds GA: Personality and Personal Illness. Caine TM (collaborator). London, Tavistock Publications, 1965

52. Horowitz LM: On the cognitive structure of interpersonal problems treated in psychotherapy. J Consult Clin Psychol 47:5–15, 1979

53. Leary T: Interpersonal Diagnosis of Personality. New York, Ronald Press, 1957

54. Lorr M, McNair DM: Expansion of the interpersonal behavior circle. J Pers Soc Psychol 2:823–830, 1965

55. Benjamin LS: Structural analysis of social behavior. Psychol Rev 81:392–425, 1974

56. Kupfer DJ, Detre TP: The KDS-15—a Marital Questionnaire. University of Pittsburgh, KDS Systems, 1974

57. Rahe RH: The pathway between subjects' recent life changes and their near future illness reports: Representative results and methodological issues. In Dohrenwend BS, Dohrenwend BP (eds): Stressful Life Events: Their Nature and Effects. New York, John Wiley & Sons, 1974

58. Holmes TH: Development and application of a quantitative measure of life change magnitude. In Barrett JE (ed): Stress and Mental Disorder. New York, Raven Press, 1979

59. Sarason EG, Johnson JH, Siegal JM: Assessing the impact of life changes. In Sarason IG, Spielberger CD (eds): Stress and Anxiety, vol 6. New York, John Wiley & Sons, 1979

60. Horowitz M, Schaefer C, Hiroto D et al: Life event questionnaires for measuring presumptive stress. Psychosom Med 39:413–431, 1977

61. Jenkins CD, Rosenman RH, Friedman M: Development of an objective psychological test for the determination of the coronary-prone behavior pattern in employed men. J Chronic Dis 20:371–379, 1967

62. Derogatis LR: Self-report measures of stress. In Goldberger L, Breznitz S (eds): Handbook of Stress. New York, Free Press, 1982

63. Garfield SL, Kurtz R: Clinical psychologists in the 1970s. Am Psychol 31:1–9, 1976

64. Korchin SJ, Schuldberg D: The future of clinical assessment. Am Psychol 36:1147–1158, 1981

7

Anton O. Kris

Psychoanalysis and Psychoanalytic Psychotherapy

The forms of treatment to be described in this chapter can be considered from several vantage points. Frequently and fruitfully an historical perspective is used to show their derivation from the work of Sigmund Freud, beginning with his collaboration with Josef Breuer on the study of hysteria in the 1880s.[1] A review of Freud's 50 years of productive investigation and treatment,[2,3] moving from hypnosis to psychoanalysis, during which he made epochal discoveries into the nature of normal and pathologic mental life, especially its unconscious components, offers a profound beginning for the study of psychoanalysis and psychoanalytic psychotherapy. Such a review would properly emphasize both his methodologic innovations, most notably the shift from hypnosis to free association, and the body of conceptual formulations he created that remains the basis of psychoanalytic theory. In addition, psychoanalysis both before Freud's death in 1939 and after it has had a host of substantial and creative contributors whose work can also be profitably studied in historical perspective.[4]

A second approach starts with present-day psychoanalytic theory and derives from it the principles and techniques of treatment—or at least it demonstrates their compatibility with the theory.[2,5–8] Freed from the task of reviewing a century of work, it can address the correlation of psychoanalytic understanding of psychiatric disorders with their psychotherapeutic treatment.

A third way to study psychoanalytic treatment begins with a descriptive account of human development, paying special attention to the development of psychopathology.[2,9–12] Psychoanalytic theory can then be seen in relation to the developmental data, and together they can provide a picture of the conditions for which psychotherapeutic treatment techniques may be indicated. Such an approach places a valuable stress on interruptions and disorders of development and the way in which psychoanalysis and psychotherapy promote the resumption of normal development and the correction of deviant development.

All these approaches and perspectives have merit, and all are important for the serious student of psychoanalysis and psychotherapy. They share a problem, however, that arises from many and substantial differences of opinion between groups of psychoanalysts and within any particular group. The line of approach to be followed here takes another course.[13] It begins with an operational statement of the central method of psychoanalysis and the psychoanalytic psychotherapies, the *method of free association,* that deliberately bypasses, at first, all but the experience-near formulations of psychoanalytic theory. In doing so it describes or formulates the basic clinical concepts of psychoanalysis in terms compatible with a number of different theoretical approaches.

After an initial statement and illustration of the method of free association and a consideration of its relationship to psychoanalytic theories of cure, the crucially important topic of the attitude and responsibilities of the doctor as an integral part of the method will be discussed. In the following section some features of the treatment process encountered in the psychoanalytic therapies are noted. In subsequent sections the range of psychoanalytic therapies from the viewpoint of the variables that distinguish between them is presented and the variables that influence choice of one or another psychotherapeutic treatment are indicated. Some problematic aspects of the psychoanalytic psychotherapies are addressed in the final section.

In this chapter attention is confined to the individual treatment of older adolescents and adults. Group therapy, family therapy, or the joint therapy of marital couples, all of which may be psychoanalytically oriented in method and in the conceptual approach of the doctor, are not considered, nor are the many forms of individual psychotherapy included that may use one or another or even several components of the psychoanalytic approach but not its central method.

The Method of Free Association

The central method of psychoanalysis and of the psychoanalytic psychotherapies is free association.[13] It is a joint venture of doctor and patient in which the patient attempts to express in words all thoughts, feelings, wishes, sensations, and memories without conscious reservation, and the doctor tries to assist the patient in the task of doing so. The doctor's attitude and responsibilities (to be described in the next section) are an integral part of the method. Although the patient aims to put all that comes to mind into words, through the *activity of free association*, the field of observation and communication includes *all* expressions and transactions, verbal and non-verbal, between patient and therapist. The complex consequences of the extended use of the method of free association is the *free association process* or *therapeutic process*.

The task of free association invariably encounters opposition owing to interferences whose origins are not within the patient's conscious awareness. Such unconscious interferences, *resistances*, impede *freedom of association*. Free association is only free in regard to the patient's attempt to suspend conscious reservation and to speak as freely as possible. This aim is sufficient, in the context of the therapeutic situation, to alter the ordinary balance of external and internal, conscious and unconscious influences and permits patient and therapist to gain access to the resistances. The immediate goal of the treatment is to help the patient to gain (or regain) greater freedom of association, manifested in an increased ability to think, to feel, to wish, to sense, to imagine, and to remember. Such gains are regularly accompanied by wider beneficial effects.

Because the method of free association is so unlike other conversations between doctors and their patients, further consideration of the relationship between the method, the disorders it is used to treat, and the formulation or theoretic conception of the therapeutic process must be postponed in favor of a brief illustration of the method of free association.

A patient who suffered from chronic depression began the first session of his psychoanalysis by saying that the couch is very comfortable. He has been terrified for several days, he continues, having strange dreams that he cannot remember, evidently to do with his treatment. He says it is too bad that he so often cannot remember his dreams. He feels stiff as a board lying on the couch. He regards his driving to the session as a cop-out, because he strongly favors using public transportation but is afraid of being seen on the way to work coming to or from the analysis, which he wants to keep secret. Another fear occurs to him: the treatment will deprive him of sleep and keep him from seeing his (young) children. He says: "Your job is tough: you have to pay attention all day." The analyst, viewing this "realistic" assessment as a resistance, an unconsciously determined interference with the expression of critical attitudes to the analyst and the analysis, points out that the patient in his new position may not feel sure of the analyst's attention. The patient acknowledges that and continues with his worries about the costs, as the tax benefits come only next year (from which the analyst silently infers a further question about whether and when the benefits of analysis may be expected). He has thought of a few things from childhood. His nickname represented a corruption of his name; he did not even know his real name when asked in first grade. In high school he had lost his football helmet. He grabbed another one, too big for him, and put it on backwards; the referee told him: "son, your helmet's on backwards." He was so nervous. Later a guy said: "go in there and show them you're not the asshole you think you are." This was the equivalent, he feels, of not knowing his own name in first grade; "the equivalent of the first day of analysis," the analyst adds. "Of course," he says, "why didn't I think of that?" "Because this *is* the first day of analysis," the analyst says (underscoring the unreasonable quality of the self-criticism, which began with the comment about not remembering his dreams).

The remainder of the hour continued in this way, with the expression of a variety of *conscious* hopes and fears, paralleled by the expression of *unconscious* hopes and fears, that is, ones of which he was initially unaware. The unconscious fear of being criticized by the analyst, which played a major part in the subsequent analysis and came to be seen both as an attribution to the analyst of the patient's current self-criticism (externalization) and as a re-experience of feeling criticized by his mother in the past (transference), was recognized first by the analyst and then by the patient in his opening session. The analyst also recognized, silently, the adumbration of a most significant theme, unconscious anal interests, in the references to doing something "backwards" and being an "asshole." Secrecy and competition also appeared.

In the small segment of the session presented here, the aim of the analyst's interventions is illustrated: helping the patient express his associations, both fearful and hopeful, hostile and friendly, conscious and unconscious, in order to promote increased freedom of association. After a brief consideration of the rationale of psychoanalytic treatment and the problem of theory, the obligations and functions of the therapist will be described further.

Free Association and Theories of Cure

The central rationale of the psychoanalytic therapies is based on the demonstration of significant limitations of freedom of association that are correlated with discontinuity in various mental functions in the disorders for which these treatments can be used. Functions that may be impaired include thought, affect, memory, sensation, relationship to the patient's own body, sense of self, sense of personal history, self-control, appraisal of reality, relationship to the environment in general, and personal relationships. The psychoanalytic therapies promote continuity in these functions and, in this way, can produce substantial therapeutic effects. The aim of expanding freedom of association is, of course, not simply to improve the patient's capacity to perform his treatment task but to bring about improvement beyond the verbal sphere and outside the confines of the consulting room. In the subsequent psychoanalysis of the patient whose first session was illustrated, for example, the gradual revision of the patient's unconscious self-criticism through increased freedom of association was accompanied by significant improvement in his mood, his capacity to work, and his relationships.

Psychoanalytic theories of cure, stated from a number of different conceptual viewpoints, correlate and attempt to explain the relationship between disorder, method, and therapeutic effect. Characteristically, psychoanalytic formulation of psychopathology, of treatment, and of cure employs a multidimensional conceptual viewpoint that encompasses a host of influences both external and internal, enduring and ephemeral, present and past, conscious and unconscious, biological and experiential.[14] Psychoanalytic theory and the theory of psychoanalytic therapy have been and continue to be the subject of revision and reformulation, extending a vigorous tradition of more than 90 years.[2,5–32]

There are, naturally, many differences among psychoanalytic therapists in regard to theory, and there are many differences, too, in the ways individuals use theory in treatment, systematically or eclectically, explicitly or implicitly, rigorously or intuitively, abstractly or concretely. The explicit statement of theory has, however, rarely expressed sufficiently the significance of differences in the way therapists use a particular theory. To some extent, but not entirely, differences in theory represent conceptual preferences rather than disagreements regarding facts of observation. The form of presentation of this chapter, with its emphasis on method, relatively free of a theory of the mind, permits articulation with a number of psychoanalytic theoretic viewpoints.[13,33] To cite only three of these, the technique of psychoanalytic treatment can be presented with an emphasis on mental conflict,[7] on object relations (the mental representation of relationships),[24,34] or on empathy (the therapist's experience of the patient's experience).[25,28] Taken to an extreme, any one of these represents a one-sided view. Taken as a point of conceptual departure, each may focus on the relationship between psychopathology and desired therapeutic effect in a way that aids the therapist in helping to achieve it.

The Attitude and Responsibilities of the Doctor in the Psychoanalytic Therapies

The psychoanalytic therapies more than any other treatments in the field of medicine involve the person of the doctor. Although rapid technological advances have significantly enhanced the diagnostic capacities of physicians in other specialties, diminishing reliance on their sensory abilities, the psychotherapist remains, as before, dependent on the impressions of the patient's history and the clinical encounter. Progress has depended on the accumulation and dissemination of knowledge of the clinical conditions to be met, greater precision in theoretic formulation, and better understanding of the nature of therapeutic processes. The training of the psychotherapist, correspondingly, must extend into the area of the therapist's personal issues.[35–37] The aim of this training is to make it possible for the therapist to operate with an "analytic stance," a blend of objectivity and involvement that can be characterized by three terms: *neutrality, anonymity, and abstinence.*[2,5,7,8,13,16,22,25,27,29,32]

Neutrality means, above all, the absolute respect for the patient's right to make decisions for himself. As the method of free association leads to the recognition and elucidation of a variety of conflicts—and nothing is more central to the psychoanalytic understanding of human behavior than its appreciation of internal conflicts—the psychoanalytic therapist remains neutral with respect to the conflicting tendencies. Holding fast to the aim of helping the patient gain increasing freedom of association, the therapist does not choose the path to be followed. The therapist assists the patient in clarifying the obstacles that stand in the chosen pathway (resistances to freedom of association) and assists the patient to recognize what is involved at points of divergence in the road (choices and dilemmas). The task of maintaining neutrality while remaining immersed in the mutual experience of the free association process requires extensive training, especially in regard to the recognition of *countertransference* reactions, unconsciously determined distorting reactions of the doctor to the patient.[6–8,22,24,34,35]

Anonymity refers to the therapist's obligation to speak only in the service of the patient's aims for enhanced freedom of association. Accordingly, in general, the psychoanalytic therapist does not intrude on the field with self-revealing commentary, though sometimes there may be a limited call for such revelation in the interest of enhancing the patient's freedom of association. Just as neutrality does not mean disinterest, indifference, or unfriendliness, so anonymity does not mean mindless secrecy. It does mean that even when the patient expresses powerful wishes for the therapist to abandon neutrality in regard to personal reticence—especially in those unconsciously fueled attempts to gratify wishes derived from past relationships that are called *transferences*—the psychoanalytic therapist maintains the analytic stance.

Abstinence is neutrality with respect to the patient's wishes in general. Although the psychoanalytic therapist aims to assist the patient in gratification of wishes in so far as the expansion of freedom of association, especially through resolution of conflict, leads to an increased capacity to gain satisfaction, the therapist does not short-cut this difficult process by providing direct gratification. Special caution is required in regard to the self-punitive wishes of patients, which often subtly invite or stimulate a punitive response from the therapist. The recognition and elucidation of such self-punitive tendencies are frequently a most important part of the psychotherapeutic process and require abstinence as a precondition. Abstinence does not, however, mean that there can be no pleasure in the therapeutic venture. On the contrary, not only is it important that the treatment lead to increased satisfaction, for frustration and dissatisfaction are inevitable concomitants of psychopathology, but also the process of the treatment must be intrinsically satisfying in order for the patient to tolerate its often arduous and painful experience.

The responsibilities of the therapist, beyond diagnostic assessment, recommendation of treatment, and adoption of an analytic stance, begin with *interpretation.* This term is sometimes used narrowly, to refer to translation from the language of unconscious mental life to the ordinary language of consciousness, but more commonly it is used broadly, as in this chapter, to refer to all interventions by the therapist. In the latter sense it refers not only to promoting the acquisition of insight, it refers to all the therapist's attempts, to increase freedom of association, including especially correlation, clarification, and confrontation. The therapist as interpreter, however, is not oracular. No matter how clearly the therapist may see and understand, the communication of the therapist's insights must produce a comparable or related effect on the patient. The authority of the therapist may ensure a hearing for interpretations, but if the interpretations are accepted uncritically, as notes in the lecture room, they cannot lead to the desired increase in freedom of association.

The therapist is also responsible for alerting the patient to problems in the treatment process and problems deriving from the treatment. For example, the therapeutic process may lead the patient so intensely to expect rejection by the therapist that the patient may avoid the treatment sessions or interrupt them altogether. Interpretive intervention may not only expand the patient's awareness of the painful expectation, it may also lead to an understanding of its basis in unconscious conflict. This is one way that increasing freedom of association may be accompanied by insight and by therapeutic effect that extends beyond the confines of the treatment situation. The therapist must also help the patient to recognize the "acting out" of unconscious fantasy, that is, the expression of (inferred) unconscious wishes and thoughts outside the treatment setting when resistances impede freedom of association within the therapy. Acting out may lead to dangerous consequences for patients, ranging from embarrassment to self-destruction, which the therapist, from the vantage point of an external but participant observer, may at times be able to foresee when the patient cannot do so.

The therapist is naturally also responsible for the requisite ancillary conditions for treatment, the provision of a suitably convenient and quiet office, scheduling of appointments, setting fees, and, especially, the assurance of confidentiality. Although these are part of every doctor's practice, they play a special role in the psychotherapies because they represent the potential point of intersection of the patient's interests and the therapist's. For example, the payment of fees or the scheduling of appointments is very frequently the focus of the patient's attention. Complaints, criticisms, objections, and disagreements must be taken both at face value *and* as part of the free association process. This obligation offers a most difficult but also a most fruitful opportunity for interpretive intervention.

Therapeutic Process

In listening to the patient's free associations, the therapist seeks to recognize their *determinants*, the conscious and unconscious, external and internal influences that promote expression and oppose it and that give the associative sequence a particular form. The therapist is guided by his own associations and by a conceptual set based on training, experience, and conceptual proclivities. The developing therapeutic process is the product of two minds. This requires that particular attention be paid to the therapist's interventions (including silence) as determinants of the patient's associations and, hence, of the evolving process. The initial agreement for a joint venture tends to develop as part of the process into an increasingly reliable and effective *therapeutic alliance*. Tolerance for ambiguity and uncertainty, sometimes for extended periods of time, is required for both participants, in order to permit unconscious determinants to become increasingly influential and recognizable. Some important components of the process are briefly presented here in, necessarily, overlapping categories.

Recognition of Unconscious Determinants and the Experience of Being Understood

For example, a very recently married 20-year-old man developed headaches and became afraid that he would injure his hand in a machine he used at work. Links and parallels to frustration, anger, and fears in his newly initiated sexual relationship with his wife appeared in the associations. That is, for example, in describing his job he used terms more appropriate to his marriage. Interpretation of the connections and patterns resulted in his recognizing that he was afraid of his wife's demands and that he felt under pressure from her. The therapist silently inferred, in addition, revival of unconscious fears of injury to him and by him in the sexual act. One week later the patient reported thinking of the therapist on each occasion at work when he became afraid of injury and thereby felt reassured. He felt less pressure at home. He was greatly relieved as he felt understood, and to some extent, understood himself better. His headaches ceased in the course of four therapy sessions over as many weeks.

Expansion of Condensation and the Development of Meaning

Among the most important functions of free association is its expansion of the hidden meanings of symptoms. The recognition of unconscious meanings expressed in symptoms, which can be discovered and made conscious through the interpretation (elucidation of the determinants) of the patient's free associations, was one of Sigmund Freud's enduring contributions. By gradually demonstrating the multiple superimposed (condensed) meanings and conflicting tendencies that determine a symptom or a characterologic disorder, use of the free association method leads the patient to gain new self-understanding. In the psychoanalysis of the patient whose first session was briefly reported earlier, his criticisms of his own intelligence proved to have several meanings. They referred to his present assessment of his competence and performance at work (a view not shared by others), to lapses of memory, and to his childhood sense of physical awkwardness and incompetence, especially in comparison to his older brother, a star athlete. They referred also to his sexual "retardation," to his unconscious anal interests, and to the lifelong reluctance to take risks and to venture forth that derived from a very early traumatic separation from his mother. Further, the criticisms were not only his own but his mother's criticisms. All these meanings gradually emerged as determinants of the associations and became, thereby, susceptible to interpretive elucidation.

Recognition of Inner Conflict and the Reacquisition of Lost Experience

Patients gain the understanding in the therapeutic process that inner conflict (often entirely unconscious) is a powerful kind of determinant of the associations. The central therapeutic paradigm of psychoanalytic theory, the lifting of repression and the acquisition of insight, is a formulation of the repeated experience of regaining access to thoughts, wishes, feelings, bodily sensations, and memories that were blocked from awareness and conscious expression by an (unconscious) inner resistance. From the perspective of inner conflict, psychoanalytic theory formulates the role of repression and related defense mechanisms as unconscious mental processes that serve to keep other mental processes from influencing action and from reaching consciousness, in order to preserve inner peace.[2,8,16–22,30] The recognition of unconscious anxieties, inner prohibitions, and restrictions, especially in loving, plays a prominent part in the therapeutic process.

Delineation and Tolerance of Affects

For many patients avoidance of particular affects, unfamiliarity with affects, or intolerance of any strong or conflicted affective experience represent significant and distressing symptoms that the free association method, with its links to unconscious determinants, can ameliorate. For example, patients who cannot bear to feel angry may come to recognize the cost to themselves in avoidance and may gradually develop new capacities to understand their fears of being angry and the matters that would make them angry if they dared to be. The expectation of painful affects is a most important influence on behavior and very often plays a major role in psychopathology and in its psychotherapeutic treatment.

Completion of Interrupted Mourning

The pathologic effects of incomplete mourning, sometimes entirely unsuspected, are particularly susceptible to reversal as free association revives that painful process. Again, here, the ubiquitous influence of unconscious conflict (*e.g.*, a conflict between the wish to maintain the illusion of permanence and the need for realistic acknowledgment) emerges as a source of resistance to freedom of association. Conflicts between affection and hostility for someone of personal importance who has died are a regular feature of interrupted mourning. They can be resolved in the therapeutic process that leads to completion of mourning.

Transference

The universal phenomenon of transference,[2,7,13,16,22,25,29,31,32,34,35] the unconscious superimposition of the *experience* of a past relationship on a present one, regularly appears in the patient's attitude to the doctor. This phenomenon, whose discovery was one of Sigmund Freud's most important contributions, may serve both as an obstacle to treatment, that is, a resistance to freedom of association, or, when it is suitably interpreted, as a uniquely valuable source of expanding freedom of association, insight, and self-understanding. Transference offers an avenue to determinants of current pathology that have their origins in the patient's distant past. Understanding of transference in the therapeutic process often contributes to regaining lost memory and regularly restores continuity to the sense of personal history. Although other sources of information, such as conscious recollection and reports from other persons, may provide valuable and irreplaceable contributions to the reconstruction of a view of the past and to the restoration of a sense of continuity, the interpretation and understanding of transference is unique in reviving the patient's past *experience*.

The self-critical patient, whose first analytic session was described earlier, became gradually acquainted with the pervasiveness of his self-criticism and to a lesser extent with his inhibited criticisms of others. A dream after 6 months of treatment brought to light unconscious memory of past experiences expressed as a transference, that is, revived in the relationship with his analyst. In the dream he is harassed by a boy from his childhood camp, and he tells the boy "it isn't nice" to be doing that. At first his thoughts lead him to the recognition that in the dream he is telling himself to stop being so self-critical (where he is represented as both figures in the dream). Further associations show, however, that the statement, "it isn't nice," is a sarcastic imitation of a parental voice, the analyst's. The analyst's attempts to demonstrate self-criticism, which have been helpful, are now experienced as being like his mother's always admonishing him to be good in his childhood. This unconsciously based feeling about his analyst is a transference that the patient can readily distinguish from his conscious appraisal.

About 6 months afterwards, the patient was recalling at age 13 being sexually seduced by his father's business partner, the year after his father's death. He had been unable, for reasons that only became clear in the analysis, to tell anyone, and he had focused on his own guilt rather than on his anger at the older man. In a dream he now identifies his analyst with Hitler and complains that a year of treatment has brought him little benefit. His analyst links this harsh criticism with the mistreatment at 13. The patient returns from a weekend interval in a state of euphoria, feeling "all my emotions were sharper, closer to the skin." During the weekend he had awakened from a frightening dream in which he was driving an ice pick into an inflated plastic toy covered with pictures and symbols of another detested political figure. He thinks it had a plastic tube behind its ear, a hearing aid. The analyst as "hearing aid" is the object of the old resentment, revived as a transference. The sense of well-being is correlated with the transference and its interpretation, with the beginning resolution of that portion of his inner conflict over hostility, and with the harmless release of anger in the dream.

Learning and Identification

The therapeutic process provides the opportunity not only for the patient's expansion of freedom of association but also for the development of the means to consolidate such gains. These include new approaches to resolution of conflicts, to mastery of unruly impulses, and to integration of capacities. In all these, the therapist may serve as a model or guide for new learning and for identification.

Some Additional Functions

Many more components of the therapeutic process can be described. The important task and opportunity of putting thought and feeling into words, in some instances for the very first time, holds a special position among them. Clarification of confusion and reversal of disorientation are often significant. Abreaction or catharsis, getting something out or off one's chest, the starting point of psychoanalytic therapy over 100 years ago,[1] often plays a beneficial part.

Termination

Just as the initiation of psychoanalytic therapy is undertaken as a joint venture, so the decision to terminate the treatment is in general made mutu-

ally. The termination phase because of its significant parallels to other experiences of separation and to past developmental achievements is an especially important part of the therapeutic process.[2,6,7,34,38,39]

The Spectrum of Psychoanalytic Therapies

The range of psychotherapies whose central method is free association can be encompassed through the enumeration of a small number of variables. With these it is possible to distinguish several qualitatively different psychoanalytic therapies.

VARIABLE FEATURES

Explicitness of the Agreement for Free Association

In establishing the working relationship, which may develop out of an initial consultative or diagnostic evaluation or may follow from a treatment whose principal method is, for example, the use of medication, the *statement* of mutual obligation in the method of free association may be more or may be less explicit. No matter how the initial "contract" is formulated, the therapist, by adopting an analytic stance, permits the patient gradually to rely increasingly on free association, that is, on the suspension of conscious direction or reservation in the sequential expression of what comes to mind.

Length, Frequency, and Regularity of Sessions and Duration of Treatment

For the most part the psychoanalytic therapies are conducted with sessions of 30 to 50 minutes. Useful therapeutic effects may be obtained in some instances with a few irregularly scheduled sessions. The most common treatment consists of once-weekly sessions of 50 minutes on a regularly scheduled basis. Psychoanalysis consists of four or five such sessions each week, without limit of time for the treatment as a whole, which tends to last several years. Short-term treatments consist of a more or less precisely defined number of sessions in a specified time frame.[39–42]

The variations in these four components serve not only the goals of treatment but also the available resources. Time of both participants, money, motivation, and a number of capacities and personality variables can be taken into account. (Relatively few psychiatrists are trained to conduct the most ''intensive'' psychotherapies and psychoanalysis, so that the therapist's training may also be a determinant in some cases, requiring referral to the specialist.) These influences on choice of therapy are considered further in the next section.

Viewed from the perspective of the method of free association, these four temporal variables can be seen to exert a significant effect as determinants of the free associations. The form and content of what the patient expresses and the patient's susceptibility to the doctor's interpretive influence will be significantly affected by them. It must not be supposed, however, that more is simply better. For example, where distrust of close involvement and great anxieties regarding intimacy pervade a patient's attitudes, occasional sessions scheduled at the patient's request may produce a therapeutic process where once-weekly therapy would invoke conflicts. On the other hand, commitment to a schedule and relatively greater frequency is required for systematic analysis of transference. Where the goals of treatment require comprehensive mobilization of the unconscious memories of past relationships as determinants of the associations, frequent full-length sessions over extended periods are required.

The Vis-à-vis Position and the Use of the Couch

The psychoanalytic psychotherapies share with other treatments a need for quiet conditions that tend to produce relaxation. Most psychoanalytic therapy is conducted with patient and doctor facing each other, comfortably seated. Psychoanalysis, from its beginnings, aimed at still greater relaxation (and substitution of words for movements in communication) by use of the couch. An additional and different effect was achieved by use of the analyst's position directly behind the patient's head, out of view. Not only does this position emphasize the role of words—especially the analyst's words, since the analyst is not seen by the patient—it limits the usually important mutual communication through facial expression, posture, and movement.

In both situations, though more so in the psychoanalytic one, the relative isolation from external stimuli promotes the influence of unconscious determinants and turns the patient's attention to inner experience. The choice of one or the other position, accordingly, is bound to affect the therapeutic process. Again, as noted earlier, more is not

necessarily better and sometimes may be worse. The relative loss of contact resulting from use of the couch may be too great for some patients to tolerate.

Speech and Silence on the Part of the Therapist

All forms of psychotherapy require silence on the therapist's part if the patient is to use free association and speech if the therapist is to have any worthwhile influence. What the therapist chooses to say and when to say it are guided by the analytic stance and the analyst's conceptual proclivities, by the patient's associations, by the patient's capacities and personality, by the goals of therapy, by the current phase of the therapeutic process, and by the external conditions of the treatment, just enumerated.

A number of alternatives regularly confront the therapist. Recognizing that every intervention on the therapist's part is a stimulus to free association in one direction and an interruption of free association in others, the therapist must also consider when the next therapy session will occur and what the effects of the interval may be on continuity of association. In psychoanalysis, where daily sessions follow one another at short intervals, the patient's activity of free association can be allowed to lead the way with far less need for interpretive closure than when sessions occur 1 week apart. The rhythm of treatment, which even in psychoanalysis is often dominated by the weekend break, is powerfully determined by the length of the intervals between sessions. Similarly, where psychotherapy of limited duration is concerned, the termination casts a far longer shadow from the first than in open-ended therapies, and the therapist's interventions must correspond.[39]

The style and content of the therapist's interventions, accordingly, are coordinated with the relative explicitness in the statement of the agreement for free association, with the temporal variables of the therapy, and with the choice of chair or couch in producing a particular form of treatment.

QUALITATIVE DIFFERENCES

Within the framework of the analytic stance and the free association method a number of qualitatively distinct psychoanalytic therapies can be described according to the variables delineated previously. The qualitative differences cannot be attributed to one or another element alone. They derive from the *interaction* among the variables outlined and the patient's characteristics. To a considerable extent these different therapies can be used sequentially. The treatment may move without interruption from lesser frequency to greater, for example, as a frightened, suspicious patient becomes more trusting and more tolerant of affect. In the opposite direction, the psychotherapy of an acutely disturbed patient may begin with daily sessions until sufficient development in the relationship between doctor and patient can provide continuity for sessions more widely spaced. Also, psychotherapy sessions once or twice weekly may be effectively used after psychoanalysis, if a further period of treatment is required after an interval.

Such shifts in therapeutic modality are, as are all transactions in psychoanalytic therapy, subject to associative inquiry. The psychoanalytic therapist does not alter the treatment modality in a unilateral fashion. Changes must be made in keeping with the mutuality of the free association method. The meaning of the modality chosen, that is, how the patient perceives the treatment selected is inevitably a determinant of the therapeutic process.

The particular features of each modality also play a role independent of their meaning that produces substantial qualitative differences in the therapeutic process. No one would expect a treatment with sessions once a week vis-à-vis to have the same impact as one that uses the couch four or five sessions weekly. Some qualitative differences between the psychotherapies are presented here. Although none of these differences can be fully considered in isolation from the problems, personality, goals, and capacities of the patient, they represent the kinds of psychoanalytic psychotherapies available.

Consultation and Extended Consultation

The psychoanalytic consultation, whether it be on referral from a primary physician or at the patient's independent request, is often, perhaps usually, a therapeutic encounter. Although the doctor must to some extent shape the initial inquiry with questions more than in an ongoing treatment, consultation sessions require no departure from the analytic stance and make significant, usually central use of the method of free association. Very often an initial consultation session may yield the patient sufficient new understanding and reorientation to provide therapeutic effects. Frequently a consultation becomes, without design, a brief therapy of several sessions in which significant therapeutic results may be achieved. For example, difficulty in taking a developmental step, such as leaving home in late

adolescence, or pathologic grief reactions may be entirely resolved in such psychotherapy. Such treatments may have a most dramatic character. On the other hand, the patient may develop a pattern of occasionally consulting the doctor over a period of years, with good effect. In other cases extended consultation may be the prelude to regularly scheduled therapy.

Short-term Therapy With Limited Number of Sessions or Time Period

Over the past 25 years a new form of psychotherapy has been developed, partly in response to the influence of third-party payers, in which either a specified number of sessions (10 to 20) or a more or less specified time period (measured in months rather than years) limits the treatment.[39–42] Some forms of such short-term treatment employ the method of free association and the analytic stance with powerful results. The pressure of impending termination combined with the doctor's attempt to clarify and formulate important dynamic foci for interpretation gives this kind of treatment a particularly intense character. In contrast to long-term treatments that are not limited in advance, especially those with frequent sessions, this form of treatment generally depends more on multiple formulations by the doctor than on the extended activity of free association by the patient.

Among those who work extensively with this form of psychotherapy the estimates of its applicability range downward from 25% of the average clinic population. The requirement for the doctor to make an early decision for applicability on the basis of relatively little information is an integral problem of such treatment.

Once-weekly Psychotherapy

Scheduled once-weekly psychoanalytic psychotherapy, without advance specification of the length of the treatment, provides a spectrum of effects between "support," due to continuing presence of the therapist's assistance, and significant internal change that yields a greater autonomy for the patient. The distinction between these two is far from absolute. All psychoanalytic psychotherapy provides support for the patient through understanding (not by reassurance, advice, and encouragement that are characteristic of other kinds of therapy). In some instances, however, external support is all that the patient is inclined to obtain or all the patient can achieve, at least at the particular time. In other instances, interrupted mourning is completed and development that has stopped or has been sidetracked is resumed in the therapeutic process. Insight, some understanding of transference experience, and resolution of conflict can be achieved. The experience for the patient may be intense and revelatory.

Once a week treatment may last no longer than a few weeks, or it may literally need to last for the patient's lifetime. In the latter case it may spell the difference between hope and despair, between life and death.

Twice and Three Times Weekly Psychotherapy

For the most part, more frequently scheduled psychotherapies aim for internal change and development of the patient's autonomy. They are used far less for support alone. Accordingly, they take for granted a certain motivation for change on the patient's part that significantly influences the doctor's interventions. In contrast to once-weekly psychotherapy, where sessions are followed by an interval of 1 week, sessions may be held on consecutive or on alternate days. The activity of free association, accordingly, plays a far greater part than in less frequent therapy, and the doctor's interventions can be directed at smaller units of the free associations, with formulations initially less global, less comprehensive. The use of the couch, with its influence on free association, is sometimes effective. The resulting free association process gains, as a consequence, a quality of great detail. Such a process offers the potential for therapeutic effects that often cannot be achieved in less frequently scheduled treatment where continuity and momentum sufficient to promote the requisite freedom of association may be lacking.

Psychoanalysis

The conditions of the patient's explicit commitment to the free association method and the use of the couch four or five times weekly for a period of years produce still greater potential for the psychoanalyst to promote the free association process in a qualitatively unique manner.[2,5,7,10,13,20,22,25,29,32,43] Absence of immediate therapeutic goals, a tolerance of uncertainty, and an emphasis on insight and on conflict resolution in producing character change are fundamental characteristics of psychoanalysis. Systematic analysis (*i.e.,* expansion in free association) of transference and of dreams to formulate reconstructions of important developmental experiences in infancy, childhood, and adolescence are essential technical ingredients. The inference of enduring unconscious fantasies as determinants of behavior and their gradual delineation and translation into consciousness through the

''lifting of repression'' can be accomplished on a far greater scale than in any other therapy. The corresponding analysis of the stable elements of character subsumed under the theoretic concepts of ego and superego can be far more complete. More so than in any other form of psychoanalytic therapy, psychoanalysis promotes the development of a capacity for self-analysis that becomes a permanent although variable characteristic of its patients.

The Choice of Psychoanalytic Therapy

The choice of psychoanalytic therapy requires not only assessment, formulation of goals, and recommendation on the part of the physician but a decision on the part of the patient that goes far beyond ''informed consent.'' In the psychoanalytic therapies, as in all rehabilitative treatment, the patient is an active participant. Accordingly, the patient's motivation, personality, capacities, goals, and social circumstances play a major role in the mutual decision of whether to use a psychoanalytic psychotherapy, when to do so, and which one to choose. Some determinants of this choice are briefly presented here. The actual process of choice is, inevitably, a part of the therapeutic process.

In the assessment, the doctor organizes the data of observation according to a multidimensional psychoanalytic framework, as indicated earlier, which correlates psychopathology, method of treatment, and theory of therapeutic effect or cure. Assessment in this sense also continues throughout the treatment, asking whether a therapeutically beneficial process can be expected to develop and how it may best be promoted by choice of one or another form of psychoanalytic therapy and by the best use of the one chosen. Naturally, in such a multivariate endeavor, there cannot be a single absolute answer to the question of whether, when, and which.

Diagnostic Considerations

Present day psychiatry identifies and distinguishes between diagnostic entities according to discontinuities that for the most part are very different from those of relevance to the psychoanalytic psychotherapies. It should not be surprising nor alarming to find only a modicum of overlap between the two approaches to assessment. The psychoanalytic therapies provide significant benefit to patients in a wide range of diagnostic groups, but within diagnostic groups there are substantial differences in the indications for using psychotherapy or for one or another form.

Although the psychoanalytic therapies may be used both for crisis and for chronic conditions, the more frequent psychotherapies and psychoanalysis are indicated for the latter, while extended consultation, once-weekly therapy, and short-term therapy are more likely to be used where the disorder is new or not yet entrenched.

It is somewhat easier to name a few contraindications than to classify the positive indications. The psychoanalytic therapies are not suitable for those with severe disorders of cognition, whether acute or chronic. They depend to some extent on a commitment to truthfulness, and, therefore, intractable dishonesty may preclude treatment in psychotherapy. Some problems of self-control (including suicidal risks), psychotic disorganization, and major affective disorders may not be treatable in psychotherapy or may require hospital confinement, medication, or both as preconditions.

Motivation and Capacities

The psychoanalytic therapies require of the patient, just as they do of the doctor, a willingness for personal involvement. The patient's motivation is a prime influence on outcome, and intermediate outcome is a powerful influence on further motivation. The patient's willingness to participate generally increases with the success of therapy, with the sense of being understood, and with the development of self-understanding. It is strained by inevitable tension induced in the treatment, and it must be sufficient to tolerate the strain. A number of capacities and attributes of personality assist in maintaining motivation and in promoting the therapeutic process and must also be included in the assessment. A few of these are presented here for illustration.

The patient's ability to recognize and to trust the therapist as a separate individual with whom to form a partnership, the *therapeutic alliance*,[8,22,34,43] although always compromised to some extent by psychopathology, is an important element in choice of therapy. A related consideration concerns the patient's realistic involvement in a life outside the therapy: substitution of a therapeutic relationship for all others is a danger for some patients. Tolerance of frustration, uncertainty, ambiguity, painful affect, and manifestations of unconscious motivation is significant in determining therapeutic progress, and verbal ability and the capacity for abstraction, although not limiting over a wide range, exert a substantial influence.

Developmental considerations also belong to this group of influences on choice of therapy. For instance, short-term therapy may be most effective where youth and wide potential can be expected to play a decisive role. However, more frequent therapy may be necessary to produce the desired effect on character for the depressed, single woman in her mid 30s who still hopes for marriage and a child if she can resolve soon enough the conflicts that arise in her love relationships.

Goals

Patients seek psychoanalytic therapy for a variety of conscious reasons: when they experience particular symptoms or painful affects from which they cannot free themselves, when they fail to achieve their ambitions (almost invariably including a component in the sphere of love), and when they are baffled or confused. Sometimes they have a clearly stated goal or chief complaint, sometimes only a vague sense of what disturbs them or what sort of help they hope to obtain. They may view their goals with apparently single-minded purpose, or they may be conflicted in regard to the treatment and what they want from it. Patients regularly need assistance in expressing and formulating their views about themselves and their disorders, since the same conflicts that contribute to the symptoms for which they seek relief may also produce interference with asking for help. The conscious statement of goals is always important but rarely complete.

The choice of psychoanalytic therapy, both whether and which, is influenced by the patient's goals of treatment. Unless they include some interest in gaining insight, the motivation for psychoanalytic therapy may be insufficient. Where relief of symptoms is narrowly defined by the patient, with no aim of understanding the relationship of the disorder to other aspects of personal experience and development, other forms of treatment may be more suitable. To undertake psychoanalysis, the patient's goals must include a very wide interest in new self-understanding.

The scope and depth of change that the patient wishes to achieve with the assistance of the doctor, however, is inevitably subject to reassessment in the course of psychoanalytic psychotherapy. New possibilities emerge during successful treatment, and unrealistic ambitions may be set aside.[44]

Time, Money, and Social Circumstances

Psychotherapy requires relatively large amounts of the doctor's time in contrast to treatments for other disorders. Accordingly, expense is a significant determinant in the choice of psychotherapy, except in the case of the very wealthy. Psychotherapy also requires large amounts of the patient's time, and this too is a significant determinant of choice of therapy. Where, for example, a patient's occupation requires irregular schedules or unpredictable travel, a regularly scheduled psychotherapy may be precluded. Similarly, a variety of social circumstances must be taken into account in considering whether a psychotherapeutic treatment can be undertaken. For instance, opposition of a marital partner may need to be addressed before therapy is started.

Combined Treatment

The selection of psychoanalytic therapy does not imply exclusive use of this modality. Several kinds of combination are regularly used.

COMBINATION WITH A SECOND PSYCHOTHERAPY.
Patients may combine an individual psychoanalytic psychotherapy with group therapy. This may be especially indicated for those whose disorder causes extreme difficulties in sustaining personal relationships. A different kind of combination increasingly in use is individual therapy and conjoint therapy of the marital couple or of the family as a whole.

COMBINATION WITH HOSPITAL TREATMENT.
For the acutely psychotic patient, the suicidal patient, or the patient out of control, inpatient hospital treatment may be, as noted previously, a necessary precondition for psychoanalytic psychotherapy. Additional services connected with the hospital or the mental health center, such as day hospital, halfway house, and rehabilitation services are also sometimes essential.

COMBINATION WITH MEDICATION.
A variety of combinations of drugs with psychoanalytic psychotherapy are standard treatment at present. This ranges from the use of minor tranquilizers through the major ones for anxiety and for psychotic symptoms. It also includes medication for affective disorders, both for depressive and for manic episodes. From the viewpoint of psychoanalytic therapy, where medication makes it possible for the patient to participate in the free association process, the combination is useful and sometimes essential.[45]

Problematic Aspects

The intense human involvement of psychoanalytic therapy is its greatest strength but, at the same time, its greatest source of vulnerability and diffi-

culty. Misapplication and mistreatment remain ever-present dangers in all fields of medicine, but in the inevitable high tension subjectivity of the psychoanalytic therapies, objectivity is hard to maintain. Training of the therapist, including personal psychoanalytic treatment, aims to strengthen the therapist's abilities, but it remains an area in need of research and improvement. As in all human affairs, the obstacles to perfectibility and predictability are likely to remain formidable if not obdurate. Fortunately, progress in the psychoanalytic understanding of psychological disorders continues to provide the psychoanalytic therapist with technical and conceptual tools of increasing power.

REFERENCES

1. Breuer J, Freud S: Studies on Hysteria (1893–1895). London, Hogarth Press, 1955
2. Freud S: The Standard Edition of the Complete Psychological Works of Sigmund Freud, 24 vols. London, Hogarth Press, 1953–1974
3. Jones E: The Life and Work of Sigmund Freud, 3 vols. New York, Basic Books, 1953–1957
4. Alexander F, Eisenstein S, Grotjahn M (eds): Psychoanalytic Pioneers. New York, Basic Books, 1966
5. Loewenstein RM: Selected Papers of Rudolph M. Loewenstein. New Haven, CT, Yale University Press, 1982
6. Langs R: The Therapeutic Interaction, 2 vols. New York, Jason Aronson, 1976
7. Brenner C: Psychoanalytic Technique and Psychic Conflict. New York, International Universities Press, 1976
8. Sandler J, Dare C, Holder A: The Patient and the Analyst. New York, International Universities Press, 1973
9. Erikson EH: Childhood and Society. New York, WW Norton, 1950
10. Freud A: Normality and Pathology in Childhood. New York, International Universities Press, 1965
11. Jacobson E: The Self and the Object World. New York, International Universities Press, 1964
12. Mahler M, Pine F, Bergman A: The Psychological Birth of the Human Infant. New York, Basic Books, 1975
13. Kris AO: Free Association: Method and Process. New Haven, CT, Yale University Press, 1982
14. Rapaport D: The Structure of Psychoanalytic Theory. Psychological Issues, Monograph 6. New York, International Universities Press, 1960
15. Klein M: The Psychoanalysis of Children. London, Hogarth Press, 1959
16. Freud A: The Ego and the Mechanisms of Defense. New York, International Universities Press, 1966
17. Hartmann H: Ego Psychology and the Problem of Adaptation. New York, International Universities Press, 1958
18. Hartmann H: Essays in Ego Psychology. New York, International Universities Press, 1964
19. Hartmann H, Kris E, Loewenstein RM: Papers on Psychoanalytic Psychology. Psychological Issues, Monograph 14. New York, International Universities Press, 1964

20. Kris E: Selected Papers of Ernst Kris. New Haven, CT, Yale University Press, 1975

21. Fenichel O: The Psychoanalytic Theory of Neurosis. New York, WW Norton, 1945

22. Greenson RR: The Technique and Practice of Psychoanalysis. New York, International Universities Press, 1967

23. Kernberg O: Borderline Conditions and Pathological Narcissism. New York, Jason Aronson, 1975

24. Kernberg O: Object Relations Theory and Clinical Psychoanalysis. New York, Jason Aronson, 1976

25. Kohut H: The Analysis of the Self. New York, International Universities Press, 1971

26. Klein GS: Psychoanalytic Theory. New York, International Universities Press, 1976

27. Schafer R: A New Language for Psychoanalysis. New Haven, CT, Yale University Press, 1976

28. Ornstein PH: On narcissism: Beyond the introduction. Ann Psychoanal 2:127, 1974

29. Blum H (ed): Psychoanalytic Explorations of Technique. New York, International Universities Press, 1979

30. Brenner C: The Mind in Conflict. New York, International Universities Press, 1982

31. Spence DP: Narrative Truth and Historical Truth. New York, WW Norton, 1982

32. Gill M: Analysis of Transference. New York, International Universities Press, 1982

33. Kris AO: The analyst's conceptual freedom in the method of free association. Int J Psychoanal 64:407, 1983

34. Meissner WW: Internalization in Psychoanalysis. Psychological Issues, Monograph 50. New York, International Universities Press, 1981

35. Greenacre P: Emotional Growth. New York, International Universities Press, 1971

36. Benedek T: Training analysis—past, present, and future. Int J Psychoanal 50:437, 1969

37. Calef V, Weinshel EM: The analyst as the conscience of the analysis. Int Rev Psychoanal 7:279, 1980

38. Bornstein M (ed): Termination. Psychoanal Inquiry 2: (No. 3), 1982

39. Mann J: Time-Limited Psychotherapy. Cambridge, MA, Harvard University Press, 1973

40. Gillman RD: Psychoanalytic perspectives on brief psychotherapy. J Phila Assoc Psychoanal 8:45, 1981

41. Winokur J, Messer SB, Schacht T: Contributions to the theory and practice of short-term dynamic psychotherapy. Bull Menninger Clinic 45:125, 1982

42. Marziali EA: Prediction of outcome of brief psychotherapy from therapist interpretive interventions. Arch Gen Psychiatry 41:301, 1984

43. Zetzel ER: The Capacity for Emotional Growth. New York, International Universities Press, 1970

44. Ticho EA: Termination of psychoanalysis: Treatment goals, life goals. Psychoanal Q 41:315, 1972

45. Lipton M: A letter from Anna Freud. Am J Psychiatry 140:1583, 1983

8

John F. Clarkin, Allen J. Frances, and Samuel W. Perry

The Psychosocial Treatments

We will begin by defining psychosocial treatment as a general category and then discuss the equally awkward problem of classifying into manageable classes the more than 200 different psychotherapies that have been identified within this rubric. It is easier to say what psychosocial treatments are not (*i.e.,* they are not medication treatment, not faith healing, and not the advice of the local bartender) than to establish a comprehensive, positive definition. For our present purposes, a *psychosocial treatment* will be defined simply and inclusively as any planned intervention offered by an expert in mental health to help a patient overcome or live with symptoms and/or impairments in functioning. In order to simplify the task of exposition, we will classify psychosocial treatments along two interacting dimensions: their orientation and their format.

The several hundred psychosocial treatments will be abstracted into four overlapping and heterogeneous "orientations": (1) psychodynamic, (2) cognitive/behavioral, (3) strategic/systems, and (4) experiential. Each orientation provides a particular way of understanding human behavior that leads to particular methods of treatment intervention. At best, each orientation provides a heuristic focus; at worst, the slavish devotion to an orientation serves as a reductionistic blinder. In actual practice, the different orientations are inextricably intertwined and are probably additively helpful. Each treatment orientation will be characterized by its history, rationale, goals, setting, techniques, and selection criteria. These aspects of a treatment co-determine one another and must be closely integrated if a treatment is to make sense. For instance, the goals of treatment cannot be established in isolation without an accompanying estimate of the patient's needs, capacities, and preferences; and all of these together help determine which techniques are likely to be possible or optimal.

We will also discuss how the various orientations influence and are influenced by the format of the treatment, that is, whether it is conducted individually, in a group, or with the family. Other dimensions that importantly characterize psychosocial treatments (*i.e.,* their setting, duration, intensity, and combination with medication) will be touched on only in passing and have been discussed by us in more detail elsewhere.[1]

There is little evidence to document that particular kinds of psychotherapy are specifically effective for particular types of patient problems. This may reflect the complex methodologic problems inherent in the research necessary to define specific psychotherapy effects or may mean that different treatments are effective more by virtue of their shared than their specific features (or both may be true depending on the circumstances). There is little justification for dogmatism among proponents of the different orientations or formats. A mastery of all of the orientations is necessary if a therapist is to gain a thorough understanding of, and the ability to intervene flexibly with, the range of patient problems described in this section of the text.

Orientation/format interactions are summarized in Table 1.

TABLE 1. Orientation/Format Interactions

Orientation	Format		
	INDIVIDUAL	GROUP	FAMILY
Psychodynamic	Psychoanalysis Focal therapy Psychodynamic psychotherapy	Insight-oriented heterogeneous group (Wolf)	Insight-oriented marital/family therapy (Ackerman, Framo)
Cognitive/behavioral	Cognitive treatment of depression (Beck) Rational-emotive therapy (Ellis) Most behavioral therapy	Group treatment of agoraphobia Assertiveness training groups	Behavioral marital/family treatment (Falloon, Jacobson, Patterson)
Strategic/systems	"Uncommon therapy" (Erikson)	Most heterogeneous group therapy	Structural family therapy (Minuchin) Strategic family therapy (Haley) Paradoxical family therapy (Palazolli)
Experiential	Client-centered (Rogers) Existential (May)	Gestalt (Perls) Psychodrama (Moreno) Most homogeneous groups	Experiential family therapy (Whitaker)

Orientations

PSYCHODYNAMIC ORIENTATIONS

The psychodynamic model and psychoanalytic treatment are discussed in detail in other chapters. Our purpose here is to distinguish briefly the three types of psychodynamic treatment (1) psychoanalytic, (2) long-term exploratory therapy, and (3) focal (*i.e.,* brief) therapy.

History and Rationale

It is often forgotten that psychoanalysis began as a relatively brief treatment focused on the one intrapsychic conflict responsible for a particular symptom. In many ways, the techniques offered by Breuer and Freud in their early cases more closely resemble current focal therapy than current psychoanalysis. Gradually, psychoanalysis lengthened and became more extensive in its scope and ambitious in its goals. This was influenced by several co-determining factors: increased therapist passivity, attempts to promote more profound transference regression, restriction to transference and resistance interpretation, and attention to character rather than to symptom pathology. Partly

in reaction to the inexorable lengthening of orthodox analysis that has occurred throughout this century, a number of clinical innovators have developed methods of applying psychodynamic technique within a brief therapy duration. The earliest contributions were made by Rank, who was interested in time-limited treatment to promote analysis of separation anxiety, and by Ferenzci, who was interested in increasing therapist activity in order to increase treatment efficiency.[2] Focal therapy was then rediscovered again and again more or less independently by Alexander and French[3] in the 1940s and by Balint, Malan,[4] Sifneos,[5] Mann,[6] and Davanloo[7] in the 1960s. Long-term exploratory psychotherapy has developed as an adaptation of psychoanalysis to meet the needs of the many patients who are unable to make the requisite commitment in time and money or meet the difficult enabling factors or tolerate the regression of a transference neurosis that are necessary for analysis. Long-term exploratory psychotherapy became the most frequently performed psychodynamic treatment as this orientation expanded (especially in the United States) outside the narrow confines of the psychoanalytic institutes to influence the training programs of all mental health professionals.

Focal therapy shares most of its basic psychodynamic assumptions with psychoanalysis but places a different emphasis on several assumptions:

1. Character change continues and expands after treatment so that all conflicts need not be resolved within the transference situation
2. Greater faith in cognitive understanding and in corrective emotional experience as facilitators of change
3. Less emphasis on the value or necessity of transference regression
4. Less attempt to achieve pervasive characterologic transformation. The model of long-term exploratory therapy shares the assumptions of psychoanalysis except for the emphasis on the necessity of transference regression to promote change.

Setting

Psychoanalysis is a long (usually 3 or more years), intense (usually three to five times per week) treatment that usually requires the patient to lie on the couch facing away from the therapist. The ambiguity of the situation allows the patient to structure the encounter, color it with his own intrapsychic fantasy, and regress in a controlled way within the transference relationship. Long-term exploratory psychotherapy is a flexible treatment that may span 1 or more years and one to three sessions per week and is usually conducted face-to-face and sitting up. Focal therapy is a brief (1 to 50 sessions), sitting up, face-to-face treatment. Psychodynamic interventions are often applicable to inpatient, day hospital, and emergency room settings, but the therapies described here most often occur in traditional outpatient encounters.

Goals

Psychoanalysis aims at pervasive character change through an extensive and intensive interpretation of the wide panoply of transference distortions that are elicited in the regression-promoting treatment situation. Focal therapy aims at circumscribed character change through the analysis of one, albeit important, intrapsychic conflict. The goals of long-term exploratory psychotherapy are intermediate in their level of ambition. All of the psychodynamic treatments differ from the other orientations to be discussed in the following sections in their much greater emphasis on character change and resolution of unconscious conflict as opposed to the provision of symptomatic relief.

Techniques

Psychoanalysis relies on the treatment setting to promote controlled regression within the transference neurosis and then permits interpretation of intrapsychic conflicts as they are manifested within the transference and resistance. Other therapist activities (interpretations outside the transference, promoting catharsis, suggestion, support, and small talk) are regarded as sometimes necessary, but less than desirable, parameters that eventually require analysis. The analyst tends to be technically neutral and relatively passive in order to allow the free flow of associations, fantasy, and regression.

Focal therapy requires a much more active therapist who quickly formulates an underlying unconscious conflict that helps to explain the patient's chief complaint, recurring patterns of behavior, early life experiences, and early transference distortions. Rather than encouraging regression, the therapist systematically undercuts it by interpreting transference distortions as soon as these occur, particularly as these are related to the focal conflict of the treatment. The therapist listens and intervenes selectively in order to focus the treatment on the central underlying conflict. Separation issues are often prominent early.

Long-term exploratory therapy includes the widest range of techniques and borders more closely on psychoanalysis or focal therapy, depending on whether its duration, frequency, and goals are closer to one or the other.

COGNITIVE/BEHAVIORAL ORIENTATION

History and Rationale

The development of the current cognitive-behavioral approach has its separate but intertwined roots in classical conditioning, in operant conditioning, and in social learning theory. In the 1950s, Wolpe[8] applied the laboratory methods of classical (Pavlovian) conditioning to the clinical situation, particularly in the treatment of phobic disorders. Wolpe's systematic desensitization promoted inhibition (or extinction) of anxiety by subjecting the patient to progressively more anxiety-provoking situations while simultaneously inhibiting the anxiety with relaxation exercises. Before long, other behavior therapists discovered that exposure alone would extinguish anxiety so long as the patient did not leave the field.

A second historical trend was the operant approach of B. F. Skinner. In the laboratory, Skinner[9] arranged an elaborate system of positive reinforcements and extinction to make pigeons perform colorful and outlandish feats. By the early 1950s, the approach was being used with psychotic patients in inpatient settings.[10] Psychotic behavior was seen as instrumental in nature, and environmental events in hospital wards were manipulated in order to extinguish or shape patient responses.

The earlier behavioral approaches ignored or downgraded the importance of cognitive processes. More recently, under the influence of Bandura,[11] Ellis,[12] Meichenbaum,[13] and Beck,[14] there has been an increased emphasis on cognitive variables and social learning. Ellis was one of the first to confront directly and attempt to change the patient's irrational cognitions. His rational-emotive therapy was used to identify specific irrational thoughts and beliefs, expose their false assumptions, and generate more realistic and positive statements. Beck emphasized the internal cognitions related to symptomatology and regarded depression as a cognitive disorder involving a negative view of the self, the world, and the future, with a tendency to set very high self-standards. The therapist uses various cognitive techniques to reexamine faulty cognitions and generate new ones.

The basic hypotheses or assumptions of the cognitive/behavioral orientation are as follows:

1. Abnormal behavior is learned and maintained according to the same behavioral principles as those governing normal behavior.
2. Emphasis is placed on the theoretic and empiric relationships between environmental stimuli and behavior exhibited by the patient.
3. Focus is placed on the current as opposed to historical relationship between the antecedent and consequent events surrounding the pathologic behaviors of the patient.
4. Focus is on definable behaviors (including explicit thoughts reported by patient) that can be counted and traced before intervention (baseline) and following intervention (change).
5. The behavioral therapist is active in using techniques that engage the patient in changing old behaviors and introducing new, more adaptive ones.

Goals

The goal in the cognitive/behavioral orientation is explicit, concrete change in definable thoughts or behaviors, the reduction and/or elimination of some behaviors, and the introduction of new behaviors. Symptom change may be amplified by positive feedback to produce more pervasive improvements in functioning, but this is not an orientation that focuses on character change.

Setting

Because of its explicit emphasis on achievement of concrete behavioral goals, the treatment tends to be brief (5 to 50 sessions). Progress (or its absence) is measured and discussed openly between therapist and patient. Although therapeutic meetings often take place in the therapist's office, there may be sessions in the specific environment in which the pathologic behaviors occur. For example, the behavior therapist may accompany an agoraphobic to a feared shopping center or observe an anorexic adolescent at the family dinner table.

Techniques

As is characteristic of the other aspects of the cognitive/behavioral orientation, the techniques are explicitly definable and easily recognized and taught. However, the clinical skill is much less definable and entails the proper timing and sequencing of the techniques and skill in eliciting the patient's active engagement and participation. The basic cognitive/behavioral techniques include relaxation training; systematic desensitization; behavioral rehearsal-modeling; reinforcement procedures (punishment, extinction, operant conditioning); problem solving (problem definition, generating alternatives, decision making); and modification of cognitive processes by way of rational restructuring, stress inoculation training, and thought-stopping.

STRATEGIC/SYSTEMS ORIENTATIONS

History and Rationale

The strategic approach to psychopathology was elaborated by Bateson,[15] Erikson, and Haley.[16] Bateson was an anthropologist of wide-ranging interests and theoretic twists who studied natives in New Guinea, dolphins in Hawaii, and schizophrenics in California. A student of cybernetics and information theory, he formulated a communication analysis in which confusing and contradictory family interactions (the "double bind") lead to schizophrenic symptomatology. Erikson, a physician who used hypnotism, made an art of therapeutically "encouraging" the patient's resistance. Ingeniously combining hypnotic techniques and paradoxic directives, Erikson creatively improvised ways of prescribing a symptom and at the same time controlling and changing it. Haley,[17] a colleague of Bateson and a student of Erikson, has enumerated strategic techniques for managing the myriad forms of resistance. In contrast to Freud, for example, Haley approaches a present-day little Hans (*i.e.,* a 6-year-old boy with a dog phobia) by asking him to find a dog that is afraid of humans and to cure it. At the same time, Haley was aware of the structural role the boy and his symptom played in the family system.

The basic assumptions of the strategic model are as follows:

1. Insight or understanding of one's problem is not a goal of treatment. In fact, insight is seen as antithetical to change unless it is imparted as part of a strategic plan.
2. The patient's present problems are not "symptoms" of illness but solutions to ordinary situations that have gone awry. Previous attempts at solution are now part of the problem.
3. There are two types of change. First-order change is a modification of behavior within a given system without a change in the system as a whole. Second-order change involves modification of the entire system.

Goals

The goal of strategic intervention is to change the problem that is presented by the patient. In contrast to the dynamic orientation that regards symptoms as the surface manifestations of underlying problems that are the real focus of intervention, strategic therapists take the problem as experienced or perceived by the patient at face value. The goal is to change that symptom as quickly as possible and then disengage from the patient or family. Mediating goals would involve changing behaviors around the problem in a stepwise fashion.

Setting

The strategic orientation is most often used with ambulatory patients who present a specific behavioral problem or impasse. The individual patient may be seen alone, but often the family members are included in the treatment in order to promote maximum impact on the whole system. Since the focus is on a sharply delimited problem, the treatment tends to be brief.

Techniques

Therapists in this orientation have generated a variety of techniques to modify, reverse, and take control of patient resistance to change. These include direct advice, paradoxic injunctions, reframing, symptom prescription, marking boundaries, and positive connotation (emphasizing the positive value of a symptom for all family members).

EXPERIENTIAL ORIENTATION

History and Rationale

Although the dynamic, cognitive/behavioral, and strategic/systems orientations were developed as innovations of clinical technique, experiential approaches developed in reaction against technology. Experiential psychotherapists often regard technology as the cause and not the cure of human ills and are concerned that we have become subordinated to mechanistic forces, which in turn have led to a depersonalized and dehumanized existence. Accordingly, any therapy that imposes directive and mechanistic methods only contributes to the basic human problem rather than solves it. Experiential therapists distrust intellectual solutions and place greater emphasis on spontaneous feelings and the immediate experiencing of events in order to acquire a sense of personal authenticity.

Of course, the importance of expressing feelings is not new. Aristotle spoke about the cathartic value of drama, and all psychotherapies provide a situation for those who are troubled to "get things off their minds." Shamanistic rituals, Catholic confessionals, Mesmer's hypnosis, and Breuer and Freud (particularly in *Studies in Hysteria*) have all depended on the therapeutic value of "abreacting," that is, ventilating feelings that had not previously been permitted direct and full expression.

At the extreme, the experiential schools view all psychopathology as the result of loculated feelings and/or inhibitions. Emotional problems are not caused by one's inheritance, constitution, or developmental trauma; they are caused by not "actualizing" one's potential. Anxiety is conceptualized as the tension between what one is and what one can become. Those with emotional distress are therefore no different than the rest of us and should not be "diagnosed" or labeled as sick. Indeed, anyone may benefit from a therapeutic experience. Experiential psychotherapy has also been influenced by Oriental religions and by Western existential philosophies. The major schools of therapy that may be labeled experiential include client centered,[19] Kohutian psychoanalysis,[20] gestalt,[21] psychodrama,[22] existential,[23] and abreactive.

The assumptions of the experiential orientation include the following:

1. The nature of man is such that he has a capacity to be aware of himself, of what he is doing, and what is happening to him. He is not passive but actively strives for meaning and strives for goals. Man is not bound by historical or unconscious

forces but rather can take responsibility for himself and make choices. Man is not a static entity but rather a being in transition, in the process of becoming.

2. Therapists provide an atmosphere in which it is possible for the patient to further his self-discovery. Therapeutic change is the result of the emotional experience itself. Behavior can be understood only from the subjective view of the patient, in the "here and now" of experience and interaction. The goal is to achieve what is "existentially real" rather than what is "abstractly true."

3. The therapist adopts an empathic observational attitude that will permit him to "experience" the patient's subjective world.

Goals

Experiential therapists are uncomfortable with the notion of specific goals of treatment. Since social and parental pressure to achieve are seen as contributing to unwarranted anxiety, every effort is made to deemphasize specific achievements such as character change or symptom removal. Instead, the client should strive to experience the therapeutic encounter as fully as possible. By not struggling and by simply allowing it to happen, the client will automatically take another step toward self-awareness, cohesiveness, and actualization.

Techniques

Experiential therapies are defined less sharply than the exploratory or directive interventions. Indeed, some proponents of the experiential method would oppose any definition of techniques, feeling that such description might become codified and would limit the necessary flexibility and intuitiveness of the therapist who is meant to be as open, receptive, empathic, and unbiased as possible when interacting with the client. Nevertheless, some experiential therapies have been articulated. The techniques of client-centered psychotherapy reflect the belief that the encounter is not designed for "treatment" but for "growth." Therapeutic maneuvers are seen as potentially destructive; instead, the emphasis is on therapeutic attitudes (empathic understanding, unlimited positive regard, and genuineness) that establish the proper conditions for growth. The psychoanalytic approach to narcissistic patients elaborated by Kohut shares many of those same values and techniques. Gestalt treatment attempts to bring the various parts of oneself into total awareness. In the belief that a holistic view—the gestalt—will give meaning to one's different ideas and feelings and experiences, the techniques are designed to overcome those barriers that prevent an individual from being totally aware of his needs. Various psychological and sensorimotor exercises are used. Psychodrama uses role-playing techniques derived from impromptu theater in order to facilitate the individual's experiencing of the true drama of his life. Various forms of abreactive treatment, sometimes including hypnosis or amobarbital (amytal) interviews, direct the patient to reexperience painful feelings and memories.

DIFFERENTIAL SELECTION CRITERIA: CHOOSING AMONG ORIENTATIONS

Certain types of patient problems lend themselves especially well to one or another of the various orientations, but very often the choice among them depends more on patient goals, capacities, and preferences and on therapist skill, training, and bias than on clearly established, specific indications. Moreover, the orientations overlap greatly and mix very well with one another. For example, psychodynamic treatments are inevitably experiential and incorporate (consciously or not) a variety of behavioral, cognitive, and strategic techniques. The choice of one particular orientation is not nearly so categorical as one might gather from the following discussion. The needs of the patient and the nature of the therapeutic alliance evolve in a way that often results in a gradual change in orientation as the treatment progresses.

Psychodynamic treatments are most indicated for psychologically minded individuals who are interested in expanded self-understanding and in changing deeply ingrained, pervasive characterologic patterns of behavior. Focal therapy requires the most from the patient in terms of previous level of functioning, psychological mindedness, motivation for autoplastic change, focality of intrapsychic conflict, ability to permit transference distortions to develop quickly and yet to analyze them with perspective, and tolerance for separation. Among psychodynamic treatments, focal therapy requires the least of the patient's time, money, or commitment to an enduring therapeutic relationship. The differential indications between long-term exploratory therapy and psychoanalysis are not well-established for patients who have the motivation, psychological ability, and the frustration and regression tolerance to participate in either. Psychoanalysis has the advantage of more thorough and deeper exploration and the possible disadvantage of encouraging greater regression and dependency. Psychoanalysis is most clearly indicated in preference to exploratory therapy for these patients who have had incomplete results or difficulty allowing the emergence of fantasy material in other less intense dynamic treatments and for those who intend to become mental health practitioners. Long-term exploratory therapy is far more flexible than either focal therapy or psychoanalysis and is the psychodynamic treatment of choice for patients who do not meet the more stringent enabling criteria for either of them.

The cognitive/behavioral approach is most indicated for patients who present with a leading symptom that is amenable to direct intervention and for whom relief of this symptom is a more important goal than more pervasive character change. This is particularly likely to be the case if the patient has not received symptom relief from previous psychodynamic treatments, if the symptom is debilitating and causing secondary demoralization, if the patient is not psychologically minded or interested in introspection, or if a rapid remission is necessary. Behavior therapy has demonstrated greatest efficiency in the treatment of anxiety, compulsive, sexual, depressive, addictive, assertiveness, and interpersonal disorders. Cognitive therapy has established its effectiveness in the treatment of depressive disorders and is now being adapted to anxiety disorders. It requires from the patient considerable cognitive ability, motivation, self-scrutiny, and ability to complete homework assignments.

The strategic/systems orientations inform all treatment but are especially important in the family and group therapy formats, as will be indicated later in this chapter. Perhaps paradoxically, an attention to treatment strategies is likely to be most necessary for those patients who have very simple problems amenable to direct advice and for those who have very complicated problems that seem impossible to resolve. Paradoxic injunctions may be the treatment of last resort for those oppositional patients who have successfully defeated all previous attempts at help.

The experiential orientation informs all treatments but is especially indicated in situations that call for catharsis, such as adjustment and post-traumatic stress disorders. This orientation also greatly informs the treatment of patients at points of developmental crisis who need tutoring in taking their next step.

Formats

THE INDIVIDUAL FORMAT

History and Rationale

Individual treatment is the most traditional and prevalent of psychotherapeutic formats. Throughout recorded history, people have found relief from suffering by private consultation with a designated authority, such as an oracle, shaman, witch doctor, priest, rabbi, village elder, or physician within a "magic circle" invested with special powers and geographically or symbolically removed from the everyday world. The relationship between psychotherapist and patient maintains elements of delegated omnipotence and confidentiality. The individual format also provides the smoothest induction into treatment with the lowest incidence of dropouts. Many patients are aware that they have emotional problems and need help but are ashamed and frightened about entering psychotherapy. The individual format is usually the easiest to accept because it provides familiarity, clear role definition, confidentiality, dyadic intimacy, flexibility, and specificity.

Setting, Techniques, and Goals

Individual therapy occurs in, and blends well with, all treatment settings, ranging from an inpatient psychiatric hospital to a family practitioner's office. It can be delivered within the widest range of frequencies and durations and provides a comfortable format for all of the orientations described previously. The goals of the individual treatment format will usually be most determined by the particular techniques employed within it rather than by the specific characteristics of the individual format. However, the individual format is most specifically useful for treatments that have as their goal the exploration and resolution of unconscious conflict and/or improvement in problems with dyadic intimacy.

MARITAL/FAMILY FORMAT

Rationale

The idea that marital or family difficulties contribute to an individual's emotional problems was well known to the ancients and informs a good part of our myth and literature. What is relatively recent is the establishment of a therapeutic format specifically designed to change marital or family behavior. Marital therapy began in the 1920s, mostly under the auspices of ministers, marriage counselors, and social workers. By the mid 1930s, psychoanalytically oriented therapists began to report treatments that combined individual and couple intervention, and soon couple treatment was performed by itself. The family format was conceived in the 1920s in child guidance clinics. It has blossomed during the last 30 years under the influence of a number of charismatic theorists and clinicians who have, in many instances, established their own families of followers.[24–27]

The basic assumptions of the family/marital approaches are as follows:

1. The individual, the marital dyad, the conjugal, and the extended family are increasingly larger organized units in a continuum of hierarchically arranged systems, each of which has its own distinctive properties of organization, homeostasis, and boundary definition.
2. Individual symptomatology can best be understood and changed in the context of the systematic, repetitive interactions of the family group. Individual symptoms have a functional role for the family, so that a change in the individual is not possible without a concomitant change in the rest of the family and vice versa.

Goals

The emphasis is on improving the functioning of the whole system or network of individuals in the marital/family unit rather than on change in any one individual. Although symptomatic behavior in an individual (the identified patient) may occasion family therapy and serve as an ultimate target for change, the mediating goals of the intervention also include improved communication, problem solving, and boundary functioning in the family as a system.

Setting

The family may assemble as a whole, or in subunits, in the therapist's office or in the home setting. Some years ago, Bowen went so far as to hospitalize whole families, but family intervention with inpatients proceeds quite well without such extreme steps. Marital/family treatment is usually brief in duration, with from 5 to 50 weekly sessions. Single sessions are often quite helpful. Several authors have described working with the entire extended family in order to learn about and influence the context in which the nuclear family problem has arisen. Most family therapists are quite flexible in their choice of particular family subunits with which to interact. Family members, particularly children and grandparents, may be included or excluded from particular sessions as the need arises.

Techniques

The marital/family format allows for the use of techniques from all the major orientations but is especially useful and specific to strategic/systems approaches. The therapist can observe first hand the family interaction and structure and provide intervention tasks intended to change the family system directly (*e.g.*, a distant father is told to teach his son who sets fires how to use matches properly while the previously overinvolved mother is told to stay out of this interchange and watch that the father does his task well). Typical systems/strategic techniques within the family format include prescribing the symptom, prescribing the interactions around the symptom, escalating stress, marking boundaries, giving intrasession and extrasession tasks, giving paradoxic injunction, giving advice, providing direction, assisting with problem solving, modeling, and teaching.

The techniques derived from the dynamic, behavioral, and experiential orientations take on an added dimension within the family format. For example, by teaching a father to use effective behavioral techniques (*e.g.*, setting limits, positive reinforcement, and proper use of punishment) with his acting-out adolescent son, the therapist helps to increase the father's power and status within the family. Psychodynamic interpretations are often particularly useful when spouses have specific transference distortion toward one another that underlie and structure their relationship problem. In the family format, there tends to be less transference distortion toward the therapist because the prominent distortions are those that occur among the family members themselves. This allows the therapist to assume the role of neutral referee and reduces the risk of transference actualizations.

HETEROGENEOUS AND HOMOGENEOUS GROUP THERAPY FORMATS

History and Rationale

Heterogeneous group therapy has achieved wide acceptance during the past 50 years. In the 1930s, social theorists and psychotherapists examined the processes generated within small groups and distinguished these from the processes that occur intrapsychically, dyadically, and in large groups. The study of the small group format was carried forth by individuals who came from radically different backgrounds: social scientists (most especially Lewin[28]), psychoanalysts (Burrow, Wender, and Shilder and later Bion,[29] Foulkes,[30] Slavson,[31] Wolf,[32] and many others), and clinical innovators (such as Moreno). These groups are called *heterogeneous* because individual members do not share one particular symptom or problem constellation and because they differ widely in strengths, ages, socioeconomic background, and personality traits and strengths. In spite of these differences, a feeling of commonality develops, and the patient realizes that he is not alone, uniquely strange, or crazy in his experiences. This realization reduces embarrassment, improves self-esteem, and promotes the sense of being acceptable.

Broadly conceived, *homogeneous* groups encompass a wide variety of shared experiences: expiation at religious communions, catharsis at Greek tragedies, and even abreaction at modern rock concerts. More narrowly and clinically defined homogeneous groups originated with the work of a Boston internist, Joseph Pratt, who in the early 1900s began speaking to groups of patients with tuberculosis. He discovered that the group began to have "a life of its own," patients were able to help one another, and the group process was psychotherapeutic in a way that meeting individually with patients was not. Before long, both within and outside the psychiatric profession, homogeneous groups became tremendously popular for combating alcoholism and drug addiction, for weight watching and stopping smoking, for consciousness raising, and for a wide variety of other disorders. Although often not labeled as "psychiatric patients," more people are engaged in one or another form of homogeneous groups than in all other outpatient psychotherapies combined.

Goals

The group format helps to create a powerful interacting network of members and provides the interpersonal world in microcosm. Mediating goals include developing group cohesion, loyalty, and support and providing an atmosphere in which typical interpersonal exchanges, dilemmas, and conflicts can emerge. The final goals include individual symptom reduction and, most especially, the resolution of interpersonal conflicts. In heterogeneous groups, the final goals tend to be more extensive and ambitious, such as the resolution of long-standing, characteristic, interactional personality traits and the emergence of more satisfying interpersonal attachments and coping styles. In contrast, the final goals in homogeneous groups are more concretely focused on the problem/symptom that brought the group together. Through mutual support and encouragement, the individuals gain group momentum for conquering or coping with their shared symptom.

Setting

Heterogeneous groups typically meet in the therapist's office on a weekly basis for 1 hour or 90-minute sessions over several years. Membership is sometimes "closed," individual patients all begin and end the group at the same time. In open groups, a complicated process occurs when new patients are added and must gain psychological admittance to an ongoing system. In contrast, homogeneous groups are less formal in their meeting locations and membership requirements. Meetings take place on hospital wards, in psychiatric outpatient clinics, in community halls, and in church basements, for example. Membership is almost always open ended, so that new patients who share the problem that is the group's focus are added, and often warmly welcomed, with an orientation to group procedures, guidelines, and philosophy. Homogeneous groups develop a life of their own. The group continues forever while the individuals come and go.

Techniques

The heterogeneous group format lends itself well to techniques derived from all of the orientations, and different group therapists focus their attention in varying degrees to psychodynamic, cognitive/behavioral, experiential, and strategic/systems techniques. In regard to psychodynamic techniques, the group has the special advantages of providing for multiple simultaneous transference relationships and for protecting therapist neutrality. The group format is especially useful in providing members with an understanding of the interpersonal roles they play in social systems. The homogeneous group format is most adapted to the experiential format. Homogeneous groups provide a structured social network for individuals who previously felt they must suffer in isolation. Within this integrated community, members are given a defined role with specified procedures, duties, rights, expectations, and responsibilities. This role definition is in itself reassuring and relieves the tension of uncertainty and alienation. A sense of belonging develops with loyalty to the group of fellow sufferers. Some homogeneous groups, such as those used in alcohol and drug rehabilitation programs, set up a hierarchy with a system of gradual promotion and the possibility of eventual leadership.

DIFFERENTIAL SELECTION CRITERIA: CHOOSING AMONG FORMATS

The choice of a particular format or combination of formats is co-determined by several interacting influences: the orientation that is most likely to guide the treatment, the patient preferences and goals and the nature of the presenting problems, and therapist comfort and training.

The individual format allows for the greatest intensity and depth of exploration in psychodynamic treatments and is a particularly good arena for uncovering and resolving problems with dyadic intimacy. Individual and family approaches are indicated in crisis situations because they are flexible and specific to the problem at hand. Although there are some reports of crisis groups in the literature, groups are usually too preoccupied with their own concerns to address successfully a new member's pressing needs. Many patients will accept nothing but individual treatment despite evidence that other formats might be more helpful or less risky. In such situations, a brief preparatory individual treatment may be indicated to provide the role induction necessary before a patient feels able or willing to participate in a family or group format. Such role induction reduces the likelihood of patient noncompliance or dropout. Individual or group treatment is also indicated for young adults or adolescents who are attempting, with difficulty, to establish a transitional base as a means of gaining autonomy from an otherwise fused family system. Individual treatment is the format most likely to preserve privacy and confidentiality and should be chosen when these are important considerations.

The disadvantages of the individual format suggest situations in which the group or family format will be chosen in preference. The therapist receives incomplete data and observes the range of patient behaviors only within the relatively limited context of the therapeutic relationship. This reduces his ability to intervene within the family system and may restrict his awareness of the full panoply of transference distortions experienced by the patient in response to the more varied interpersonal triggers encountered in everyday life. Moreover, some patients regress within the individual format and develop actualized, intense, infantile transferences

that are not amenable to interpretation. This is less likely to occur within the more diluted transferential atmosphere of a family or group format.

Marital/family therapy is the treatment of choice for marital/family problems when these are presented as the chief complaint. Sexual dysfunctions, marital conflict, communication problems, and threatened dissolution of the marriage can all be foci for intervention. Marital/family treatment may also be indicated even when an individual patient presents with symptoms if these are clearly related to current, structured problems in the family relationship and functioning, with each member contributing overtly or covertly to the difficulties. Such families may display marked projective identification (each member blames the other for all problems), collective cognitive chaos, excessively fused or distanced relationships, poor boundary functioning, and amorphous communication patterns. This is also a useful format when the patient's strongest transferential distortions are directed toward other family members and are not readily transferable to the therapist. Family treatment may be indicated when another form of therapy has reached a stalemate, when the reduction in symptomatology of one member is accompanied by an increase in that of another, to undercut secondary gain, or when there is a family crisis.

Family/marital treatment is relatively contraindicated when one or more family members insist on the privacy of individual treatment (*e.g.*, because of a ''valid'' family secret), when the individuation of one or more family members would be compromised, and when the family is well along into a breaking-up process and members have little or no motivation or need for collaboration.

A heterogeneous group format is specifically indicated for those patients who are relatively comfortable within dyadic relationships but who fear establishing new interpersonal relationships or dealing with established ones. The heterogeneous group provides an arena for exploring maladaptive interpersonal behaviors and for learning new social skills. The format is also indicated when it is necessary to ration therapist time or to provide the patient with a relatively economical treatment. It is useful for patients who have failed or are likely to fail in the individual format (*e.g.*, they become too dependent, intellectualize excessively, cannot tolerate dyadic intimacy or interpretations from an authority, or elicit harmful and unmanageable countertransference within individual therapy). This may be the format of choice for adolescents or young adults with separation problems who are having difficulty establishing a new social network.

Symptom or problem constellations that may be an indication for homogeneous group therapy include *impulse disorder* (such as obesity, smoking, alcoholism, drug addiction, gambling, or criminal behavior); a *medical disorder* (cardiac ailments, ileostomy, terminal illness, or deafness); a particular *developmental phase* (childhood and adolescence or geriatrics); or a *psychiatric disorder* (agoraphobia, schizophrenia, somatoform disorder) and many others.[33] The homogeneous group format has the highest level of patient acceptance and probably successful outcome for this wide variety of symptoms and problems that have served as an immediate badge of admission and a target for intervention. Because the content and process of these groups are focused on a specific problem area, the range of interactions among members tends to be more constricted than in heterogeneous groups. Patients who desire or need increased insight and characterologic change are less likely to find this in the homogeneous group than in the other formats that have been discussed.

Concurrent or sequential combinations of different formats are often desirable. Typical examples include combined individual and family formats for an emancipating young adult or individual and group formats for an avoidant patient who has difficulty entering new situations alone.

Conclusions

Although some patients who meet criteria for the personality disorders and neuroses will benefit from medication treatment, the treatment of choice is usually one or a combination of various psychosocial interventions. The selection of one particular orientation or format of treatment, or particular combinations, remains largely uninformed by systematic research, but no one has suggested that such decisions are trivial or should be made randomly. In the absence of scientifically confirmed selection criteria, the choice of treatment and its delivery rely on the therapist's art and clinical experience and on the patient's capacities and preferences. In most instances, the *Diagnostic and Statistical Manual of Mental Disorders*, 3rd ed. (*DSM-III*) diagnosis does not by itself provide enough data to predict which particular combination of orientation, format, duration, and setting is the most indicated for a particular patient. Negotiation with the patient is a crucial step in treatment selection. There is no evidence in the available literature to support dogmatic assertions from proponents of

particular schools. The time has come to eliminate stridency of discourse and to draw from what is necessary and valuable in each orientation and format.

REFERENCES

1. Frances A, Clarkin JF, Perry S: Differential Therapeutics in Psychiatry: The Art and Science of Treatment Selection. New York, Brunner/Mazel, 1984

2. Ferenczi S, Rank I: The Development of Psychoanalysis. New York, Nervous and Mental Disease Publishing Co, 1925

3. Alexander F, French T: Psychoanalytic Therapy. New York, Ronald Press, 1946

4. Malan DH: A Study of Brief Psychotherapy. New York, Plenum, 1963

5. Sifneos PE: Short-term Psychotherapy and Emotional Crisis. Cambridge, MA, Harvard University Press, 1972

6. Mann J: Time-limited Psychotherapy. Cambridge, MA, Harvard University Press, 1973

7. Davanloo H: Basic Principles and Techniques in Short-term Dynamic Psychotherapy. New York, Spectrum Books, 1978

8. Wolpe J: Psychotherapy by Reciprocal Inhibition. Stanford, CA, Stanford University Press, 1958

9. Skinner BF: The Behavior of Organisms. New York, Appleton-Century-Crofts, 1938

10. Lindsley OR: Operant conditioning methods applied to research in chronic schizophrenia. Psychiatry Res Rep 5: 118–139, 1956

11. Bandura A: Principles of Behavior Modification. New York, Holt, Rinehart & Winston, 1969

12. Ellis A: Reason and Emotion in Psychotherapy. New York, Lyle Stuart, 1962

13. Meichenbaum D: Cognitive-Behavior Modification: An Integrative Approach. New York, Plenum Press, 1977

14. Beck AT: Cognitive Therapy and the Emotional Disorders. New York, International Universities Press, 1976

15. Bateson G: Steps to Ecology of Mind. New York, Ballantine Books, 1972

16. Haley J: Uncommon Therapy: The Psychiatric Techniques of Milton H. Erikson. New York, WW Norton & Co, 1973

17. Haley J: Strategies of Psychotherapy. New York, Grune & Stratton, 1963

18. Freud S: Studies in hysteria. In Strackey J (ed): The Standard Edition of the Complete Works of Sigmund Freud, vol. 2. London, Hogarth Press, 1955

19. Rogers CR: Counseling and Psychotherapy. Boston, Houghton Mifflin, 1942

20. Kohut H, Chessick R: The Technique and Practice of Intensive Psychotherapy. New York, Jason Aronson, 1974

21. Perls FS, Hefferline RF, Goodman P: Gestalt Therapy. New York, Julian Press, 1951

22. Moreno JL: Psychodrama and group therapy. Sociometry 9:249–253, 1946

23. Yalom I: Existential Psychotherapy. New York, Basic Books, 1980

24. Ackerman NW: Treating the Troubled Family. New York, Basic Books, 1966

25. Bowen M: Family Therapy in Clinical Practice. New York, Jason Aronson, 1978

26. Minuchin S: Families and Family Therapy. Cambridge, MA, Harvard University Press, 1974

27. Framo J: Integration of marital therapy with sessions with family of origin. In Gurman A, Kniskern D (eds): Handbook of Family Therapy. New York, Brunner/Mazel, 1981

28. Lewin K: Field Theory in Social Science. New York, Harper & Bros, 1951

29. Bion WR: Group dynamics: A re-view. Int J Psychoanal 33:235–247, 1952

30. Foulkes SH: Therapeutic Group Analysis. New York, International Universities Press, 1964

31. Slavson SR, Schiffer M: Group Psychotherapies for Children. New York, International Universities Press, 1975

32. Wolf A: The psychoanalysis of groups. In Rosenbaum M, Berger M (eds): Group Psychotherapy and Group Function. New York, Basic Books, 1963

33. Frances A, Clarkin JF, Marachi J: Selection criteria for group therapy. Hosp Community Psychiatry 31:245–250, 1980

9

James H. Kocsis and J. John Mann

Drug Treatment of Personality Disorders and Neuroses

Recent introduction of potentially effective therapeutic interventions for psychiatric conditions classified as "personality disorders" and "neuroses" has stirred up a good deal of attention and controversy. Development of effective treatments makes reliable and valid diagnoses in these areas of more than academic concern.

There have been considerable problems because of the lack of generally accepted criteria for many of these conditions, of obvious overlap among them, and of absence of demonstrable predictive validity for many of the diagnoses. Undoubtedly, development of operational criteria for diagnosis, as exemplified by the *Diagnostic and Statistical Manual of Mental Disorders* (*DSM-III*), and preliminary reports of effectiveness for psychotherapeutic, behavioral, and pharmacologic approaches to treatment, will prompt further scientific and clinical advances in these areas and redress some of the existing problems in the near future.

As a general principle, however, it is not always necessary to have a valid diagnosis in order to initiate effective treatment. Certain guidelines can be outlined that can help clinicians in conducting treatment trials, pharmacologic or otherwise, for these disorders. In the following sections we will discuss types or subtypes of personality disorders or "neuroses" for which drug treatments have been reported to have efficacy. *DSM-III* diagnostic nomenclature will be employed. Other types (*e.g.*, narcissistic or masochistic personality disorders) are not discussed because they have not as yet been suggested to have effective pharmacologic therapies. It is important for clinicians to learn about these subtypes and to make efforts to apply medications only when indicated. Furthermore, it is clear that certain drugs may have higher therapeutic indices or possess less potential risk for serious adverse effects such as addiction or tardive dyskinesia. These issues should be considered in evaluating possible drug trials. Perhaps most important as a general issue is that careful accounting of target symptoms or behaviors be made prior to initiating therapy, that changes in these be carefully measured over time, and that the need for continuing drug therapy be evaluated and reevaluated on this basis. More important than avoidance of exposing patients to ineffective treatments is the importance of discontinuing potentially toxic treatments that are ineffective.

With these general considerations as background, the following sections are intended to guide the reader by summarizing existing psychopharmacologic studies of treatment of these conditions and making some practical suggestions relevant to the decision to treat and to the management of specific disorders.

We will discuss only aspects of diagnosis that pertain to making a decision about indications for pharmacologic treatment. Similarly, details about dosing and other practical issues of drug trials will not be given, unless they differ from standard practice for these medications. More extensive descriptions of various personality disorders and "neuroses," as well as the various psychotropic medications, are included in other chapters in this text.

Borderline Personality Disorder

The diagnosis of borderline personality disorder (BPD) has been used to refer to the chronic presence in adult life of various syndromes of disturbance in behavior, affect, and interpersonal relationships. Although in quite popular clinical use in recent years, considerable controversy has been focused on the nature and significance of this diagnosis. An important aspect of these controversies has been the question of degree of overlap both with other personality disorder diagnoses and with major functional psychoses (i.e., schizophrenia and affective disorders). It seems reasonable at present to view BPD as described in *DSM-III* as a heterogeneous group of conditions and not as a distinct entity. It is certain that manifestations of these disorders show considerable interindividual variability. Such considerations are important background to an examination of the potential role of psychotropic agents in the treatment of BPD.

Thus far, few studies have been conducted on the use of drugs for treatment of BPD. Some of these have been motivated by observations of similarities between BPD patients and patients with functional psychotic disorders or by hypotheses that a particular affective state or behavior (e.g., depression or aggressive outbursts) would be improved by the drug therapy being instituted. Other studies have included patients with BPD among populations of psychiatric patients being examined for effectiveness of various drug therapies. In the latter category is the study of Klein,[1] who randomly assigned 295 inpatients to placebo, imipramine, or chlorpromazine regardless of diagnosis. Although conducted prior to the development of *DSM-III* criteria, two groups, those with "pseudoneurotic schizophrenia" and those with "character disorders," appear to overlap with the *DSM-III* description of BPD. Pseudoneurotic schizophrenics were reported to respond significantly more favorably to imipramine but not to chlorpromazine than to placebo, although the magnitude of the difference was quite modest. Patients with character disorders as a group responded more favorably to chlorpromazine, particularly those in the "emotionally unstable" subgroup. A small subgroup of "retarded" character disorders responded favorably to imipramine.

Brinkley and co-workers[2] published a report of five cases of BPD, diagnosed by criteria similar to those of *DSM-III*, who were helped by low-dose treatment with various antipsychotic drugs. They noted improvement especially in patients who demonstrated mild forms of thought disorder or brief psychotic episodes, which presumably places them on the "schizotypal" end of the borderline spectrum. They also noted the importance of careful dosage titration, their patients' intolerance of side-effects when doses are too high, and a preference for high-potency antipsychotic agents.

Klein and colleagues[3-5] have suggested that subgroups of BPD patients who may respond to various pharmacologic interventions can be recognized by certain clinical characteristics. Thus "emotionally labile" inpatients have been found, in a double-blind, placebo-controlled trial, to respond to lithium carbonate with dampening of their mood swings.[6] Another subgroup of so-called rejection-sensitive or "hysteroid dysphorias" have been described as responsive to the monoamine oxidase (MAO) inhibitor phenelzine but not to imipramine.

Finally, in a series of studies conducted by Wender and associates,[7,8] it has been found that a group of patients with "attention deficit disorder" and a history of childhood "hyperactivity" responded favorably to treatment with the psychostimulant drugs pemoline and methylphenidate. Although it is specified that patients fulfilling *DSM-III* criteria for BPD were excluded from this study, it is stated that many seem similar to patients with "emotionally unstable character disorders" as described by Rifkin and co-workers[6] and to patients with "atypical" depression. This raises the possibility that there may be some overlap between BPD and "attention deficit disorder." In instances of BPD in which attention-deficit symptoms exist and childhood hyperactivity has been present, intervention using psychostimulant drugs might be considered.

Based on the previously detailed considerations and available research data certain recommendations can be made for drug therapy of BPD. It is important to maintain awareness that many BPD patients are refractory to any form of intervention, somatic or behavioral, and that BPD probably represents a heterogeneous group of disorders overlapping with other personality disorders and functional psychotic states. In instances where certain target symptoms are present for which drug treatments have been reported to have efficacy, a trial of such treatment may be undertaken. It is important to document pretreatment target symptoms, monitor clinical change, and discontinue drug therapy if no significant improvement occurs. Subtypes of BPD that have been suggested to be responsive to drug intervention (and the indicated drugs) include pseudoneurotic schizophrenia (imipramine), schizotypal disorders (low doses of antipsychotic drugs), emotionally labile character disorders (chlorpromazine, lithium), hysteroid dysphorics (MAO inhibitors), and adults with attention deficit disorders and history of childhood hyperactivity (psychostimulants).

Experienced clinicians may have strong opinions about potential side-effects and toxicities, including psychological side-effects, from administration of drugs to these patients; however, little systematic data have as yet been gathered to address these issues. Clinical wisdom would dictate a healthy degree of skepticism and a watchful attitude toward the possibility that some patients with BPD may react badly to the "drug-taking" experience. However, with sufficient attention to diagnostic subgroups and careful pharmacologic management, it is likely that a considerable number of patients with BPD may benefit at certain times and to some degree from medication trials. Because of the chronicity of these disorders and the tendency of these patients to be intolerant to side-effects, doses of most psychotropics should be increased more slowly and may be generally lower than for treatment of psychotic states.

Antisocial Personality Disorder

Many of the same general considerations that apply to pharmacotherapy of BPD pertain to antisocial personality disorders (APD). Antisocial behavioral syndromes are heterogeneous and overlap with other personality disorder diagnoses, neurologic conditions, and major functional psychotic disorders. APDs are generally characterized by early age at onset, chronicity, and some incidence of spontaneous remission during adult life. Although certain subtypes of APD may be helped by pharmacotherapy, drug abuse and noncompliance are major obstacles.

The medical and psychiatric literature contains numerous anecdotal and uncontrolled reports, as well as a small number of controlled systematic studies, of pharmacologic interventions for patients who have been described as being within the purview of the APD concept. These can be roughly divided into three categories: (1) those focusing on hostility, aggression, and impulsive behavior; (2) those pertaining to persistence of syndromes akin to childhood "hyperactivity" or "minimal brain dysfunction"; and (3) those involving abnormalities of an electroencephalogram in conjunction with behavioral disturbance.

Lithium and neuroleptics have shown some usefulness in the management of patients with hostile, aggressive, or "explosive" behavioral syndromes. Sheard and associates[9] randomly assigned aggressive, acting-out prisoners to lithium carbonate or placebo and found a marked reduction in "infractions" during a 3-month, double-blind trial in the lithium-treated subjects only. Among neuroleptic

drugs, thioridazine has been recommended for treatment of aggression because of few side-effects and low potential for tardive dyskinesia, although presumably all antipsychotic drugs might be expected to be equally effective for this purpose. Patients with personality disorders can be expected to be particularly intolerant to side-effects of these drugs, and compliance is a major issue. These considerations generally would dictate use of doses considerably below those used for treatment of schizophrenia. Presence of seizure disorder or epileptic focus on an electroencephalogram would constitute relative contraindications to the use of lithium or neuroleptics for such patients.

Wender and associates[7,8] have reported the effectiveness of psychostimulants (methylphenidate, pemoline) in the management of patients with "attention deficit disorder" and history of childhood "hyperactivity." Many of the characteristics described for this patient population, such as impulsivity, stress intolerance, impaired interpersonal relationships, and inability to complete tasks, overlap with characteristics of APD. Therefore it seems reasonable to attempt this type of therapy in selected cases.[10] History of stimulant abuse and prominent aggression should be considered relative contraindications to such a trial.

Use of anticonvulsant drugs for treatment of behavior disorders with and without electroencephalographic abnormalities has been well reviewed.[11,12] The weight of evidence tends to suggest a role for carbamazepine in the management of paroxysmal behavior disturbances, especially in epileptics. The only antiepileptic drug to be studied in controlled trials for treatment of aggression and hostility in delinquents and sociopathic personalities has been phenytoin. Although reported effective in several anecdotal and open studies, phenytoin has not outperformed a placebo in controlled studies. Benzodiazepines may also be useful for paroxysmal behavioral disturbances of ictal origin, although their abuse potential must be considered. Finally, recent case reports have suggested a role for beta-adrenergic blocking agents such as propranolol in patients with episodic aggression.[13]

In summary, APD syndromes are heterogeneous and often poorly responsive to any form of intervention. Subgroups of APD for which drugs may have a role (and the indicated drugs) include hostile, aggressive, "explosive" types (lithium, neuroleptics), those with adult "attention deficit" disorders and history of childhood "hyperactivity" (psychostimulants), and those with seizure disturbances (anticonvulsants, benzodiazepines). It is important to document pretreatment target symptoms, monitor clinical change, and discontinue treatment if no significant improvement occurs. Numerous obstacles and relative contraindications should be kept in mind with regard to the drug treatment of APD. These include noncompliance, drug abuse, the tendency of some drugs to lower seizures thresholds, and the possible paradoxic aggravation of target behaviors by the drugs.

Schizotypal and Paranoid Personality Disorders

Schizotypal and paranoid personality disorders have received relatively little recent systematic investigation. Data are sparse about course, family history, and prevalence, and we know of no studies of drug therapy for these disorders. The point is made in *DSM-III*[14] that it is unclear whether these conditions should be considered to be formes fruste of paranoid schizophrenia and other more severe psychotic conditions or whether they are stable personality configurations that should be regarded as distinct entities and unlikely to progress to more severe forms.

In terms of pharmacologic interventions, Klein and co-workers[5] have suggested a possible role for antipsychotic drugs to reduce referential ideas and psychoticlike symptoms in paranoid and schizoid personality disorders. We agree that this possibility makes sense, and it is supported by the case reports of Brinkley and associates,[2] who found "schizotypal" borderlines to be helped by low doses of antipsychotic drugs. Similarly, an open trial of low doses of haloperidol in 13 schizotypal patients diagnosed according to *DSM-III* criteria found improvement in schizotypal symptoms.[15] This question deserves further investigation in other patient samples in placebo-controlled trials.

Depressive Personality (Dysthymic Disorder, Depressive Neurosis, Chronic Depression)

Chronic depression or dysphoria is common among patients presenting for psychiatric treatment. One recent epidemiologic survey found a 5% incidence of depressive personality.[16] It is likely that chronic dysphoria may present as a feature of several types of psychiatric disorders including primary affective illnesses, personality disorders, chronic stress reactions and depressions secondary to severe chronic medical illnesses, or other primary psychiatric disorders such as alcoholism or schizophrenia. Review of the psychiatric literature reveals few systematic studies of the clinical characteristics or treatment of chronic depression.

Chodoff used the term *depressive personality* to refer to personality characteristics such as oral or obsessional traits that predisposed to clinical depression.[17] Schildkraut and Klein delineated two types of chronic dysphoria. *Chronic characterologic depression* is seen as an inherent part of a life-long personality problem in which minor stresses precipitate depressive symptomatology. A specific type of character pathology is not viewed as necessary, but the diagnosis is based on a characteristic symptom pattern (*i.e.*, reactivity, demanding manipulativeness, irritability, self-pity, and lack of vegetative symptoms). A second type of chronic dysphoria, which they call *demoralization,* is seen as a chronic attitude of helplessness in the face of even normal life tasks, which stems from real experiences of life defeat (including repeated episodes of psychiatric illness), again without vegetative symptoms.[18] Akiskal and co-workers have pointed out a number of characteristics shared by both a subgroup of chronic depressives and patients with primary affective disorders, including favorable response to antidepressant medications. They have proposed that some chronic depressives have milder or subaffective forms of unipolar depression, in the same sense in which cyclothymic personality can be considered to represent an attenuated form of bipolar disorder.[19] This conceptualization heavily influenced the inclusion of chronic mild depression under the term "dysthymic disorder" in the affective disorder section of *DSM-III*.[20]

Thus, it appears that chronic depression overlaps with or is superimposed on a number of *DSM-III* Axis I or Axis II diagnoses. Clinicians should pay attention to this issue when formulating treatment plans for such patients. Family history of psychiatric illness and prior responses of patients and family members to psychotropic drugs may provide additional clues when deciding on pharmacologic approaches.

Several recent studies have reported efficacy of antidepressant medications for treatment of chronic depression.[19,21,22] Numerous types of tricyclics and monoamine oxidase (MAO) inhibitors, as well as lithium, have been employed. Although a substantial portion of chronic depressives appear to respond to drug therapy, specificity of any particular drug for this purpose has not been established. According to Akiskal and co-workers, favorable response predictors include family history of affective illness and a prior history of typical episodes of affective disorders in the patient. Substance abuse and "unstable" personality characteristics, on the other hand, tend to predict poor response to drugs. Dosages used for this kind of patient have been generally equivalent to those used for typical depression.

Finally, although it is discussed elsewhere in this volume, we will say a word about brief reactive, nonendogenous or neurotic episodes of depression. Such conditions should be distinguished from acute endogenous depression (major depression with melancholia) and chronic depression (dysthymic disorder). Generally speaking, no drug therapy is indicated for brief reactive depression. An exception to this may be the recurrent tendency to develop depression in response to romantic rejection, which has been labelled as rejection-sensitive or "hysteroid" dysphoria by Klein.[4] Such patients may benefit from prophylactic therapy with the MAO inhibitor, phenelzine, in doses of 45 mg to 60 mg per day.

Generalized Anxiety Disorder

Generalized anxiety disorder (GAD), a primary disorder occurring in the absence of panic attacks, a depressive disorder, obsessive-compulsive disorder, other major psychiatric disorder, or some situational stress, usually presents to family practitioners rather than in hospital or office psychiatric practice. In fact, it is difficult to find systematic studies confirming GAD as a primary disorder.

The role of pharmacotherapy in this condition is to provide transient relief while nonpharmacologic treatments are used to achieve longer term or more lasting benefit.

Almost all classes of psychotropic drugs have been used to treat GAD. Among the earliest classes of medication used were the barbiturates. Disadvantages of this group of drugs include the potential for tolerance and dependency, an abstinence syndrome, and the danger of overdosage.

More recently the benzodiazepines have been widely used for treatment of GAD. These drugs have been shown in controlled studies to be effective compared with a placebo. They vary principally with respect to half-life and the tendency for accumulation. They are less prone to produce tolerance and dependency than barbiturates, although the risk is still present. They are safer in overdosage than barbiturates. Because of the potential for tolerance and dependency, it is suggested that the period of use of these drugs should be less than 8 to 12 weeks. Although some anxiety relief is often prompt, within 1 to 2 hours, benefit may increase over the first 3 to 5 days of usage. Most benzodiazepines are metabolized to methyldiazepam, a long-acting benzodiazepine, and should therefore be prescribed only once or twice daily. These drugs should not routinely be taken more frequently than three times daily, particularly in the elderly, because of the risk that the drug may accumulate and result in excessively high plasma and tissue levels. The benzodiazepines should be tapered slowly in patients treated for longer than 3 to 4 weeks to avoid withdrawal symptoms such as irritability, agitation, and psychophysiologic symptoms.

Because of concern over the potential for dependency on minor tranquilizers, clinicians have explored other alternatives. The tricyclic antidepressants, particularly those with greater sedative properties such as doxepin and amitriptyline, have been used as minor tranquilizers. There are controlled studies demonstrating tricyclic antidepressants to be as effective as benzodiazepines for GAD.[23]

Another alternative drug class has been the antipsychotic agents. Low doses of drugs such as chlorpromazine, trifluoperazine, and haloperidol have been prescribed for GAD. However, placebo-controlled studies do not support their use as anxiolytics,[24] and their neurotoxic potential makes them undesirable for this use.

Newer nonbenzodiazepine drugs with anxiolytic properties are urgently required. Buspirone may be one such drug. Its mechanism of action is unclear. It acts on the dopaminergic system as a mixed agonist-antagonist. However, it is a proven effective anxiolytic in placebo-controlled studies, with comparable efficacy to the benzodiazepines and, thus far, no evidence of tolerance or withdrawal effects. Clearly more studies are required to evaluate the presence or absence of the potential for tolerance and dependency with buspirone, which is not marketed in the United States.

Propranolol may have a beneficial effect for some patients. Its other main area of application has been in social phobias.[25]

Clonidine is of theoretic interest only since it has been found in pilot studies to have transient benefit for both panic attacks and anxiety.[24,26]

Panic Disorder and Agoraphobia with Panic Attacks

Panic disorder and agoraphobia with panic attacks are grouped together because the principal difference between them is the presence of widespread avoidance behavior involving a significant impairment of the patient's ability to travel outside the home.

Two classes of drugs have been shown in multiple controlled studies to be effective for the treatment of panic attacks: the MAO inhibitors and the tricyclic antidepressants.[27–33]

The tricyclic antidepressants desipramine and imipramine have been most widely studied. The dose range is similar to that used in depression, 150 mg to 300 mg/day. Often it is necessary to begin with a lower dose, such as 25 mg or 50 mg/day, because some of these patients are exquisitely sensitive to side-effects such as anticholinergic effects, feeling stimulated, or paradoxic insomnia. In such patients escalation of the dose should proceed slowly. It is occasionally worthwhile to check the plasma level of the drug to verify that the patient is not a slow metabolizer with excessive levels of drug on a low oral dose. It takes 2 to 6 weeks to see a beneficial effect.

In some patients, benefit may take months to appear. Since this condition tends to wax and wane, it is not clear in the latter cases whether there was a definite pharmacologic effect. These drugs can abolish or reduce the frequency of the panic attacks and/or ameliorate the severity of attacks that may occur. In the latter case the patient will often say that he feels the symptoms of panic attack begin but it does not progress to a full-blown panic attack.

Controlled clinical trials have verified the efficacy of imipramine and desipramine in panic disorder. Similar studies have not been published for most of the other tricyclic antidepressants, and thus their relative efficacy is an open question.

The MAO inhibitors are at least as effective as tricyclic antidepressants for the treatment of panic attacks. The dose range of the MAO inhibitors is the same as for depression (*e.g.*, 45 mg to 90 mg/day for phenelzine). Although controversial, it does not appear that the efficacy of MAO inhibitors and tricyclic antidepressants in treating panic attacks can be related directly to an antidepressant effect in these patients,[24,34] since these drugs were shown to be effective in a patient population that excluded significantly depressed patients.[35] As with the tricyclic agents it takes several weeks for the full therapeutic effect of MAO inhibitors to develop.

Control of the panic attacks is only part of the treatment for agoraphobia. The anticipatory anxiety and avoidance behavior that develop secondarily to the panic attacks must also be treated. Tricyclic antidepressants and MAO inhibitors have some effect, but sometimes benzodiazepines are required in addition. Avoidance behavior is best managed by nonpharmacologic means, which is discussed elsewhere in this text.

Other drugs that have been examined for the treatment of panic disorder include alprazolam, a triazolo-benzodiazepine[36]; propranolol[18]; the major tranquilizers; and the new generation antidepressants, such as buproprion, trazodone, and fluoxetine. Preliminary studies show propranolol, antipsychotics, and buproprion to be ineffective. Further controlled studies proving the efficacy of alprazolam, propranolol, trazodone, and fluoxetine are required; therefore these medications are not currently first-line drugs in the treatment of panic attacks.

Agoraphobia Without Panic Attacks

Whether agoraphobia without panic attacks responds to MAO inhibitors or tricyclic antidepressants is not settled, and the literature is in disagreement. Nevertheless a trial of tricyclic agents or MAO inhibitors seems indicated since these medications do not carry the risk of dependency. It may be argued that tricyclic antidepressants and MAO inhibitors work best by controlling panic attacks and therefore have little role in this disorder. This is an oversimplification. It is not uncommon to find that such patients actually do experience panic attacks that are either atypical or poorly described by the patient, who may not be a good historian. Second, both tricyclic antidepressants and MAO inhibitors do appear to relieve the anticipatory anxiety as well as the panic attacks. Thus there is a potential role for these drugs in this condition. Behavior modification is the appropriate alternative to pharmacologic treatment in agoraphobia without panic attacks since it is the superior treatment of avoidance behavior, which is the predominent psychopathology in this condition.[37] Furthermore, there may be a significantly lower rate of relapse after behavior therapy than after medication.[37,38]

Although behavioral treatment is equally effective in agoraphobic patients with high or lower anxiety levels, this treatment is less effective in patients with significant associated depression. In these patients, antidepressants should be combined with behavior modification.

Social Phobias

Social phobias include fear associated with public speaking, performing, eating, urinating, and so on. Two classes of drugs are most commonly prescribed: the benzodiazepines and propranolol. Their efficacy has been confirmed by controlled studies. Propranolol seems to help the physiologic concomitants of anxiety rather than the affect itself.[25] Propranolol, given in doses of 20 mg to 40 mg, acts within 30 minutes, and the benefit lasts 4 to 6 hours. Artists and public speakers may derive considerable benefit from low doses of beta-adrenergic blockers taken 30 minutes before a performance or speech. Behavioral treatments may also be effective for social phobias.

Simple Phobias

Simple phobias involve fear of common objects such as spiders, snakes, and mice. Medication has little specific role to play in their management.[39]

Obsessive-Compulsive Disorders

Two treatment modalities have been shown to be effective in the traditionally treatment-resistant obsessive-compulsive disorders (OCD): (1) behavior therapy involving exposure and response-prevention[40,41] and (2) antidepressants.[41-44]

Although anecdotal case reports suggest that a number of tricyclic antidepressants, MAO inhibitors, and perhaps electroconvulsive therapy (ECT) may be effective for OCD, the relatively limited number of studies carried out have largely involved one tricyclic antidepressant, clomipramine.

Clomipramine has been shown to be effective for OCD in controlled studies.[42,44] Other antidepressants, particularly those with serotonergic effects, may also be effective.[43] Doses employed in the treatment of OCD are similar to those used for depressive disorders. As in the case of panic disorders, this raises the question of whether these somatic treatments work because of their effect on an associated depressive disorder or whether they work independently and specifically on the OCD.[44] The time course for response of obsessional symptoms to drug treatment may actually be slightly longer than that for depressive symptoms in the same patient.[44] Furthermore, there does not seem to be a clear correlation between the degree of amelioration of obsessional symptoms and the amelioration of depressive symptoms. Thus, available data suggest a dissociation between the pharmacologic effects on obsessional symptoms versus depressive symptoms. Further studies are required to test this point. In summary, tricyclic antidepressants such as clomipramine appear to be indicated in OCD, even in the absence of significant depression. In the United States clomipramine is not a marketed antidepressant. Therefore, largely based on clinical impression we suggest the use of imipramine or amitriptyline for OCD. The usual antidepressant dose range should be used.

Although behavioral techniques are effective for OCD, their efficacy is reduced in the presence of significant depression.[37] In such patients, tricyclic antidepressants are therefore more clearly the treatment of first choice or at least should be combined with behavioral treatments.

Posttraumatic Stress Disorder

At least two open studies in the literature describe beneficial results in posttraumatic stress disorder with the use of MAO inhibitors. Therefore, when symptoms do not appear to be abating with time, a trial of an MAO inhibitor may be warranted. The usual antidepressant doses are given, and benefit may take 1 to 3 weeks and longer in isolated cases to appear.

Acute Conversion Disorder

Treatment and diagnosis of this condition involve anxiety-reducing strategies such as minor tranquilizers or hypnosis combined with suggestion, interpretation, or direction. There is a lack of data from controlled studies involving minor tranquilizers. However, rapid improvement has been reported after the administration of intravenous amytal combined with an interpretative and directive-oriented interview.[45,46] It is not clear that this strategy is superior to the use of hypnosis other than the fact that not all clinicians are well trained in hypnosis.

Oral use of benzodiazepines is probably just as effective as intravenous sodium amytal, although, it is clearly a less dramatic form of treatment. The use of benzodiazepines should aim for initial acute anxiety control through use of, for example, 5 mg to 20 mg of diazepam orally. Initial dosage depends on the patient's level of anxiety, recent level of sedative or alcohol use, medical health, and age. When the patient appears relaxed, a psychotherapeutic interview process is essential to abolish the conversion symptom. There may be no need for further medication unless the patient's recovery is partial or if symptoms return. In that event, the procedure is repeated. Benzodiazepine use should be limited to several acute doses. Longer term treatment must address the characterological and social issues that combined to generate the acute conversion symptoms.

REFERENCES

1. Klein DR: Importance of psychiatric diagnosis in prediction of clinical drug effects. Arch Gen Psychiatry 16:118–126, 1967
2. Brinkley JR, Beitman BD, Friedel RO: Low-dose neuroleptic regimens in the treatment of borderline patients. Arch Gen Psychiatry 36:319–326, 1979
3. Klein DF: Pharmacologic treatment and delineation of borderline disorders. In Hartocollis P (ed): Borderline Personality Disorders, pp 365–384. New York, International Universities Press, 1977
4. Klein DF, Shader RI: The borderline state: Pharmacologic treatment approaches to the undiagnosed case. In Shader RI (ed): Manual of Psychiatric Therapeutics, pp 281–293. Boston, Little, Brown & Co, 1975
5. Klein DF, Gittelman R, Quitkin F et al: Diagnosis and Drug Treatment of Psychiatric Disorders, 2nd ed, pp 568–571. Baltimore, Williams & Wilkins, 1980
6. Rifkin A, Quitkin F, Carillo C et al: Lithium carbonate in emotionally unstable character disorders. Arch Gen Psychiatry 27:519–523, 1972

7. Wood DR, Reimherr FW, Wender PW et al: Diagnosis and treatment of minimal brain dysfunction in adults: A preliminary report. Arch Gen Psychiatry 33:1453–1460, 1976
8. Wender PH, Reimherr FW, Wood DR: Attention deficit disorder ("minimal brain dysfunction") in adults. Arch Gen Psychiatry 38:449–456, 1981
9. Sheard MH, Marini JL, Bridges CI et al: The effect of lithium on impulsive aggressive behavior in man. Am J Psychiatry 133:1409–1413, 1976
10. Stinger AY, Josef NC: Methylphenidate in the treatment of aggression in two patients with antisocial personality disorder. Am J Psychiatry 140:1365–1366, 1983
11. Cloninger CR: Antisocial behavior. In Hippuns H, Winokur G (eds): Psychopharmacology, Part 2, Clinical Psychopharmacology, chap 25. Amsterdam, Excerpts Medica, 1983
12. Kellner R, Rada RT: Pharmacotherapy of personality disorders. In Davis JM, Greenblatt D (eds): Psychopharmacology Update: New and Neglected Areas, chap 3. New York, Grune & Stratton, 1979
13. Ratey JJ, Morill R, Oxenkrug G: Use of propranolol for provoked and unprovoked episodes of rage. Am J Psychiatry 140:1356–1357, 1983
14. Diagnostic and Statistical Manual of Mental Disorders, 3rd ed, pp 307–311. Washington, DC, American Psychiatric Association, 1980
15. Hymowitz P: Unpublished study, 1983
16. Weissman MM, Myers JK: Affective disorders in a US urban community. Arch Gen Psychiatry 25:1304–1311, 1978
17. Chodoff P: The depressive personality. Arch Gen Psychiatry 27:666–673, 1972
18. Schildkraut JJ, Klein DF: The classification and treatment of depressive disorders. In Shader RI (ed): Manual of Psychiatric Therapeutics, pp 39–61. Little, Brown and Co, Boston, 1975
19. Akiskal HS, Rosenthal TL, Haykal RF, et al: Characterologic depression. Arch Gen Psychiatry 37:777–783, 1980
20. Frances A: DMS-III personality disorders section, commentary. Arch J Psychiatry 137:1050–1054, 1980
21. Ward NG, Bloom VL, Friedel RO: The effectiveness of tricyclic antidepressants in chronic depression. J Clin Psychiatry 40:1–4, 1979
22. Rounsaville BJ, Sholomskas D, Prusoff BA: Chronic mood disorders in depressed outpatients. J Affective Disord 2:73–88, 1980
23. McNair DM, Kahn EJ: Imipramine vs. a benzodiazepine for agoraphobia. In Klein DF, Rabkin JG (eds): Anxiety: New Research and Changing Concepts, pp 69–80. New York, Raven Press, 1981
24. Klein DF: Medication in the treatment of panic attacks and phobic states. Psychopharmacol Bull 18:85–90, 1982
25. Cole JO, Altesman RI, Weingarten CH: Beta-blocking drugs in psychiatry: Psychopharmacological update. McLean Hosp J 4:40–68, 1979
26. Hoehn-Saric R, Merchant AF, Keyser ML et al: Effects of clonidine on anxiety disorders. Arch Gen Psychiatry 38:1278–1282, 1981
27. King A: Phenelzine treatment of Roth's calamity syndrome. Med J Aust 6:879–883, 1962
28. Zitrin CM, Klein DF, Woerner M: Behavior therapy, supportive psychotherapy, imipramine, and phobias. Arch Gen Psychiatry 35:307–316, 1978
29. Tyrer P, Candy J, Kelly D: A study of the clinical effects of

phenelzine and placebo in the treatment of phobic anxiety. Psychopharmacologia 32:237–254, 1973

30. Klein DF, Fink M: Psychiatric reaction patterns to imipramine. Am J Psychiatry 119:432–438, 1962

31. Kelly D, Guirguis W, Frommer E et al: Treatment of phobic states with antidepressants. Br J Psychiatry 116:387–398, 1971

32. Mountjoy CQ, Roth M, Garside RF et al: A clinical trial of phenelzine in anxiety depressive and phobic neuroses. Br J Psychiatry 131:486–492, 1977

33. Sheehan DV, Ballenger J, Jacobsen G: Treatment of endogenous anxiety with phobic, hysterical, and hypochondriacal symptoms. Arch Gen Psychiatry 37:51–59, 1980

34. Marks IM: Are there anticompulsive or antiphobic drugs? Psychopharmacol Bull 18:78–84, 1982

35. Zitrin CM, Klein DF, Woerner MG: Treatment of agoraphobia with group exposure *in vivo* and imipramine. Arch Gen Psychiatry 37:63–72, 1980

36. Sheehan DV: Panic disorders: A treatment overview. Presented at the Annual Meeting of the American Psychiatric Association, Toronto, Canada, 1982

37. Mavissakalian M, Michelson L: Agoraphobia: Behavioral and pharmacological treatments, preliminary outcome, and process findings. Psychopharmacol Bull 18:91–103, 1982

38. Tyrer P, Steinberg D: Symptomatic treatment of agoraphobia and social phobias: A follow-up study. Br J Psychiatry 127:163–168, 1975

39. Klein DF, Gittelman R, Quitkin FM et al: Diagnosis of anxiety, personality, somatoform, and factitious disorders. In Diagnosis and Drug Treatment of Psychiatric Disorders: Adults and Children, pp 493–521. Baltimore, Williams & Wilkins, 1980

40. Foa EB, Goldstein A: Continuous exposure and complete response prevention treatment of obsessive-compulsive neurosis. Behav Ther 9:821–830, 1978

41. Marks IM, Stern RS, Mawson D et al: Clomipramine and exposure for obsessive-compulsive rituals. Br J Psychiatry 136:1–25, 1980

42. Thoren P, Asberg M, Cronholm B et al: Clomipramine treatment of obsessive-compulsive disorder: A controlled clinical trial. Arch Gen Psychiatry 37:1281–1289, 1980

43. Insel TR, Murphy DL: The psychopharmacological treatment of obsessive-compulsive disorder: A review. J Clin Psychopharm 1:304–311, 1981

44. Insel TR, Alterman I, Murphy DL: Antiobsessional and antidepressant effects of clomipramine in the treatment of obsessive-compulsive disorder. Psychopharmacol Bull 18:115–117, 1982

45. Lambert C, Rees WL: Intravenous barbiturates in the treatment of hysteria. Br Med J 2:70–73, 1944

46. Maris DP: Intravenous barbiturates: An aid in the diagnosis and treatment of conversion hysteria and malingering. Military Surgeon 96:509–513, 1945

Psychotherapy Outcome Research

The contemporary course of psychotherapy outcome research has been characterized by two parallel yet seemingly incongruent developments: (1) increased conceptual and methodologic sophistication and (2) increased skepticism regarding the meaningfulness of the accumulating mass of assessment evidence. The general field of psychotherapy—research and practice—now is confronted by an undeniable crisis of credibility, and research evidence has not served to reduce it. Indeed, recent research reports claiming to demonstrate psychotherapy's promiscuously positive effects appear, instead, to have exacerbated latent skepticism and incredulity.

Over the past 10 to 15 years, the field of psychotherapy research has been the beneficiary of such useful technical advances as a revised and potentially more reliable diagnostic classification scheme,[1] more useful research instruments,[2–4] and improved individualized measures.[5] With the development of treatment "manuals" describing the critical and differentiating elements of therapies it has become more feasible to train therapists to predetermined criterion levels of mastery and to increase the opportunities for replication of treatment assessment studies. Expanded knowledge of the biochemical and genetic predispositions, bases, concomitants, and consequences of mental disorders permits a broader range of interventions and measurements of effective treatment.[6,7] Among the conceptual advances, two are particularly noteworthy: investigators of both outcome and process research have all but abandoned their earlier search for single variables to explain the complex phenomena of treatment and its effects; however, the change that is potentially of most significance is the greater willingness of researchers representing all schools of psychotherapy to draw on insights derived from the full range of psychotherapies. Such pooling of knowledge promises to advance understanding and, thereby, ultimately to increase the efficacy of psychotherapy.[8–10]

Seemingly independent of these advances, a usually well-mannered internecine struggle continues between the psychotherapy researcher and practitioner. As in all fields of health care, research on the efficacy of treatments is more avidly pursued by the innovators of new treatments than by the practitioners of "established" and "accepted" ones. With the advent of militant behavior therapy, and more recently cognitive therapy, the hegemony of the preceding psychologic treatment approaches has been challenged. The new schools of psychotherapy earnestly set about to supplant what they perceive to be an era of mysticism, superstition, and outright buffoonery by attempting to enlighten through the use of rigorous experimental science and its products—hard evidence. Their influence has also resulted in some refinements in at least a small portion of research in psychodynamic therapies.

Psychodynamically oriented therapy, despite its initial aspirations to establish itself as a behavioral science, has rarely found experimental evidence as compelling as the authority of its "standard and accepted" theories and practices. A shadowlike struggle between the old and the new therapies is acknowledged but never fully joined. Although a steady stream of research reports on behavior therapy spewed from the battlements of academia's ivory towers, the psychodynamic protagonists on the whole have chosen not to respond with their own research findings, electing instead to catapult heavy slogans. Ultimately, the battle of words counterposed the antagonists' preferred values and concepts. What more congenial weapons for psychotherapists?

Epithets such as these were regularly exchanged: reality versus symbols, determinism versus freedom, events versus meanings, logic versus intuition, standardization versus spontaneity, and measurement versus understanding. The wisdom of seeking valid explanations of meanings, purposes, and motives by means of intuition and inference was pitted against the logic of seeking to isolate utility and "cause" by means of measurement and quantification. The scientist-clinician was accused by the practitioner-theoretician of callous disregard for the complexity of psychotherapy and of irreverently attempting to unravel harmonious wholes into arbitrary parts. Investigators who claimed to seek truth by adherence to the tenets of the scientific method were dismissed as simply lacking the imagination to do otherwise.

In turn, practitioners who persisted in describing psychotherapy as consisting primarily of the creative interplay between therapist and patient were charged by critics with merely encouraging their patients to play more imaginatively with their "mental blocks." The war of words continues, but its impact has been slight. Some members of each camp have come to recognize the cogency of some of the criticisms leveled against them, but most prefer to view such commentary as a mischievous test of the strength of their faith.

In this context a large body of controlled research evidence regarding the efficacy of the psychotherapies has emerged. This paper undertakes to summarize such findings and then to identify the major inferences that have been drawn from them. Finally, those inferences are discussed in order to highlight salient research problems that continue to require attention.

Summary of Research Evidence

Findings have been organized to indicate the answers provided to the seven questions most often asked of the field of psychotherapy:

1. Is psychotherapy effective?
2. What forms of psychotherapy are most effective in the treatment of what kinds of problems/patients?
3. Is psychotherapy safe?
4. Is psychotherapy cost-effective?
5. Is there a positive relationship between outcome and length of treatment?
6. Is there a positive relationship between length of therapist experience and outcome?
7. Do the effects of treatment endure?

IS PSYCHOTHERAPY EFFECTIVE?

It is puzzling that after more than 80 years of ever-expanding psychotherapy practice so patently naive a question continues to be raised. Perhaps even more puzzling is the fact that the field continues its efforts seriously to answer it. Other treatment approaches are not similarly importuned. Such undifferentiated and unqualified questions as "Does surgery work?" or "Are drugs effective?" do not invite serious response. Clearly, there is something about the "talking therapies" that provokes a persistent skepticism relieved neither by their reported benefits nor by the authoritative claims of the psychotherapy professions.

The question "Is psychotherapy effective?" implies the erroneous assumption that the field is a homogeneous entity. It is not. Psychotherapy now encompasses about five major theories (psychodynamic, behavioral, cognitive, humanistic-experiential, and transpersonal) and over 250 forms of psychotherapy.[11] These are available for the treatment of over 150 discrete diagnostic categories described in the *Diagnostic and Statistical Manual of Mental Disorders*, 3rd ed (*DSM-III*).[1]

Before examining the responses offered by research to the question "Is psychotherapy effective?" it is appropriate to identify the concerns that provoke the query. The evident disquietude may be traced in part to the earlier equivocal appraisals of psychological treatments.

Prior to the 1970s serious doubts were expressed about whether the effects of psychotherapies then available were demonstrably more beneficial than the effects of "spontaneous remission," that is, the mere passage of time.[12-17] In 1970, however, Meltzoff and Kornreich[18] reviewed 101 studies in order to determine, "Whether or not anyone has been able to demonstrate satisfactorily that individuals with emotional disturbances (of any type) can be more benefited by psychotherapy (of any variety) than by lack of it over the same time span." They found that 80% of the studies yielded positive findings (statistically significant differences in favor of the treated group).

After reviewing 57 studies of psychotherapy outcome, Bergin[19] reported: "It now seems apparent that psychotherapy, as practiced over the past 40 years, has had an average effect that is modestly positive."

Yet another literature review was undertaken by Luborsky and associates[20] in 1975. This survey included psychodynamic, client-centered, and behavior therapies (exclusive of analogue studies or investigations involving volunteer subjects). The "box score" method was used to summarize findings: a frequency tally was made of the number of studies in which (1) significant differences between groups favored the treated group, (2) significant differences favored the comparison group, or (3) no significant differences were found between the treatment and comparison groups. The authors concluded that a "high percentage of patients who go through any of these psychotherapies gain from them."

By 1978 Bergin and Lambert[21] offered their revised estimate of the research evidence and stated that outcome data "look more favorable. . . These findings generally yield clearly positive results when compared with no-treatment, wait-list, and placebo or pseudo-therapies."

For all practical purposes, the fear that psychotherapy effects did not exceed those attributable to spontaneous remission had been set to rest. Psychotherapy is better than its absence!

Of course, none of these surveys escaped criticism. First, each reviewer included studies in accordance with his own highly selective standards of what constituted adequate and appropriate research evidence. In addition, special criticism was leveled at the "box score" method, which had the unfortunate effect of giving equal weight to all studies regardless of the size of the involved samples. This practice failed to correct for the dependence of statistical significance on sample size.[22–24]

Furthermore, despite positive evidence in support of psychotherapy, treatment effects continued to be viewed as clinically insubstantial. As recently as 1979, Frank[25] reexamined the research output and offered the following judgment: "Psychotherapy [is] . . . more effective than informal, unplanned help. Unfortunately . . . these efforts are not impressively more effective." It was not until researchers adopted a new methodology for reviewing and integrating the outcome findings derived from independent studies that the psychotherapy efficacy evidence emerged as impressive.

The new method is meta-analysis, a statistical procedure designed to reduce all measures of outcome to a common metric, thereby permitting the results of independent studies to be combined. The procedure provides statistically defensible bases for estimating the magnitude of the treatment effect (*i.e.*, the effect size). One of the major advantages of this procedure was that it shifted emphasis away from the earlier preoccupation with the assessment of statistical significance of group mean differences to the more clinically relevant concern with determining the magnitude of the effects of treatment. The effect size is expressed in terms of standard deviation units and is independent of the size of the sample on which it is calculated.

The most comprehensive survey of the psychotherapy outcome literature ever undertaken was conducted by Smith and associates[26] using the meta-analysis approach. To avoid the problem of biased selection of studies, they attempted to include all published and unpublished studies that had compared at least one therapy treatment group to an untreated or waiting-list control group or to a different therapy group. They found 475 studies that met this criterion. A total of 1766 separate outcome comparisons were made, and their effect sizes were calculated. These findings are summarized here in conjunction with another recent survey that applied the meta-analysis method to an additional set of outcome studies.

Shapiro and Shapiro[27] adopted more rigorous selection criteria than those used by Smith and co-workers, requiring that eligible studies must have involved the assignment of patients to two or more treatment groups and to one or more control groups. Reviewing research published from 1974 through 1979, the Shapiros identified 143 eligible studies—about 10% of all outcome studies actually published during that interval. Only 21 of the studies identified by the Shapiros overlapped with those of Smith and co-workers. Thus, *in toto*, 597 controlled studies assessing the outcome of the psychotherapies have been analyzed by the meta-analysis procedure.

Based on an examination of the effect sizes calculated (.85 standard deviation units), Smith and co-workers reported that the average person who received therapy was better off (on some outcome measure of well-being) at the end of treatment than were 80% of the patients who did not receive such treatment. When instances of "placebo treatment" and "undifferentiated counseling" were removed from the data set, the average effect size increased, revealing that the average person who receives psychotherapy was better off at the end of it than about 85% of the prospective patients who did not receive such treatment. In effect, patients at the 50th percentile of the untreated population could be expected to rise to the 80th or 85th percentile of that group after undergoing treatment. The results of the Shapiro and Shapiro review of outcome research were even more supportive of the potency of treatment. The mean effect size found in their more carefully controlled sample of studies approached 1 standard deviation unit.

Another yardstick for evaluating the effects of the psychotherapies tested was offered by Rosenthal and Rubin.[28] Their calculations indicate that the psychotherapy effect size reported by Smith and co-workers would be equivalent to reducing an illness or death rate from 66% to 34%. It appears, then, that by any reasonable standard applied to the field of treatment efficacy, the overall therapeutic impact of the psychotherapies tested must be viewed as clinically important.

Do these massive surveys of the best-controlled psychotherapy outcome research finally provide a definitive answer to the layman's question "Is psychotherapy effective?" For reasons to be detailed later, probably not.

WHAT FORMS OF PSYCHOTHERAPY ARE MOST EFFECTIVE IN THE TREATMENT OF WHAT KINDS OF PROBLEMS/PATIENTS?

Adequate research evidence does not now exist on which to base decisions regarding the comparative efficacy of each of the existing psychotherapies in the treatment of each of the problems now deemed eligible for its services. Moreover, it is unlikely that complete and systematic research evidence will ever exist. The methical research approach theoretically would require the testing of each of the various psychotherapies now on the market with each of the more than 150 disorders and problems described by the *DSM-III*. The number of classes of patients and problems accepted for treatment is actually greater than the number catalogued in the *DSM-III* since some therapists treat not just patients suffering from disorders, dysfunctions, and malfunctions but also problems of daily living—miseries of normalcy and the human condition.

If researchers were guided by the simple matrix of 150 disorders and Herink's listing of 250 forms of therapy,[11] approximately 4.7 million separate comparative studies would be required. Of course, this example is facetious. Herink's listing included many "fringe" therapies that are mere curiosities; the numerous professionally recognized therapies could conceivably be grouped into more manage-

able numbers; and the *DSM-III* disorders can be considered in clusters.[29] Nevertheless, any reasonable matrix would still involve thousands of comparisons, and that number would be multiplied manyfold if attempts were made systematically to investigate the effects of varying treatment "dosage" (frequency, length, total duration, maintenance sessions), therapist characteristics (nature and length of training and experience, demographic and personality characteristics), patient characteristics (demographic and personality), treatment settings, test–retest intervals, and the criteria and measures used in assessing change. All of these variables may be critical, since they may greatly influence findings and the conclusions that may be drawn.

On the bases of their reanalyses of outcome research, Smith and co-workers conclude that the reported benefits of psychotherapy are a function of (1) the outcome criteria used, (2) the kind of measuring instruments employed, (3) the time of assessment, and (4) the kinds of patients treated. They found that independent of form of therapy, the largest effects were associated with the measurement of anxiety or fears, global adjustment, emotional-somatic complaints, and vocational or personal development. The smallest treatment effects were found on measures of adjustment, physiologic stress, work or school achievement, and personality traits. The largest treatment effects were routinely associated with (1) measurement by paper-and-pencil questionnaires completed by the patients, (2) measurement of outcome immediately after completion of therapy, and (3) treatment of monosymptomatic phobic or depressed patients.

Since behavior therapies are more likely than verbal therapies to be used to treat monosymptomatic patients, to assess change in terms of what have been identified as the more highly reactive measures, and to make outcome assessments close to the end of therapy, it is not surprising to find reports of the superiority of behavior therapy.[24,30] In the review of Smith and co-workers, when comparisons between behavioral and "verbal" therapies were made on measures that were "less susceptible to influence," the differences observed between these treatment approaches were negligible. Similarly, the findings of Shapiro and Shapiro, when corrected for the nature of the problems treated and the kinds of measures used, revealed that the seeming advantage of behavioral therapies over the nonbehavioral therapies diminished or the results were equivocal.

The meta-analysis finding of "no difference" between therapies is, of course, consistent with the earlier surveys of research based on narrative summaries and "box score" analyses. The consistent finding of comparable effectiveness of the various forms of psychotherapy has been so widely reported (if not universally accepted), that it is referred to as the "Dodo verdict": "Everybody has won and all must have prizes."[20]

The inference that all forms of psychotherapy are equally effective—or, more properly, have not been shown to differ in effectiveness—is derived from research that focuses on the treatment of the following: nonpsychotic depressions, mild-to-moderate anxieties; fears and simple phobias; compulsions; sexual dysfunctions; reactions to life crises of adolescence, midlife, and aging; and problems of everyday life such as vocational and marital adjustment.

With the more severe and chronic disorders we may again find that all forms of psychotherapy are equally effective or, more properly, equally ineffective, for that appears to be the overall assessment in the *Report of the President's Commission on Mental Health.*[31] A few examples from that report are shown in the chart on this page.

Thus, in the collective opinion of a highly qualified panel of experts (clinicians and researchers) the currently available forms of psychotherapy play only a modest role in the treatment of some of the most disabling disorders. Psychotherapies may provide important supportive, habilitative, and rehabilitative functions, but the sizable body of accumulated research evidence has failed to provide useful guidance for the matching of particular therapies for particular problems.

IS PSYCHOTHERAPY SAFE?

As in all forms of treatment, psychotherapy practitioners and professional societies are concerned with offering assurances that their techniques and procedures are safe, but not absolutely safe. To this end they make ostentatious efforts to establish ethical, professional, and technical standards that purport to protect the public interest.

Overall, psychotherapy has devoted more attention to establishing its benefits and to creating mechanisms for protecting the public against harm than to documenting the need for such protections. Its publicly voiced concerns regarding the likelihood of psychonoxious consequences resulting from the bumblings of improperly trained therapists, or the dangers of inappropriate or inadequately administered techniques, are discounted by critics of psychotherapy as evidence of self-aggrandizement and idle puffery.[32,33]

SCHIZOPHRENIA

"Treatment [of schizophrenia] by various types of psychotherapy is as yet of unestablished efficacy, although in combination with drug treatment psychotherapy may facilitate recovery and social adaptation."

ALCOHOLISM

"Follow-up studies generally indicate that failure or success appears independent of the type of treatment received, whether inpatient or outpatient." "It is a general impression that self-help groups such as Alcoholics Anonymous (AA) offer the most successful treatment, but scientific evidence is lacking. What is clear, however, is that many alcoholics are unsuited for AA."

DRUG ABUSE

The effectiveness of psychological treatments independent of drug treatment is not established.

OBSESSIVE-COMPULSIVE DISORDERS

". . . there is very little evidence suggesting that drugs or psychotherapy are successful with severe obsessions or compulsions."

INFANTILE AUTISM

"Clearly, no great or even modest treatment promise can be held by mental health professionals for children with Infantile Autism."

ANTISOCIAL DISORDERS

"So far, short of removal from an antisocial family, no early psychiatric intervention has been shown to alter the course of this serious disorder."

HYPERACTIVE CHILDREN

Behavioral treatment programs have been of some use, but medication has repeatedly been shown to be more effective in dramatically reducing the most disabling symptoms of hyperactive children. "There is no cure nor prevention for the disorder."

For the purposes of this chapter the question regarding the safety of psychotherapy is limited to an inquiry about evidence of the worsening of patients' condition as a direct consequence of having undergone psychotherapy. The scope of inquiry is further limited here by considering empiric studies on only the recognized psychotherapies, excluding encounter groups, growth groups, and so forth.

In 1971, Bergin reported his conclusion, based on a careful examination of psychotherapy research studies, that approximately 10% of those entering psychotherapy had been damaged by the treatment. In contrast, only about 5% of untreated control group patients showed negative effects.[19] This judgment followed Bergin's series of literature reviews aimed at testing the hypothesis that the previously published assessments of the efficacy of psychotherapy may have underestimated the positive effects for some patients and the negative effects experienced by others. The practice of reporting averaged scores for the treatment and control groups might represent the averaging of positive effects for many patients and negative effects for an appreciable but far smaller number of patients.[34,35] Consistent with the implications of his hypothesis, he found that some groups of treated patients showed a significant increase in the variability of criterion scores at posttreatment retesting. In contrast, untreated subjects in control groups showed less variability. He inferred that studies that showed increased dispersion of criterion scores in treated groups could be interpreted as direct evidence that some patients had "deteriorated" as a consequence of their treatment.

The inference that increased variance scores provided convincing evidence of deterioration has been appropriately challenged.[36,37] In addition, methodologic errors were readily identified in the original studies cited to support the deterioration hypothesis, raising further doubts about the adequacy of Bergin's method for testing the deterioration hypothesis.

Subsequently, Lambert, Bergin, and Collins presented 48 studies to support the contention that some patients were harmed by psychotherapy.[38] They reported that negative effects were found with varying frequency among a range of patients treated by a range of therapists using a variety of psychological treatment approaches. Strupp and colleagues[39] undertook to reexamine the 48 studies cited by Lambert and associates and reported that all but one of these studies were so flawed that no inferences regarding deterioration effects were warranted. Strupp and colleagues concluded that the body of research failed to provide a credible test of the hypothesis and did not demonstrate that psychotherapy produced negative effects at a rate greater than the 3% to 6% observed in untreated wait-list patients.

Smith and co-workers state that they too failed to find evidence of negative effects in their review of 475 outcome studies. In support of this conclusion they reported that only 9% of the 1766 effect sizes analyzed were negative. This inference may reflect a semantic confusion, since by negative effect Smith and co-workers refer to those instances where the mean of the control group was found to be higher at the end of treatment than the mean of the psychotherapy group. This observation does not require that the treated patients have deteriorated. Consider, too, that research on negative effects based on group means rather than individual cases would require that the aversive effects of a particular treatment approach be so pervasive or so severe as to be reflected in the overall group mean. It is of small comfort to learn from the paucity of evidence of negative group-averaged effects that entire patient groups are not regularly savaged by their treatment.

Strupp and colleagues were not content with reanalyzing the findings of Lambert and associates and conducted their own questionnaire survey, eliciting responses from approximately 70 expert clinicians, theoreticians, and researchers. Almost unanimously, the respondents agreed, "there is a real problem of negative effects in psychotherapy."[39] Despite the inconsistent empiric evidence, there does seem to be a clinical consensus that psychotherapy, if inappropriately administered, can produce psychonoxious effects.

IS PSYCHOTHERAPY COST-EFFECTIVE?

It is self-evident that treatments providing relief from symptoms and syndromes that are debilitating and disruptive of social functioning afford both direct and indirect financial benefit to the individual, family, community, and ultimately to the nation. However, precise estimates of cost-effectiveness and cost-benefit of psychotherapy remain elusive.

Underlying the concept of cost-effectiveness is the idea that treatments that can achieve the goals of therapy at the least cost are the most efficient and therefore the most desirable. At present no standard method for calculating these costs has been adopted. Although it is theoretically feasible to calculate the cost-effectiveness of psychotherapies, the conceptual and methodologic issues that beset this field are no less complex than those of the field of psychotherapy assessment itself.[40] Even more difficult is the determination of "cost-benefit" of treatments because this involves the arbitrary translation of psychological benefits into monetary units.

Some investigators have attempted to finesse the complexities of cost assessment by focusing instead on the possible "cost offset" values of psychotherapy. Usually this has involved efforts to demonstrate that psychotherapy contributes to the reduced rate of use of medical care facilities and services (e.g., office visits, laboratory tests, and days of hospitalization). The circumstances under which such cost-offset analyses are most compelling are those in which it has been clearly demonstrated that the physical health services had been misused prior to psychotherapy. The judgment of misuse must include not only overuse but also underuse of necessary health services. Misuse also includes evidence that the medical care was inappropriate or inadequate for the care of the patient. Furthermore, the possible cost-offset value must consider the fact that emotional and physical disorders are inextricably intertwined, so that proper medical care may be expected to provide a cost-offset value in reducing the overuse of psychotherapy in particular cases.

Careful surveys of cost-offset studies have been done by two sets of investigators: Jones and Vischi[41] and Mumford and colleagues.[42] Both groups concluded that the optimistic claims made by the authors of the original studies must be tempered. All the studies suffered from gross methodologic, statistical, and interpretive errors. The best estimates of the probable reduction in use of medical facilities attributable to the patients' exposure to psychological treatment range from zero to a maximum of 19%.

Other investigators have attempted to determine the impact of psychotherapy on medical use by individuals who concurrently suffered from physical and emotional disorders. Mumford and colleagues reported that such patients tend to reduce their medical use more quickly than do patients diagnosed as suffering the identical physical disorder alone.[43] They further reported that the use of "psychologically informed" mental health services with surgical or coronary patients tended to reduce their required periods of hospitalization.

Thus, evidence is gradually accumulating to the effect that attending to the psychological needs of patients may reduce their inappropriate use of medical care facilities and may also shorten the period of use of such services. However, only cautious inferences are warranted from these limited data.

IS THERE A POSITIVE RELATIONSHIP BETWEEN OUTCOME AND LENGTH OF TREATMENT?

The meta-analysis reviews of nearly 600 studies found no appreciable relationship between the size of the treatment effect and the duration of psychotherapy.[26,27] Interpretation of these findings is restricted because the range of treatment length in the studies reviewed was narrow: the average treatment in the study of Smith and co-workers was 16 hours, and it was only 7 hours in the Shapiros' survey. Furthermore, the negligible relationship found between average length of treatment and average effect size is derived from a between-study analysis. This may have obscured any relationships existing between duration and benefit within each of the studies.

Orlinsky and Howard[44] reviewed 55 studies on this subject and reported that the association between treatment length and outcome was erratic. Of 33 studies investigating the effect of the number of treatment sessions, 20 (60%) showed a positive association between amount of therapy and outcome; 6 reported a curvilinear relationship; and 7 found no significant relationship. Of 22 studies dealing with time in treatment, 12 (55%) showed positive relations between outcome and duration, 1 reported a negative relation, and 9 found no significant relationship. The reviewers chose to interpret these findings as indicating that the sheer number of sessions is likely to be less important than the intensity of treatment. Of particular interest is the curvilinear relationship, which suggests that there may be a point of diminishing returns in some treatment situations.

The usefulness of conclusions that may be drawn regarding the length and amount of treatment will be limited until careful attention is also paid to the specification of the patients/problems treated and the adequacy of measurement of relevant treatment goals.

IS THERE A POSITIVE RELATIONSHIP BETWEEN LENGTH OF THERAPIST EXPERIENCE AND OUTCOME?

Repeated surveys of the available evidence fail to demonstrate a reliable relationship between the therapist's level of experience and patient benefit. Contrary to the conclusions of earlier reviewers that "experience does seem to make a difference,"[18,19,45] more recent surveys inspire less conviction. Auerbach and Johnson,[46] after a comprehensive review of the area of therapist experience level, concluded: "the view that experienced therapists achieve better results, while it may be true, does not find the unequivocal support that we expected." A subsequent intensive examination of the research literature by Parloff and associates led to this statement: "Our conclusions are even more pessimistic than those of Auerbach and Johnson . . . the body of data available is not sound enough to permit us to draw any firm conclusions."[47]

DO THE EFFECTS OF TREATMENT ENDURE?

With regard to the durability of treatment effects, again reviewers have drawn different conclusions from their research findings and surveys. Frank[48] has reported that whatever the form of therapy, most patients who show initial improvement maintain it. Moreover, when two therapies yield differences in outcome at the close of treatment, with rare exceptions these differences disappear over time. The closing of the gap seems to depend more on patients who received the less successful therapy catching up than on both groups regressing equally toward the mean.

Quite the opposite inference is drawn by Mash and Terdal[49] from their survey of the effects of behavior therapies. The size of treatment effects appeared to decrease over time, with the patients who had initially shown the greater benefit apparently not maintaining their benefits. This finding is consistent with that of Smith and co-workers,[26] who found that the average effect size decreased from about .9 standard deviation units found immediately after therapy to around .5 units 2 years later. Andrews and Harvey[50] reanalyzed 81 of the studies of Smith and co-workers, which represented patients who had sought treatment for neuroses, phobias, or emotional-somatic complaints. A comparison of effect sizes of outcome measured at the conclusion of therapy and at intervals ranging to about 9 months after treatment revealed: "the benefits are stable for many months but decline slowly thereafter at an average estimated .2 effect size units per annum."

Despite Frank's judgment, there is thus considerable evidence that the effects of the most frequently tested forms of therapy tend to diminish over time. To this, Smith and co-workers proffer

solace: "The benefits of psychotherapy are not permanent, but then little is."[26]

Discussion

The discussion of major criticisms leveled at the outcome research findings is organized around two indictments: (1) the positive effects may be artifacts and (2) the research evidence is inadequate to support the sweeping generalizations being made. Following the presentation of these criticisms, their implications will be analyzed.

THE POSITIVE EFFECTS OF PSYCHOTHERAPY MAY BE ARTIFACTS

Arguments presented for this position center around two related issues: (1) psychotherapy effects may be due simply to placebo effects or (2) they may be due to "nonspecific" elements common to all therapeutic interventions.

The overall concern that psychotherapy lacks specificity also involves a tacit assumption that some mechanisms of change are, *ipso facto*, less acceptable than others, whether they are considered specific or nonspecific. If the seemingly positive effects of psychotherapy are attributable primarily to such mechanisms as "suggestion," "placebo effects," "attention effects," or "commonsense" advice, then the credibility of psychotherapy as a professional procedure is automatically impugned.

Placebo Effects

The term *placebo* (literally, "I shall please") is typically used in medicine to characterize any intervention (medication, procedure, device) believed to lack ingredients specific to the amelioration of the condition (usually physical) thought to require treatment.[51] Nonetheless, patients frequently report either positive or negative effects associated with the administration of the supposedly inert placebo. In this sense the placebo, while physically inactive, may be psychologically quite active. Such effects are treated as artifacts and are attributed to so-called nonspecific psychological factors. The term *nonspecific* is generally used as a synonym for "suggestion," attention, hope, faith, and patient compliance with the demand nature of the situation.

Placebos may serve a useful function in placating the patient and allaying anxieties attendant to the primary disorder. Placebo effects may also be associated with known "active" therapeutic interventions and may act therefore to enhance or inhibit their effects. In assessing the effects of active treatments, it is necessary to control for possible placebo influences. Should an individual's disorder be effectively and enduringly benefited by a known placebo treatment, suspicion arises regarding the accuracy of the original diagnosis and the patient's "need" for treatment.

The medically based concept of placebo is difficult to transpose directly to the broad field of psychotherapy, where neither the theories of disease, illness, and disorder nor the specificity of treatment are generally accepted or understood. Some schools of psychotherapy also question the validity of the distinction made between symptoms and underlying disorder. The different schools of psychotherapy espouse different theoretic and conceptual views regarding who and what needs treating, which therapeutic processes, mechanisms, and interventions are "active," and which are likely to be "inert." Further confusion arises because in medical treatment placebos are considered to have only "psychological" effects. Since psychotherapy is a psychological treatment, the question arises of how much of its effects might be "placebo."

In the field of psychotherapy, the term *placebo* is used in its most pejorative sense to characterize interventions that in the judgment of the proponents of a competing theoretic orientation lack the essential ingredients for effecting meaningful change. Whether an intervention is inert or active apparently cannot be convincingly demonstrated by the examination of the differential changes associated with the different treatments (*i.e.,* their nature, degree, durability, scope, and speed of action). The invective *placebo* is also used among psychotherapists in its conventional medical sense to refer to procedures believed to depend for their effects on suggestion, confidence, faith, and so forth.

Another problem arises in the effort to apply the term *placebo* to psychotherapy research. Unlike drug research, the feasibility of creating placebo groups as controls in comparative psychotherapy outcome studies is sharply limited.[52] Designing placebo control therapies would require the omission of all elements currently believed to have therapeutic value by one or another of the current therapeutic approaches; this is very likely impossible.

If the condition of qualifying as a placebo inheres in the supposition that a given procedure does not address the core problem as conceived by an alternate theory, then almost any set of contrasting therapeutic approaches may serve as placebos for each other. This view has permitted some researchers to justify the use of "client-centered" psychotherapy groups as a placebo control in behavior therapy studies.[26] Similarly, the comparison of theoretically disparate approaches to the treatment of major depressive disorders, such as interpersonal therapy versus cognitive behavior therapy,[53] may provide an adequate placebo control condition.

Nonspecific Effects

The nonspecificity hypothesis states that if different forms of psychotherapy, using apparently different "specific" techniques and procedures, achieve equivalent effects, then the potency of psychotherapy may be attributable to shared "nonspecific" elements common to all psychological treatments.[54–56] The research challenge is to identify these common elements and to use them more purposefully to enhance further the efficacy of psychotherapy. These nonspecific components are not "artifacts" to be dismissed but active elements to be understood.

Special emphasis must be given to the work of Frank,[55] who has elaborated the nonspecificity hypothesis most fully. However, frequently overlooked in the discussions of Frank's conceptions is the implicit differentiation of different phases of treatment and the specific heuristics proposed as particularly appropriate for each. Frank's approach to nonspecificity is linked with his clinical inference that the nonspecific factors he has identified are uniquely effective in the treatment of a syndrome commonly shared by patients seeking help: demoralization. Frank argues that demoralization—a sense of helplessness, inability to cope, self-blame, feelings of worthlessness, alienation—can be found in most patients regardless of their specific "disorders" or the nature of their presenting complaints.

Before considering the nonspecificity hypothesis further, it must be emphasized that therapy techniques are the most conspicuous aspects of different therapies. If these various techniques bear no distinctive relationship to specific effects of such treatment (*i.e.,* nature, quantity, breadth, speed of action, durability), then the legitimacy of the authority granted to the various treatment approaches is in question.

The nonspecificity hypothesis also invites the interpretation that the major qualification of psychotherapists is to be well-intentioned "nice guys" who confidently offer palliatives and treacly relationships instead of "specific" treatments for specific disorders. Criticism of this kind implies that psychotherapists may be witting or unwitting "faith healers."

However, I believe that further study of Frank's exposition is reassuring. Frank has identified four major shared elements[57]:

1. Therapists offer a special type of relationship: they show concern for the patients' welfare, and encourage the formation of a trusting, confiding, emotional relationship with them.
2. The treatment setting is special: efforts are made to establish an aura about the psychotherapy institution or office that encourages patients to believe they are in a safe place—a sanctuary—that is "presided over by a tolerant protector."
3. The therapist provides a conceptual schema: the patient is offered an explanation for his "inchoate or bewildering subjective states and behaviors" and told how the treatment will relieve the problems. The formulations must be convincing to the patient, that is, linked to the "dominant cosmology of his culture." The acceptability of these formulations is enhanced by the therapist's mantle of science or religion.
4. Therapy provides a prescribed set of procedures based on the conceptual scheme. These procedures provide the vehicle and the justification for the maintenance of the therapeutic relationship. Techniques may provide the patient with further evidence of the therapist's knowledge and competence. Techniques that are dramatic or produce dramatic effects such as alterations of the patient's subjective state or state of consciousness are particularly useful for their morale-building function.

Frank further states that all psychotherapies produce similar experiences in the course of treatment, such as a degree of emotional arousal, which may be a state necessary for change to occur in attitudes and behaviors; increasing patient awareness of options available to them; and arousal and maintenance of patients' hope for improvement (this is achieved initially through the attitude of the therapist and later on the basis of evidence of the patient's success in treatment and life settings).

The term *nonspecific* is infelicitous because it tends to obscure the concept's *positive* formulation regarding the active ingredients of all therapies. The full hypothesis implies at least two phases of treatment and suggests that in the initial phase the cultivation of the patient's hope and favorable expectations of receiving help is critical. Patients in a state of demoralization require some assurance of the potential usefulness of the treatment and particularly of the ability of the therapist to provide it. Initially, specific techniques for establishing treatment as an appropriate option are less important than the nontechnical aspects of therapy, such as the nature and quality of the relationship offered, the characteristics of the therapist, the context in which treatment is to be provided, and evidence of the therapist's skills. Patients seeking help wish to be assured that the therapist is an expert (knowledgeable, competent, capable) but of equal importance, they wish to be assured that the therapist is a person to whom they can relate with some degree of ease and intimacy.

Frank's formulations recognize that the strategies and goals commonly pursued in all forms of psychotherapy after the initial phase are less dependent on "suggestion":

1. *Reality-testing strategies.* The therapist provides the patient with the opportunity to learn that the feared consequences of the patient's carefully avoided thoughts and behaviors do not in fact occur, or if they do occur they are not accompanied by the anticipated disaster. The therapist encourages the patient, in the context of a relatively safe setting, to test out new ways of behaving. The patient is thus helped to recognize that a wider range of behaviors are available to him.
2. *Cognitive and experiential learning opportunities.* In the context of an affective relationship with the therapist, the patient is helped to learn new ways of formulating problems and to recognize the validity of alternate interpretations of events and their potential consequences. Treatments aim at assisting the patient to gain new information about self and others, which will enable the patient to behave more appropriately and adaptively to the actual rather than imagined situation.
3. *Promotion of the development of self-esteem.* This is usually accomplished by helping the patient achieve a reality-based sense of mastery and competence consistent with actual success experiences in the treatment setting and ultimately in the "real world."

In effect, treatment may begin by artificially instilling in patients a sense of confidence in the therapist and ends with the patients developing a realistic sense of mastery and confidence in themselves.

All schools of therapy recognize that these elements are relevant to their own approach and represent to some degree their own procedures and aims, but they differ, of course, in their judgment of crucial elements that might be missing from Frank's conceptualization. Since there are no research data on those possibly "missing" elements, the most relevant point here is that the hypothesis is silent regarding what specific techniques and mechanisms of change are most appropriate in achieving the stated goals. Whatever they are, Frank's hypothesis does not assert that they are "nonspecific."

Thus, the nonspecificity hypothesis does not require that the common elements be viewed as the "necessary and sufficient" conditions for the treatment of all patients but does hold that the "initial conditions" are necessary to begin all treatment. Perhaps for the treatment of the "nonspecific" problems of interpersonal relationships, the nonspecific human relationship established with a wise and skilled psychotherapist may serve not only as a potent element of therapy but also as the uniquely appropriate corrective medium of treatment. Where the nature of the problem may not be obviously interpersonal (*e.g.*, simple phobias, agoraphobia, compulsions, obsessions) or is secondary to a "severe, unrelieved biological illness such as chronic panic disorders or melancholia,"[58] the nonspecific treatment may not be sufficient. However, even in these instances it may be useful in providing relief from the associated symptoms of demoralization and enable the patients to comply with any more useful "specific" treatment techniques and procedures.

In summary, the nonspecificity hypothesis, as elaborated, may provide a basis for resolving some of the contentiousness of earlier efforts to differentiate sharply between the claimed primacy of "techniques" and "therapeutic relationships." It proposes that psychotherapy is implemented by its technology but is not dependent for its effects simply on its technology. Techniques can support the development of the essential therapeutic relationship, which in turn may trigger therapeutic processes; conversely, a therapeutic relationship can set the stage for the introduction of what may be therapeutic techniques. Technology and relationships are, therefore, interdependent in effective treatment.

THE RESEARCH EVIDENCE IS INADEQUATE TO SUPPORT SWEEPING GENERALIZATIONS

Two principal arguments are here subsumed: (1) it is premature to subject psychotherapy treatment approaches to a rigorous model of investigation, and (2) the body of outcome research evidence accumulated is unrepresentative of psychotherapy practice.

Rigorous outcome research is premature

This argument has been used unblushingly for the past 30 to 40 years by practitioners and "process" researchers alike. Included among the protagonists are at one extreme those who simply dismiss the possibility that the art of psychotherapy can ever be appropriately subjected to rigorous scientific models of study and at the other those who ardently embrace the paradigm of measurement and replicability but would apply it first to the identification of critical mechanisms of change.

The "anti-science" position and the related view that the treatment of each patient is unique (an atypical experience that cannot be measured) are in a sense matters of belief that are beyond discussion. The only comment that might be proffered here is that all treatment is, at some level, based on patterns of diagnosis and behavior. The critical issue is how these patterns are recognized (intuitively, subjectively, on the basis of individual experience, through exposure to a professional culture, or through attempts at precise definition and measurement). The persuasiveness of different kinds of evidence—whether one is talking about the relationship of cigarettes to cancer, the best way to avoid nuclear war, or the effectiveness of various kinds of psychotherapy—remains a function of personal factors.

The other argument regarding the prematurity of outcome research is that comparative efficacy studies, as usually conducted and summarized, do not specify the procedures and processes that are causally connected to outcomes. In the absence of the prior clear identification of the critical elements that may be effecting particular kinds of change, the argument continues, research does not contribute to the advancement of the field. Under these circumstances proper controls cannot be implemented, and therefore findings based on possibly inconsistent and improperly applied procedures cannot be usefully compared or interpreted.

This criticism has received renewed attention in the light of the current preference for multilevel and multidimensional analyses of many small interaction units that can be subjected to comprehensive coding systems. If there is any agreement among the range of process investigators, it is that the gross units represented by psychotherapy approaches and procedures are unsuitable for discovery. Since psychotherapy is conceived to be sequential steps toward intermediate goals, which are hypothesized to lead to ultimate therapeutic goals, each step must be systematically investigated. However, it is unlikely that such steps can be usefully studied in isolation from the particular patterning of relationships among symptoms and syndromes occurring in the context of particular personality structures; the quality and strength of the relationship (working alliance) between the therapist and patient; the patient's capacities, particularly those that limit accessibility to specific therapy tasks; and the appropriateness of the therapist's interventions and style, both overall and on a moment-to-moment basis during the course of treatment.

Such enormous complexities require the development of new strategies of research, including, perhaps, the development of miniature theories of process.[59-64] The technical advances of the past 40 years (tape recorders, audiovisual recordings) have greatly assisted process research, and now computer-facilitated analysis increases the investigators' capability for performing multidimensional descriptions and calculations.

Formidable obstacles remain, however, to the conduct of process studies. Here are a few examples: The "Rashomon" effect—the different perceptions and interpretations of selected events in therapy by the therapist, patient, and researcher—cannot readily be resolved by soliciting descriptions from each of these perspectives. The units selected for intensive study may not be the units responded to by the patients. No direct and reliable measure of a patient's subjective experience is yet available. Similarly, the development of measures of individualized change acceptable to clinicians as possessing an adequate degree of "sensitivity" remains an elusive goal. Process studies are appropriately more concerned with interaction effects than "main" effects; however, traditional experimental designs and procedures cannot readily accommodate the number of interactions generated by three or more variables.

It remains an act of faith that findings based on the meticulous microlevel analyses currently undertaken can be extrapolated to the macrolevels of actual treatments and their outcomes. The half-life of "laws" developed in the field of process studies is notoriously short, because the systems studied are open-ended. The more open-ended the context, the less generalizable are the findings.

With rare exceptions, investigators now agree that the strategy of separating process studies from outcome research (intermediate or ultimate goals)

has not been useful. The dogged investigation of the processes associated with a course of actual treatment independent of clear criteria of the nature of its benefits to patients contributes little to an understanding of the mechanisms of therapeutic change. Although outcome research can be conducted without knowledge of the "process," process research cannot meaningfully be pursued without reference to outcome.

Since process research is ultimately aimed at answering basic questions, its scientific justification is self-evident. Nevertheless, process research that deals satisfactorily with the obstacles enumerated has yet to be designed.

Outcome Research is Unrepresentative of Psychotherapy Practice

Because psychotherapy outcome research now increasingly attempts to produce carefully controlled studies, it tends to be limited to material amenable to such control. Consequently, contemporary psychotherapy research is based largely on the investigation of behavior therapies, although psychodynamically oriented therapies remain the dominant force in American psychiatry and clinical psychology.[65]

Although precise measures of the relative proportions of psychotherapy practice represented by psychodynamic and behavioral therapies are not yet available, reasonable inferences may be drawn from preliminary evidence provided by a survey of members of the American Psychological Association.[66] Only 14.4% of respondents classified themselves as behavior therapists, while 30.0% considered themselves psychodynamically oriented and 30.9% "eclectic." It is plausible to expect that even fewer psychiatrists would subscribe to behavior therapy practice and a far greater proportion would describe themselves as psychodynamically oriented.

Of the nearly 500 studies reviewed by Smith and co-workers, only about 13% may be classed as psychodynamic or insight therapies, even when the most flaccid criteria of classification are used (6% psychodynamic, 6% dynamic eclectic, and 1% Adlerian). In the Shapiros' survey, only 5% of the treatment groups received a form of dynamic or humanistic psychotherapy. About half of the treatment effects reported were derived from group rather than individual therapy.

These integrators of outcome research recognize that in the scant instances where insight therapies were included in comparative outcome studies they were intended to serve merely as "straw man" treatment groups. The investigators clearly favored the behavior therapy approaches and made no serious attempt to ensure that the dynamic therapies were properly conducted or that their specialized goals were appropriately measured.

The therapists in the studies included in both meta-analysis surveys were predominantly novices who had not yet completed their doctoral training or their psychiatric residencies. The patients treated in the studies reviewed were predominantly recruited by the investigators and had not actively sought treatment. The Shapiros report that only 17% of the patient–subjects had requested treatment or presented problems of "clinical severity." Typically, problems of general anxiety and depression are characteristic of patients who seek psychotherapy; yet the Shapiros found that only 7% of the patients in the studies they reviewed reported having such problems. In contrast, complaints of phobias and performance anxiety (*e.g.*, test anxiety, public speaking anxiety) were highly represented. As mentioned, the average duration of treatment was 16 hours in the Smith survey and about 7 hours in the Shapiros' review.

Only 56 of the 475 studies reviewed by Smith and co-workers directly compare various treatments in the same study. As a result the comparability of outcome measures was not strict. These 56 studies provided comparisons of "verbal" and behavioral therapies by using the same measures and comparable patients. It is not clear how many psychodynamic therapies were represented in the class of "verbal" therapies, which included rational-emotive, "other cognitive," reality therapy, transactional analysis, client-centered, and gestalt therapies. The Shapiros' survey included so few dynamic therapies (and the quality of these was so dubious) that reliable conclusions regarding comparative efficacy based even on the restricted measures used cannot be derived.

Measures of "internal" dynamic changes, so valued by the analytically oriented, were not adequately represented or assessed in these studies. On the basis of the available research the generalization that there are no differences in the effectiveness of psychotherapies can appropriately be made only for the behavior therapies.

A further limitation of the data is that research focused primarily on the *classes* of therapies tested rather than on the *techniques* actually used. It cannot be assumed that professed adherence to any school or form of therapy guarantees that specific techniques associated with that treatment were exclusively or even predominantly used.

Another difficulty with the meta-analytic inte-grations of an array of independent studies is that patients treated by the diverse therapies may differ systematically. It cannot be assumed that persons seeking psychotherapy assort themselves randomly in behavioral, psychodynamic, cognitive, and gestalt therapies. As a result, any reported differences or lack of differences in therapeutic effectiveness of the psychotherapies compared may be a function of interactions with patient as well as measurement characteristics. Such errors cannot be partialled out statistically to study treatment impact if the type of disorder, form of measurement, and type of treatment provided are inherently confounded.

On the basis of the limitations of the data base, the fundamental conclusion that *all* psychotherapies produce comparable effects seems at best premature. The door should not be closed, therefore, on the possibility that more careful research might yet uncover differences among therapies in effecting different kinds and degrees of change when applied to well-defined "disorders." There may also be significant differences in patient acceptability of particular interventions. In addition, particular strategies, procedures, or techniques may produce differential effects with different speeds and degrees of durability.

In summary, while the body of research investigations analyzed does seem to represent the existing population of outcome studies, that population does not adequately represent the field of psychotherapy practice, typical patients and problems, or fully trained and experienced psychotherapists.

IMPLICATIONS OF RESEARCH CRITICISMS

The many problems associated with psychotherapy research may give the impression that psychotherapy is a uniquely impalpable and imprecise field, uniquely unsuited to the scrutiny of experimental research. To maintain perspective it may be useful to identify assessment problems that inhere in all psychiatric treatment (and in all medical treatment) and to indicate those aspects that may present special problems for the psychotherapy researcher.

Limited Generalization of Efficacy Findings

Studies conducted under rigorously controlled conditions cannot readily be generalized to the "naturalistic" world of practice. This is less of a problem in the field of drug administration, because the medication is itself standardized even if the therapist's styles and skills are not. Psychotherapists tend to dismiss findings derived from laboratory or "ivory tower" efficacy studies as having little practical value for their day-to-day work.

Generalizations regarding the efficacy of particular interventions and procedures are routinely qualified by specifying the nature and range of problems or disorders to be so treated. It is rare, however, that generalizations also specify the level of expertise and skill required of the therapist. Although therapist competence is assumed, psychotherapy outcome findings have often been based on the efforts of novices. This may have operated systematically to underestimate the potency of particular treatment approaches and may contribute to the apparent lack of differences found in the efficacy of the various psychological treatments investigated.

Limited Scale of Research

Research on the efficacy of drug treatments is usually undertaken and underwritten by private organizations and institutions. The impetus for such research (aside from conformance to the requirements of regulatory agencies) is the potential to the drug industry of large profits. Opportunities for such benefits do not exist in the field of psychotherapy, and no comparable large-scale psychotherapy industry has developed. Psychotherapy research remains a "cottage industry,"[67] conducted by relatively few individuals or small groups whose work is dependent on the uncertain support of public agencies and cannot provide more definitive answers to basic and applied questions.

Difficulty of Clarifying Goals

What needs treating appears to be more ambiguous and in some ways more ambitious in the field of psychotherapy than in the somatic therapies. The need for health care is usually based on the presence of a recognized illness that is beyond the patient's control or responsibility. The need for mental health care is similarly justified in many instances of "mental disorders"; however, the need is less self-evident in persons seeking assistance with problems of "daily living" or seeking personal growth and self-fulfillment. Many psychotherapists, too, see their function as going beyond symptom amelioration or removal to assisting patients in achieving the benefits of "positive mental health"—joy, zest, creative expression, social skills, and the capacity to function more effectively in all aspects of life. These goals pose special problems of measurement.

Difficulty of Standardizing Interventions

Problems surrounding the specification and reliable measurement of treatment goals are shared by all treatment outcome research; however, special problems arise in psychotherapy outcome assessment with regard to the specification and standardization of "treatment interventions." Debate still rages about what research should measure, such as the therapeutic relationship or working alliance, microunits of moment-to-moment interactions between therapist and patient, interpretations of transference, encouragement of emotional release, and so forth.

The conceptual ambiguity regarding the nature and units of psychotherapy makes it difficult for investigators to conduct rigorous studies and even more difficult for practitioners to take seriously the findings of such research.

Recommendations

The primary recommendation of this review is that academicians, researchers, and clinicians further examine and attempt to remedy the circumstances that have created and threaten to maintain the striking imbalance among the forms of therapy that are subjected to systematic and scientifically credible research. Research that appears increasingly to focus its attention on the study of a narrow band of therapies threatens to restrict the opportunities for identifying the effects and potential of alternate strategies and procedures. By the systematic omission of psychotherapies that are thought to be based on contrasting theories, the field restricts its chances of identifying other possible useful mechanisms of change.

More systematic research is needed on psychotherapies such as the psychoanalytically oriented, which maintain that they achieve far-reaching durable effects, different from those limited to symptom reduction, by procedures that contribute something beyond suggestion and persuasion. Researchers owe the dynamic psychotherapies more than the current minimal courtesy of sullen indifference.

Although it is difficult to be sanguine about the possibility that further research will identify "specific" psychological interventions, techniques, and procedures that produce specific effects, the continued effort in that direction seems necessary. As Smith and co-workers comment, those who choose to pursue the grail of specificity must "hunt with better measuring instruments. . . The measurement of results is currently the most poorly executed."[26] The need to develop refined instruments remains a high priority.

Instead of waiting for the Godot of a new and more congenial research paradigm, the field will be best served by extending its search for possible specific mechanisms of change and attempting to relate them to specific patient classes and problems. Like Klein and Rabkin,[58] I believe that the identification of such processes may be facilitated by comparing therapies that differ markedly, or appear to differ, in their theories, their assumptions and, above all, their actual procedures. If real differences in the speed, nature, quality, and durability of changes produced by different forms or classes of psychotherapies can be identified, and there is clinical evidence and lore suggesting that such differences exist, then it will become far easier to identify any associated specific mechanisms of change. The valuable store of knowledge in the psychodynamic therapies should not be left unmined.

REFERENCES

1. Diagnostic and Statistical Manual of Mental Disorders, 3rd ed. Washington, DC, American Psychiatric Association, 1980

2. Feighner JP, Robins E, Guze SB et al: Diagnostic criteria for use in psychiatric research. Arch Gen Psychiatry 26:57, 1972

3. Spitzer RL, Endicott JE, Robins E: Research Diagnostic Criteria (RDC) for a Selected Group of Functional Disorders, 3rd ed. Rockville, MD, National Institute of Mental Health, Clinical Research Branch Collaborative Program on the Psychobiology of Depression, 1978

4. Endicott J, Spitzer RL: A diagnostic interview: The schedule for affective disorders and schizophrenia. Arch Gen Psychiatry 35:837, 1978

5. Mintz J, Kiesler DJ: Individualized measures of psychotherapy outcome. In Kendall PC, Butcher JN (eds): Handbook of Research Methods in Clinical Psychology. New York, John Wiley & Sons, 1982

6. Wender PH, Klein DF: Mind, Mood, and Medicine: A Guide to the New Biopsychiatry. New York, Farrar, Straus, & Giroux, 1981

7. Rosenthal D: Genetic Theory and Abnormal Behavior. New York, McGraw-Hill, 1970

8. Goldfried MR (ed): Converging Themes in Psychotherapy: Trends in Psychodynamic, Humanistic and Behavioral Practice. New York, Springer, 1982

9. Marmor J, Woods SM (eds): The Interface Between the Psychodynamic and Behavioral Therapies. New York, Plenum Press, 1980

10. Wachtel PL: Psychoanalysis and Behavior Therapy. New York, Basic Books, 1977

11. Herink R (ed): The Psychotherapy Handbook. New York, New American Library, 1980

12. Eysenck HJ: The effects of psychotherapy: An evaluation. J Consult Psychol 16:319, 1952

13. Eysenck HJ: The Effects of Psychotherapy. New York, International Science Press, 1966

14. Levitt EE: The results of psychotherapy with children: An evaluation. J Consult Psychol 21:186, 1957

15. Levitt EE: Psychotherapy with children: A further evaluation. Behav Res Ther 1:45, 1963

16. Rachman S: The Effects of Psychotherapy. Oxford, Pergamon Press, 1971

17. Truax, C, Carkhuff R: Toward Effective Counseling and Psychotherapy. Chicago, Aldine, 1967

18. Meltzoff J, Kornreich M: Research in Psychotherapy. New York, Atherton Press, 1970

19. Bergin AE: The evaluation of therapeutic outcomes. In Bergin AE, Garfield SL (eds): Handbook of Psychotherapy and Behavior Change. New York, John Wiley & Sons, 1971

20. Luborsky L, Singer B, Luborsky L: Comparative studies of psychotherapies. Is it true that "Everyone has won and all must have prizes"? Arch Gen Psychiatry 32:995, 1975

21. Bergin AE, Lambert MJ: The evaluation of therapeutic outcomes. In Garfield SL, Bergin AE (eds): Handbook of Psychotherapy and Behavior Change: An Empirical Analysis, 2nd ed. New York, John Wiley & Sons, 1978

22. Cohen J: Statistical Power Analysis for the Behavioral Sciences, rev ed. New York, Academic Press, 1977

23. American Psychiatric Association Commission on Psychotherapies: Psychotherapy Research: Methodological and Efficacy Issues. Washington, DC, American Psychiatric Association, 1982

24. Rachman SJ, Wilson GT: The Effects of Psychological Therapy, 2nd ed. New York, Pergamon Press, 1980

25. Frank JD: The present status of outcome studies. J Consult Clin Psychol 47:310, 1979

26. Smith ML, Glass GV, Miller TI: The Benefits of Psychotherapy. Baltimore, Johns Hopkins University Press, 1980

27. Shapiro D, Shapiro D: Meta-analysis of comparative therapy outcome studies: A replication and refinement. Psychol Bull 92:581, 1982

28. Rosenthal R, Rubin DB: A simple, general-purpose display of magnitude of experimental effect. J Educ Psychol 2:166, 1982

29. Parloff MB: Psychotherapy research evidence and reimbursement decisions: Bambi meets Godzilla. Am J Psychiatry 139:718, 1982

30. Agras WS, Kazdin AE, Wilson GT: Behavior Therapy: Towards an Applied Clinical Science. San Francisco, Freeman, 1979

31. President's Commission on Mental Health: Report to the President, vol 4. Washington, DC, US Government Printing Office, 1978

32. Gross M: The Psychological Society. New York, Random House, 1978

33. Zilbergeld B: The Shrinking of America. Boston, Little, Brown & Co, 1983

34. Bergin AE: The effects of psychotherapy: Negative results revisited. J Counsel Psychol 10:244, 1963

35. Bergin AE: Some implications of psychotherapy research for therapeutic practice. J Abnorm Psychol 71:235, 1966

36. Braucht GN: The deterioration effect: A reply to Bergin. J Abnorm Psychol 75:293, 1970

37. May PRA: For better or for worse? Psychotherapy and variance change: A critical review of the literature. J Nerv Ment Dis 152:184, 1971

38. Lambert MJ, Bergin AE, Collins JL: Therapist-induced deterioration in psychotherapy. In Gurman AS, Razin AM (eds): Effective Psychotherapy: A Handbook of Research. New York, Pergamon Press, 1977

39. Strupp HH, Hadley SW, Gomes-Schwartz B: Psychotherapy for Better or Worse. New York, Jason Aronson, 1977

40. Office of Technology Assessment: The Implications of Cost-Effectiveness Analysis of Medical Technology, background Paper No. 3, The Efficacy and Cost-Effectiveness of Psychotherapy. Washington, DC, US Government Printing Office, 1980

41. Jones KR, Vischi TR: Impact of alcohol, drug abuse and mental health treatment in medical care utilization: A review of the research literature. Med Care 17(12):1, 1979

42. Mumford E, Schlesinger HJ, Glass GV: Problems of analyzing the cost offset of including a mental health component in primary care. In Institute of Medicine: Mental Health Services in General Health Care. Washington, DC, National Academy of Sciences, 1979

43. Mumford E, Schlesinger HJ, Glass GV: The effects of psychological intervention on recovery from surgery and heart attacks: An analysis of the literature. Am J Public Health 72:141, 1982

44. Orlinsky DE, Howard KI: The relation of process to outcome in psychotherapy. In Garfield SL, Bergin AE (eds): Handbook of Psychotherapy and Behavior Change: An Empirical Analysis. New York, John Wiley & Sons, 1978

45. Luborsky L, Chandler M, Auerbach AH et al: Factors influencing the outcome of psychotherapy. Psychol Bull 75:145, 1971

46. Auerbach AH, Johnson M: Research on the therapist's level of experience. In Gurman AS, Razin AM (eds): Effective Psychotherapy: A Handbook of Research. New York, Pergamon Press, 1977

47. Parloff MB, Waskow IE, Wolfe BE: Research on therapist variables in relation to process and outcome. In Garfield SL, Bergin AE (eds): Handbook of Psychotherapy and Behavior Change: An Empirical Analysis. New York, John Wiley & Sons, 1978

48. Frank JD: Therapeutic components shared by all psychotherapies. In Harvey JH, Parks MM (eds): Psychotherapy Research and Behavior Change. Washington, DC, American Psychological Association, 1982

49. Mash EJ, Terdal LJ: Follow-up assessments in behavior therapy. In Karoly P, Steffen J (eds): Improving the Long-term Effects of Psychotherapy. New York, Gardner Press, 1980

50. Andrews G, Harvey R: Does psychotherapy benefit neurotic patients? Arch Gen Psychiatry 38:1203, 1981

51. Shapiro AK, Morris LA: The placebo effect in medical and psychological therapies. In Garfield SL, Bergin AE (eds): Handbook of Psychotherapy and Behavior Change: An Empirical Analysis. New York, John Wiley & Sons, 1978

52. O'Leary KD, Borkovec T: Conceptual, methodological, and ethical problems of placebo groups in psychotherapy research. Am Psychol 9:821, 1978

53. Waskow IE, Parloff MB, Hadley SW et al: NIMH Treatment of Depression Collaborative Research Program: Background and research plan. Arch Gen Psychiatry (in press)

54. Rosenzweig S: Some implicit common factors in diverse methods of psychotherapy. Am J Orthopsychiatry 6:412, 1936

55. Frank JD: Persuasion and Healing, rev ed. Baltimore, Johns Hopkins University Press, 1973

56. Marmor J: The nature of the psychotherapeutic process. In Psychiatry in Transition: Selected Papers. New York, Brunner/Mazel, 1974

57. Frank JD: General psychotherapy: The restoration of morale. In Freedman DX, Dyrud JE (eds): American Handbook of Psychiatry, 2nd ed., vol 5. New York, Basic Books, 1975

58. Klein DF, Rabkin JG: Specificity and strategy in psychotherapy research and practice. Paper presented at annual meeting of the American Psychopathology Association, New York, March 1983

59. Greenspan SI, Sharfstein SS: Efficacy of psychotherapy. Arch Gen Psychiatry 38:1213, 1981

60. Rice LN, Greenberg LS (eds): Patterns of Change: Intensive Analysis of Psychotherapy Process. New York, Guilford, 1983

61. Benjamin LS: Use of structural analysis of social behavior (SASB) and Markov chains to study dyadic interactions. J Abnorm Psychol 88:303, 1979

62. Dahl HA: A quantitative study of a psychoanalysis. In Holt RR, Peterfreund E (eds): Psychoanalysis and Contemporary Science, vol 1. New York, Macmillan, 1972

63. Horowitz MJ: States of Mind: Analysis of Change in Psychotherapy. New York, Plenum, 1979

64. Bordin ES: Research Strategies in Psychotherapy. New York, John Wiley & Sons, 1974

65. Davison G, Neale J: Abnormal Psychology: An Experimental Clinical Approach. New York, John Wiley & Sons, 1978

66. Norcross JC, Prochaska JO: A national survey of clinical psychologists: Characteristics and activities. Clin Psychol 35:1, 1982

67. London P: The future of psychotherapy. Hastings Center Rep 3:11, 1973

Robert E. Hales and Robert J. Ursano

The Brief Psychotherapies

Interest in brief psychotherapy has flourished in recent years. In a 4-year period alone, from 1980 to 1984, over 200 articles on brief psychotherapy appeared in American medical journals. This number is equal to the total number of articles published on this same subject during the 10 years between 1969 and 1979. Following World War II, interest in psychoanalysis resulted in a rapid growth in the demand for psychotherapy. This, in turn, increased the pressure on psychiatrists to develop briefer forms of psychotherapy. In addition, the community mental health movement and, more recently, the increasing cost of psychiatric care have stimulated efforts to find briefer forms of psychotherapy. Today, brief psychotherapy is a necessary part of the psychiatrist's armamentarium. Brief psychotherapy is not a replacement for long-term psychotherapy but rather is an additional technical skill available to the psychiatrist for treatment of appropriate patients and illnesses.

Psychotherapy has been defined by Sullivan as primarily a verbal interchange between two persons: one of these persons is an expert and the other a help-seeker. They work together on the patient's life problems in hope of achieving behavioral change.[1] All psychotherapies, including brief psychotherapy, share the importance of nonspecific curative factors in their anticipated outcome. These factors—abreaction, new information, and success experiences—guide all forms of medical treatment in which clinicians are striving to increase the probability that patients will experience relief of pain and suffering. However, brief psychotherapy, like long-term psychotherapy and psychoanalysis, also identifies specific technical interventions and procedures that are directed toward behavioral change above and beyond that caused by nonspecific curative factors. Brief psychotherapy is distinguished from longer-term treatments by the time limits placed upon the endeavor. It is the time limit in brief psychotherapy that gives unique characteristics to the treatment and distinguishes it from long-term psychotherapy and psychoanalysis.[2]

Although psychotherapy is often described as beginning as soon as the physician sees the patient, this hyperbole is intended to emphasize the importance of interpersonal and transferential elements in the initial session. In fact, it is extremely important to distinguish the diagnostic interviews from the ongoing treatment. Interventions and technical procedures performed during the evaluation phase are substantially different from the technical aspects of the psychotherapeutic process. During the evaluation, the physician must consider the interaction among the diagnosis, the patient's ego strength, physical health, and other selection criteria and the various treatment options. Through negotiation with the patient, a treatment decision is reached and psychotherapy begins. Many patients do not make it through the evaluation phase of seeking help. Brief psychotherapy is not the panacea for this population of patients, and it is inaccurate to consider them as having been in brief psychotherapy. Clearly, some of the "dropout" patients experience benefit during their short contact with mental health professionals, some through the nonspecific curative factors of help seeking, and others through guidance and crisis intervention. In addition, many may drop out because they did not receive what they were looking for.

This chapter looks at brief psychotherapy from the perspective of patient selection criteria, technique, and duration of treatment. Individual psychotherapies that rely less on psychodynamic techniques, including interpersonal psychotherapy and cognitive therapy, are summarized briefly, as well as brief group psychotherapy. In addition, research issues for the brief individual psychotherapies are reviewed. Finally, the application of brief therapies in various treatment settings and the economic pressures that are decreasing reimbursement for outpatient psychotherapy are discussed.

Brief Individual Psychodynamic Psychotherapies

HISTORICAL PERSPECTIVE

As is true for most psychotherapeutic treatments, the brief dynamic psychotherapies began with the work of Sigmund Freud. His earliest psychoanalytic treatments lasted only several months. Freud reported a successful six-session cure of the hysterical arm paralysis of the conductor, Bruno Walter, and a single 4-hour session was used to resolve Gustav Mahler's sexual impotence. Freud was not shy about giving advice and interacting actively with his patients, a point that was lost during debates on the analyst as a "mirror." In recent times, psychoanalysis and psychoanalytic psychotherapy have increased in length. The goals of treatment have become more ambitious, focusing on character pathology rather than symptom neuroses.

Ferenczi was the first psychoanalyst to shorten therapy with his technique of "active" therapy. Ferenczi saw his approach as a natural refinement of Freud's conclusion that active measures sometimes had to be taken by the therapist to cause the patient to deal with the source of his anxiety. Freud used the setting of a termination date with the "Wolf Man" as a parameter in treatment to mobilize unconscious conflicts. Among Ferenczi's techniques were restrictive methods, such as forbidding masturbation, and "reparative" approaches, including kissing and hugging. Rank tried setting a termination date in advance in order to focus therapy on the anxieties and conflicts around termination of therapy and separation from the therapist. As a result, the length of therapy was shortened considerably.

In 1946 Alexander and French published *Psychoanalytic Therapy*, which, although controversial

at the time, eventually led to a great expansion in the application of psychoanalytic principles to short-term dynamic psychotherapy. Alexander's and French's book summarized research conducted at the Chicago Institute for Psychoanalysis.[3] This work continued that of Rank and Ferenczi on the development of techniques to shorten psychotherapy. Among Alexander's and French's contributions were the importance of flexibility, manipulation, suggestion, and abreaction. Specific patient selection criteria and techniques and the duration of treatment distinguish brief individual psychodynamic psychotherapy from other forms of individual psychotherapy, both short- and long-term.

MALAN AND THE TAVISTOCK GROUP: FOCAL PSYCHOTHERAPY

The work of David Malan was influenced by Michael Balint, with whom he worked at the Tavistock Clinic in London. From their workshops developed the idea of focal psychotherapy as an example of applied psychoanalysis.[4] Malan has subsequently carried on Balint's work.[5] Previous attempts to develop brief forms of psychoanalytic psychotherapy involved primarily the use of "activity." However, Malan underscores the importance of choosing and maintaining a narrow focal area to be dealt with in a brief period of time. Rather than increasing "activity," which was frequently equated with manipulation, Malan emphasizes the importance of "finding the appropriate focus from what the patient offers" and "consistently approaching the focal problem with interpretative activity alone." Through selective attention and neglect, the therapist maintains the focus and completes a brief psychotherapy. The importance of determining the focus underscores the value of the diagnostic process, including the psychodynamic assessment of the patient, prior to the initiation of psychotherapy.

Malan identified the following factors as leading to the lengthening of treatment: resistance, overdetermination, a need for working through, the roots of conflict in early childhood, transference, dependence, negative transference connected with termination, and the transference neurosis. In addition, some therapist characteristics may lengthen treatment. These include a tendency toward passivity, a sense of timelessness conveyed to the patient, therapeutic perfectionism, and a preoccupation with deeper and earlier experiences. All of these factors must be dealt with in order to maintain a brief therapy.

For Malan, identifying a focal conflict acceptable to the patient is of critical importance to a successful outcome. In addition, the patient must have a capacity to think in feeling terms, demonstrate a high motivation, and exhibit a good response to trial interpretations made during the evaluation phase. Patients who have had serious suicidal attempts, drug addiction, "convinced" homosexuality, long-term hospitalization, more than one course of electroconvulsive therapy (ECT), chronic alcoholism, incapacitating severe chronic obsessional symptoms, severe chronic phobic symptoms, or gross destructive or self-destructive acting out are excluded from treatment.

The patient is also rejected if the therapist anticipates certain problem areas, including the following:

1. An inability to make contact with the patient
2. A necessity for prolonged work in order to generate motivation in the patient
3. A necessity for prolonged work in order to penetrate rigid defenses
4. An inevitable involvement in complex or deep-seated issues
5. A severe dependence or other forms of unfavorable intense transference
6. An intensification of depressive or psychotic disturbances

Malan groups these areas into several specific dangers. Numbers one through three impair the ability to form an effective therapeutic working alliance within a short time; numbers four and five indicate possible difficulties at the time of termination; and number six is taken as a warning of a possible depressive or psychotic breakdown during treatment. Thus, Malan takes seriously the time limitation in a brief therapy, which requires the rapid establishment of a therapeutic alliance and an ability to terminate without the development of unexpected serious symptomatology.

Malan is not as concerned as other practitioners that the patient manifest nonserious psychopathology. In fact, several of the cases that he presents show significant degrees of pathology. Rather it is the balance between motivation and focality that is important. A patient with only moderate motivation but a highly focal conflict might be accepted into treatment. Similarly, a patient with high motivation but not as focal a conflict might also be accepted into treatment with the hope that clarification of the focus would occur in a short period of time.

Identifying the precipitating factors, early traumatic experiences, or repetitive patterns can point to the area of internal conflict present since childhood and to the focus for treatment. The congruence between the current conflict and the "nuclear" or childhood conflict should be seen by the therapist during the evaluation phase. The patient's response to interpretations about aspects of this conflict may lead to acceptance into treatment. According to Malan, the greater the probability that the conflict area will manifest itself in the transference, the more positive the outcome will be. Furthermore, he reported that transference interpretations correlated with character change and that character change endured 2 to 10 years later.

Malan is much less concerned with technique than with the importance of choosing the focus. He employs all the usual technical procedures of psychoanalytic psychotherapy and emphasizes the importance of making interpretations of the transference and connecting these to current and past relationships. This "triangle of insight" (the transference, the current relationship, and the past relationship) leads to the patient's cure. Overall, the goal is to clarify the nature of the defense, the anxiety, and the impulse that the patient is experiencing and to link these to the present, the past, and the transference. Once the defense and the anxiety are clarified, the link to the past can be made. The interpretation that links to the past may be experienced as reassuring by the patient because of its emphasis on the conflict belonging to the world of fantasy rather than to the world of the present. Malan emphasizes transference interpretations as the most therapeutically effective interpretations because of their here-and-now character.

In the brief therapy unit at the Tavistock Clinic, a time limit was almost always imposed. With trainees this was frequently 30 sessions. However, in his publications, Malan indicates a mean of 20 sessions for those cases with favorable outcomes. The longer time for trainees gives the opportunity to correct mistakes that might occur. In some cases, therapy has extended up to one year (46 sessions). In general, Malan advocates the importance of a definite date rather than a set number of sessions. Practically speaking, this eliminates the need for the patient and therapist to keep count of the number of sessions and eliminates complications related to whether or not to make up sessions that the patient has missed. Such a time limit gives a definite beginning, middle, and end to the therapy, helps to concentrate the patient's material and the therapist's work, maintains the focus, and decreases diffuseness, which might lead into long-term work.

SIFNEOS: SHORT-TERM ANXIETY-PROVOKING PSYCHOTHERAPY

At the same time that David Malan was undertaking his research at the Tavistock Clinic, Peter Sifneos was studying brief psychotherapy at the Massachusetts General Hospital in Boston.[6] Many of his conclusions are similar to those of Malan. However, there are some differences.

Sifneos emphasizes the importance of patient selection because of the anxiety-provoking nature of the brief psychotherapy techniques he uses. He distinguishes anxiety-provoking therapy from anxiety-supressing therapy, commonly referred to as supportive psychotherapy. For short-term anxiety-provoking psychotherapy (STAPP), the patient must be of above average intelligence and have had at least one meaningful relationship with another person during his lifetime. The patient who has had such a relationship will be able to withstand the anxiety produced by the therapy and to develop a mature relationship with the therapist. This criterion tends to exclude the narcissistic disorders. In addition, the patient must be highly motivated for change, not only for symptom relief.

Sifneos also identifies several criteria for patient selection based on the presentation of the patient during the evaluation. The patient must have a specific chief complaint. Sifneos asks the patient which of his complaints is of top priority. The patient's ability to identify one conflict area and to postpone work on others is taken as an indication of the patient's ability to tolerate anxiety. Sifneos looks for patients with anxiety, depression, phobias, conversion, and mild obsessive–compulsive features or personality disorders involving clear-cut interpersonal difficulties. During the evaluation, the patient must show an ability to interact with the evaluating psychiatrist, to express feelings, and to show some flexibility.

Sifneos is one of the few authors who clarifies his assessment of motivation. He defines motivation as including the patient's ability to recognize symptoms as psychological, a tendency to be introspective and honest about emotional difficulties, and a willingness to participate in the treatment situation. In addition, motivation includes curiosity, a willingness to change as well as a willingness to make reasonable sacrifices, and a realistic expectation of the results of psychotherapy.

Sifneos focuses on the oedipal conflict and does not expect a good outcome in dealing with other than oedipal-conflict areas. The majority of failures using STAPP have occurred in patients who complained of reactive depression following the loss of a loved one. He believes that this failure is due to the dyadic, nontriangular (nonoedipal) origins of the ambivalent feelings in some patients. In such cases, when the issue of termination arises, the patient regresses and an impass is reached.

During the initial phase of psychotherapy, the therapist must establish good rapport with the patient in order to create a therapeutic alliance. The therapist uses anxiety-provoking confrontations in order to clarify issues around the patient's early life situation and present-day conflict. The therapist avoids areas such as passivity, dependence, and acting out, which might lead to extensive regression. The use of anxiety-provoking confrontations in a direct attack on the patient's defenses distinguishes STAPP from other brief psychotherapies. Although it is made clear to patients during their evaluation that the psychotherapy is expected to last only a few months, no specific number of sessions or termination date is given. Interviews are held weekly and are 45 minutes long. The vast majority of treatments last from 12 to 16 sessions, and none goes beyond 20 sessions. The aggressive confrontational style of this treatment underscores the importance of excluding preoedipal problems and the importance of observing countertransference reactions in the therapist, frequently related to being too aggressive.

MANN: TIME-LIMITED PSYCHOTHERAPY

James Mann has focused upon the specific limitation of time in brief psychotherapy. Mann sees the variable of time as a specific operative factor in psychotherapy as well as an element in its curative effect.[7] The experience of the timelessness of treatment and of the treatment's termination is a significant element in Mann's view of the psychotherapeutic process.

Usually there are two to four evaluation meetings prior to beginning psychotherapy. Mann limits psychotherapy to a total of 12 treatment sessions. He admits having chosen this number somewhat arbitrarily; however, his clinical experience indicates that somewhere between 10 and 14 sessions is a sufficient number. Mann also emphasizes the importance of a uniform number of sessions for evaluating the psychotherapeutic process among different therapists. In this way the relationship between the presenting problems of the patient and psychotherapeutic technique can be studied more easily. Frequently, the provision of a specific number of sessions can also be more easily accepted by the patient as a typical medical "prescription." Although Mann indicates that the 12 sessions may be "prescribed" in any form (e.g., two visits per week for 6 weeks or one half hour each week for 24 weeks), in practice he almost always schedules one session per week for 12 weeks. The setting of a specific last session in the initial contract with the patient allows the therapy to have a clear beginning, middle, and end.

Mann, to some extent, minimizes selection as a central issue for brief psychotherapy. He does indicate a number of exclusionary criteria: serious depression, acute psychosis, borderline personality organization, and the inability to identify a central issue. Mann sees Sifneos' criteria as excluding primarily borderline patients. He does not agree with Sifneos' emphasis on superior academic or work performance.

In a more recent publication and in contrast to earlier work, Mann expands his selection criteria by emphasizing the importance of the patient's ego strength as measured by prior work performance and past relationships.[8] Patients who may have difficulty engaging and disengaging rapidly from treatment are excluded. This includes schizoid patients, certain obsessional patients, patients with strong dependency needs, some narcissistic patients, some depressive patients who will not be able to form a rapid therapeutic alliance, and some patients with psychosomatic disorders who do not tolerate loss well.

According to Mann, the selection of the central issue for the psychotherapy is the critical event. It is the vehicle through which the patient is engaged in the work of therapy and on which a successful outcome depends. Mann looks for a central issue that is developmentally and adaptively relevant and has been recurrent over time. He describes this issue as the patient's "present and chronically endured pain" and characterizes it as a preconscious element. The therapist's statement of the central issue is a clarification that can be readily recognized, felt, and held onto by the patient. Time-limited psychotherapy is intended to resolve this present and chronically endured pain. The therapist frames the central issue to the patient in terms of a general statement about feelings.

Mann goes into substantial detail on the phrasing of the central issue to the patient. In the phrasing of the central issue, the therapeutic contract and the goal of the therapy are specified. In the case of a 41-year-old-depressed woman who was preoccupied with her husband and children being even one minute late, Mann suggested the central issue: "You've encountered extreme life situations and have managed them remarkably well. . . yet you fear and have always feared that despite your best efforts you will lose everything." In a 31-year-old married man attempting to obtain a college degree who was consumed with a fear of failing, Mann suggested the central issue: "Because there has been a number of sudden and very painful events in your life, things always seem uncertain, and you are excessively nervous because you do not expect anything to go along well. Things are always uncertain for you."[8]

Mann makes use of the usual psychoanalytic psychotherapy techniques: defense analysis, transference interpretation, and genetic reconstruction. Transference is interpreted from within the central identified conflict area and in terms of the adaptive processes of the patient. However, he does not confront the patient. In general, his interventions are very close to the conscious material provided by the patient. Mann identifies specific dynamic events that unfold during the 12 sessions. The opening sessions are understood as representing a "surge of unconscious magical expectations" that past pains will now be resolved. During the initial phase the therapist makes few comments and accepts the positive transference of the patient. Important aspects of the current problem, defense mechanisms, coping styles, and genetic roots of the central issue become clearer during this phase. In the middle four sessions, resistance is likely to appear, as well as the negative transference. The patient begins to experience the frustration that all of the wished for changes may not occur. In the ending phase of treatment, termination and the patient's resistance to termination in the face of unresolved problems in other areas of life are prominent.

Mann sees the importance of confronting separation and termination issues as critical to the success of brief psychotherapy. Frequently the patient unconsciously reveals an awareness that the midpoint of treatment has come. The patient experiences separation from the transference-invested therapist as a separation from an ambivalently experienced person from the past, without having achieved the fantasied magical resolution. The goal is to enable the patient to separate from the transference-invested therapist less ambivalently than he had done from this earlier important figure. Consequently, both the resolution of the central issue and the unfolding of an attachment/separation process in the 12-session treatment contract are intimately related through the development and interpretation of the transference.

DAVANLOO: BROAD-FOCUS SHORT-TERM DYNAMIC PSYHCOTHERAPY

Habib Davanloo writes about broad-focus, short-term dynamic psychotherapy.[9] His selection criteria include patients with an oedipal focus, a loss focus, and patients with multiple foci. Davanloo is particularly interested in patients suffering from long-standing obsessional and phobic neuroses. His research data indicate that 30% to 35% of the psychiatric outpatient population can benefit from this mode of therapy. Unfortunately, Davanloo's research work has not been published in a systematic manner. Most information about his technique is derived from the publication of cases, presentations, and brief descriptions of his research that accompany case presentations.

The initial evaluation is a specific, focused interview in which the patient's defenses against "true feelings" are "gently but relentlessly confronted." Davanloo says that this is not a universal technique for the initial interview and cautions on its use with patients with severe psychopathology. Selection is based on psychological-mindedness, the quality of the patient's interpersonal relations, and, in particular, on the presence of at least one meaningful relationship in the patient's past. The patient's ability to tolerate and experience anxiety, guilt, and depression is important. The patient must be motivated to complete the treatment process and to resolve neurotic problems. The patient's ability to respond to interpretation is an important selection criterion. In particular, response to transference interpretations that link the transference with the present and the past is a critical feature in the assessment for broad-focus, short-term dynamic psychotherapy. Davanloo finds no value in criteria based on severity and duration of illness. Finally, the presence of flexibility in the ego's defensive pattern and a lack of use of the primitive defenses of projection, splitting, and denial are important factors in selecting patients.

Davanloo emphasizes that the therapist should have the answers to the following questions by the end of the evaluation procedure:

1. What is the central neurotic structure of the patient's problem?
2. Does the patient respond to interpretation?
3. Is it possible to make links between the present and the past?
4. Does the patient relate in a meaningful way to the interviewer?
5. Have there been some meaningful relationships in the patient's past?
6. Does the patient's history indicate the ability to face the uncovering process of therapy without serious adverse effects, such as psychotic decompensation or suicide?
7. Is the patient motivated to look at himself/herself and to go through the uncovering process?

The technique Davanloo uses in therapy is a continuation of that used in the initial interview. The patient is "gently but relentlessly" confronted about his defenses against feelings in the transference relationship and in the past. All the usual techniques of psychoanalytic psychotherapy are employed: defense analysis, transference interpretations, and genetic reconstruction. Dreams and fantasy material are also used. Transference interpretations tend to be made early. Because of the confrontive style, a strong therapeutic alliance is necessary. Davanloo warns therapists that passive dependent and obsessional characters may develop a symbiotic transference relationship. This may be avoided through active confrontation and selection of patients.

Davanloo recommends 5 to 40 sessions, depending on the patient's conflict area (oedipal versus multiple foci) and other selection criteria. In general, his treatments fall between 15 and 25 sessions. Davanloo notes the appearance of transference resistance by the second interview. This rapid mobilization of transference and defenses may be a result of the confrontational style and the early use of transference interpretation. The emotional experiences of the patient in the transference are emphasized in the treatment.

COMPARISON OF THE BRIEF INDIVIDUAL PSYCHODYNAMIC PSYCHOTHERAPIES

The work of Malan, Sifneos, Mann, and Davanloo shows substantial overlap in their goals, selection criteria, technique, and duration of treatment. These authors tend to agree with Bennett,[10] who describes the goals of brief psychotherapy as facilitating health-seeking behaviors and mitigating obstacles to normal growth. From this perspective, brief psychotherapy focuses on the patient's continuous development throughout adult life and the context-dependent appearance of conflict, depending upon environment, interpersonal relationships, biological health, and developmental stage. This picture of brief psychotherapy supports modest goals, which require the therapist to refrain from perfectionism. Malan, Sifneos, Mann, and Davanloo also seem to agree with Stierlin's[11] contrast between brief psychotherapy's use of the "propitious moment" and long-term treatment's emphasis and use of "a shared past" between therapist and patient. Both the "propitious moment" and the "shared past" carry psychotherapeutic advantages and disadvantages, emphasizing certain technical possibilities and limiting others.

Many of the selection criteria emphasized by the above authors are common to all types of psychodynamic psychotherapy. However, unique selection criteria are required because of the brief duration of treatment. Patients in brief psychodynamic psychotherapy must be able to engage quickly with the therapist, terminate in a short period of time, and be able to carry on much of the working through and generalizing of the treatment effects on their own. The necessity for greater independent action by the patient mandates high levels of ego strength, motivation, and responsiveness to interpretation. Sifneos' rather unique emphasis on intelligence as a criterion may be related to his anxiety-provoking interpretations, which require a broader educational context in order to be understood. The importance of the rapid establishment of a therapeutic alliance underlies a substantial number of the selection and exclusion criteria.

The central importance of a focus in brief psychotherapy is mentioned by all authors. They also emphasize the importance of the evaluation sessions to determine this focus. Mann formulates the focus to the patient in terms of the patient's fears and pain. However, Mann would probably agree with Malan, Davanloo, and Sifneos in the importance of constructing the psychodynamic focus at a deeper level in one's own understanding of the work being done. Maintaining the focus is the primary task of the therapist. This enables the therapist to deal with complicated personality structures in a brief period of time. Resistance is limited through "benign neglect" of potentially troublesome but nonfocal areas of the personality.

The authors also discuss the importance of transference interpretations. However, the manner and rapidity in which transference is dealt with vary considerably. Malan takes a more typical psychoanalytic approach of waiting for transference to become resistance before it is interpreted. Sifneos, in his emphasis on the oedipal relationship, is more aggressive in handling the deep conflictual areas of transference material. Davanloo is confrontational in developing a transference experience. This confrontational style may at times confuse the patient's experience of the real and the transferential therapist. However, Davanloo's focus on the treatment of severe obsessional disorders, where the need to "stir affect" is high, may be where this particular technique is most useful. Malan's emphasis on the importance of making the transference/parent link for the successful outcome of treatment is significant and requires further exploration.

Strupp's studies of college students in brief psychotherapy tend to confirm the importance of interactional variables.[12,13] He found the quality of the therapeutic interaction and the handling of the transference and countertransference to be critical to success or failure in treatment. Strupp's studies indicate that patients treated by nonprofessionally trained therapists, on the average, are as much improved as patients treated by professional therapists. However, they also show that such nonexperienced therapists run out of relevant material and soon become unwilling to continue to treat patients over an extended period of time.[14] One of the important tasks of training in psychotherapy may be the development of the ability to "endure" with the patient and, over time, with numbers of patients. Technical training and a theoretical framework may allow the therapist to maintain a sense of competence, direction, and interest in the work that the nonprofessional therapist cannot.

The role of countertransference in brief psychotherapy is as complicated as it is in long-term treatment. Countertransference issues related to the aggressive techniques used by Sifneos and Davanloo have been observed. Countertransference experiences related to termination are emphasized by Mann. The goal-directed techniques of brief psychotherapy limit the development of regressive countertransference responses.

There is remarkable agreement on the duration of brief psychotherapy. Although the duration ranges from 5 to 40 sessions, authors generally favor 10 to 20 sessions. The duration of treatment is critically related to maintaining the focus within the brief psychotherapy. Shilien[15] has found in Rogerian therapy a correlation between the number of sessions and recovery. In general, he reports an increasingly successful outcome (measured by the patient's self-concept) up to about 20 sessions. After 20 sessions, little improvement is noticed until 40 or more sessions. When treatment extends beyond 20 sessions, the therapist frequently finds himself enmeshed in a broad character analysis without a focal conflict. Change after 20 sessions may be slow. Clinical experience generally supports the idea that brief individual psychodynamic psychotherapy should be between 10 and 20 sessions unless the therapist is willing to proceed to long-term treatment of greater than 40 or 50 sessions.

Brief psychodynamic psychotherapy for depression[16] and narcissistic disturbances[17] has been described. Bellak and Lazarus perform an important role by describing the techniques most effective for specific diagnostic categories. Horowitz has described brief psychotherapy focused on the stress responses evidenced by various personality styles.[18] He emphasizes that this psychotherapy is directed toward dealing with the process of the stress response and not character change. However, his outcomes indicate that selected character changes are possible in some areas. The distinction between recovery from a disruption in homeostatic balance, reconstitution of self-esteem and self-concept, and changes in character structure require further exploration.

The identification of critical points during brief psychotherapy at which the "danger" of becoming a long-term treatment emerges will further clarify the technical handling of brief psychodynamic psychotherapy. Amada[19] has identified phenomena that characteristically appear in the interlude between a short- and a long-term treatment. He notes an increasing vagueness with respect to the goals of the treatment, decreased activity by the therapist, and the emergence of the transference as a central element. These variables indicate the potential of a short-term psychotherapy becoming a long-term treatment. Prelinger[20] has identified the fourth to sixth hours of once a week therapy as a point at which incipient or potential regression may suddenly appear. The patient at this time is testing the boundaries of the treatment. Action by the therapist is required if a brief psychotherapy is to remain "exactly that"—brief. The study of technical interventions to be used at these critical moments will further elucidate the handling of limited regression in brief psychodynamic psychotherapy.

EDUCATION

The importance of brief psychodynamic psychotherapy to the practicing clinician makes mandatory the inclusion of instruction on brief psychotherapy in psychiatric residency training. Learning long-term psychotherapy is not the equivalent of learning brief psychotherapy. However, it may be true that the long-term psychotherapist is best prepared for using brief psychotherapy where there are fewer opportunities to make mistakes and correct them. Psychiatric residents must develop the skills to apply all psychotherapeutic treatment modalities: crisis intervention, brief psychodynamic psychotherapy, long-term psychodynamic psychotherapy, and supportive psychotherapy. The understanding of which patient for which treatment at which time is as critical for the prescription of psychotherapy as it is for the prescription of psychopharmacologic agents.

Brief psychotherapy is best taught in conjunction with a discussion of the principles of long-term psychotherapy. In the context of learning psychodynamic formulations of pathology and the ways in which defense, transference, and countertransference appear in the psychotherapeutic dyad, the resident can begin to learn the unique constraints and advantages that accrue with a brief time period. Through contrasting short- and long-term psychotherapy, the psychiatry trainee can learn appropriate patient selection and technical procedures to accomplish brief psychodynamic psychotherapy. Such training requires both a familiarity with brief psychotherapy literature and supervised clinical experiences of brief psychodynamic cases.

In learning brief psychodynamic psychotherapy, residents gain a better understanding of the importance of the evaluation procedure as a separate, distinct element in the management of their approach to patients. Seeing psychotherapy as a modality that must be prescribed in duration, focus, and intensity, and with a plan similar to any pharmacologic management of a patient enhances the resident's sense of mastery, accomplishment, and competence in dealing psychotherapeutically with a broad range of patients.

Other Brief Individual Psychotherapies

INTERPERSONAL PSYCHOTHERAPY

Short-term interpersonal therapy (IPT) has been developed by Klerman, Weissman, and collegues.[21] IPT is brief—12 to 16 weeks in duration—and focuses on current interpersonal problems in outpatient nonbipolar, nonpsychotic depressed patients. IPT has been the major psychotherapeutic modality used in combined psychotherapy and pharmacologic treatment studies. IPT derives from the interpersonal school of psychiatry originating with Adolf Meyer and Harry Stack Sullivan. The understanding of social supports and of attachment provides further theoretical underpinning for this form of psychotherapy. IPT focuses on reassurance, clarification of feeling states, improvement in interpersonal communication, testing of perception, and interpersonal skills rather than personality reconstruction.

IPT has been used primarily in the treatment of depressed patients. In the opening phase of IPT, a detailed symptom history is taken, usually using a structured interview. The symptoms are reviewed with the patient, and the patient receives explicit information about the natural course of depression as a clinical condition. There is an emphasis on legitimizing the patient in the sick role. A second major task of this phase is the assessment of interpersonal problem areas. There is an attempt to identify one or more of four problem areas: grief reaction, interpersonal disputes, role transition, or interpersonal deficits. Each of these areas is felt to be related to depression. The middle phase of treatment is directed toward resolving the problem area or areas. Clarification of positive and negative feeling states, identifying past models for relationships, and guiding and encouraging the patient in examining and choosing alternative courses of action constitute the basic techniques for handling each problem area. The focus is kept on current dilemmas and not past interpersonal relationships. Interpersonal events rather than intrapsychic or cognitive events are the focus of IPT.

Much of IPT is based upon psychodynamic theory. Applying the dictum of working "from the surface to the depths" results in psychodynamic psychotherapy resembling IPT. However, Klerman and colleagues have found it useful to highlight the differences between these approaches in order to standardize a psychotherapeutic technique. Collaborative clinical trials have demonstrated the advantage of maintenance IPT in enhancing social functioning in recovery from depression and in reducing symptoms and improving functioning during the acute phase of a depressive episode. These effects require 6 to 8 months to become apparent and do not appear in the first 4 months of treatment. Patients on combined pharamacologic and IPT therapy have the best outcomes.[22]

COGNITIVE THERAPY

Cognitive therapy has been developed and refined by Aaron Beck[23] and A. John Rush.[24] Cognitive therapy is a short-term psychotherapy in which specific cognitions (thoughts or images) or schemata (silent assumptions) account for the onset and persistence of symptoms. The first part of treatment is directed toward reducing symptoms (often depression or anxiety) that are derived from these cognitions. This is accomplished by having the patient recognize and record cognitions and learn to develop new cognitions that will not produce dysphoric affects. In the later part of treatment the focus is on identifying and modifying the silent assumptions or schemata that determine the content of the cognitions.

Three important concepts are defined in cognitive therapy. *Cognitions* are thoughts or images that are immediately brought to consciousness when a person is faced with a situation. As Rush emphasizes, cognitions "are what a person thinks *in* a situation," not what he thinks *about* a situation.[24] The cognitions play a direct role in affect and behavior. *Schemata* are silent assumptions derived from a patient's early experience that determine the content of cognitions employed in certain situations. Schemata form the basis for how one evaluates, categorizes, and distorts experiences. *Logical errors* are the *consequences* of negative cognitions. They are the incorrect inferences or conclusions derived from events. Logical errors include personalization (giving personal meaning to a neutral event), selective attention (ignoring the positive aspects of a situation), overgeneralization, and magnification.[23] Situations may cause a person to formulate cognitions, which reflect negative views of oneself, the world, or the future, and which are derived from schemata. Negative cognitions lead to the development of symptoms and result in logical errors, which may further distort the situation and intensify symptoms.

The objectives of cognitive therapy are summarized in Table 1.[23,24] The therapist guides the pa-

TABLE 1. Objectives of Cognitive Therapies for Patients

Early stages
    Awareness of stereotyped views that they bring to situations
    Recognition and correction of these views to conform more to objective reality
Later stages
    Identification of schemata
    Development and application of new cognitive responses to situations
Generation of new schemata and their application to anticipated and actual situtations

tient through a multitude of diverse experiences in order to teach the patient to recognize dysfunctional cognitions and to assist the patient in developing more adaptive patterns of thinking and behaving.

Cognitive therapy is indicated for those patients capable of forming a therapeutic relationship in a brief period of time. A number of the criteria developed by Sifneos, Malan, and Davanloo and discussed earlier in this chapter are applicable to the cognitive therapies. Patients who are psychotic (as a result of schizophrenia, bipolar disorder, major depression with psychotic features, schizoaffective disorder, and others), who exhibit severe cognitive or memory deficits (as a result of a variety of organic mental disorders), or who have a borderline personality disorder usually do not respond to treatment.[25]

Cognitive therapy has been used to treat a wide range of psychiatric disorders: generalized anxiety disorders, phobic disorders, obesity, drug and alcohol abuse, chronic pain syndromes, and depression. However, it has been used successfully most often to treat patients with relatively acute, non-psychotic depressions of mild to moderate severity. Depressions with endogenous and melancholic features have not been adequately studied to determine the efficacy of cognitive therapy alone.[25] Patients with a diagnosis of major depression secondary to a physical disorder often respond well to cognitive techniques. Those with organic affective syndromes secondary to medication or physical illness do not.

Patients with moderate to severe depressions are seen twice a week for up to 14 sessions. If significant relief of symptoms is not achieved at the end of 7 weeks, modification of treatment to include the addition of tricyclic antidepressants is considered. Patients with mild to moderate depressions may benefit from only weekly sessions. Following acute treatment, the clinician may schedule the patient for once or twice a month maintenance treatment for 6 to 12 months to consolidate therapy gains and to decrease the probability of relapse.

Brief Group Psychotherapy

Group psychotherapy is often brief. The length of therapy and frequency of sessions per week are related to the setting in which the therapy takes place and the goals of therapy. For instance, group therapies for inpatient psychiatric patients or for patients hospitalized on a medical ward are usually of brief duration, meeting one or more times per week with a limited goal of reestablishing sufficient functioning to allow for discharge. Outpatient groups, frequently with more ambitious goals, reflect a wider range of total sessions and frequency. Psychotherapy groups used in a general hospital or on an inpatient psychiatric service are usually open groups, in which members are replaced as they leave the hospital to maintain a selected group size. In outpatient settings, closed groups are more frequently used. A closed group meets for a specified period of time and accepts no new members nor replaces departing members once the sessions begin.

The literature on brief group psychotherapy is limited, but in many areas it parallels the literature on general group psychotherapy. Group psychotherapies can be characterized as either heterogeneous or homogeneous. Homogeneous groups are composed of patients with similar psychiatric or medical disorders. They are frequently used to help hospitalized medical inpatients deal with issues related to their treatment. Groups have been used for patients with cancer, chronic pain, myocardial infarction, and those undergoing dialysis. Brief psychotherapy groups of homogeneous composition have also been used successfully with health care providers, oncology fellows, intensive care unit nurses, and residents from a variety of medical specialties. Homogeneous groups are often of short duration (20 sessions or less) but may be longer and may even last a lifetime (Alcoholics Anonymous). Heterogeneous groups include patients with a variety of psychiatric disorders, ego strengths, personality traits, and interpersonal difficulties. Heterogeneous groups are most frequently used by psychiatrists practicing in outpatient settings.

Groups are also defined by the technical focus of treatment: individual, interactional, or group as a whole. Those focusing on individual issues apply the principles of psychodynamic psychotherapy to individual–therapist transference issues. Interactional groups emphasize individual interactions with other group members and the therapist. These groups focus on immediate events that occur in the group. Those whose focus is the group as a whole emphasize the individual members' unconscious transference toward the therapist as reflected in the group dynamics. Individual and interactional issues are minimized, and group-wide interpretations predominate. All types and combinations of foci have been used successfully in homogeneous and heterogeneous patient groups.[26]

TECHNICAL ISSUES

The optimal length of a single group session is usually 90 minutes. Sessions lasting for shorter or longer periods of time are associated with diminished benefits. Brief group therapy sessions may be held once or twice weekly, and, by definition, are time-limited, the number of sessions usually being determined by the goals of treatment. Treatment goals vary greatly depending upon the group's composition. For instance, brief group psychotherapy for recently discharged schizophrenic patients emphasizes learning social and interpersonal skills. Brief oncology patient groups may emphasize adjustment to the hospital setting or resolution of emotional conflicts related to their diagnosis or prognosis. In general, they are goal-directed and frequently have an educational quality.

Yalom[27] has defined the therapist's roles as the following: constructing and maintaining the physical system, constructing the therapeutic culture, and emphasizing here-and-now interactions. With regard to the physical system, the psychiatrist determines who will join the group and when it will meet, outlines its goals, and attempts to minimize outside influences that may undermine the group's work. The therapist, through example and explanation, establishes the behavioral rules that guide the group's interaction and that constitute the therapeutic culture. Finally, the group leader focuses the group's attention to material generated from within the group and not outside it.

PATIENT SELECTION

The selection of patients for brief group therapy varies widely, depending upon the type of group (homogeneous versus heterogeneous; individual, interactional or group as a whole), goals of the group, and setting (inpatient versus outpatient). Generally agreed upon selection criteria for psychiatry groups include psychological-mindedness, motivation for treatment, a minimum level of interpersonal skills, expectancy of therapeutic gain, psychiatric symptoms (especially anxiety), and reasonably good premorbid adjustment.[26] Patients who should not be included in heterogeneous outpatient groups include those with the following diagnoses: organic mental disorders, drug or alcohol addiction, paranoid disorders, narcissistic and antisocial personality disorders, and hypochondriasis. Patients who are acutely psychotic or suicidal should also be excluded. On the other hand, several of these same patients, especially those with alcohol- and drug-abuse disorders, do well in ho-

mogeneous, goal-oriented groups. Also, selected narcissistic patients may benefit from group therapy. Brief group psychotherapy with a homogeneous patient composition has been shown to be effective for the following medical and psychiatric conditions: alcoholism, drug abuse and dependence, myocardial infarction, posttraumatic stress disorder, peptic ulcer disease, asthma, diabetes, seizure disorders, chronic pain syndromes, arthritis, headaches, and postamputation.[26]

CONCURRENT TREATMENT

An important clinical question is whether to combine brief individual psychotherapy with brief group treatment. A concurrent approach may be beneficial for patients with personality disorders, especially the borderline and narcissistic types.[27] For these patients, the group may reduce fears of engulfment and retaliation and temper aggressive feelings that are frequently projected on the therapist during individual therapy. Also, the group provides a setting for multiple transferences to develop, hence diluting the overwhelming dependency needs, regression, and destructive affects (especially anger and hostility) that may impede progress in individual therapy. From a practical standpoint, the group provides most patients with a sense of belonging and an opportunity for reality testing. Other group members may give direct and helpful feedback that patients may use in regulating their interpersonal relations. In other words, a group experience helps patients to adapt their behavior to social reality while individual therapy assists them in resolving intrapsychic conflicts. In practice this is a very common inpatient treatment combination, although its advantages and disadvantages have rarely been studied.

Concurrent treatment is not without risks. Yalom contends that group therapy may impede the development of transference and a therapeutic alliance in individual therapy, which at the same time may decrease involvement and participation in the group.[27] Also, some borderline or schizophrenic patients may find the addition of group therapy destabilizing by promoting regressed behavior and by causing dysphoric affects, especially anxiety and depression.

The literature provides no clear guidelines for clinicians to follow in deciding which patients would benefit from concurrent brief group and brief individual therapy. However, a concurrent approach generally appears to work best for patients with preoedipal conflicts and primitive ego defenses (especially borderline and narcissistic patients) and for patients who may benefit from the interpersonal relationships and reality testing that the group provides (especially schizophrenic patients not currently psychotic). However, as emphasized above, patients with these diagnoses are the same one who may have the most difficulties with concurrent group treatment.

Research in Brief Psychotherapy

EMPIRICAL OUTCOME STUDIES

Research of psychotherapy outcome is reviewed comprehensively by Parloff elsewhere in this volume. Consequently, only a few major studies that pertain to the outcome of brief psychotherapy are discussed here.

Interest in psychotherapy outcome studies was greatly stimulated by Eysenck's critical review.[28] He reviewed studies (mostly uncontrolled) that reported on outcomes in a wide range of psychotherapeutic modalities, including psychoanalytic, "eclectic," and brief forms of therapy. All the "eclectic" therapies described by Eysenck satisfy usually accepted criteria in length (less than 40 sessions) for brief therapies. His controversial conclusion that psychoanalytic psychotherapy was not an effective technique and that behavioral therapies were more effective than no treatment was subsequently criticized by a number of investigators. The first comprehensive response was published by Meltzoff and Kornreich,[29] who reviewed 101 controlled outcome studies to determine whether patients with a variety of mental disorders would benefit more from psychotherapy than from no treatment. They characterized studies as either adequate or questionable and judged results as positive, null (no difference between control and treatment groups), and negative. Meltzoff and Kornreich found that 84% of the adequate studies demonstrated positive outcomes, 54% considered major or multiple positive outcomes, and 30% showed minor or limited positive outcomes. These findings led them to conclude that controlled research had, in fact, demonstrated significantly more behavioral and social adjustment improvement in patients with various disorders treated with a wide range of psychotherapeutic techniques. Their work also led to the refinement of

criteria by which to evaluate outcome studies and contributed to an increase in the numbers of outcome reports and their research sophistication. In a comprehensive survey of brief and crisis-oriented therapies, Butcher and Koss[30] concluded that 60% to 70% of treated patients improved. Improvement was measured both by patients and therapists.

Luborsky and colleagues[31] reviewed eight studies in which time-limited treatment was compared with time-unlimited treatment. In five studies, there was no difference in outcome. In two reports, time-limited therapy produced more favorable outcomes and in one, poorer results. One of the problems with this review is that the studies include mostly college students with relatively minor problems in whom significant improvement would not be expected. In spite of these and other methodological problems, Luborsky and associates concluded that there was no difference in outcome between the short- and long-term therapies. A different conclusion was reached by Reid and Shyne,[32] who, in a relatively well-designed study, referred patients to either time-limited (eight sessions) or time-unlimited (open-ended) therapy. They concluded that time-limited therapy produced better results. However, they failed to specify the treatment techniques or selection criteria used. Such studies are highly dependent upon what outcome measures are chosen to be studied.

The Temple study[33] compared outcomes in outpatients suffering from neurotic or personality disorders referred to one of three groups: behavioral therapy; brief, psychodynamically oriented psychotherapy; and a waiting list group. Therapists, patients, and, in some cases, an informant rated symptoms, general adjustment, and overall improvement. Approximately 80% of both treatment groups improved, and the treatment groups showed more improvement than the untreated controls.

The explosion of psychotherapy research has led to a pressing need to develop criteria for evaluating outcome studies. Two important methods have been developed recently for use in evaluating psychotherapy outcome studies: the box-score method and meta-analysis. The box score method was first applied to psychotherapy research by Luborsky and colleagues.[31] This method is simply a way of analyzing numerous psychotherapy studies, which use different therapeutic techniques, in terms of the outcomes that they produce. Three outcomes are possible: positive effects from treatment, no significant effect, or negative effects. Studies that evaluate a particular form of psychotherapy are simply tallied according to these three outcomes, with the "winner" being the outcome that was reported by the majority of the studies; in other words, the outcome with the highest "box score." Meta-analysis also integrates large numbers of research studies through statistical analysis of the data of individual studies. It was first used by Smith and Glass[34] to evaluate 375 psychotherapy outcome studies. To be included in a meta-analysis, a study must have at least one therapy treatment group that is compared with a control group or different therapy group. Smith and colleagues calculated the relative magnitude of the effect of the therapy called "effect size," which can be computed regardless of the sample size. In each study effect size could be calculated for a number of outcome variables–depression, anxiety, self-esteem–and aggregated with effect sizes computed from other studies. The reviewers found that the average person on the 50th percentile who received psychotherapy of any type was better off at the end of therapy than 80% of persons who were in the control group. Most of the therapies that they reviewed were short-term and were applied to young people. Finally, they concluded that duration of therapy and experience of the therapist were unrelated to outcome.

The brief psychotherapies have been shown to be beneficial with a number of patient populations. For patients hospitalized on the medical or surgical services of a general hospital, brief psychotherapy, usually employed by consultation/liaison psychiatrists, has resulted in fewer days of hospitalization. When used to treat patients in health clinics or health maintenance organizations, brief psychotherapy, in comparison with controls, has been shown to decrease visits to primary health care providers, reduce visits for laboratory and x-ray studies, decrease the number of prescriptions given, and generally reduce direct health care costs.[35] One recent study[36] compared 72 patients found to have significant emotional problems and treated only by internists working in a general medical clinic with 62 patients also found to have emotional difficulties but who, in addition to being treated by internists for medical problems, received 10 weekly psychotherapy visits. Both groups had an approximately equal degree of emotional disturbance. At 4-month and 1-year follow-ups, the brief psychotherapy–treated group reported significantly more global improvement than the nonpsychotherapy-treated group. Also, more patients unemployed at screening in the brief psychotherapy–treated group became employed at 1-year follow-up than in the non-psychotherapy-treated group. This study tends to suggest specific beneficial effects of brief psychotherapy when used in a medical setting by skilled psychotherapists.

The brief psychotherapies have proven themselves efficacious in the military. Since World War II, military psychiatrists have incorporated the principles of combat psychiatry—proximity, immediacy, simplicity, and expectancy—into their brief psychotherapy techniques when treating soldiers with combat-related psychiatric disorders. The brief treatments are effective not only in combat situations, but also in the noncombat military post environment. In this setting, pressing training requirements and frequent personnel reassignments often make long-term treatment untenable. Also, shortages of military psychiatrists and other mental health workers frequently make brief psychotherapy the treatment of choice. Reductions in health care visits, similar to that achieved in the civilian community, have been reported.[35]

The brief psychotherapies have been shown particularly effective on college campuses. Adolescents often require treatment approaches that include active involvement by the therapist in setting protective limits, providing emotional support and guidance, and teaching psychological-mindedness. These approaches, frequently incorporated in the brief therapies and using either an individual or group approach, enable the college student to try out new feelings, thoughts, and actions.[37] In one study, time-limited approaches have produced more favorable outcomes than no treatment in college students.[38] This study and others document the utility of a brief therapeutic approach for adolescents in resolving earlier developmental issues and contributing to the formation of an autonomous ego identity.

FUTURE RESEARCH

A number of unanswered research questions persist for evaluating both the process and outcome of brief psychotherapy. Empirical research is needed to determine how patient characteristics relate to outcome. Certain affective, cognitive, and personality characteristics in patients ("capacity for therapy variables") can limit their ability to participate in particular types of brief therapies. Yet very few of these variables have been investigated. Brief psychodynamic psychotherapy, IPT, and cognitive therapy have very different foci. Patients can be expected to vary in their ability to respond to these different perspectives. Similarly, there is an urgent need to identify therapist characteristics that either enhance or impede the effectiveness of a particular brief psychotherapy technique and the rapid formation of the therapeutic alliance. Since some studies have shown the therapeutic relationship to be the most powerful predictor of outcome, the identification of the characteristics of the physician–patient relationship (roles, expectations, communication, and time) that determine a favorable outcome is needed. Research is also needed to determine which brief psychotherapy technique is most effective for which psychiatric condition and yields what outcomes.

Precise definition of the various brief therapies is necessary for research and clinical practice. The development of treatment manuals and the more detailed explanation of specific techniques have improved this situation, but much work remains. Finally, in today's economic climate, empirical studies are needed to assess the relative costs and benefits among various brief psychotherapy techniques with selected psychiatric conditions and to determine when brief psychotherapy is not cost-effective and when long-term psychotherapy is indicated. The cost-offset benefits of brief psychotherapy in reducing general medical health care costs for third-party carriers are of particular importance. Outpatient psychiatric benefits have undergone a considerable decline in the last decade and will continue to fall unless tangible cost savings to insurers can be demonstrated.

Economic Concerns

From 1955 to 1977, the number of inpatient- and outpatient-care episodes in specialty mental health facilities nearly quadrupled, from 1.7 million to 6.4 million. However, from 1963 to 1977 there was a tenfold increase in patient-care episodes occurring in outpatient settings. The percentage of all psychiatric patient-care episodes being treated in outpatient settings increased from 25% in 1955 to 75% in 1977. Furthermore, the costs associated with this tremendous growth in psychiatric services also increased dramatically, reflected in part by the rise in health care expenditures as a percentage of gross national product from 6% in 1965 to 10.3% in 1982. Cost-containment pressures from the federal government, states, and private insurers have been enormous, and psychiatry, as a specialty, has suffered from discriminatory insurance provisions. For instance, a recent survey revealed that of 137.7 million persons under age 65 with employment-related insurance coverage, 77.8% were covered

for some outpatient psychiatric care, but only 7.7% had coverage identical to other outpatient medical benefits.[39] A direct indication of the degree of discrimination toward psychiatric care was shown in a 1981 U.S. Department of Labor study of over 1500 businesses with insurance coverage for 24 million workers. Although 90% of the employees were covered for some outpatient psychiatric treatment, over half of the employees were in plans that required 50% copayment by the patient.[39] Finally, another study revealed that over 55% of insurance plans surveyed in 1982 with dollar limits on eligible charges for each visit limited the per session charge for psychotherapy to under $30.[39]

The implications for brief psychotherapeutic treatments are direct and considerable. First, proponents of various brief psychotherapy techniques need to demonstrate their effectiveness in treating psychiatric disorders associated with selected medical conditions. As Mumford and colleagues have recently summarized from their meta-analysis of the cost-offset effects of outpatient mental health treatment (the majority of which were short-term), outpatient psychotherapy resulted in a 33% average reduction in medical care utilization. Furthermore, these reductions occurred mostly in more expensive, inpatient medical services.[33] Second, since outpatient psychiatric patients are paying more of the costs of their treatment, they probably will continue to demand shorter and more goal-directed therapies. Third, prospective payment for outpatient treatment of selected psychiatric disorders is expanding greatly and will probably become even more of a factor within the next decade. Consequently, it seems likely that in the future satisfactory reimbursement may be provided only for the time-limited therapies and that this will strongly tilt the pattern of care toward this form of treatment. Empirical studies are needed to determine the most effective brief therapy for various psychiatric conditions treated in outpatient settings. A better understanding of the cost-benefit effects of brief psychotherapy will also clarify the role of long-term psychotherapy as a necessary and beneficial treatment for selected patients and will strengthen arguments for its appropriate use in those situations for which brief psychotherapy is shown ineffective. Finally, in spite of excellent arguments to the contrary, future reimbursements may be limited to treatments of proven efficacy *and* cost-effectiveness. Advocates of particular brief psychotherapies would be wise to document their efficacy and cost-effectiveness for selected mental disorders.

REFERENCES

1. Sullivan HS: The Psychiatric Interview. New York, Norton, 1954

2. Ursano RJ, Dressler DM: Brief versus long-term psychotherapy: A treatment decision. J Nerv Ment Dis 159:164–171, 1974

3. Alexander F, French TM, Bacon EL et al: Psychoanalytic Therapy: Principles and Application. Lincoln, University of Nebraska Press, 1974

4. Balint M, Ornstein P, Balint E: Focal Psychotherapy. Philadelphia, JB Lippincott, 1972

5. Malan DH: A Study of Brief Psychotherapy. New York, Plenum Press, 1975

6. Sifneos P: Short-Term Psychotherapy and Emotional Crisis. Cambridge, Harvard University Press, 1972

7. Mann J: Time-Limited Psychotherapy. Cambridge, Harvard University Press, 1973

8. Mann J, Goldman R: A Casebook in Time-Limited Psychotherapy. New York, McGraw Hill, 1982

9. Davanloo H (ed): Short-Term Dynamic Psychotherapy. New York, Jason Aronson Press, 1980

10. Bennett MJ: Brief psychotherapy in adult development. Psychotherapy 21:171–177, 1984

11. Stierlin H: Short-term versus long-term psychotherapy in the light of a general theory of human relationship. Br J Med Psychol 41:357–367, 1968

12. Strupp HH: Success and failure in time-limited psychotherapy. Arch Gen Psychiatry 37:595–604, 1980

13. Strupp HH: Success and failure in time-limited psychotherapy: Further evidence. Arch Gen Psychiatry 37:947–954, 1980

14. Strupp HH, Hadley SW: Specific versus non-specific factors in psychotherapy: A controlled study of outcome. Arch Gen Psychiatry 36:1125–1136, 1979

15. Shilien JM, Mosik HH, Dreikurs R: Effective time limits: A comparison to psychotherapy. J Counsel Psychol 9:31–34, 1962

16. Bellak L: Brief psychoanalytic psychotherapy of non-psychotic depression. Am J Psychother 35:160–172, 1981

17. Lazarus LW: Brief psychotherapy of narcissistic disturbances. J Psychother Theory, Res, Pract 19:228–236, 1982

18. Horowitz MJ, Marmar C, Krupnick J et al: Personality Styles in Brief Psychotherapy. New York, Basic Books, 1984

19. Amada G: The interlude between short- and long-term psychotherapy. Am J Psychother 37:357–364, 1983

20. Prelinger E: Some recurrent phenomena in brief psychotherapy. Unpublished manuscript. New Haven, Yale University, 1975

21. Klerman GL, Weismann MM, Rounsaville BJ et al: Interpersonal Psychotherapy of Depression. New York, Basic Books, 1984

22. Weissman MM, Klerman GL, Prusoff BA et al: Depressed outpatients: Results one year after treatment with drugs and/or interpersonal psychotherapy. Arch Gen Psychiatry 38:51–55, 1981

23. Beck AT, Rush AJ, Shaw BF et al: Cognitive Therapy of Depression. New York, Guilford Press, 1979

24. Rush AJ: Cognitive therapy. In Grinspoon L (ed): Psychiatry Update, vol 3, pp 44–55. Washington, DC, American Psychiatric Press, 1984

25. Rush AJ: The therapeutic alliance in short-term directive therapies. In Hales RE, Frances AJ (eds): The American Psychiatric Association Annual Review, vol 4, pp 562–572. Washington, DC, American Psychiatric Press, 1985

26. Fuchs RM: Group therapy. In Karasu TB (ed): The Psychiatric Therapies, pp 415–438. Washington, DC, American Psychiatric Association, 1984

27. Yalom I: The Theory and Practice of Group Psychotherapy. New York, Basic Books, 1975

28. Eysenck HJ: The Effects of Psychotherapy. New York, International Science Press, 1966

29. Meltzoff J, Kornreich M: Research in Psychotherapy. New York, Atherton Press, 1970

30. Butcher JN, Koss MP: Research on brief and crisis oriented therapies. In Garfield SL, Bergin AE (eds): Handbook of Psychotherapy and Behavior Change: An Empirical Analysis, 2nd ed, pp 723–767. New York, John Wiley & Sons, 1978

31. Luborsky L, Singer B, Luborsky L: Comparative studies of psychotherapies: Is it true that "everyone has won and all must have prizes"? Arch Gen Psychiatry 32:995–1008, 1975

32. Reid WJ, Shyne AW: Brief and Extended Casework. New York, Columbia University Press, 1969

33. Sloane RB, Staples FR, Cristol A et al: Psychotherapy Versus Behavior Therapy. Cambridge, Harvard University Press, 1975

34. Smith ML, Glass GV: Meta-analysis of psychotherapy outcome studies. Am Psychol 32:752–760, 1977

35. Mumford E, Schlesinger HJ, Glass GV et al: A new look at evidence about reduced cost of medical utilization following mental health treatment. Am J Psychiatry 141:1145–1158, 1984

36. Meyer E, Denogatis LR, Miller MJ et al: Addition of time-limited psychotherapy to medical treatment is a general medical clinic. J Nerv Ment Dis 169:780–790, 1981

37. Austin L, Inderbitzin LB: Brief psychotherapy in late adolescence: A psychodynamic and developmental approach. Am J Psychother 37:202–209, 1983

38. Keilson MV, Dworkin FH, Gelso CJ: The effectiveness of time-limited psychotherapy in a university counseling center. J Clin Psychol 35:631–636, 1979

39. Sharfstein SS, Muszynski S, Myers E: Health Insurance and Psychiatric Care: Update and Appraisal. Washington, DC, American Psychiatric Press, 1984

SUGGESTED READING

KLERMAN GL, WEISSMAN MM, ROUNSAVILLE BJ et al: Interpersonal psychotherapy for depression. In Grinspoon L (ed): Psychiatry Update, Vol. 3. Washington, DC, American Psychiatric Press, 1984

MALAN DH: The Frontier of Brief Psychotherapy. New York, Plenum Press, 1976

RUSH AJ (ed): Short-Term Psychotherapies for Depression. New York, Guilford Press, 1982

Introduction to Personality Disorders

The provision within the official nomenclature of the American Psychiatric Association of a separate axis specifically for the diagnosis of personality disorders illustrates the growing interest in personality disorders and recognition of their importance. Indeed, the principle reason for introducing the multiaxial system into the *Diagnostic and Statistical Manual of Mental Disorders*, 3rd ed (*DSM-III*), was the realization that personality disorders often coexist with and influence the treatment of the other more acute psychiatric syndromes. Many recent studies have investigated the possible contribution made by personality disorders to the predisposition, presentation, course, and treatment response of Axis I conditions.[1] This has generated accumulating evidence of important interactions between personality disorders and unipolar,[2,3] bipolar,[4] dysthymic,[5] cyclothymic,[6] schizophrenic,[7,8] addictive,[9] and cardiovascular[10] disorders. Moreover, every clinician knows, often from painful personal experience, the degree to which personality features in both the physician and the patient shape the treatment relationship and influence compliance and outcome.

It should, therefore, occasion no great surprise that we will devote considerable attention to the personality disorders and that, for the most part, we have followed the *DSM-III* Axis II system of notation. Several caveats are in order before we proceed. The personality disorders comprise the least reliable, least researched, and least well defined section of *DSM-III*. Only three personality disorders—the antisocial, borderline, and schizotypal—have received systematic study and, even for these, the available data are relatively sparse and their interpretation is subject to controversy. The other personality disorders have been the subject of considerable, and often vivid, clinical description but they are supported by little or no systematic evidence. Most of what is known about personality disorder rests on the weight of untested, if extensive, clinical observation (with all the strengths and weaknesses such evidence entails). Furthermore, there is little reason to believe that the particular 11 personality categories chosen for description in *DSM-III* form the most useful selection or even that the *DSM-III* method of categorical diagnosis is well suited to personality classification. This section is organized around the *DSM-III* terminology and categorical method, not because these are expected to endure in their current form, but rather because *DSM-III* serves as a convenient lingua franca and there is no better established or more reasonable system available.

This introduction has several additional tasks. A definition of personality disorder is provided and the reasons why the concept is inherently difficult to define in an operational and reliable fashion is illustrated. Next, the concept that specific personality disorders may reside on a spectrum with specific Axis I conditions is discussed. Finally, the advantages and disadvantages of a categorical system of personality diagnosis are outlined and compared to the less familiar prototypal and dimensional approaches. We hope to convey the sense that personality diagnosis is intellectually interesting and clinically crucial, even if its scientific underpinnings are insubstantial and difficult to establish.

Definition

Personality disorder is a kind of "will-o'-the-wisp" concept that eludes precise definition and merges imperceptibly at its boundaries with a number of close and difficult to distinguish neighbors. The introduction to the personality disorders section of *DSM-III* begins with a carefully worded paragraph that provides a series of crucial definitions. This constitutes a nice try at precision and covers the right territory but, for reasons that are unavoidable, certain key terms remain vague and lack operational usefulness.

"Personality traits are enduring patterns of perceiving, relating to, and thinking about the environment and oneself, and are exhibited in a wide range of important social and personality contexts. It is only when personality traits are inflexible and maladaptive and cause either significant impairment in social or occupational functioning or subjective distress that they constitute personality disorders. The manifestations of personality disorders are generally recognizable by adolescence or earlier and continue throughout most of adult life, though they often become less obvious in middle or old age."[11]

Although not labelled as such, this definition is really an attempt to set operational boundaries around the personality disorders as a group, just as the separate sets of diagnostic criteria for each of the individual personality disorders are meant to distinguish each of them from one another. In fact, the clear definitions and operational criteria included in *DSM-III* and its provision of separate axes to reduce confusion between clinical syndrome and personality disorder have increased the reliability of personality diagnosis far beyond what had been achieved by any previous system.[12]

Nonetheless, serious problems remain that may resist easy solution because they inhere in the nature of personality disorder. Although the overall reliability of personality diagnosis has been substantially improved by *DSM-III*, the level achieved still remains much lower than what has been achieved for most of the Axis I disorders. Personality disorders are difficult to classify within a categorical system of nomenclature because they lack clear boundaries and instead overlap with one another, with normality, and with Axis I conditions.[13]

A close textual analysis of the *DSM-III* definition recorded above illustrates the difficulties encountered in placing boundaries around the personality disorders. The *DSM-III* definition distinguishes between personality traits and personality disorders

on just one parameter—the personality disorder must cause significant impairment. This seems sensible enough, but there are no criteria offered to specify what constitutes significant impairment. This judgment is likely to vary considerably depending on the eye (and tolerance) of the beholder. This is not a problem that resulted from careless definition but is rather inherent in the situation. There is no suitable marker to delineate the boundary between normality and disorder and any assignment of border individuals must be arbitrary and unreliable.

Personality disorders are defined in *DSM-III* as conditions with an early onset and a long, enduring course. This seems clear enough on paper, but in practice it is often difficult to acquire an accurate history that is unbiased by the patient's current state and attitudes. If the symptoms that characterize the individual's personality disorder are present or accentuated only when he or she is in the midst of an Axis I condition, this should not be considered personality disorder and only the Axis I condition should be diagnosed. However, the sharp separation of state and trait is not always possible and this confound leaves room for unreliable assignments. Furthermore, the *DSM-III* definition of personality disorder requires that the maladaptation be present "in a wide range of social and personal contexts" and thus not be an isolated reaction to one particular stressor. For example, this means that many army trainees are incorrectly labelled as passive aggressive personalities. Instead, they should be diagnosed within the category of adjustment disorders, unless the behaviors in question preceded boot camp, characterize a considerable range of the individual's experience, and have not arisen as a response to just this one particularly stressful situation. It is not always possible, however, to distinguish the extent to which the variance in a given behavior is best assigned to trait or to situational factors.

In summary then, the definition of personality disorders is difficult and made with relatively low reliability because these conditions cannot be sharply delineated from normality, intercurrent morbid states, and situational role assignments. This lack of clear boundaries imposes an unavoidable vagueness on the *DSM-III* definition of personality disorders and prevents the provision of easily followed operational criteria for the following crucial defining terms: *significant impairment* (at the boundary with normality), *enduring patterns* (at the boundary with states), and *wide range* (at the boundary with adjustment disorders). In a later section we shall also note that the various personality disorders overlap a great deal with one another. Although the lack of sharp boundaries surrounding personality disorders may result in part from the insufficient knowledge we have about them and may be clarified by further research, we must recognize that this is in part an inherent and unavoidable problem. Everyone has at least a few maladaptive personality traits and there is little reason to expect that a clear severity marker will emerge to indicate when these warrant the label *disorder*. It is also in the nature of things that state *versus* trait and trait *versus* role are similarly incapable of being distinguished dichotomously and instead are inherently confounded at least in some people in some situations. The implications of this issue for reliability and methods of classification are discussed in more detail in a later section.

Spectrum Disorders

The concept that certain longstanding temperaments might correlate with and predispose to acute disorders originated with the ancient Greeks (if not earlier) and has informed the work of descriptive psychiatrists and of psychoanalysts. *DSM-III* has taken the position that clinical syndrome and personality disorders are sufficiently distinguishable from and independent of one another that it is useful to provide separate axes with which each might be designated. There is, however, a widely held expectation that certain personality disorders correlate significantly and meaningfully with certain Axis II conditions (likely examples are compulsive personality with anxiety disorders, histrionic personality with somatoform and dissociative disorders, and a schizotypal personality with schizophrenic disorders.)

Four types of relationships are possible between a personality disorder and a clinical syndrome when both occur together in the same patient. These possibilities follow from the fact that correlations provide no information about causality. For example, if A and B are significantly correlated with one another, A may be partly causing B, or B may be partly causing A, or A and B may both be partly caused by another variable C or by interacting variables C, D, E; or the correlation may be due to a chance association that implies nothing about causality. The implications of each of the possibilities for the relationship between personality disorders and Axis I syndrome are discussed briefly below.

There have been many suggestions by both descriptive and psychoanalytic observers that certain personality traits increase the vulnerability and predispose to certain Axis I conditions. In this model, the personality is seen as an etiologic factor partly causing the emergence of the clinical syndrome. Recently, the reverse direction in etiology has been emphasized by more biologically oriented psychiatrists. Perhaps certain personality features are the muted, chronic expression or residue of the more florid clinical syndrome. The best researched examples are the personality features that may express or result from affective disorder. The third type of relationship would imply that the personality feature (*e.g.*, compulsiveness) and the clinical syndrome (*e.g.*, depression) may arise from some yet unknown but shared background of constitutional and environmental interaction. In the fourth type of relationship, the joint occurrence of the personality disorder and the clinical syndrome has resulted from coincidence and implies no etiologic connection. It is clear, however, that even such chance association may dramatically complicate the treatment and influence prognosis.

The concept that certain personality disorders are on a spectrum with major clinical syndromes was suggested by Kraepelin and has received considerable recent research attention.[14,15] The most suggestive evidence pertains to the affective spectrum personality disorders (*i.e.*, cyclothymic, dysthymic, and perhaps borderline) and to the schizophrenic spectrum personality disorders (*i.e.*, schizotypal and perhaps schizoid and paranoid) and it seems likely that anxiety spectrum personality disorders (perhaps avoidant, compulsive, and dependent) will be studied next. The *DSM-III* handling of spectrum personality disorders is inconsistent and illogical. The proposed affective spectrum disorders (*i.e.*, cyclothymic and dysthymic) appear in the Affective Disorder section and are treated as Axis I, not Axis II, conditions. In contrast, schizotypal personality disorder was introduced by *DSM-III* as an Axis II condition although it has equal supporting claim to spectrum status. These alignments perhaps reflect *DSM-III's* overreaction to past American diagnostic sins and its resulting overinclusiveness in regard to affective disorder and restrictiveness with regard to schizophrenia.

Although the spectrum concept of personality disorder is venerable, plausible, and has received support from recent research, we must recognize that our available evidence is limited and difficult to interpret. Much more must be learned about the pathogenesis of personality disorders and of clinical syndromes before we will understand what are likely to be their complicated and varied interactions with one another.

Category, Prototype, or Dimension

As Kendall points out, the ideal classes of the logician require the satisfaction of such stringent criteria as to defy frequent attainment in the empirical world.[16] Ideal classes are defined to be homogeneous, mutually exclusive, and jointly exhaustive. All the criteria for class membership must be met completely by all qualifying members. Each defining attribute is always totally present or totally absent, never partially expressed, and members must meet criteria for placement into one, and only one, class.

These requirements are sometimes satisfied in everyday tasks of classification (*e.g.*, in sorting geometric shapes), but less often than is commonly realized. Recent work by philosophers, linguists, and psychologists suggests that a more probabilistic conception of categories is necessary in most situations. Only rarely is it possible to establish categories that are completely homogeneous, with absolute defining features, and no borderline cases. Most commonly, categories are prototypal, that is, each member is considered to be no more than an approximation of the prototype.[17,18]

The classification of psychiatric disorders is difficult even with the use of the most flexible categorical systems. Psychiatric diagnoses are polythetic rather than monothetic, that is, they are usually not defined by the presence or absence of a single, necessary, and pathognomonic attribute. Instead, the patient need display only some or most of several attributes (*e.g.*, symptoms, signs, course *etc.*), none of which is sufficient in itself. Moreover, most psychiatric phenomena are not simply present or absent, but instead they are capable of a continuous distribution. Membership in one diagnostic class generally does not restrict membership in other classes. Patients may, and often do, satisfy simultaneously the requirements of several different diagnoses even on the same axis.

DSM-III is an innovatively prototypal system and is vastly more flexible than *DSM-I* and *II*, both of which were more rigidly categorical in spirit. The introductory section of *DSM-III* acknowledges that there are no sharp and natural boundaries to separate mental disorders from normality and from one another. *DSM-III* disclaims the assumption that mental disorders are discrete entities and cautions against the common misconception that a classification of disorders is also a classification of individuals. Nonetheless, the flexible categorical system embodied in *DSM-III* is much more effective in rendering Axis I conditions than Axis II personality disorders. All typological classifications require the presence of points of rarity separating the conditions to be classified. When patients are distributed continuously, one must be arbitrary in establishing boundaries between groups or even in deciding how many separate groups to define. Any effort to type a continuum must result in relatively low reliability and validity at the boundaries. Two similar patients who happen to fall on adjacent but opposite sides of the artificial boundary are forced arbitrarily into quite different categories. As we have seen, this problem of continuities especially bedevils the categorical classification of personality disorders and accounts for their comparatively low reliability.

A dimensional system of personality diagnosis may have advantages over the categorical system in use in *DSM-III*. In this system, patients would receive numerical ratings on each of several personality features rather than being placed in diagnostic categories. The common situations in which dimensional classifications have supplanted the categorical classifications are those that involve standardized measurements (*e.g.*, height, weight, intelligence) of continuously distributed features that lend themselves to numerical expression. Many problems in classification must be simultaneously addressed from both points of view and dimensional measurements can often be conveniently converted back into typologies (*e.g.*, all men over 6 ft tall could be typed together as "tall").

The advantages and disadvantages of the dimensional approach suggest some general indications for its use. Dimensional is superior to typological classification in its ability to describe reliably and precisely those phenomena that follow a continuous distribution. Dimensional systems are better in describing border cases. These are described accurately and information is saved rather than artificially forcing the patient into one or another poorly fitting category. Dimensional systems reduce the halo effect, that is, the tendency to ignore atypical cases and to see things in stereotyped ways that conform to preconceived categorical definitions. By using a dimensional system, one can manipulate complex data mathematically and include many variables. In reducing dimensions to typologies, information with important predictive value may be lost.

There are also disadvantages in the use of dimensional systems that account for the fact that most classification in everyday life, in medicine, and in psychiatry remains categorical. Dimensional descriptions are often too complex and too unwieldy for ordinary purposes. They may provide too much or inconveniently expressed information and a more accurate but less vivid picture of what is described. Moreover, a surface continuum may conceal underlying discontinuous categories (*e.g.,* different viruses produce similar overlapping symptom pictures, but the disorders can be distinguished on immunologic grounds). Categorical classification is most appropriate when the phenomena to be classified are sharply discontinuous in their distribution (*i.e.,* with points of rarity between groups) or incapable of being reduced to numerical measurement.[19]

How do the advantages and disadvantages of the categorical and dimensional systems balance in the diagnosis of personality disorders? Historically, the standard method of classification of medical and psychiatric disorders has been categorical. The medical nomenclature consists of a variety of conditions considered to be more or less discrete and separable from one another. The process of differential diagnosis is an effort to sort patients into one of the typological categories. Atypical patients are either left undiagnosed or are sorted into the category that provides the closest fit.

DSM-III recognizes the limitations of the categorical approach in classifying personality disorders and the fact that different disorders are not mutually exclusive. The introduction to the personality disorders section explicitly encourages the use of multiple personality diagnoses when the patient meets criteria for more than one diagnosis.

Indeed, it has been shown empirically that two thirds of carefully studied patients who met criteria for any one personality disorder met criteria for two or more diagnoses. In fact, one third of patients met criteria for three or more personality disorders.[20] This degree of overlap suggests that there is likely to be an eventual tilt toward the dimensional diagnosis of personality disorders, and several promising systems will be described in another chapter. For some purposes and some diagnoses, the categorical method may retain its usefulness and, as mentioned above, the two systems are complementary, not inherently contradictory. For the reasons detailed above, a categorical classification of personality disorders must be flexible, prototypal, and probabilistic.

The study of personality disorders lies in waters that are mostly uncharted from a scientific point of view but are nonetheless familiar from clinical work, literature, and everyday experience. Although much remains to be learned, a keen appreciation for personality diagnosis usually pays rich rewards in all sorts of clinical encounters.

The psychiatric literature on personality disorders heretofore has been insufficiently cognizant of the methods and results generated by psychometrically sophisticated psychologists who have generally used a dimensional approach to investigate personality functioning. Another chapter in this set summarizes this work and further discusses the specific personality disorders.

REFERENCES

1. Hirschfield R, Klerman G: Personality attributes and affective disorders. Am J Psychiatry 136:67–70, 1979
2. Weissman M, Prusoff B, Klerman G: Personality and prediction of long term outcome of depressions. Am J Psychiatry 135:797–800, 1978
3. Bielski R, Friedel R: Prediction of tricyclic antidepressant response. Arch Gen Psychiatry 33:1479–1489, 1976
4. Taylor M, Abrams R: Acute mania: Clinical and genetic study of responders and nonresponders to treatments. Arch Gen Psychiatry 32:863–865, 1975
5. Akiskal HS, Rosenthal TL, Hayka RF et al: Characterological depressions. Arch Gen Psychiatry 37:777–787, 1980
6. Akiskal HS, Djenderedjian AH, Rosenthal AH et al: Cyclothymic disorder: Validating criteria for inclusion in the bipolar affective group. Am J Psychiatry 134:1227–1233, 1977
7. Garmezy N: Process and reactive schizophrenia, some conceptions and issues. In Katz M, Cole J, Barton W (eds) Classification in Psychiatry and Psychopathology. Chevy Chase, US Department of Health, Education and Welfare, 1975
8. Gittelman-Klein R, Klein D: Premorbid asocial adjustment and prognosis in schizophrenia. J Psychiatr Res 7:35–53, 1969
9. Treece C, Nicholson DS: DSM III personality type and dose levels in methadone maintenance. J Nerv Ment Dis 168:621–628, 1980
10. Haynes SG, Feinleib M, Kannel WB: The relationship of psychosocial factors to coronary heart disease in the Framingham study. Am J Epidemiol 111:37–51, 1980
11. American Psychiatric Association: Diagnostic and Statistical Manual of Mental Disorders (3rd ed), p 305. Washington, D.C., 1980
12. Spitzer R, Forman J, Nee J: DSM III Field trials: Initial interrater diagnostic reliability. Am J Psychiatry 136:815–817, 1979
13. Frances A: The DSM III personality disorders section: A commentary. Am J Psychiatry 137:1050–1054, 1980
14. Akiskal HS: Subeffective disorders: Dysthymic, cyclothymic, and bipolar II disorders in the "borderline realm." Psychiatr Clin North Am 4:25–46, 1981
15. Stone M: The Borderline Syndromes: Constitution, Personality, and Adaptation. New York, McGraw–Hill, 1980

16. Kendall RE: The Role of Diagnosis in Psychiatry. Oxford, Blackwell, 1975

17. Clarkin JF, Widiger TA, Frances A et al: Prototypic typology and the borderline personality disorder. J Abnormal Psychology 92:263–275, 1983

18. Cantor N, Smith EE, French R et al: Psychiatric diagnosis as prototype categorization. J Abnorm Psychol 89:181–193, 1980

19. Frances A: Categorical and dimensional systems of personality disorder: A comparison. Compr Psychiatry 23:516–527, 1982

20. Frances A, Clarkin J, Gilmore M et al: Reliability of criteria for borderline personality disorder. A comparison of DSM III and DIB. Am J Psychiatry 1984

13

Robert Plutchik and Hope R. Conte

Quantitative Assessment of Personality Disorders

Psychiatrists are constantly involved in the assessment and diagnosis of patients. These activities simultaneously serve the goal of understanding the individual's dynamics and provide guidelines for treatment. Such assessment and diagnostic skills are complex and multidimensional and require a fairly long apprenticeship for successful acquisition.

Appropriate assessment makes good communication possible between the doctor and his patient and among clinicians. To maximize effective communication, the participants must share a common intellectual framework and agree on certain conceptual dimensions of assessment.

Because the need for mutually understood conceptual systems is particularly acute in the diagnosis of mental disorders, psychiatrists have evolved a way of describing patients in relatively explicit diagnostic terms, as exemplified in the *Diagnosis and Statistical Manual of Mental Disorders* (*DSM-III*) system. Although the major disorders are clearly explicated, there is less agreement on exact definitions of personality disorders. For example, the definition of borderline personality disorder is still in dispute, and the differences between borderline and schizotypal disorders are still not clear.[1]

In such ambiguous situations it is helpful to supplement clinical judgment with additional sources of information: projective test results, rating scale data, and patient self-reports. The psychiatrist may use such information to expand his evaluation, just as he uses data obtained from family members, schools, or social agencies. However, to use quantitative data optimally, something must be known about how the test was constructed, the population on which it was standardized, and how to interpret standard scores.

In this chapter we provide such information about quantitative sources of data and suggest a conceptual framework for considering diagnostic issues in general. This chapter will present a brief historical overview evaluating the use of projective tests, rating scales, and self-report tests. There will then be a discussion of basic psychometric concepts (such as reliability, validity, standardization, norms, and the role of theory in the development of tests) that are necessary for the understanding of the published descriptions of quantitative tests. Two empirically based tests of personality disorders and three theoretically based tests of personality disorders will be then discussed, and an integrating model of personality diagnoses based on the circumplex as an organizing principle will be proposed.

Historical Overview

During the past 50 years there has been a gradual increase in the number of quantitative measuring instruments used by psychiatrists or others in psychiatric settings. These instruments include projective measures, rating scales, and self-report tests. There has been simultaneous increase in the sophistication of both the constructors and users of such instruments.

Ideally, these measuring devices serve three functions: (1) they provide the psychiatrist with information to supplement the data traditionally gathered about each patient; (2) they provide information on a variety of content areas in a standard fashion to minimize any biases a clinician might have; and (3) when the measuring instrument is based on a theoretic model, it can integrate information pertaining to broad and diverse areas.

PROJECTIVE TESTS

Projective instruments are based on either ambiguous stimuli or settings that require a relatively unstructured response. The oldest and best known of the projective measures is the Rorschach Inkblot Test. Also widely used by clinicians are the Thematic Apperception Test (TAT), based on interpretations of ambiguous drawings, and the figure drawing test, based on an individual's freehand drawings of a male and a female figure. The assumption is made that both content and style of response reveal something of an individual's personality traits and dynamic conflicts.

Projective tests, however, suffer from a number of serious weaknesses from the point of view of psychiatrists' concerns with diagnosis. First, because projective techniques are considered to be a specialty of clinical psychology, psychiatrists must either refer patients to trained psychologists or have them available on staff to administer, score, and interpret the tests. Second, the process of administration, scoring, and interpretation is often so lengthy that many psychologists have developed abbreviated, idiosyncratic ways of administering these tests (*e.g.*, giving 5 of the 10 Rorschach cards), so that whatever norms are available are no longer appropriate. Third, many investigators have raised questions about the reliability and the predictive validity of projective tests as measures of personality and adjustment, and although some recent efforts have attempted to remedy this situation,[2,3] such standardization applies only to a small part of the total number of currently administered tests. For example, there are currently at least five reasonably distinct Rorschach systems of scoring and analysis. Finally, projective tests do not provide clear cut information on all the *DSM-III* personality disorders. In a recent attempt to standardize both scoring and interpretation for the Rorschach test, Perline[4] has provided computer-interpreted Rorschachs based on the Klopfer system. Such computer-interpreted Rorschachs still require a trained psychologist to administer and score the test in a standard fashion in order to produce reliable, consistent narratives for a given input; they do not deal explicitly with standard personality diagnostic labels or with the problem of the questionable validity of the Rorschach test.

RATING SCALES

Rating scales have been used by psychiatrists for many years as a mode of assessment and for research. They have been of particular value in epidemiologic surveys of large populations when the concern was with identifying psychiatric symptomatology during a brief interview. Among the better-known rating scales for psychiatry are those developed by Spitzer and his associates at the Rockland Research Center,[5] which have been widely used. Scales for rating adjustment are exemplified by the Structured and Scaled Interview to Assess Maladjustment (SSIAM).[6] A well-known unidimensional scale is the Hamilton Rating Scale for Depression.[7] More recently, a partially structured interview technique has been developed to identify major affective disorders and schizophrenia. This is the Schedule for Affective Disorders and Schizophrenia (SADS), which uses criteria based directly on those published in the *DSM-III*.[8]

To ensure reasonably consistent interactions with the patient, such rating scales generally require administration by an experienced clinician. In practice, relatively few psychiatrists feel comfortable with rating scale questionnaires that "put words into their mouths." There have been two results: (1) that most such scales are administered by trained research assistants and (2) that new questionnaires have been devised that reduce interviewer training needs to a minimum.

The most recent example of a fully structured interview schedule that minimizes the need for experienced raters is the National Institute of Mental Health Diagnostic Interview Schedule (DIS).[9] The aim of this interview is to provide a computer-scorable instrument that can be administered by persons not trained in psychiatry that will provide standard *DSM-III* diagnoses equivalent to those made by a clinician.

The DIS interview is completely precoded, although certain questions can be omitted if, in the judgment of the interviewer, sufficient responses have been obtained to define a criterion set of symptoms. The computer combines the item responses according to predetermined *DSM-III* criteria and prints out a "definite" or "probable" diagnosis. However, there are still several questions that have not yet been unequivocally answered:

Are the diagnoses obtained by computer in fact equivalent to those provided by a trained psychiatrist?

Do varied combinations of items produce the same diagnosis, as would be the case when the *DSM-III* categories are used in a qualitative way?

Why is the computer unable to distinguish among the schizophrenia subtypes?

Why is the computer only able to provide diagnoses on two (compulsive personality disorder and antisocial personality disorder) of the 11 Axis II personality disorders?

One other important point needs to be made. Rating scales have become increasingly explicit sets of questions with precoded answers. Once the questionnaire has been constructed, the questions can be asked by a college student or nurse, who simply records answers. In fact, the logical extension of this approach—to have a computer ask the questions, record the answers, and then immediately print out a diagnosis—has already begun and is illustrated most clearly in the use of self-report scales or tests. This seems to leave little or no role for the experienced clinician, except in the sense of constructing the questions and answers of the schedule in advance. However, such a development does not render the experienced clinician obsolete. Rather, it should greatly assist the psychiatrist by making the gathering of information about patients more efficient. Furthermore, only the trained clinician can integrate data from different sources.

SELF-REPORT SCALES

Self-report scales, when appropriately developed, represent ways to obtain comprehensive samples of a patient's behavior, feelings, or thoughts in a systematic way. They are based on the assumption that a patient can read and understand the items of the scale; certain patients, however, may need to have someone read them the items, as in an interview.

Over the years, an elaborate body of psychometric theory has been developed by psychologists to guide the construction, use, and evaluation of self-report scales or tests. (The terms *tests, scales, inventories,* and *indexes* may be used interchangeably.) This theory applies with equal relevance to ratings and projective tests but was most fully elaborated in the context of self-report instruments.

Psychometricians point out that self-report tests have been used for many functions: assessment of intellectual levels, assessment of personality, differential diagnosis, vocational guidance, prognosis, and treatment planning. In order to serve these multiple functions adequately, tests have to have certain properties, most importantly internal reliability, stability, validity, relevance, standardization, and norms. A test may have some of these characteristics but not others; for example, it may be reliable but not valid, or it may be standardized and possess norms but be irrelevant for a given purpose. Thus, each test instrument must be considered in a given context and for a given type of patient population. A test may sometimes give the illusion of precision because exact scores can be obtained, but the extent of error or inapplicability may be unknown. However, when well constructed and relevant, a test may provide much useful supplementary information to the psychiatrist.

Psychometric Concepts

To follow the discussion of self-report measures soon to be presented, a brief explanation of some key psychometric concepts may be helpful. The internal *reliability* of a test or scale is a measure of the degree to which the items of the scale correlate with one another. This in turn reflects the extent to which the items of the test measure the same underlying dimension. Internal reliability may be measured by means of the split-half correlation between two randomly selected halves of the test, or in a more sophisticated way, by means of coefficient alpha. Reliabilities are measured on a scale from 0 to 1.0 and values below .6 are not usually considered to demonstrate adequate internal reliability. Each subscale or dimension of a test has its own reliability, and it is possible for different subscales to vary greatly in their degree of reliability.

Test validity is a complex idea, and psychologists have identified several different kinds. *Content validity* refers to the extent to which the items of the test adequately cover all the facets or aspects of the domain of interest. For example, a test designed to measure borderline personality disorder should cover impulsivity, heightened affectivity, mild psychotic experiences, identity disturbances, and disturbed close relationships.[1] The content domain of a test is determined by experts in the field (clinicians), and the extent to which the items reflect the many facets of a concept is also determined by expert clinical judgment. This procedure is designed to ensure the clinical relevance of a scale.

The terms *predictive validity* and *concurrent validity* (sometimes referred to as *convergent validity*) are used to refer to related ideas; that is, the extent to which the scores obtained on a test correlate with scores obtained on some other measure that is assumed (on the grounds of independent evidence) to be a valid measure of the concept. For example, the concurrent validity of a new test for measuring depression might be established by showing that it correlated highly with the Hamilton Rating Scale for Depression or the Beck Depression Inventory. The predictive validity of a suicide potential scale would be established by correlating scores on the test with actual future incidents of suicide or attempts. It is possible for a test to have content validity but not predictive validity.

Discriminative validity refers simply to the idea that a valid test of a concept should be able to disciminate individuals who exemplify that concept from those who do not. A test designed to measure suicide potential should be able to discriminate those people who have made a suicide attempt from comparable individuals who have not. A test designed to measure hysterical personality should be able to distinguish between clinically identified hysterical patients and other kinds of patients or normal individuals. However, since no test has perfect discriminating power, it is desirable to be given the number of true and false positives and true and false negatives identified by any given cutoff score of the test.

Construct validity is the most controversial of the concepts that have been identified. The basic idea is that any theoretic dimension (such as schizophrenia) has a number of derivative implications that can be tested indirectly. For example, if a patient is diagnosed as schizophrenic, this would imply evidence of an attention deficit, of certain abnormal eye movement tracking patterns, and of higher than normal use of ego defenses. These implications are based on previous research and theory related to the schizophrenic syndrome and may be used here as derived hypotheses. To the extent that such derived hypotheses are confirmed, the construct validity of the test designed to identify schizophrenic patients is enhanced. It should be evident that construct validity is a matter of degree and that one may gradually accumulate evidence for the construct validity of any particular test.

Obviously it is incorrect to talk about *the* validity of a test, because each test may be described in terms of many different types of validity that are often independent of one another. In addition, each type of validity is a matter of degree that depends on many factors: the sizes of the groups used in establishing validity, the types of persons used in each group, the extent of verification by independent investigators, the conditions of testing, and others. The establishment of test validity may be thought of as an ongoing process rather than as an all-or-nothing condition.

Several other test characteristics should be briefly mentioned. Once a test has been constructed, it is assumed that it will be administered in a standard or consistent way. Scoring of self-report instruments is generally quite routine and automatic with no inferences or judgment required and can generally be better done by a computer than a person. Test scores, however, must be compared with norms and interpretations made; this is where clinical judgment and experience are necessary. Most tests of psychiatrically relevant concepts use several subscales, resulting in complex patterns of scores with highs and lows in many different combinations. Humans are still the best and most efficient pattern analyzers. There is no reason why psychiatrists cannot learn to become expert test interpreters of measures produced by computer scoring of self-report tests.

There is one final point to be made about test construction issues. Tests can be designed on purely empiric or on theoretic grounds. For example, it may be discovered by trial and error that schizophrenic patients prefer the color green while normal individuals prefer the color red. If this is a fairly general finding, then the item may be used as part of a test to discriminate schizophrenic patients from others, particularly in doubtful cases, but the item has no theoretic significance. In contrast, in tests designed on theoretic grounds, psychoanalytic theory might be used to define ego defenses and then to construct a test to measure these theoretic constructs. Such a procedure is illustrated in the development of the Life Style Index, which is designed to measure such ego defenses as repression, displacement, and intellectualization.[10]

Although many tests such as the Minnesota Multiphasic Personality Inventory (MMPI)[11] or Cattell's 16 Personality Factor Questionnaire (16-PF)[12] have been developed empirically, there are advantages to tests that have been constructed on the basis of theoretic models. Such theoretically derived tests have a network of relations implied by the theory. These relations can suggest testable hypotheses that, if confirmed empirically, provide both a degree of construct validity for the test and support for the theory. In addition, tests based on theory have a coherence and elegance that is more aesthetically satisfying than the somewhat haphazard quality of tests constructed solely on discrimination between two or more populations. Tests developed empirically on the basis of factor-analytic studies may also be questioned on the grounds that different factor-analytic techniques often produce different clusters of items.

In the following two sections we will describe empirically and theoretically derived tests. The first considers the empirically based MMPI,[11] and the

Clinical Analysis Questionnaire (CAQ).[13] The second section briefly evaluates three theoretically based tests of personality disorders. One is the Personality Research Form (PRF),[14] the second is the test developed by Benjamin called the Structural Analysis of Social Behavior Test (SASB),[15] and the third is the Millon Clinical Multiaxial Inventory (MCMI).[16]

Empirically Based Tests of Personality Disorders

MINNESOTA MULTIPHASIC PERSONALITY INVENTORY

The MMPI was originally developed in 1939 as a way of discriminating between hospitalized psychiatric patients and normals, using relatives of hospitalized patients as the "normal" group. Eventually 566 items were selected to make up the test, with 16 items repeated. Respondents are asked to indicate whether each statement is true of them or false as applied to them. Examples of statements on the test include: "At times I feel like swearing," "I have a good appetite," "I work under a great deal of tension," and "I believe in a life hereafter." In most cases the selection of items was based simply on the fact that they discriminated a normal from a patient group. Many of the items are scored on more than one scale.

The MMPI provides measures on ten clinical scales: Hypochondriasis, Depression, Hysteria, Psychopathic Deviate, Male Sexual Inversion, Paranoia, Psychasthenia, Schizophrenia, Hypomania, and Social Introversion. In addition, several so-called validity scales were constructed to provide some indices of whether the test was completed in a reasonable way (not whether the test itself is valid); these scales are labeled: cannot say, lie scale, confusion scale, and suppressor factor. Most college students can complete the test in 1 to $1\frac{1}{2}$ hours, but patients often take much longer.

Scores on the test are converted into "standard scores," and a profile is obtained based on the norms obtained in 1940. These norms consisted of Minnesota adults from rural and semirural areas with an average eighth grade education. Interpretations are made by experienced clinicians or more commonly by computer.

The various scales differ considerably in internal reliability. Some are quite high, while others are

unacceptably low (e.g., .36, .43) with a median reliability for all scales of .70. Despite the relatively low reliabilities of some of the scales, thousands of studies have been published that use the MMPI, often with the presumption that the test is valid. However, literature reviews[17] have indicated that the individual diagnostic utility of the test is questionable and that its ability to discriminate various diagnostic groups is limited. Recent research has demonstrated that various brief versions of the MMPI (e.g., a selection of 168 items of the 566) produced scale scores that correlated very highly with those obtained from the total test and that also discriminated various diagnostic categories more effectively than did the full test.[18] A recent evaluation of the test states, "Undoubtedly the best instrument of its generation, it has assumed an almost mystical impregnability as a function of its age . . . Unfortunately, enthusiastic users have often exceeded the intent of the test developers, misreading meaning into unreliable data and applying the instrument in appropriate settings."[19] One aspect of its outmoded structure is the fact that most of the scales of the MMPI have little relevance to the personality disorders as now defined by the *DSM-III*.

THE CLINICAL ANALYSIS QUESTIONNAIRE (CAQ)

The CAQ was developed by Krug[13] for use in the clinical diagnosis of neurotics and psychotics, for evaluating therapeutic progress, and for clinical research. The CAQ had its origins in studies that used factor analysis to identify basic underlying dimensions of personality.

The test consists of 28 primary scales and 9 secondary or derived scales that will not be discussed here. Part I consists of 16 scales that measure "normal" personality dimensions previously included in Cattell's 16-PF test.[12] The 12 newer scales of Part II deal specifically with the psychopathologic domain. Descriptions of the 16 essentially normal personality scales are as follows: Warmth, Intelligence, Emotional Stability, Dominance, Impulsivity, Conformity, Boldness, Sensitivity, Suspiciousness, Imagination, Shrewdness, Insecurity, Radicalism, Self-Sufficiency, Self-Discipline, and Tension. The 12 scales designed to detect psychopathology are Hypochondriasis, Suicidal Depression, Agitation, Anxious Depression, Low Energy Depression, Guilt and Resentment, Boredom and Withdrawal, Paranoia, Psychopathic Deviation, Schizophrenia, Psychasthenia, and Psychological Inadequacy. No scales are provided to detect faking or random responding. There are 8 items per scale for the 16 scales of Part I and 12 items per scale for the 12 Part II scales, making a total of 272 items.

For each item, there are three possible responses; an "a" response means "yes, true, very much so," and a "c" answer means "no, false, never," and so on. The "b" answer indicates uncertainty. For example, a Dominance item such as "I like to be the one who tells others what to do" may be answered (a) yes, (b) uncertain, or (c) no. Similarly, for the Suicidal Depression item "I think about death, which ends all our problems," an individual may respond (a) a lot, (b) sometimes, or (c) hardly ever. The total test is said to require about $1\frac{1}{2}$ to 2 hours for completion and may be hand or machine-scored.

Raw scores are converted to standard scores, and norms are available for large adult and college male and female populations. CAQ profiles are also available for various neurotic groups, schizophrenic groups, alcoholics, narcotic addicts, and convicts.

Reliabilities for the 28 scales (expressed as test–retest correlations) average .73, ranging from .51 to .74 for the personality dimensions and from .67 to .90 for the pathology scales.

Krug[13] claims "concept validity" for the CAQ. By this he means that items of the CAQ for any given scale cluster when factor analyzed and that the items of a given scale (or factor) load higher on that scale than they do on other scales of the test. This is an idiosyncratic and seldom-used concept of validity. Data on more traditional measures of validity are quite limited. The test has been reported to discriminate successfully between drug addicts and alcoholics. Correlations are also given between CAQ scales and MMPI scales, which are, however, relatively low. In addition, the dimensions that are measured by the CAQ have little relevance to *DSM-III* diagnoses.

Theoretically Based Tests of Personality Disorders

PERSONALITY RESEARCH FORM (PRF)

The PRF, developed by Jackson,[14] provides multidimensional assessment of normal persons. The most frequently used edition has parallel forms (A and B), each of which provides scores for the 14 content scales, and an infrequency scale to detect nonpurposeful, or random, responding. The PRF is based on 14 of the 20 variables of personality proposed by Murray[20] in 1938. Murray's schema was a theoretic classification of personality dimensions based partly on psychoanalytic theory.

The 14 basic scales of the PRF are Achievement, Affiliation, Aggression, Autonomy, Dominance, Endurance, Exhibition, Harm Avoidance, Impulsivity, Nurturance, Order, Play, Social Recognition, and Understanding. A true–false response format is used. Each of the PRF's 15 scales consists of 20 items, 10 worded in a positive manner and 10 negatively. The trait of Affiliation, for example, is represented by responding "true" to such positive statements as "I believe that a person who is incapable of enjoying the people around him misses much in life" and "false" to such negative statements as "I think a man is smart to avoid being talked into helping his acquaintances." The Social Recognition scale has items such as "I very much enjoy being complimented" and "I give thought to the impression I make on others." The 15 scales of the PRF have a total of 300 items that most college students can complete in about 45 minutes.

Norms, expressed in both standard scores and percentile equivalents of raw scores, are based on large separate samples of male and female college students. However, no discussion is provided in the manual concerning profile interpretation. The internal consistency data that are presented for the 14 basic PRF scales of forms A and B are high, with an odd–even median reliability of .92. No test–retest data are provided for these forms.

Evidence is provided for both convergent and discriminative validity of the PRF scales, based on correlations with behavior ratings by peers and with tests designed to tap similar types of data (*e.g.*, the Strong Vocational Interest Blank[21] and the California Psychological Inventory).[22] The evidence for convergent validity would have been considerably strengthened, however, had the PRF been compared with other measures that actually have overlapping scales, such as the Edwards Personal Preference Schedule,[23] which attempts to measure 12 of the same dimensions.

The development of the PRF shows considerable methodologic sophistication and would appear useful for research with a college population. However, from a psychiatric point of view, it possesses several drawbacks. First, it appears to have been developed primarily for personality research, and the restricted nature of its norms makes its use somewhat problematical in applied settings among psychiatrists, psychologists, and counselors. Potential test users are urged to "exercise caution" when applying the norms to a noncollege population, but since almost no demographic correlates of the PRF scales are given, this leaves the potential user in something of a quandary. Furthermore, the names of the scales are generally unfamiliar to clinicians working with psychiatrically ill patients and the scales themselves do not clearly relate to *DSM-III* diagnostic concepts.

BENJAMIN'S STRUCTURAL ANALYSIS OF SOCIAL BEHAVIOR (SASB) TEST

The SASB test is a theoretically constructed instrument that is based explicitly on a theory of interpersonal behavior.[15] It assumes the following: that most psychiatric diagnoses are made on the basis of observed clusters of interpersonal behaviors, that diagnostic labels have both prognostic and therapeutic implications, and that one may best describe the relations among personality traits by means of a circumplex. The circumplex, which is described in detail later in this chapter, implies that trait descriptions may be ordered around a circle, with similar behaviors near one another and opposite behaviors placed at opposite locations. Benjamin assumes that the initiation of action may come from the *self* as well as from an *other*. When the focus is on the self, a separate circumplex of self-initiated actions is presented. In this case "flee, escape" is opposite "follow, maintain contact," while, "detach" is adjacent to "refuse assistance." When the focus is on the other, Benjamin[24] postulates that the behaviors of "warmly welcome" and "tender sexuality" are next to one another and opposite the behaviors of "approach menacingly" and "annihilating attack."

In order to apply the theory to a patient, the patient must complete a questionnaire consisting of 612 items that concern feelings about himself and his mother, father, and other important people in his life. Patients rate each question on a 0 to 100 scale representing the range of "never" to "always." Examples of questions are: Does your significant other person "angrily leave (you) out, absolutely refuse to have anything to do with (you);" Your mother, when you were 5 to 10 years old, "stimulated and taught (you), showed (you) how to understand, do;" Your mother in relation to your father "warmly, happily kept in contact with him."

The model makes detailed predictions about what behaviors are most likely to be associated with each other (based on the circumplex); it specifies how interpersonal behaviors are likely to affect one's self-concepts, and it suggests what the psychotherapist should do to maximize the possibility of producing desirable behavior changes. Scoring and analyses are currently done by a computer program.

Benjamin[25] reports high internal consistency for the scales of the questionnaire on the order of .90. She also describes the clinical usefulness of her system in exploring family dynamics, in developing a treatment plan, and for measuring changes in therapy. However, the questionnaire has gone through five different revisions, and the theory is so complex that considerable study is required before a potential user will feel comfortable with it. In addition, with the exception of Benjamin's 1979 paper,[15] few studies have been published demonstrating its validity in the contexts cited above.

MILLON CLINICAL MULTIAXIAL INVENTORY

The primary intent of the MCMI, developed by Millon,[16] is to provide a multidimensional diagnostic profile for persons with emotional and interpersonal difficulties. In addition, it was designed to provide scales that are consonant with the official diagnostic system, the *DSM-III*. The MCMI is not meant to be used with persons who do not evidence psychological symptoms or with those who are neither in psychotherapy nor undergoing psychodiagnostic evaluation.

The 20 clinical scales of the MCMI were developed on the basis of Millon's[26,27] theoretic system. Among the basic assumptions of this system are the following: syndromes should be differentiated according to severity; where appropriate, each diagnostic syndrome should be shown to be an extension or disruption of a patient's basic personality pattern; and the content of different syndromes overlaps to varying degrees.

The scales themselves reflect this theoretic framework. With regard to severity, for example, the first 8 basic personality scales tap mild severity. These are Schizoid, Avoidant, Dependent, Histrionic, Narcissistic, Antisocial, Compulsive, and Passive-Aggressive. The next 3 scales, Schizotypal, Borderline, and Paranoid, reflect moderate or marked levels of impairment. These 11 scales correspond to the personality disorders listed in *DSM-*

III Axis II. Similarly, the remaining 9 scales differentiate Axis I clinical syndromes, which are usually of briefer duration than personality disorders. Those of moderate severity are labeled Anxiety, Somatoform, Hypomanic, Dysthymic, Alcohol Abuse, and Drug Abuse. Those of marked severity are called Psychotic Thinking, Psychotic Depression, and Psychotic Delusion. These last nine syndromes are conceived as disruptions of basic personality patterns that occur during stress. Two additional scales are employed to correct for "denial versus complaint" attitudes (Scale W) and to detect careless, confused, or random responding (Scale V).

The MCMI's scales contain from 16 to 47 items. The entire inventory consists of only 175 items; therefore, many items are used in more than one scale. This is consonant with Millon's theory, inasmuch as all syndromes are considered to be composed to some degree of overlapping symptoms. Most items are written very simply: "Lately, I've begun to feel lonely and empty," and "I will often do things for no reason other than they might be fun." The entire test may be completed in about 30 minutes. It must be computer scored, and both a profile report and an automated interpretive report are provided.

Normative data, based on large samples of both nonclinical and patient populations, are available. Rather than being expressed as customary standard scores, these norms are obtained by an innovative procedure of transforming raw scores in terms of the known prevalence of personality and syndrome base rates.

Reliability data are provided for both retest stability and internal consistency. The median coefficient for test–retest reliability over the period of a week is .83, and that for internal reliability is .90.

The relations between the MCMI's clinical scales and scales of other, comparable diagnostic inventories provide an index of convergent validity. These inventories include the MMPI and two relatively new instruments, the Psychological Screening Inventory (PSI), developed by Lanyon,[28] and the Symptom Distress Checklist (SCL-90), developed by Derogatis and co-workers.[29]

The MCMI appears to be a very promising instrument for psychiatric use, both for diagnostic assessment and research. It has high internal reliability and stability, has satisfactory evidence of validity, and is relatively short. Perhaps most important is that the descriptive categories of the test are directly related to the official *DSM-III* categories.

The Circumplex Model As An Integrating Framework for *DSM-III* Axis II Diagnoses

A model that depicts a two-dimensional circular ordering of concepts, based on their degree of similarity, has been called a *circumplex*.[30] Over approximately the past 30 years, various investigators have endeavored to demonstrate that the structure of personality traits, when defined by an individual's interpersonal behavior, may best be represented in terms of this circumplex model.

The circular ordering of personality variables proposed by most investigators in the 1950s and 1960s was largely theoretic. For example, in 1951 Freedman, and colleagues[31] hypothesized 16 modes of interpersonal interaction that they believed could best be represented by a circular model. The modes included such ways of behaving as dominating, loving, trusting, and complaining. The circular continuum defines the relations among the variables: the closer two variables are to one another, the more similar they are (*e.g.*, supportive, loving); the farther the separation, the more dissimilar are the variables. Theoretically, variables opposite one another on the circle should represent bipolarities (*e.g.*, dominating, submissive).

According to Leary's[32] theory of the interpersonal personality system, these 16 modes of interaction reflect eight broader categories that are used in interpersonal diagnosis. Each category has a moderate (adaptive) and an extreme (pathologic) intensity (*e.g.*, "competitive-narcissistic" at a moderate level and "aggressive-sadistic" at an extreme level). The sequence in which these eight categories is presented reflects both their similarities and their polarities. As a simple example, "self-effacing-masochistic" is next to "docile-dependent" and opposite "managerial-autocratic."

In a particularly important study, Schaefer[33] reanalyzed data from a number of studies of parent–child interactions. Despite the different methods and conceptual schemes used in these studies, they all gave similar circumplex organizations of social and emotional behavior. The theoretic circumplex he constructed to represent his conclusions clearly shows such similar behaviors as "neglecting," "indifferent," and "detached" to be opposite the equally similar behaviors of "accepting," "overindulgent," and "protective."

Further evidence of a circular ordering of traits related to interpersonal interaction is presented by Lorr and McNair.[34,35] In 1963 they reported the development of an "interpersonal behavior circle." A factor analysis of clinicians' ratings of both psychiatric patients and normal individuals on an inventory of statements describing various kinds of interpersonal behavior was interpreted as reflecting nine clusters of variables. In 1965, they replicated their study on another large group of patients and normals and derived a similar but expanded circular order of personality clusters in which the circular sequence was as follows: sociability, affection, nurturance, agreeableness, deference, submission, abasement, inhibition, detachment, mistrust, hostility, recognition, dominance, and exhibition. Although no theoretic rationale is given for the choice of these particular trait terms, it is evident that neighboring terms are similar to one another and that there exist such bipolarities as dominance–submission and hostility–agreeableness.

The circumplex models described thus far have been theoretic; that is, the variables or concepts identified by the investigators have been placed equal distances apart on the perimeter of a circle. No attempt has been made to find empiric placements. In addition, for each study the sequence of variables has been identified through the use of only one method. Subsequent to these studies, however, Conte and Plutchik[36] demonstrated by two independent methods that a circumplex model provides a valid representation of the structure of interpersonal personality traits.

Similarity ratings of 223 trait terms, obtained using a modified paired-comparison method, empirically located the angular position of each of these terms on a circle. An independent method, using factor analysis of semantic differential ratings of a sample of 40 of these terms, produced an essentially identical empiric circular ordering when the terms were plotted on the basis of their loadings on the first two factors. The angular placement of terms based on the method of semantic differential profile similarity is shown in Figure 1. As inspec-

FIG. 1. Angular placement of 40 personality trait terms based on a semantic differential profile similarity analysis. (Conte HR, Plutchik R: A circumplex model for interpersonal personality traits. J Pers Soc Psychol 40:706, 1981. Copyright 1981 by the American Psychological Association. Reprinted by permission of the authors)

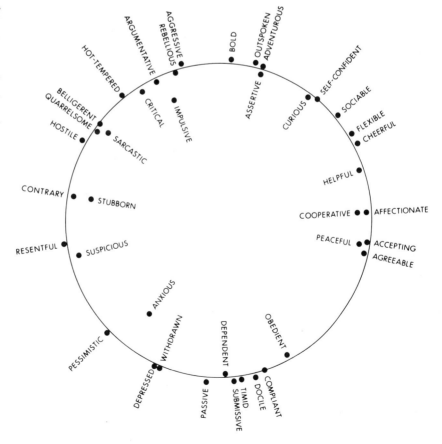

tion of the figure indicates, the ordering of the trait terms demonstrates the properties of similarity and bipolarity.

The main clinical applications of a circumplex model of interpersonal traits have been in the areas of diagnosis and assessment. Wiggins,[37] for example, presents an excellent discussion of the relevance of circumplex models for depicting the relations among psychiatric diagnoses. Among the studies cited are one by Plutchik[38] and another by Plutchik and Platman.[39] In the first study (1967), the domains of affective states and diagnoses were related to one another. Clinicians were presented with a list of diagnostic terms such as *hysteric, psychopathic,* and *paranoid* and were asked to indicate to what extent they believed each diagnostic label to be related to such emotions as anger, sadness, fear, and so on. Ratings between pairs of diagnostic labels were correlated. The resulting matrix was factor-analyzed, and the diagnostic labels were plotted on the basis of their factor loadings. An approximate circumplex resulted in which, on an empiric basis, extraverted was opposite introverted, psychopathic was opposite dependent, and well-adjusted was opposite a grouping of obsessive, compulsive, and schizoid labels.

Using another method for examining the question of whether diagnostic concepts form a circumplex order, Plutchik and Platman[39] gave 20 psychiatrists a list of *DSM-II* personality disorders, such as paranoid, schizoid, hysterical, and cyclothymic, and asked them to indicate what personality traits were typically associated with each disorder. A factor analysis of the ratings again showed a circular configuration of relative similarity among the different diagnoses. With some exceptions, the results were fairly similar to those of the 1967 study, indicating that a circular model is appropriate for at least a subset of diagnostic labels.

We have conducted a study of the similarity structure of the 11 personality disorders listed in *DSM-III,* and the results are presented here for the first time. The disorders are as follows: paranoid, schizoid, schizotypal, histrionic, narcissistic, antisocial, borderline, avoidant, dependent, compulsive, and passive-aggressive. To these was added the label "well-adjusted."

The methodology followed was similar to that employed in the study of Conte and Plutchik.[36] For the direct similarity scaling method, three reference terms (*compulsive, antisocial,* and *histrionic*) were chosen. All 11 personality disorder terms, plus well-adjusted, were then rated by 10 psychiatrists in terms of their perceived similarity to each of the reference words. These ratings were translated into

angular placements relative to each of the reference terms, and an average angular placement on a circle was then determined for each disorder. The diagnostic terms were found to be relatively well distributed around the circle, and the ordering suggested the circumplicial characteristics of similarity and bipolarity. *Borderline* and *narcissistic,* for example, were approximately opposite *compulsive.* The terms *schizoid, schizotypal, avoidant,* and *passive-aggressive* clustered together and were opposite *well-adjusted.*

Since the possibility of bias exists in relation to any one method, an attempt was made to replicate these angular placements using an entirely different and independent method. This method, semantic differential profile similarity scaling, was based on a factor analysis of semantic differential ratings for each of the 12 personality diagnoses. The method may be briefly described in the following way: 12 psychiatrists rated, on seven-point scales, the extent to which each of 20 adjectives such as *dependable, active,* and *strong* described patients given each of the Axis II diagnoses.

The data provided a semantic profile for each disorder in terms of its connotative meaning. These profiles were then intercorrelated, and the resulting matrix was factor-analyzed. When the disorders were plotted on the basis of their loadings on the first two factors, a circular ordering was obtained that appeared highly similar to that which emerged in the direct similarity scaling analysis. In order to determine the equivalence of the two orderings (*i.e.,* to determine the validity of these placements), a Pearson product–moment correlation was computed between the angular locations based on the first method and those based on the second method; this correlation was found to be +.91, indicating high validity of the placements. On the basis of this high correlation, the angular locations obtained by each method for each of the disorders were averaged.

The similarity and bipolarity characteristics of the data are shown in Figure 2. Borderline, narcissistic, and antisocial cluster together opposite dependent; histrionic is opposite compulsive; and the schizoid, schizotypal, avoidant cluster is on the opposite side of the circle from well-adjusted.

It is of considerable interest to note that the ordering around a circle of these *DSM-III* personality disorders is highly similar to that obtained by Plutchik and Platman,[39] using *DSM-II* diagnoses and an entirely different method.

The fact that exceptionally similar orderings of personality disorders were found by three different, independent methods has a number of implica-

FIG. 2. A circumplex structure of *DSM-III* Axis II personality disorders based on direct similarity scaling and semantic differential profile similarity.

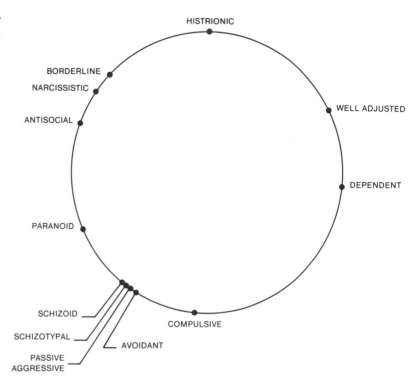

tions. First, it provides evidence for the convergent validity of the specific locations of the disorders on a circle; more importantly, it provides strong evidence for the construct validity of the circumplex structure of personality disorders. Second, it implies that a circumplex structure is applicable for the representation of the domains of emotions, personality traits, and disorders. If, as Plutchik[40] has claimed, personality traits represent mixtures of basic emotions that have frequently occurred together over time, and if personality disorders may be conceptualized as extremes or exaggeration of certain personality traits, then these personality disorders may be seen as derivatives of emotion. This conclusion places diagnostic concepts in a larger conceptual domain and suggests connections that might not otherwise be noticed. For example, a person who frequently experiences strong feelings of anger and disgust may eventually be described as a paranoid personality type. This same person, if psychologically disturbed, would probably be given the diagnosis of paranoid personality disorder. These findings may be interpreted to mean that psychiatrists carry in their heads a set of abstractions about the kinds of people to whom diagnostic labels of particular types are applied. Diagnosis may be thought of as attempts to develop well-organized, discrete schemas for making sense of the overlapping traits actually observed in patients.

Conclusions

This review of quantitative issues in the assessment of personality disorders suggests a number of conclusions. One is that multidimensional self-report measures, particularly those based on a theoretic framework, have distinct advantages over other forms of data gathering. They provide useful supplementary information to assist the psychiatrist in making diagnostic and treatment decisions. They are relatively cost-effective in the sense that the data can be easily obtained by testers with a minimal amount of training. Self-report instruments, more than other forms of assessment, are more likely to have gone through a process of psychometric development and refinement. In addition, they greatly diminish the possible influence of interviewer bias. Finally, the increased availability of interactive computers makes possible highly standardized administration, scoring, and interpretation of tests.

A second general conclusion is that tests based on explicit theoretic models are more likely to be useful than tests based simply on empiric determinations of discrimination between two or more groups or on the basis of factor-analytic studies. Theoretic models have greater generalizability and imply a network of relations. In addition, test dimensions that relate directly to well-known psychiatric constructs such as the disorders described in *DSM-III* are more likely to find general acceptance by psychiatrists than those that use other principles of classification. From this point of view, the MCMI developed by Millon holds great promise as a diagnostic tool.

The third major conclusion of this chapter is that the circumplex model of personality and of personality disorders is a useful conceptualization of the data concerning Axis II diagnoses. Empiric evidence reveals that psychiatrists do in fact have an implicit model in their minds of the relations among personality diagnoses. This model, which in part fits the criteria for a "fuzzy set,"[37] implies that some diagnoses are relatively more similar than others and that some diagnoses may be conceptualized as nearly bipolar. When a diagnosis is made, reference is made to an implicit prototypic image; the characteristics of an actual patient are only an approximation to this prototype. Diagnoses, therefore, represent probabilistic classifications that are related to these prototypic images.

From a broad theoretic point of view it is important to emphasize that, just as the circumplex model has been reported to be an integrating idea for the description of both personality traits and emotions,[36,40] so, too, may it be an integrating model for nonpsychotic personality disorders.

REFERENCES

1. Conte HR, Plutchik R, Karasu TB et al: A self-report borderline scale: Discriminative validity and preliminary norms. J Nerv Ment Dis 168:428–435, 1980

2. Exner, JE Jr: The Rorschach: A Comprehensive System. New York, John Wiley & Sons, 1974

3. Koppitz EM: Psychological Evaluation of Children's Human Figure Drawings. New York, Grune & Stratton, 1968

4. Perline IH: Computer Interpreted Rorschach. Tempe, AZ, Century Diagnostics, 1979

5. Spitzer R, Endicott J: An integrated group of forms for automated psychiatric case records. Arch Gen Psychiatry 24:540–547, 1971

6. Gurland BJ, Yorkston NJ, Stone AR et al: The structured and scaled interview to assess maladjustment (SSIAM). Arch Gen Psychiatry 27:259–263, 1972

7. Hamilton M: Development of a rating scale for primary depressive illness. Br J Soc Clin Psychol 6:278–296, 1967

8. Spitzer RL, Endicott J: Schedule for Affective Disorders and Schizophrenia. National Institute of Mental Health, Clinical Research Branch, May 1978

9. Robins L, Helzer J, Croughan J et al: The NIMH diagnostic interview schedule: Introduction and history. Unpublished report of the Division of Biometry and Epidemiology, National Institute of Mental Health, 1980

10. Plutchik R, Kellerman H, Conte HR: A structural theory of ego defenses. In Izard CE (ed): Emotions, Personality, and Psychopathology. New York, Plenum, 1979

11. Hathaway SR, McKinley JC: Manual of the Minnesota Multiphasic Personality Inventory, rev ed. New York, Psychological Corporation, 1951

12. Cattell RB, Eber HW, Tatsuoka MM: Handbook for the Sixteen Personality Factor Questionnaire (16PF). Champaign, IL, Institute for Personality and Ability Testing, 1970

13. Krug SE: Clinical Analysis Questionnaire Manual. Champaign, IL, Institute for Personality and Ability Testing, 1980

14. Jackson DN: Personality Research Form Manual. Goshen, NY, Research Psychologists Press, 1967

15. Benjamin LS: Structural analysis of differentiation failure. Psychiatry 42:1–23, 1979

16. Millon TM: Millon Clinical Multiaxial Inventory Manual, 2nd ed. Minneapolis, Interpretive Scoring Systems, 1982

17. Adcock CJ: Review of the MMPI. In Buros OK (ed): The Sixth Mental Measurements Yearbook, pp 313–316. Highland Park, NJ, Gryphon Press, 1965

18. Poythress NG Jr: Selecting a short form of the MMPI: Addendum to Faschingbauer. J Consult Clin Psychol 46:331–334, 1978

19. Green CJ: Psychological assessment in medical settings. In Millon T, Green C, Meagher R (eds): Handbook of Clinical Health Psychology. New York, Plenum, 1982

20. Murray HA: Explorations in Personality. Cambridge, MA, Harvard University Press, 1938

21. Strong EK Jr: Strong Vocational Interest Blank. Stanford, CA, Stanford University Press, 1966

22. Gough HG: California Psychological Inventory. Palo Alto, CA, Consulting Psychologists Press, 1960

23. Edwards AL: Edwards Personal Preference Schedule. New York, Psychological Corporation, 1959

24. McLemore CW, Benjamin LS: Whatever happened to interpersonal diagnosis? A psychosocial alternate to DSM-III. Am Psychol 34:17–34, 1979

25. Benjamin LS: Validation of structural analysis of social behavior (SASB), Unpublished manuscript

26. Millon T: Modern Psychopathology. Philadelphia, WB Saunders, 1969

27. Millon T: Disorders of Personality: DSM-III, Axis II. New York, John Wiley & Sons, 1981

28. Lanyon RI: Psychological Screening Manual. Goshen, NY, Research Psychologist Press, 1973

29. Derogatis LR, Lipman RS, Covi L: An outpatient rating scale. Psychopharmacol Bull 9:13–28, 1973

30. Guttman L: A new approach to factor analysis. In Lazarsfeld PT (ed): Mathematical Thinking in the Social Sciences. Glencoe, IL, Free Press, 1954

31. Freedman MB, Leary TF, Ossorio AG et al: The interpersonal dimension of personality. J Pers 20:146–161, 1951

32. Leary TF: Interpersonal Diagnosis of Personality: A Functional Theory and Methodology for Personality Evaluation. New York, Ronald Press, 1957

33. Schaefer ES: Converging conceptual models for maternal behavior and child behavior. In Glidewell JC (ed): Parental Attitudes and Child Behavior. Springfield, IL, Charles C Thomas, 1961

34. Lorr M, McNair DM: An interpersonal behavior circle. J Abnorm Soc Psychol 67:68–75, 1963

35. Lorr M, McNair DM: Expansion of the interpersonal behavior circle. J Pers Soc Psychol 2:823–830, 1965

36. Conte HR, Plutchik R: A circumplex model for interpersonal traits. J Pers Soc Psychol 40:701–711, 1981

37. Wiggins JS: Circumplex models of interpersonal behavior in clinical psychology. In Kendell PC, Butcher JN (eds): Handbook of Research Methods in Clinical Psychology. New York, John Wiley & Sons, 1982

38. Plutchik R: The affective differential: Emotion profiles implied by diagnostic concepts. Psychol Rep 20:19–25, 1967

39. Plutchik R, Platman SR: Personality connotations of psychiatric diagnoses. J Nerv Ment Dis 165:418–422, 1977

40. Plutchik R: Emotion: A Psychoevolutionary Synthesis. New York: Harper & Row, 1980

14

Larry J. Siever and Kenneth S. Kendler

Schizoid/Schizotypal/Paranoid Personality Disorders

Schizoid, schizotypal, and paranoid personality disorders constitute the "odd cluster" of Axis II diagnoses in the *Diagnostic and Statistical Manual of Mental Disorders* (*DSM III*). As such, they characterize individuals whose chronic maladaptive patterns are marked by peculiarities of behavior that may attract less attention than the "dramatic cluster" and are often accompanied by less apparent subjective distress than is frequently observed in the "anxious cluster." All of these disorders are marked by a degree of social isolation and guardedness. Beyond these commonalities, distinctions between these disorders are largely based on the presence of psychoticlike symptoms in the schizotypal individual and the presence of extreme suspiciousness and guardedness in the paranoid individual. Criteria for each of these disorders are based in part on very different historical rationales. There has been remarkably little empiric study of these disorders, although they are beginning to be more systematically investigated. Thus, although much of the information available represents clinical description or formulation, relevant recent empiric studies will be emphasized.

Schizoid Personality Disorder

HISTORICAL BACKGROUND

The central characteristic of schizoid individuals is their social isolation and emotional distance from others. These characteristics were frequently noted by German descriptive psychiatrists in schizophrenics, both prior to the onset of their psychosis and when in remission from their psychosis, as well as in the relatives of schizophrenics. The concept and term thus evolved in the context of an attempt to better understand the nature and genetic basis of schizophrenia. Over time it came to be applied in a psychodynamic context to a less specific population marked by difficulty with intimacy and even became a term for a broad range of behavioral peculiarities. The *DSM-III* definition of schizoid personality disorder falls into the intermediate range of specificity in between the broad psychoanalytically oriented use of *schizoid* and the narrow psychogenetically oriented use, which tended to include characteristics of eccentricity and suspiciousness. The latter clinical picture is now diagnosed as schizotypal personality disorder.[1]

DEFINITION

The *DSM-III* inclusion criteria for schizoid personality disorder are (1) emotional coldness and aloofness and absence of warm tender feelings for others; (2) indifference to praise or criticism or to the feelings of others; and (3) close friendships with no more than one or two persons, including family members. The other criteria are exclusionary: individuals meeting criteria for schizotypal personality disorder, schizophrenia, paranoid disorder, or, if under 18, schizoid disorder of childhood or adolescence, may not be diagnosed as having schizoid personality disorder.

These items are derived from clinical experience rather than from empiric studies. They are difficult to rate reliably, particularly in the absence of operationalized criteria, and reliability has been reported as low in rating a small sample of schizoid personality disorders by *DSM-III* criteria.[2] The central characteristic of this disorder is social isolation, which must be discriminated from avoidance of relationships due to fear of rejection, as in avoidant personality, or the solitary life style of the schizotypal individual, which is often accompanied by suspiciousness and eccentricities. The creation of these two new diagnostic categories, that is, the schizotypal and the avoidant personality disorders, has substantially reduced the applicability of this diagnosis. Future studies are required to delineate the boundaries of this disorder in relation to other personality disorders and to determine whether it may not more meaningfully be combined with schizotypal personality disorder into one category.

EPIDEMIOLOGY

Data regarding epidemiology of the personality disorders in general is meager, and we are not aware of any studies examining the prevalence of *DSM-III* diagnosed personality disorders in the general population. In psychiatric settings, particularly inpatient settings, this disorder appears to be rare.[2] It may be somewhat more frequently observed in the outpatient clinic and may occur in males more frequently than females.[3] More definitive epidemiology will depend on reliable operationalized interviews for these disorders.

CLINICAL DESCRIPTION

The following case report illustrates some of the characteristics of schizoid personality disorder:

> A 46-year-old single white male accountant sought professional consultation on the advice of a colleague because of persistent feelings of dissatisfaction and depression following a change in his work situation. Although he retained his position at his firm, where he had worked for 20 years, many of his more important responsibilities had been shifted to a younger colleague. He had always worked well in a rather autonomous position in the firm but now felt that his daily work routine had been disrupted and he no longer had meaningful tasks to accomplish. It turned out that he had always been socially isolated, with social contacts limited to acquaintances at work, and followed a rather prescribed pattern of reading the newspaper and watching television as his evening recreation. He at times saw a married sister and her family on weekends. This limited life style had been tolerable for him for some time and he appeared rela-

tively indifferent to the opinions of co-workers as long as he could count on being assigned his quota of accounts. His redefined position left him with less work to do and an unclear role in the firm. He felt as if "the rug had been pulled out from under me." In the consultation, he was a quiet man who although cooperative was difficult to engage affectively. He spoke with little emotion and mumbled at times, exhibiting no sense of attachment to other people in his life, but only to his "way of doing things," which he had great difficulty in changing.

Although this patient did not present with a complaint of social isolation, which is rarely an explicit source of concern for the schizoid individual, the central feature of his personality was his stable solitary existence. He appeared indifferent to others' opinions of his life and work, as long as he was allowed to continue "undisturbed" in his work and personal life. Although this rigidity is often observed in individuals with compulsive personality disorder, they usually have the capacity for more intimate relationships and are more disturbing to others in their controlling behavior.

It seems unlikely that schizoid individuals entirely lack tender feelings or are completely indifferent to others' opinions. Clinical experience, however, suggests that, in contrast to, for example, avoidant personality disorder, in which isolation is a defense against disappointment in relationships, schizoid individuals have often not been able to attain mutually gratifying relationships in their lives, even with parental or other early caretaking figures. Thus, they have not had the experience of having the expectations for relationships that the individual with avoidant personality disorder may have had prior to their disappointments. As relationships are not experienced as a potential source of gratification but still pose the threat of frustration or disruption, they are avoided by the schizoid individual except in their most attenuated forms.

The course of schizoid personality disorder has been investigated primarily to examine the issue of whether it is the premorbid personality picture of individuals who go on to develop schizophrenia. Evidence has been mixed in this regard and suggests that a variety of clinical profiles characterize preschizophrenic individuals, including unsocialized aggressive behavior. However, when schizoid personality disorder is observed prior to the onset of schizophrenia, most studies suggest it is associated with a poorer outcome.[4] One study suggests that most children with schizoid personality disorder as children go on to manifest a schizoid personality as adults.[5] However, careful longitudinal studies are lacking, particularly using *DSM-III* criteria for this disorder, which has now been demarcated from schizotypal personality disorder.

ETIOLOGY

Although there is theoretic speculation regarding schizoid personality disorder, there has been little empiric study of the etiology of this disorder. Genetic studies suggest that social isolation in childhood and adulthood may be observed in the relatives of schizophrenics, although results are not uniform in this regard. As discussed earlier, the hallmark of these individuals is the apparent lack of gratification derived from human relationships. Some formulations emphasize genetic or constitutional predispositions, while others emphasize defensive characteristics evolving from inadequate caretaking. Some etiologic factors to be considered are as follows:

A constitutionally determined anhedonia or lack of pleasure derived from interpersonal relationships[6]

A social aversiveness based on a predominance of aversive versus appetitive systems[6]

Impaired attachment behavior secondary to attentional or broader neurointegrative slippage,[6,7] resulting in dysynchrony between the parent and developing child

Inadequate or unreliable mothering, leading to a sense of isolation and fear of being overwhelmed by others[8,9]

These theories are not necessarily incompatible, and there exists few empiric studies to support any of them. The association of social isolation and smooth pursuit eye movement dysfunction,[7] possibly reflecting an impaired capacity for attentional focusing, might be considered consistent with the third hypothesis, although this hypothesis is perhaps more applicable to schizotypal personality disorder. In any case, it seems likely that schizoid individuals do not experience satisfying relationships from early childhood on as a result of an interaction between constitutional predispositions and early relationships with caretaking figures.

DIAGNOSIS AND DIFFERENTIAL DIAGNOSIS

The diagnosis of schizoid personality disorder should be applied when there is evidence that social isolation has been part of a long-term pattern rather than a temporary state due to a change in life circumstances or loss.

It is to be distinguished from avoidant personality disorder where a fear of rejection and disappointment may lead to a pattern of withdrawal from close social relationships. In schizotypal personality disorder, social isolation is usually accompanied by suspiciousness or eccentricity in behavior or speech. Individuals with other personality disorders such as compulsive personality disorder or narcissistic personality disorder may show marked impairment in their capacity for intimacy, a relative sparseness of truly close relationships, and emotional distance in face-to-face interactions. However, in these disorders, the social isolation is less pervasive and difficulties in intimacy are more observed in the character of these individuals' relationships rather than in their absence. For example, individuals with compulsive personality, when questioned, will usually speak warmly of their children or pets (in contrast to their descriptions of, for example, co-workers). Individuals with narcissistic personality disorder may speak of others as if they were "things" to be exploited, but important, if limited, relationships are usually present. Paranoid personality disorder is characterized by emotional coldness as well, but this characteristic must be accompanied by pervasive suspiciousness and mistrust. However, restricted emotional expression is a criterion for three other personality disorders (paranoid, schizotypal, and compulsive) and lack of close relationships for two others (schizotypal and avoidant). Thus, it is likely that schizoid personality disorder will coexist with other personality disorders, except in the case of schizotypal personality disorder, where it is by definition excluded. Schizoid personality disorder of childhood or adolescence and the psychotic disorders such as schizophrenia or paranoid disorder also exclude the diagnosis of schizoid personality disorder but should not present problems of differential diagnosis.

As the applicability of schizoid personality disorder has been substantially eroded by the creation of the two new personality disorders, schizotypal and avoidant personality disorder, its clinical prevalence and usefulness as well as its demarcation from these other two disorders need to be empirically examined. Schizoid individuals may be less likely to present in a psychiatric setting due to their often stable, if restricted, adaptation, making such investigation difficult in a psychiatric setting.

TREATMENT

Because of the rarity with which these people present for treatment, there exists a paucity of clinical studies regarding their treatment. In the absence of some painful shift in their life circumstances, it is unlikely that these individuals would be amenable to clinical intervention. When they seek treatment following a crisis, intervention may be based on the nature of the acute symptomatology rather than aimed at effecting a long-lasting change in social adaptation. However, limited shifts in the direction of decreased withdrawal may be possible if the therapist accepts the patient's withdrawal but is able to slowly develop a reconstructive relationship with them.[9]

Schizotypal Personality Disorder

HISTORICAL BACKGROUND

In contrast to the other two diagnoses in this cluster, *schizotypal personality disorder* was introduced as a diagnostic entity in the process of formulating *DSM-III*. The term itself is based on conceptions of the "schizotype" by Rado[10] and Meehl,[6] who were interested in characterizing individuals with a genetic predisposition for schizophrenia who were not overtly psychotic. The impetus for the delineation of schizotypal personality disorder came from an attempt to differentiate within the context of the *DSM-III* the chronic instability of borderline personality disorder, in which regressions may be accompanied by loss of reality-testing, from "borderline schizophrenia," in which psychoticlike symptoms are presumably based on a phenomenologic and perhaps genetic relatedness to schizophrenia. Spitzer and co-workers[11] established a new diagnosis of "schizotypal personality disorder" based largely on characteristics of "borderline schizophrenic" relatives of schizophrenics and included it in the "odd cluster" with schizoid and paranoid personality disorder.

DEFINITION

There are eight *DSM-III* criteria for schizotypal personality disorder,[2] and four of these must be satisfied for the diagnosis to be applied. Three of these criteria represent aspects of social dysfunction and are included as criteria for other personality disorders as well: (1) social isolation, (2) inadequate rapport in face-to-face interaction, and (3) undue social anxiety or hypersensitivity. The other five

represent symptoms that are psychoticlike but more attenuated and less pervasive than observed in the major psychoses: (1) magical thinking, (2) ideas of reference, (3) recurrent illusions, (4) odd speech, and (5) suspiciousness or paranoid ideation (also observed in paranoid personality disorder). The former are more akin to the "negative symptoms" of schizophrenia, while the latter might be considered attenuated "positive symptoms" of psychosis.

There is some empiric basis for these criteria, since they were selected on the basis of an examination of the case records of those relatives of adopted-away schizophrenics and controls who were considered to have characteristics related to schizophrenia.[11] Such characteristics were observed significantly more frequently in the biological relatives of schizophrenic probands than in their adopted relatives or the biological relatives of controls.[12] Thus these characteristics might be expected to characterize individuals with a genetic relationship to schizophrenia, as well as perhaps some other individuals without such an established relationship. However, as these criteria were selected originally according to the diagnostic scheme of the investigators involved, it is not clear that they represent the most sensitive or best characterizations of such individuals. Studies suggest that, in fact, the "negative symptoms" may be more characteristic of these individuals than the "positive symptoms."[1,13,14] Although suspiciousness or referential ideation is not infrequently observed in the relatives of schizophrenics, items such as magical thinking and recurrent illusions may not be as discriminating for a genetic relatedness to schizophrenia. One study found somatization and serious scholastic or occupational dysfunction to also characterize the schizotypal relatives in the adoptive studies.[13] Thus as empiric studies such as these increase our knowledge of this disorder these criteria will undoubtedly be refined.

The establishment of schizotypal personality disorder raises some important general considerations regarding the personality disorders. This is the only personality disorder in *DSM-III* to have been derived in part from empiric studies, rather than from the clinical consensus of the *DSM-III* architects. As such, it represents a considerable methodologic advance in an attempt to formulate criteria for the personality disorders more scientifically. However, several important caveats are in order here. The first is that this diagnosis was not developed without preconceived clinical notions as to its nature. The case records of preselected "schizophrenia spectrum"–disordered relatives defined on the basis of clinical tradition were reviewed to generate the criteria for this disorder. The formalization of criteria depended on Spitzer and colleagues' sense of what characterized these relatives. They were able to validate these criteria, but this does not, however, imply that numbers of other criteria sets might also distinguish schizophrenic relatives from controls. Another problem arises because this set of criteria was not formulated as a means of distinguishing relatives of schizophrenics from controls but as identifying a personality disorder that, in some people, is related to schizophrenia. It is, of course, an *a priori* assumption that identifying individuals on the basis of a genetic relatedness to an Axis I diagnosis is the most rational means of identifying such personality disorders. For example, clinical utility (*e.g.,* treatment responsiveness) is another basis, which may not be directly correlated with genetic factors. However, with the caveats noted, this approach does allow for validators external to the clinical characteristics selected. It is interesting that the use of such a validator, in this instance a genetic relatedness to schizophrenia, leads to the selection of individuals with enduring dysfunction in the social sphere.[13] This finding raises the possibility that underlying genetic or psychobiological predispositions may more likely be associated with longer-term adaptational characteristics of an individual, which may result in a cohesive perceived ''personality'' rather than transient psychoticlike symptoms, which do not seem such good discriminators for these disorders. Analogously, studies suggest that long-term characteristics, such as clinical course as well as social and affective functioning, may better distinguish schizophrenic from affective disorder patients than does the presence or absence of psychotic symptoms.[15] However, more careful delineation of the character of such psychoticlike symptoms in schizotypal personality disorder may provide them with greater discriminative power.

EPIDEMIOLOGY

Only clues exist as to the prevalence of schizotypal personality disorder in the general population. Kendler and colleagues[16] found only two cases in 138 interviewed biological relatives of control adoptees from the Copenhagen Adoption Studies.[12]

Thus, the prevalence of this personality disorder in the general population is likely to be rather low. However, in several studies in psychiatric clinics the prevalence is likely to be higher than that of many of the other personality disorders. For example, Mellsop and colleagues[2] found that schizotypal personality disorder is one of the more frequently diagnosed of the personality disorders, along with borderline, histrionic, and avoidant personality disorder, and was diagnosed in almost half of their inpatients receiving a personality disorder diagnosis. The *DSM-III* field trials found a prevalence of schizotypal personality disorder in only 5% to 10% of outpatients with specific personality disorders.[3] Thus prevalence and frequency of diagnosis in relation to other diagnoses is likely to vary with clinic populations and diagnostic practices. However, available evidence suggests that schizotypal patients, usually with concomitant Axis I and/or Axis II diagnoses, may be observed in inpatient populations more frequently than outpatient populations. In the outpatient setting, they may be observed less commonly than borderline personality disorder, but more commonly than schizoid personality disorder.[3]

CLINICAL DESCRIPTION

A representative case history of an individual with schizotypal personality disorder is as follows:

> A 22-year-old college student was referred by his school counselor because of persistent academic difficulties and behavioral peculiarities that brought him to the attention of his teachers. He lives with his parents where he spends most of his time alone in his room reading or solving crossword puzzles. He has no close friends, although he does have several ''nodding acquaintances'' at school. His performance at school is inconsistent despite his relatively high IQ on testing, and he has experienced several ''slumps'' where he has had to drop courses, thus delaying his graduation. Teachers note he is often preoccupied in class and is difficult to engage. On mental status examination, he walked in awkwardly in somewhat disheveled clothes, avoided eye contact, spoke almost inaudibly with few words, and did not develop a comfortable rapport with the interviewer. When he responded to questions, they were not always ''on the mark'' responses. He noted feeling concerned that others in his class might be ''against him'' and perhaps causing him to have difficulty on his tests, although he was not sure exactly how. He often interpreted smiles on the face of classmates as ridiculing him and thus shunned them further. When these feelings would worsen, he was unable to perform adequately academically. He, however, experienced no hallucinations or specific delusions.

In this example, symptoms of social isolation combined with eccentricity of both appearance and ideation establish the diagnosis of schizotypal personality disorder. This young man is not only isolated, but affectively constricted with poor rapport, hypersensitivity, suspiciousness with referential ideation, and somewhat odd speech.

There may be several types of clinical presentation of individuals with schizotypal personality disorder. A subgroup presents with more prominent psychoticlike symptoms. Of these, some may have recurrent illusions bordering on hallucinations but too ill-defined to be considered "true hallucinations" (e.g., an intermittent whispering sound that sounds like the patient's mother saying "watch it" only heard in the presence of such sounds as those of the wind whistling or a passing subway). Persistent referential ideation and suspiciousness are common in this truly schizotypal presentation. Others of this subgroup develop psychoticlike symptoms episodically in the context of a loss of an important person in their life and are frequently considered borderline. The speech of these patients is often productive and digressive. They may or may not be dramatically socially isolated, although it is rare to see such individuals who have sustained close relationships. In a second subgroup, there may be more prominent symptoms of social isolation without clear-cut psychoticlike symptoms, although the suspiciousness and eccentricity of appearance of these individuals suggest schizotypal rather than schizoid personality disorder. Although the patient with psychoticlike symptoms may be apparently more "ill," a presentation with psychoticlike symptoms may be observed in some individuals with an underlying affective instability and a greater degree of social relatedness, often coexisting with borderline personality disorder, as well as in more severely disturbed schizotypal patients. The latter presentation of social isolation is more typical of the clinical picture of the biological relatives of chronic schizophrenics.

It has not been determined empirically what the clinical course of schizotypal personality disorder is. Studies suggest that some but not all schizophrenics have a premorbid clinical picture similar to schizotypal personality disorder. However, most individuals with schizotypal personality disorder do not go on to develop schizophrenia but maintain their schizotypal characteristics for most of their life. These individuals do not usually seek treatment except when experiencing a crisis that precipitates dysphoria or even a clinical depression. These acute episodes can often be treated without altering these individuals' long-term character structures. Thus, the prognosis for schizotypal personality disorder remitting is poor, but deterioration is also not likely.

ETIOLOGY

It appears that genetically determined psychobiological abnormalities shared with schizophrenia may contribute to the psychopathology of at least a subgroup of individuals with schizotypal personality disorder. Kendler and colleagues[16] found schizotypal personality disorder to be significantly more prevalent in the interviewed biological relatives of schizophrenics than in their adoptive relatives or the biological relatives of controls. Reider[17] found that "borderline schizophrenia," as diagnosed by the *DSM-III* criteria for schizotypal personality disorder, using a cut-off of three rather than four criteria as in *DSM-III*, was observed with a prevalence of 73% in a mixed sample of relatives of schizophrenics from three different samples. Kendler and colleagues also found an increased prevalence of certain schizotypal symptoms in the relatives of the Iowa 500 schizophrenics compared with controls.[14] These studies cumulatively support the hypothesis that schizotypal personality disorder is observed more frequently in the relatives of schizophrenics than nonschizophrenics, although, as noted previously, negative symptoms (e.g., social isolation, constricted affect, or poor rapport) appeared to be more sensitive discriminators than positive symptoms (e.g., perceptual distortions, magical thinking). No studies have been published with a schizotypal proband group, so that at present it may only be concluded that a subgroup of such individuals share a genetic relationship with schizophrenia. Whether this subgroup is well represented among patients who present to psychiatric clinics with schizotypal personality disorder is not yet known.

Psychobiological "markers" that are observed with increased prevalence in schizophrenics may also be observed in individuals with schizotypal personality disorder. Baron and colleagues found that biological relatives of schizophrenics had an increased prevalence of schizotypal personality disorder compared with relatives of controls and that these schizotypal relatives, like the schizophrenics, had decreased activity of plasma amine oxidase.[18,19] Siever and associates[7,20,21] found that impaired smooth pursuit accuracy was associated with schizotypal personality disorder in a college volunteer population selected by virtue of their eye-tracking accuracy. Again, negative symptoms rather than positive symptoms appeared to characterize the low accuracy trackers. Other psychophysiologic tests measuring information processing have also found deficits in schizotypal patients.[22,23] These studies complement genetic studies in suggesting that schizotypal individuals may share psychobiological abnormalities with schizophrenic individuals.

It is possible that these genetically determined vulnerabilities related to schizophrenia may be associated with the social withdrawal and eccentricities observed in schizotypal individuals. For example, individuals with defects in "cognitive centering" or attentional focusing may have greater difficulty in establishing mutually gratifying attachments to others and thus find them unrewarding. They may have difficulty in communicating in a focused, appropriate way and be more susceptible to cognitive and perceptual distortions. Although these considerations are speculative, they illustrate a possible mechanism by which such genetically determined characteristics may, in interaction with psychosocial influences, lead to the development of schizotypal personality disorder. However, further research is required to define the specificity and character of such hypothetic mechanisms. Studies identifying a group of schizotypal probands are needed to determine whether a psychobiological predisposition to affective abnormalities may also in some individuals lead to transient psychoticlike symptoms, as is suggested by clinical experience.

DIAGNOSIS AND DIFFERENTIAL DIAGNOSES

At present, there are no clinical validators of the diagnosis of schizotypal personality disorder other than the *DSM-III* criteria applied as described previously. The psychobiological abnormalities described previously, such as eye tracking abnormalities or low plasma amine oxidase, have not been sufficiently studied to be diagnostically useful. Psychologic testing has not yielded sufficiently specific test profiles to characterize these individuals at this point, although attempts in this direction are underway.[24]

Individuals with schizotypal personality disorder may present with major depressive disorder as an Axis I diagnosis. When the depression is treated with antidepressants and/or psychotherapy as appropriate, depressive symptoms may remit, while schizotypal symptoms will usually remain. Exacerbation of psychoticlike symptoms may result in a transient psychotic episode (*e.g.*, schizophreniform or atypical psychosis).

Individuals with schizophrenia in remission may present clinically like patients with schizotypal

personality disorder (*e.g.*, with chronic asociality, eccentricity, and perceptual distortions). In these individuals, it is only by establishing the history of a previous schizophrenic episode that the schizotypal diagnosis can be excluded. Since schizotypal and schizophrenic individuals are often very guarded with high degrees of denial, a tactful but comprehensive history taking, coupled with a thorough search for previous records, may be required to rule in or out schizophrenia. Similarly, schizotypal personality may precede the onset of schizophrenia, thus requiring revision of the diagnosis after the psychotic episode.

Schizotypal personality disorder frequently overlaps with borderline personality disorder, in which case both disorders should be diagnosed. It is important, however, in the formulation of a treatment plan to recognize that borderline patients with a primary affective disturbance may show transient psychotic symptoms episodically such that they satisfy criteria for schizotypal personality disorder without a very close phenomenologic relationship to schizophrenia. Other individuals with schizotypal pathology combined with impulsive features may also satisfy both criteria sets. More knowledge is required with regard to the etiology of these disorders and their relationship to the Axis I syndromes to develop more valid criteria. The character of the psychoticlike symptoms, that is, associated with mood shifts, reactivity to availability of important others (perhaps more related to affective instability) versus pervasive, generalized symptoms (perhaps more related to schizophrenia) needs to be clarified in relation to such possibly different etiologies. Such an approach has been useful in ascertaining that many patients previously diagnosed as schizophrenic or schizoaffective have family and treatment histories similar to affective disorder patients.

The line between schizoid personality disorder and schizotypal personality disorder also requires clearer delineation. As negative symptoms such as social isolation seem to characterize the biological relatives of schizophrenics more than positive symptoms, the rationale for dividing the two disorders as they are currently divided is not clear. Schizotypal personality disorder was actually formulated in contradistinction to borderline personality disorder, and thus its empiric relationship to schizoid personality disorder needs to be established. It is possible the two disorders may be more validly included as one category.

Schizotypal personality disorder may overlap with other personality disorders, such as compulsive or histrionic personality disorder, and, in these instances, the diagnoses should thus be made concomitantly.

TREATMENT AND PREVENTION

Although systematic studies of the treatment of schizotypal personality disorder have not been undertaken, clinical experience suggests that these patients may have a chronic course, although they may gain limited benefit from psychotherapy. Stone[25] suggests helping such patients accept their solitary life-style and employing a reliable, cautious, and systematic approach to therapy without unduly great expectations. He has found that in a mixed group of schizotypal and borderline patients diagnosed by *DSM-III* criteria the greater the schizophrenialike symptoms such as suspiciousness or social aversiveness, the less likely were these patients to improve. However, in the absence of marked impairment in their reality testing, they were unlikely to worsen either.

There is little empiric study of treatment response to pharmacologic agents in this disorder as diagnosed by *DSM-III*, although patients with similar characteristics have been reported to respond to neuroleptics when psychotic symptoms were prominent and to antidepressants when depressed.[25] However, these interventions in most cases relieve only the acute symptomatology, leaving the underlying character pathology relatively untouched.

There is no known prevention for this disorder, although children diagnosed as ''schizoid'' who may have had characteristics currently considered schizotypal may go on to show similar pathology as adults and might be identified at school age.[5] In general, too little is known about this newly formulated disorder to guide interventions empirically.

Paranoid Personality Disorder

HISTORICAL BACKGROUND

The outstanding clinical characteristic of individuals with this personality disorder is a life-long suspiciousness and an exaggerated attribution of malicious intent to the actions of others. Descriptions of such individuals can be seen in works of 19th century descriptive psychiatry and in literature from even earlier times. However, paranoid personality disorder first entered the official psychiatric nomenclature in the United States in 1942, as a subtype of psychopathic personality in the 10th edition of the *Statistical Manual for the Use of Hospitals for Mental Diseases.*[26]

DEFINITION

The *DSM-III* has three groups of inclusion criteria for the diagnosis of paranoid personality disorder under the categories of (1) pervasive, unwarranted suspiciousness and mistrust of people; (2) hypersensitivity, and (3) restricted affectivity. Each of these three categories, which must be characteristic of the individual's long-term functioning, have from four to eight specific inclusion criteria. The *DSM-III* has a single exclusion criterion for paranoid personality disorder, which is that the symptoms rated as present for the disorder must not be due to another mental disorder, especially schizophrenia or paranoid disorder.

To our knowledge, the 16 specific inclusion criteria for paranoid personality disorder in the *DSM-III* are without empiric basis. It is not clear that so many items, especially ones such as ''inability to relax'' or ''lack of a true sense of humor,'' which are highly inferential, will improve the reliability or validity of this clinical syndrome. It is hoped that future studies will address the utility of the specific diagnostic criteria for this disorder proposed in the *DSM-III*.

EPIDEMIOLOGY

Data about the population prevalence of paranoid personality disorder are meager. Results from a midtown Manhattan study indicate that ''paranoid ideation'' is very common in an urban US population.[28] For example, 23.2% of respondents answered yes to the following question: ''Do you sometimes feel people are against you without any good reason?'' Using a definition of paranoid personality disorder as one who was ''consistently hostile, not only to the interviewer but also to acquaintances, neighbors and hospital staff,'' Stephens and co-workers[29] found three cases (4.3%) among 69 personally interviewed relatives of control subjects. Applying *DSM-III* criteria, Kendler and Gruenberg[30] found one case (0.7%) in 138 personally interviewed biological relatives of control adoptees. No epidemiologic risk factors for paranoid personality disorder have yet been identified, but our clinical experience suggest that this disorder is more common in males. The *DSM-III* field trials support this possibility and also suggest that paranoid personality disorder, like the other diagnosis in the "odd" cluster, is diagnosed less frequently (approximately 5%) than "dramatic" cluster diagnosis such as borderline personality disorder.[3]

CLINICAL DESCRIPTION

The following is a representative case history of an individual with paranoid personality disorder:

> A 36-year-old, single white male engineer was referred for psychiatric evaluation, with his grudging cooperation, by his project manager. He described his current work situation as very tense because his co-workers had been "ganging up" on him, giving him the most difficult assignments and sometimes removing the crucial information he needed from the relevant files. He said they did this "because they like to see me sweat." He had changed jobs four times in the past 6 years because of similar problems at previous jobs. Aside from his frequent contact with a sibling, the patient was socially isolated. He stated, "I've never trusted people. All they want to do is take advantage of you." On mental status examination he was tense, aloof, and obviously very angry at his co-workers. He was hypervigilant and made several comments indicating that he felt that the interviewer might not "see things my way." There was no evidence of psychosis or depression.

From a clinical and historical perspective, the persistent, inappropriate mistrust of others has been the core feature of the syndrome of paranoid personality disorder. Other commonly associated features are social isolation and a "hypervigilant" combative style. Although some individuals with this syndrome are emotionally aloof and restrained, others are labile and often initiate arguments and physical fights. A subgroup of these patients may be very litiginous, a factor that should be considered in their clinical assessment. Although individuals with paranoid personality disorder rarely function well in social situations, their occupational performance can be good, especially if their work does not require extensive cooperation with others.

No systematic studies have been made of the course and prognosis of paranoid personality disorder. By definition, this diagnosis is not applied to individuals who demonstrate the features of this disorder for only brief periods of time. Clinical experience indicates that the intensity of the symptomatology in individuals with paranoid personality disorder can wax and wane over time. Often the change in symptoms are associated with the presence or absence of environmental stress. Retrospective data have suggested that individuals with paranoid personality disorder may be at increased risk to develop schizophrenia.[31]

ETIOLOGY

Little systematic data exist regarding possible etiologic factors in paranoid personality disorder. Three studies have suggested that familial-genetic factors may play an etiologic role in this disorder. Using the definition noted above, Stephens and co-workers[29] found that paranoid personality disorder was present in 9.0% of interviewed first-degree relatives of schizophrenic versus 4.3% of interviewed first-degree relatives of controls. This difference was not, however, statistically significant. Using *DSM-III* criteria, Kendler and Gruenberg[30] found that paranoid personality disorder was significantly more common in interviewed biological relatives of schizophrenic adoptees (3.8%) than in the interviewed biological relatives of control adoptees (0.7%). No excess of paranoid personality disorder was found among the adoptive relatives of the schizophrenic adoptees. These two studies suggest that paranoid personality disorder may have a familial relationship to schizophrenia. Furthermore, the results of the adoption study suggest that genetic and not environmental factors are responsible for the familial link between schizophrenia and paranoid personality disorder.

In one study* the following definition of paranoid personality disorder was used: "consistent pattern of suspiciousness or distrustfulness inappropriate to social circumstances, evidence of paranoid ideation, with undue social anxiety and hypersensitivity to imagined criticism."

Using this definition in a blind, family history study, the risk for paranoid personality disorder was 0% in 119 first-degree relatives of controls, 0.8% in 330 first-degree relatives of schizophrenics, and 4.8% in 100 first-degree relatives of patients with nonschizophrenic paranoid psychosis (delusional disorder). The risk for paranoid personality disorder was significantly greater in the relatives of the patients with a paranoid psychosis than in either the relatives of the controls or the schizo-

---

* Kendler KS, Masterson CC, Davis KL: Unpublished data.

phrenics. These results suggest that the familial link between paranoid personality disorder and paranoid psychosis may be stronger than the familial link between paranoid personality disorder and schizophrenia.

Several psychological theories for "paranoid ideation" have been postulated but not, to our knowledge, empirically tested. According to Colby,[32] there are four major theories:

1. Homosexual theory. Paranoid phenomena result from the repression, reaction formation, and projection of homosexual wishes.
2. Hostility theory. Paranoid phenomena result from the projection of the intense unconscious hate and hostility. A related broader psychoanalytic theory suggests that paranoid symptomatology derives from the projection outward of a variety of unwanted internal affects.
3. Homeostatic theory. Paranoid phenomena result from the attempts of the organism to pursue internal equilibrium. To restore equilibrium, any internal threat such as feelings of guilt or inadequacy are transformed into the belief that "others threaten me."
4. Shame–humiliation theory. Paranoid phenomena result from a discordance between a person's ideal self and experienced shame and humiliation. Rather than permitting the unpleasant affect of shame and humiliation to be experienced, this theory postulated that in the "paranoid mode," the individual blames others for wronging the self.

From the perspective of its explanatory power, Colby regards the shame–humiliation model as providing the broadest and most clinically relevant explanation of "paranoid phenomena."

DIAGNOSIS AND DIFFERENTIAL DIAGNOSIS

Under conditions of stress, individuals can develop features of paranoid personality disorder that will remit when the stress is removed. Such reactions are better considered a form of adjustment disorder than a personality disorder.

Many cases meeting *DSM-III* criteria for paranoid personality disorder will also meet criteria for other personality disorders as defined in *DSM-III*. This is particularly true for schizotypal personality disorder. Of the eight criteria for schizotypal personality disorder, four of them are very similar to certain *DSM-III* criteria for paranoid personality

disorder. Individuals meeting criteria for paranoid personality disorder also frequently meet criteria for schizoid or antisocial personality disorder.

The differential diagnosis between paranoid personality disorder and paranoid disorder can sometimes be difficult and hinges on the phenomenologic distinction between paranoid "ideation" and paranoid "delusion." Clinical experience indicates that patients with paranoid personality disorder maintain suspicions but not firm beliefs. Compared with patients with psychotic disorder, the ideation in paranoid personality disorder is usually not elaborated into organized "plots" or "conspiracies."

TREATMENT

To our knowledge no controlled studies exists about the treatment of paranoid personality disorder. Clinical experience indicates that these patients are often difficult to treat in psychotherapy and rarely acquire psychological insight into the origins of their personality difficulties. However, if even a modicum of trust can be established, some patients with paranoid personality disorder can benefit from a psychotherapeutic relationship. Since many patients with paranoid personality disorder fear intimacy, a distinct "professional" attitude on the part of the therapist is often the most beneficial. Although it can be helpful to assist the patient in "checking out" his suspiciousness in certain situations, it rarely is useful to confront the patient's ideas more directly. Some therapists recommend explicitly discussing with such patients the possibility that they may become suspicious of the therapist and suggesting that such suspicions should be examined and not result in a premature termination of treatment.[33] Patients with paranoid personality disorder are probably not good candidates for group therapy. Our experience indicates that low doses of neuroleptic medication can sometimes be of help to individuals with a paranoid personality disorder. However, the benefit derived from this therapy must be carefully balanced against the possible long-term risks, especially tardive dyskinesia.

REFERENCES

1. Siever LJ, Gunderson JG: The search a for schizotypal personality: Historical origins and current status. Compr Psychiatry 24:199–212, 1983
2. Mellsop G, Varghesi F: The reliability of Axis II of *DSM-III*. Am J Psychiatry 139:1360–1361, 1982

3. Kass F, Spitzer RL, Williams JBW: An empirical study of the issue of sex bias in the diagnostic criteria of *DSM-III* Axis II personality disorders. Am Psychologist 38:799–801, 1983

4. Siever LJ, Schizoid and Schizotypal Personality Disorders, pp 32–64. Baltimore, Williams & Wilkins, 1981

5. Wolff S, Chick J: Schizoid personality in childhood: A controlled follow-up study. Psychol Med 10:85–100, 1980

6. Meehl PE: Schizotaxia, schizotypy, schizophrenia. Am Psychologist 17:827–838, 1962

7. Siever LJ, Haier RJ, Coursey RD et al: Smooth pursuit eye movements in non-psychotic populations: Relationship to other "markers" for schizophrenia and psychological correlates. Arch Gen Psychiatry 39:1001–1005, 1982

8. Guntrip H: Schizoid Phenomena, Object-Relations and the Self. Sutherland JD (ed). London, Hogarth Press, 1968

9. Appel G: An approach to the treatment of schizoid phenomena. Psychoanal Rev 61:99–113, 1974

10. Rado S: Theory and therapy: The theory of schizotypal organization and its application to the treatment of decompensated schizotypal behavior. In Rado S (ed): Psychoanalysis of Behavior, vol 2, pp 127–140. New York, Grune & Stratton, 1962

11. Spitzer RL, Endicott J, Gibbon M: Crossing the border into borderline personality and borderline schizophrenia: The development of criteria. Arch Gen Psychiatry 36:17–24, 1979

12. Kety S, Rosenthal D, Wender PH et al: The types and prevalence of mental illness in the biological and adoptive families of adopted schizophrenics. In Rosenthal D, Kety SS (eds): The Transmission of Schizophrenia. Oxford, Pergamon Press, 1968

13. Gunderson JG, Siever LJ, Spaulding E: The search for a schizotype: Crossing the border again. Arch Gen Psychiatry 40:15–22, 1983

14. Kendler KS, Gruenberg AM, Tsuang MT: The specificity of *DSM-III* schizotypal symptoms. Abstracts of the 136th Annual Meeting of the American Psychiatric Association, 1983

15. Pope HG, Lipowski JF: Diagnosis in schizophrenia and manic-depressive illness: A reassessment of the specificity of "schizophrenic" symptoms in the light of current research. Arch Gen Psychiatry 35:811–828, 1978

16. Kendler KS, Gruneberg AM, Strauss JS: An independent analysis of the Copenhagen sample of the Danish adoption study of schizophrenia: II. The relationship between schizotypal personality disorder and schizophrenia. Arch Gen Psychiatry 38:982–987, 1981

17. Reider RO, Rosenthal D, Wender PH et al: The offspring of schizophrenics: Fetal and neonatal deaths. Arch Gen Psychiatry 32:200–211, 1975

18. Baron M: Schizotypal personality disorder: Family studies. Abstracts of the 136th Annual Meeting of the American Psychiatric Association, 1983

19. Baron M, Asnis L, Gruen R et al: Plasma amine oxidase and genetic vulnerability to schizophrenia. Arch Gen Psychiatry 40:275–282, 1983

20. Siever LJ, Coursey RD, Alterman IS et al: Smooth pursuit eye movement impairment: A vulnerability marker for schizotypal personality disorder in normal volunteer population. Am J Psychiatry, in press

21. Siever LJ, Coursey RD, Lees R et al: Physiologic and psychologic correlates of deviate-eye tracking. In Hanin I, Usdin E (eds): Biologic Markers in Psychiatry and Neurology, pp. 359–370. New York, Pergamon Press, 1982

22. Braff DL: Impaired speed of information processing in non-medicated schizotypal patients. Schizoph Bull 7:499–508, 1981

23. Simons RF, MacMillan FW III, Ireland FB: Reaction-time crossover in preselected schizotype subjects. Abnorm Psychol 91:414–419, 1982

24. Golden R, Meehl P: Detection of schizoid taxon with MMPI indications. J Abnorm Psychol 88:217–233, 1979

25. Stone M: Psychotherapy with schizotypal borderline patients. J Am Acad Psychoanal 11:87–111, 1983

26. Klein DF: Importance of psychiatric diagnosis in the prediction of clinical drug effects. Arch Gen Psychiatry 16:118–126, 1967

27. Lewis NC: Outlines for Psychiatric Examination, 3rd ed, p 114. Albany, New York State Department of Mental Hygiene, 1943

28. Langner TS, Michael ST: Life Stress and Mental Health, p 44. London, Free Press of Glencoe, 1963

29. Stephens DA, Atkinson MW, Day DWK et al: Psychiatric morbidity in parents and siblings of schizophrenics and nonschizophrenics. Br J Psychiatry 127:97, 1975

30. Kendler KS, Gruenberg AM: Genetic relationship between personality disorder and the "schizophrenic spectrum" disorders. Am J Psychiatry 139:1185, 1982

31. Kay DWK, Roth M: Environmental and hereditary factors in the schizophrenias of old age and their bearing on the general problem of causation in schizophrenia. J Ment Sci 107:649, 1961

32. Colby KM: Appraisal of four psychological theories of paranoid phenomena. J Abnorm Psychol 86:54, 1977

33. Bullard DM: Psychotherapy of paranoid patients. Arch Gen Psychiatry 2:137, 1960

Borderline Personality Disorder

History of the Term *Borderline*

THE ERA BEFORE PSYCHOANALYSIS

About 100 years ago, psychiatry had been developed and refined to the point where the traditional, institution-based alienists had begun to describe more subtle forms of the major "psychoses" (*e.g.*, manic-depression and dementia praecox); other practitioners, particularly the hypnotists, were gaining in popularity among ambulatory patients. The psychiatric profession was beginning to situate certain forms of abnormal behavior *in between* the then current notions of sanity and insanity. These are the beginnings of a *borderline* concept. One of the very first uses of the term is credited to Hughes[1]: "The borderline of insanity is occupied by many persons who pass their whole life near that line, sometimes on one side and sometimes on the other." In a similar vein, Rosse[2] defined *borderline insanity* as relating to patients who drifted between reason and despair.

At the dawn of the psychoanalytic era, hospital-based psychiatrists were beginning to notice subtle distinctions—atypical and attenuated forms of the classic psychoses. Kraepelin and Bleuler did not use the term *borderline*, but each was aware of milder versions of the conditions they sought to delineate. Kraepelin[3] outlined the "temperaments" (depressive, manic, irritable, and cyclothymic)— each a collection of presumably innate personality tendencies—that were found abundantly either as premorbid manifestations of manic-depressives themselves or as personality abnormalities among their close relatives. Bleuler recognized that not all patients with dementia praecox (or schizophrenia, as he renamed it) showed the deteriorating course Kraepelin believed was their fate: milder, nondeteriorating forms also existed.

AT THE BEGINNING OF THE PSYCHOANALYTIC ERA

Freud distinguished between the "transference neuroses" and the "narcissistic neuroses"[4]: the former, manifesting often as hysterical or obsessional disorders, were amenable to the psychoanalytic process; the latter involved paranoid or schizophrenic patients whom Freud believed were unable to form a transference and were hence not amenable to analysis. As the psychoanalytic pioneers grappled with the distinction essential to them of neurosis versus psychosis, they soon realized that there were patients with disorders that did not fit neatly into these categories. This might also be true even if a patient's problem did fit fairly well into one of the characterologic subtypes (hysterical, obsessional, narcissistic, phobic) that psychoanalysis had explored in depth. Still, throughout the 1910s and 1920s there are only scant references to "borderline" cases. Moore[5] described a number of patients who were borderline with respect to the psychoses, particularly to manic-depression. He believed hereditary predisposition contributed to these borderline states. In the meantime others had begun to push the frontiers of psychoanalysis toward the realm of the classic psychoses: Maeder[6] and Bjerre[7] applied psychoanalytic methods to the treatment of ambulatory schizophrenics and also to paranoid patients, who were certainly "borderline" with respect to analyzability, although neither author used the term.

As psychoanalysis flourished, familiarity with the clinical region between analyzability and nonanalyzability broadened and so did the catalog of terms used to label these in-between cases, since *borderline* did not become popular as a diagnostic term until the late 1930s, and then only in the United States. At first analysts were more impressed by the likelihood that if there were any linkage between these scarcely analyzable cases and one of the classic psychoses, the linkage was to schizophrenia. Sometimes such a connection was alluded to by the new label itself: "borderline schizophrenia,"[8] "latent schizophrenia,"[9] or "pseudoneurotic schizophrenia."[10] In other instances, the supposed proximity to schizophrenia is implied in the textual description although not in the label: "impulsive character,"[11] "as-if personality,"[12] or "psychotic character."[13] Throughout the middle of this century *borderline* was thus used in two senses at once to designate (1) a condition seemingly analyzable at first glance that proved refractory on closer examination, even though no glaring psychosis was present and (2) a condition allied in some way to schizophrenia, as an incipient,[12] attenuated,[8] or atypical[14] form.

Those most influential in popularizing the term *borderline* in mid century were Stern, Knight, and Grinker. The contributions of Kernberg, who also was influential, are discussed more fully later in this chapter. The description of Stern[15] was intuitive and clinical, stressing such qualities as inordinate hypersensitivity, narcissism (manifested as alternating idealization and devaluation of the analyst), constitutional feeling of inferiority, projective mechanisms (a tendency toward externalization, sometimes close to the point of delusion), and difficulties in reality-testing. Knight[16] stressed the "regressive position of the ego forces" despite the dramatic display of healthier-appearing neurotic symptoms of hysterical, obsessional, or other type. Deutsch[12] had earlier stressed the disturbance in internalized objects in her "as-if" cases; Knight emphasized the severe weakness in ego functions and primitivity of defense mechanisms. Although Knight inclined to the view that these *borderline* cases were within the penumbra of schizophrenia, he used the label more as an independent entity. His work appears to have set the trend for this tendency[17]: in the 30 years after Knight's paper, *borderline* has come to be used increasingly to denote a separate nosologic entity with no particular rela-

tionship to schizophrenia. This tendency remained in effect even though "borderline" cases were no longer the exclusive preserve of office-based psychoanalysts but were encountered in hospitals as well. Many cases were suspected of being "borderline to psychosis," a point made by Frosch, who also speculated that among etiologic factors, one might find in these "non-decompensating" conditions some predisposition to manic-depression as well as to schizophrenia or else merely a "chaotic early environment."

During the 1960s Grinker and colleagues took a step further toward establishing *borderline* disorder as a separate syndrome.[18] As diagnostic guidelines, they used such criteria as fear of criticism, fear of closeness, low self-esteem, primitive defenses (denial, projection), suspiciousness, and problems with aggression. They studied patients with these characteristics who had been hospitalized, often for gestures at suicide or outbursts of rage. Their research design focused on observable data relating to ward-behavior, affect, and so on. The study of Grinker and colleagues isolated several features of borderline patients that were particularly common: anger as the predominant affect; serious defects in close relationships; absence of consistent self-identity; and a strong tendency toward depression, a depressive cast to one's life. Factor analysis of their data suggested the existence of four subtypes: (1) the border with psychosis (reality sense was deficient; behavior strikingly inappropriate); (2) the "core" borderline syndrome (inconsistent sense of identity; acting-out of angry impulses); (3) affectless, as-if persons (behavior more adaptive but relationships lacking in genuineness and spontaneity); and (4) the border with neurosis (anaclitic depression; narcissistic character).

At the end of the 1960s, impressions about the essence of borderline states had begun to converge into a clinical picture of an angry, depressed, and impulsive person who might, or might not, be simultaneously near the "border" of a classic psychosis, but if so, the latter need not necessarily be schizophrenia.

Additional material on the evolution of *borderline* as a diagnostic concept is available in the reviews of Mack,[19] Millon,[20] Perry and Klerman,[21] and Stone.[17]

Current Definitions of *Borderline*

Although it is beginning to dominate other definitions in popularity, the diagnosis of *borderline per-*

sonality disorder in the *Diagnostic and Statistical Manual of Mental Disorders (DSM-III)* is difficult to understand or appreciate fully without some knowledge of its origins and of its relationships with competing systems.[22]

There are at least six different usages of the term *borderline:*

1. A level of function or psychic organization
2. A syndrome
3. A personality disorder
4. A dynamic constellation
5. A prognostic statement
6. An adjective denoting inclusion within the spectrum of either of the two classic psychoses: manic-depression or schizophrenia.

BORDERLINE AS LEVEL OF FUNCTION

Writing within the psychoanalytic tradition, Kernberg[23,24] has drawn elements from the works of Frosch (altered relationship to reality but adequate reality testing capacity), Hoch and Polatin (overvalued ideas rather than frank delusions), Deutsch (disturbances in internalized images of self and other), Erikson[25] (identity diffusion), and the British objects-relations School (levels of psychic structure; splitting and projective identification as primitive defenses) and has woven them into a tighter and more coherent definition of *borderline* than had hitherto been formulated within the psychoanalytic community. Kernberg saw the patient with a borderline personality disorder as being at one of three levels of psychic function (between the neurotic and the psychotic), each of which tended to be stable over long periods, if not over the lifetime, of any given person. These levels of function, to the extent that they could be defined in mutually exclusive ways, constitute three categories of diagnosis. Because they also define regions of relative sickness or health, they may be seen as having a dimensional quality, relating to the continuum between the psychiatrically most impaired and the most healthy. Since the correlation between these levels and one's overall life adaptation is not perfect (*e.g.*, some chronically delusional persons perform fairly well occupationally), the borderline "category" also defines a region, along a continuum of adaptation, *most* of whose members function better, socially and occupationally, than those with psychotic structure and worse than those with neurotic structure.

As chief characteristics and necessary conditions of the borderline level, Kernberg posited severe impairment in ego-integration (analogous to the Eriksonian concept of ego-diffusion) and adequate capacity to test reality. Presence of the first quality distinguished the borderline level from the healthier neurotic level (where ego-integration was intact); presence of the second quality demarcated the borderline level from the psychotic level (where reality-testing capacity was lost). In addition, Kernberg drew attention to the borderline patient's primitivity of defenses (that might include denial, splitting, projective identification, omnipotent control or devaluation, and primitive idealization) as well as to certain nonspecific signs: low anxiety tolerance (*i.e.*, high vulnerability to ordinary stresses), poor impulse control, and poor sublimatory capacity (manifested customarily as poor performance in work, school, or hobbies).

The detection of a patient's status with regard to ego-integration and reality-testing capacity depends on a psychoanalytically oriented interviewing technique, outlined by Kernberg,[24] designed to ferret out contradictions and sharp discrepancies in the patient's habitual view of his own self and of the personalities of those close to him. Since there are some discrepancies in every person's self-image compared with how others see him (*e.g.*, the bigot who thinks of himself as a fine, upstanding citizen; the philanthropist who does not tip cab drivers), the distinction concerning identity integration is not always made easily. One looks for multiple, pervasive, and glaring contradictions, as well as the complaint, made by many borderline level patients that, "I don't know who I really am." The coexistence of sharp contradictions in self-image is sometimes apparent in the difference between one's self-assessment and one's behavior or between one's behavior and one's dress: a prudishly dressed woman who disclaims any interest in sex but who is actually promiscuous and who, furthermore, sees herself as ugly while others find her attractive would show the kind of identity disturbance Kernberg equates with borderline function.

Kernberg's criteria relate particularly to the area of interpersonal relationships, the realistic appraisal of which is, of course, much more subtle and difficult than evaluating the reality of the external world. It is consistent with borderline functioning to manifest some serious distortions in evaluation of self and others, but reality-testing capacity is preserved. This means that, when confronted with the nature of his contradictions, the borderline person can grasp, and begin to agree with, the other person's point of view: his distortion had only the force of an "overvalued idea," in other words, and lacked the fixity of a true delusion.

The advantages of the Kernberg system lie in its relative precision, compared with other psychoanalytic approaches to the "borderline." Although derived from psychoanalytically oriented therapy with selected ambulatory and hospitalized patients, the Kernberg criteria, when reflected back into the population as a whole, are seen to apply to a large percentage (perhaps 10%) of people. Many patients diagnosed under other, more restrictive labels, such as pseudoneurotic schizophrenia and hysteroid dysphoria,[26] and others whose clinical features seem to defy conventional nosology (undiagnosed illness[27]) satisfy Kernberg criteria.

The disadvantages of the Kernberg system concern the breadth of applicability just mentioned and the relative difficulty in its objectification, compared with several of the more recent systems. The large number of patients exhibiting borderline function are not homogeneous etiologically: some are young persons whose conditions evolve later into more sharply defined entities (e.g., recurrent depression, cyclothymia); others show concomitant sociopathy or severe substance abuse, conditions not amenable to modified psychoanalytic techniques, and who might best not be given a diagnostic label that is traditionally associated with treatability by those techniques.

From an epidemiologic or research standpoint, the Kernberg system, depending as it does on a sophisticated psychoanalytic interview, is not as easy to teach and use when one is attempting to assess large numbers of patients and to achieve good reliability between raters.

Since most patients, apart from rapid-cycling manic-depressives or women with severe premenstrual changes of state, do show a habitual level of function the Kernberg system is an excellent approach to measuring this function and serves as a separate axis of diagnosis, alongside axes relating to personality type and to symptom type.

BORDERLINE AS SYNDROME

The currently most widely used syndromal definition of *borderline* is that created by Gunderson[28] and his collaborators. The Gunderson system may be seen as a refinement of the approach used by Grinker and colleagues, inasmuch as emphasis is placed on a collection of symptoms and traits that are fairly readily observable clinically or fairly easy to ascertain through routine anamnesis. To minimize uncertainty, however, Gunderson and coworkers have devised an extensive questionnaire, the Diagnostic Interview for Borderlines (DIB), whose items relate to the six main attributes on which diagnosis of borderline personality disorder rests:

1. Lowered achievement (diminished work capacity)
2. Impulsivity (*viz.,* drug abuse, promiscuity)
3. Manipulative suicidal threats (*viz.,* wrist cutting)
4. Mild or brief psychotic episodes
5. Good socialization (mostly a superficial adaptiveness, beneath which is a disturbed identity camouflaged by rapid and shifting identifications with others)
6. Disturbances in close relationships
   a. A tendency to be depressive in the presence of one's love object and to be enraged or suicidal should the latter threaten to leave; tendency to have psychotic reactions when alone (and lonely)
   b. In general, a predominance of rageful affect rather than emotional warmth

In distinguishing borderline personality disorder from neighboring diagnostic concepts, the key attributes are good socialization, which discriminates borderlines from (core or nuclear) schizophrenia, and lowered achievement, discriminating from psychoneurotics, who for the most part show adequate work histories. The final appraisal of borderline personality disorder depends on scores obtained (0, 1, or 2) in the five main categories (impulsivity and manipulative suicidal threats are reduced to one category for scoring purposes). A score of 7 or higher is required. For this a score of 1 or 2 must be present in at least four of the main categories: a patient must show almost all the features enumerated to be diagnosed as having a borderline personality disorder. The presence of disturbed close relationships and lowered achievement would not in and of themselves suffice to make the diagnosis. Gunderson and coworkers further stipulate that severe chronic (as opposed to mild and occasional) substance abuse excludes the diagnosis, warranting a different diagnosis (*e.g.,* alcoholism). The diagnosis of sociopathy also excludes the diagnosis of borderline personality disorder.

From this resumé, some of the advantages of the Gunderson system should already be apparent. In comparison with the Kernberg system, it is less inferential, more easily used by non–psychoanalytically trained clinicians, and more objectifiable, in the sense that it permits interrater reliability to be tested more readily and adapts easily to the demands of computerization. If one is considering psychoanalytically oriented psychotherapy for a patient who may have a borderline personality disorder, the Gunderson system may have some advantage insofar as it is a narrower, more restrictive definition: sociopathic and alcoholic patients (who would not be good candidates for that method of treatment) are excluded. This very restrictiveness may constitute a disadvantage, however: the Gunderson definition covers fewer patients whose clinical features lie in the borderland between neurosis and clear-cut psychosis, perhaps only a third of those who would be identified as borderline by Kernberg criteria. Clinicians for whom it was important to have available a convenient label for the multitude of patients in this diagnostic borderland might be better served by the Kernberg system. Although some schizotypal patients satisfy Gunderson criteria, the typical patient with a borderline personality disorder is, like the cases of Grinker and co-workers, depressed, angry, and impulsive.

BORDERLINE AS PERSONALITY TYPE

The borderline personality disorder is listed in the *DSM-III* among the types of personality disorders. The definition represents an amalgam of the Kernberg (K) and Gunderson (G) systems. An effort was made by Spitzer and his colleagues[29] to distill and objectify the elusive definitions of borderline in a form that would be comprehensible and usable to the broadest range of clinicians. Since *borderline* has been used, traditionally, to designate attenuated forms of schizophrenia, just as it had been used to refer to angry, chaotic, narcissistic, and depressed patients, Spitzer fashioned a checklist with key items related to both uses of *borderline:* the "schizotypal" and the other, which he called the "unstable." The eight items of the "unstable" borderline personality are as follows (their derivation is designated by K or G where applicable):

1. Identity disturbance (K)
2. Unstable and intense interpersonal relationships (G)
3. Impulsivity (K, G)
4. Inappropriate intense anger (G)
5. Physically self-damaging acts (G)
6. Affective instability (G)
7. Chronic feelings of emptiness or boredom (K)
8. Problems tolerating being alone (G)

Item 7 is not alluded to directly among Kernberg's criteria but is mentioned in many of his more detailed clinical descriptions.

These "unstable" items constitute the list that became incorporated into the *DSM-III* as "borderline personality" (minus the adjective "unstable"). The eight items that made up the schizotypal borderline checklist were likewise incorporated into the *DSM-III,* only as "schizotypal personality" (minus the word "borderline"). By *DSM-III* criteria, at least five of the eight items listed previously are required for the diagnosis of borderline personality.

The advantages of the *DSM-III* approach consist of simplicity and objectifiability, which are greater even than what is afforded by the Gunderson system.

A disadvantage of the *DSM-III* approach concerns the fact that, although derived from important sources in the literature on borderline cases, the *DSM-III* definition reflects this tradition with only a modest degree of accuracy. It is possible for a patient to exhibit five *DSM-III* items that do not include identity disturbance (in which case the Kernberg system would not have considered the patient "borderline") or that do not include, for example, impulsivity and unstable relationships (which would lead to rejection by the Gunderson system).

Borderline, in the earlier psychoanalytic literature, could refer to schizotypal as well as to the "unstable" patients, whose symptoms are predominantly affective; in many instances, there was a pronounced intermingling of these different characteristics. Now that the term *borderline* in *DSM-III* is reserved for the former "unstable" variant, the *DSM-III* has led to a redefinition of *borderline* along more affective lines, thus severing the term, partially, from the borderline concept as it existed up to the time of the *DSM-III*'s publication. There is a possible disadvantage here, too, in the sense that the schizotypal qualities of certain "mixed" borderlines (by K or G criteria) might be overlooked, if one uses the *DSM-III* as one's reference point or would else require a second diagnosis (of schizotypal personality), which is cumbersome. Again, it is the depressed, angry, and impulsive type of borderline patient who satisfies the criteria of all the systems thus far outlined (if identity disturbance is also present) and who emerges as the least equivocal "borderline" case.

BORDERLINE AS A DYNAMIC CONSTELLATION

A number of authors, writing in the psychoanalytic tradition, have approached borderline disorders from the vantage point of psychodynamics, searching for abnormal patterns of development that might be characteristic. Masterson[30] and Rinsley[31] give special weight to dynamic considerations even with respect to diagnosis. These authors draw attention to disturbances in the mother–child relationship during the second and third years of life, when the child's major tasks concern individuation and the mastery of separation anxiety. Masterson regards a separation–individuation phase disturbance as the specific factor engendering a borderline condition in later life and speaks of the "borderline triad": problems in separation-individuation leading to depression, which in turn mobilizes defenses (viz., those enumerated by Kernberg).

The advantage to this focus of psychodynamics relates to the importance dynamic factors play in understanding and in treating borderline patients. In the matter of diagnosis, however, there are some serious drawbacks. Diagnosis depends on evaluation of historical data and of signs and symptoms discernible within the initial consultation. The details of psychodynamics unfold gradually over the course of psychotherapy and do not, therefore, provide a convenient basis for diagnosis. Second, although the bulk of borderline patients do show signs of not having mastered the tasks pertaining to the phase of separation-individuation, this was not always because of pathologic parenting and some borderlines have become ill owing to factors unrelated to problems peculiar to that phase (see section on etiologic factors). Finally, attention to psychodynamic issues, which tend to be similar for many borderline patients, if not amplified by attention to possible differences in symptom type, might fail to distinguish between affective, schizotypal, and organic variants within this diagnostic domain. These distinctions, however, have important implications for treatment.

BORDERLINE AS A PROGNOSTIC STATEMENT

Kohut and his followers constitute an important and highly influential school of psychoanalytic thought. Their concern has been to adapt the techniques of psychoanalytic therapy to the needs of patients with serious problems in the self, that is, along the narcissistic, as opposed to object-relational, path of development. The term *borderline* is employed frequently by Kohut, but in a manner that differs from the usages thus far described. In order to understand the Kohutian literature, one must be aware of this difference: *borderline* has not

evolved into a separate entity but has retained one of the connotations it had acquired among the psychoanalytic pioneers, namely, that of proximity to psychosis. Kohut[32] writes, for example, of the "differentiation of the analyzable narcissistic personality disturbances from (unanalyzable) schizophrenic psychoses, especially from the veiled or fended-off instances of the latter disorders which are often referred to as 'borderline cases.' "

The Kohutian usage of *borderline* thus becomes not a diagnostic term but rather a term indicating prognosis and a particular response to psychoanalytic therapy. The disadvantage of this usage lies in its lack of overlap with the more popular usages, including the official one in conformity with the *DSM-III.*

BORDERLINE AS DENOTING A SPECTRUM CASE OF SCHIZOPHRENIA OR MANIC-DEPRESSION

One of the original meanings of *borderline* concerned the periphery of the concept of psychosis (*i.e.*, an attenuated or incipient form of some psychotic disorder). At first, schizophrenia was the disorder of reference. Bleuler's idea of a *latent schizophrenia* approximates what others had begun to call *borderline schizophrenia*. These terms were described imprecisely, having been diagnosed intuitively, until efforts were made to extract from these descriptions the most salient features. The first step was made by Kety and his co-workers.[33] The biological relatives of (adopted-away) schizophrenics were examined and compared with adopted relatives. Among the former were a number of persons ill with conditions that resembled schizophrenia but that failed to fulfill strict criteria for the more severe illness. Some of the qualities that characterized borderline schizophrenia included strange or atypical mentation (short of gross delusion); vague, murky speech; brief episodes of cognitive distortion; anhedonia; chaotic sexuality; multiple "neurotic" manifestations; and severe widespread anxiety.

More recently, Spitzer and associates[29] sought to objectify this diagnosis further, developing a convenient checklist for borderline schizophrenia (called "schizotypal borderline" in their study), in the same manner as the checklist organized for the "unstable" type of borderline. The resultant list, of which four of the eight items are required for positive diagnosis, has now been incorporated into the *DSM-III*[22] as "schizotypal personality disorder."

Taken in the aggregate, these eight items (odd communication, ideas of reference, suspiciousness, recurrent illusions, magical thinking, inadequate rapport, undue social anxiety, and social isolation) belong to a diagnostic concept that means in essence borderline with respect to nuclear schizophrenia, in the spectrum, that is, of this heredofamilial psychosis.

The idea that there could be borderline instances of manic-depression (manic-depressive psychosis [MDP]) was, despite Kraepelin's outline of MDP-related temperaments, slower to develop. Acceptance has been growing of the proposition that a significant percentage of patients diagnosed as borderline by Kernberg, Gunderson, or *DSM-III* criteria may be viewed simultaneously as borderline, in the spectrum sense, to the heredofamilial conditions subsumed under the heading of MDP.[17] The hysteroid dysphoric patients described by Klein[26] and the subaffective dysthymic patients described by Akiskal[34] are similarly (in most instances) borderline in two or three senses at once: functional (Kernberg), syndromal (*DSM-III* and, in some cases, Gunderson), and spectrum (*i.e.*, attenuated forms of MDP).

Epidemiology

OCCURRENCE AND DISTRIBUTION

There has been some question whether borderline conditions have become more common than they once were. Because of the changes that have taken place in how these conditions have been defined and because of the paucity of epidemiologic studies related even distantly to the topic, no definitive answer can be made. Many patients diagnosed as borderline by functional or syndromal criteria are borderline also in the spectrum sense (much more often in the MDP spectrum, only rarely in the schizophrenia spectrum).[17] In some series half or more *DSM-III* borderline patients show "soft signs" and a family history of *MDP*.[34] Because the classic psychoses and their "core" or unequivocal forms have not changed in incidence over many generations, one could speculate that their dilute or "borderline" variants might exist also in approximately equal percentages of the population from one decade to the next. There has been more attention paid to borderline conditions in recent years; the term

has enjoyed greater popularity; many older terms (*viz.*, pseudoneurotic schizophrenia, as-if personality) have fallen into disuse and been replaced by one or another definition of *borderline*. This may account for the apparent increase in borderline conditions in our era.

Estimates of prevalence depend on whether broad or restrictive definitions are used. The Kernberg criteria constitute a broad definition, more so than the *DSM-III* criteria; the Gunderson criteria are much narrower. Kernberg has estimated that perhaps 10% or more of the general population functions at the borderline level. Gunderson has noted that data on consecutive admissions to a general psychiatric hospital yield a prevalence of 13% ($\pm$5%) for borderline conditions.

Borderline inpatients generally have strong affective (especially, depressive) features: many will have been admitted because of gestures of suicide made in the aftermath of rejection in a love relationship. These patients are often (one third to two thirds, depending on the series) in the MDP spectrum as well. Schizotypal borderline patients, unless there is some admixture of affective disturbance, are seldom seen in the hospital. The latter are usually marginal loners, working below their potential, troubled by loneliness, yet only rarely resorting to suicide gestures. They are seen predominantly in office practice or in the clinic.

SEX RATIO

Although the male-female ratio is nearly even among schizotypal borderlines, in samples of the more common affective borderlines there is a strong female preponderance (of the order of 2 : 1 to 3 : 1). The hysteroid dysphorics of Klein are almost all female.

A striking overrepresentation of females of this sort is hard to explain purely on the basis of psychodynamics connected with separation-individuation, because there is no inherent reason why daughters should have more difficulty negotiating this phase of development than sons. The explanation would appear to rest on other factors, peculiar to the biology and psychology of being female. On the biological side, there is the matter of predisposition to the depressive types of MDP, where a 2 : 1 female excess has been noted.[3,35] Since many female patients with atypical or borderline (spectrum) variants of MDP are also borderline by syndromal and functional criteria, their number alone tends to make the sex ratio uneven in samples selected by *DSM-III* or other criteria. Furthermore, about 4% of women experience premenstrual tension of such severity as to engender a borderline clinical state (with depression, irritability, and at times gestures of suicide) at least transiently; some exhibit borderline function even in the follicular phase.[36] Finally, on the psychological side, it is becoming more known that incest is much more common than was once thought: it has been estimated that 5% of women in the United States have experienced incestuous relations with an older male relative or with a brother. Daughters are much more vulnerable to incest than sons. However, many of the daughters victimized in this situation develop precisely the sort of ambivalent attitude toward men and the impulsivity, as they grow older, that becomes transformed into the traits of dependency, anger, irritability, low self-esteem, and disturbances in close relations that make up the borderline syndrome. It is noteworthy that in preliminary studies the incidence of incest in populations of borderline women is much higher (15% in office patients; 30% or more in a hospitalized sample) than in the general population.[37]

Clinical Description

AGREEMENT AND DISAGREEMENT BETWEEN DIAGNOSTIC SYSTEMS

To understand better the ways in which the various definitions of *borderline* may either overlap or be discordant, it is useful to consider clinical material. Of the two vignettes offered here, the first shows concordance; the second, disjunction.

A 27-year-old woman was married and had two small children. She had had a stormy adolescence, having been forced into sexual relations with a brother 6 years her senior whom she at first idolized and later feared. Their relationship continued until just before she left home for college, when she told her parents of it. In the ensuing emotional turmoil, she made a gesture of suicide (overdose of aspirin) but was not hospitalized. Although attractive, she lacked confidence in her appearance, insisting to others that she was "ugly," the word her hypercritical mother had often used in taunting her when she was a child. She was confused about her academic goals, having entered college more to extricate herself from her family than to pursue any particular career. Outwardly flirtatious, although inwardly shy and ill at ease, she felt intensely lonely and went through a period of mild alcohol abuse and brief sexual affairs in

an effort to cope with her anxiety and sense of inner emptiness. At age 19, she married a classmate and dropped out of school.

Fairly at ease in the first years of her marriage, she became anxious, bored, and given to fits of sadness and tearfulness after the birth of her second child. Her mood fluctuated widely from hour to hour, day to day, but negative feelings were greatly intensified on the 3 or 4 days before her period. Her husband had grown less attentive as the family expanded, in response to which she became increasingly irritable, provocative, and at times abusive (smashing plates, hurling insults). Her husband began to carry on an extramarital relationship, which she eventually discovered. At that point, she became seriously depressed, lost sleep and appetite, began to abuse alcohol and sedatives, and made several gestures of suicide, including one instance of cutting her wrist. On two occasions she hid for several nights in motels without informing anyone where she was. Each time she took her 8-year-old daughter with her, as though to protect her from the "designs" she imagined her husband had on their elder girl. After the wrist-cutting incident, when she had also left a note apologizing for being a "failure" as a wife and mother, she was hospitalized. She understood the unrealistic nature of her suspicions, as she explained to the hospital staff, but could not shake off the morbid doubts she experienced.

This patient is the "archetypal" borderline. She exhibits all eight *DSM-III* items for borderline personality, satisfied the Gunderson criteria, and demonstrates the poor ego-integration but adequate reality-testing capacity (despite her "overvalued ideas" concerning her husband, her appearance, and so on) required by the Kernberg system.

A 20-year-old college student was referred for psychotherapy because of difficulty concentrating on his studies. He had felt increasingly isolated from his classmates and was becoming markedly irascible and, at times, violent. On weekends he frequently drank to excess in his dormitory room and on several occasions, in a fit of rage, would tear up books and smash furniture. His dreams were often grotesque, filled with scenes of murder and dismemberment, and so disturbing as to awaken him in a panic. Twice he dreamed of being dead and was surprised to wake up still alive. He had no close male friends; a girlfriend, with whom he had had sexual relations a few times had recently rejected him, stating she "couldn't get through to him" and could not tolerate his extreme touchiness over the most minor criticisms. He then alternated between suicidal ruminations and outbursts of rage but meantime felt lost and unable to do his schoolwork. The previous year he had "gone through" two brief relationships with women, each characterized by a blind infatuation that soon gave way to jealous scenes, recriminations, and rejection.

After the second of those he suddenly took a leave of absence and sailed on a freighter to South Africa, wondering if it might not be better to abandon his studies completely and live perpetually on the sea "without home or country." He returned 3 months later, no longer certain of what courses to enroll for or what career to pursue, so long as it was something other than his original plan of joining his father's business.

During the initial interviews he was aloof, taciturn, ill at ease, and suspicious. Dressed impeccably and in a manner too old for his age, he had the appearance of a stern executive. He was preoccupied with fantasies of cruel and diabolical revenge against the women who had "wronged him" and against various students in adjoining rooms at the dormitory who made "too much noise." He had fantasies of killing both his father, who expected "too much of him," and his mother, who seemed to favor him above the four younger children and to behave toward him in a seductive fashion.

This patient demonstrated five *DSM-III* items for borderline personality (identity disturbance, impulsivity, unstable relations, intense anger, emptiness) but also four of the items for schizotypal personality (poor rapport, suspiciousness, hypersensitivity to criticism, and social isolation). He was thus a "mixed" borderline, with both unstable and schizotypal features. By Kernberg criteria he was also borderline, but he just failed to meet the Gunderson criteria (his scores on socialization, brief psychotic episodes, and impulsivity were too low).

This patient may be seen as situated along a continuum with "typical" cases, as in the first example, at one end and equivocal cases and cases positive in only one system at the other. In any large series, a varying number of patients will be positive in only the Kernberg or *DSM-III* system.

NATURAL HISTORY AND PROGNOSIS

At present only a few methodical follow-up studies of borderline patients are available. These are comparatively short term (2 to 5 years). The study of Carpenter and colleagues[38] compared Gunderson-criteria borderlines with schizophrenics and neurotics over a 5-year period. The borderline group resembled the schizophrenics in many aspects of course and outcome, with the exception that some social deterioration was noted in the schizophrenics but not in the borderline patients. Symptomatically the borderline patients were often between neurotic and psychotic depression; many responded favorably to antidepressants.

A series of 51 Kernberg-criteria borderline office patients, some of whom dropped out of treatment after 3 months but some of whom (12) remained in psychotherapy 5 years or more and were followed up 2 to 10 years later, showed the following results: 11 (22%) were dramatically improved, functioning on a level superior to their best premorbid level; 19 (37%) showed only modest gains, whose relationship to psychotherapy was not easy to determine; and 21 (41%) either were no better or were worse, often dropping out of treatment or requiring hospitalization. Two of the four who needed hospital care made good recoveries later on.[39]

When borderline patients are first diagnosed in late adolescence or their early 20s, some will develop recurrent major depressive illness (the depressive type of MDP); a small percentage will develop bipolar illness. The number who will become schizophrenic is very small (<5%), unless the original diagnostic criteria leaned toward schizotypal features. Males diagnosed "borderline" in adolescence often have explosive personalities and may have subtle organic deficits ("minimal brain damage") or temporal lobe epilepsy.[40] Their prognosis is guarded; they respond more favorably to appropriate medications, including anticonvulsants, than to insight-oriented psychotherapy.

Personality factors play an important role in prognosis. In general, borderline patients with predominantly histrionic, depressive, obsessive, or phobic features respond well to psychotherapy or have a favorable outcome with respect to social and occupational adjustment. Those who are predominantly narcissistic or paranoid respond less favorably or poorly. Schizotypal patients are slow to respond and often seem neither worse nor better even after prolonged psychotherapy. A few improve dramatically, especially if they are not particularly odd or eccentric.[41] Similarly, cyclothymic patients, some of whom are concurrently borderline (Kernberg or *DSM-III* criteria), are not good candidates for psychotherapy, although they may respond favorably to lithium. The presence of serious antisocial features is ominous and is almost always associated with a poor outcome.

Despite the frequency with which gestures of suicide are encountered in a borderline population (especially if selected by Gunderson or *DSM-III* criteria; pure schizotypals are less prone to self-damaging acts), the rate of completed suicides is low (<5% in a hospitalized group). Deaths are more likely to occur in males than in females, although some borderline patients of either sex literally throw their lives away in reckless acts not consciously intended as suicide, yet in other respects the equivalent of suicide.[42]

Borderline is a term applied most often to people within the age range of 18 to 40, despite the relatively unchanging nature, the "stable instability," of the condition. The paradox becomes resolved when one takes into account that in the usual definitions *borderline* represents a mixture of personality traits and symptoms (*viz.,* suicide gestures, brief psychotic episodes). The abnormal traits tend to persist throughout life. However, certain symptoms characteristically subside as middle life is approached: impulsivity lessens, gestures of suicide are less often resorted to, relationships either have by then grown more stable or else have been given up in favor of a solitary life that, however lonely, is less chaotic. Hence the same patient whose clinical picture warranted a borderline diagnosis at age 20 or 30 will have calmed down to the point of manifesting, at age 40 or 50, only a (severe) personality disorder.

Etiologic Factors

Each of the currently popular definitions of *borderline* is unified by a sameness of traits, symptoms, behavioral patterns, or dynamics. This homogeneity is no longer present with respect to etiology. Although in some cases only one major causative factor seems to be operative, the majority of cases stem from the interaction of complex factors: hereditary, constitutional, and psychosocial. A number of these factors have already been alluded to. Significant affective symptoms figure in half or more borderline patients, especially in an inpatient series. Depressive symptoms will be much more common than the hypomanic, although some borderline patients present with a picture closely resembling the bipolar-II form of MDP.[34] Unfavorable life circumstances may suffice to account for the depressive features in perhaps half the affective ("unstable") borderline patients. However, in the other half, the illness may be understood as a spectrum or "borderline" instance of MDP. The family history in these cases is often positive for a close relative with MDP or alcoholism.[17] The symptoms share many of the features of "endogenous" depression.

Among schizotypal borderline patients, one might expect an increase in family incidence of nuclear schizophrenia, analogous to the heightened incidence of "borderline schizophrenia" noted in the close relatives of nuclear schizophrenics. This correlation was not noted in the small sample available to Kety[33] in the Danish Adoption Study but has been noted in a methodologically less precise study based on schizotypal borderline patients seen in private practice.[41] Evidence linking schizotypal borderline patients to nuclear schizophrenics by way of common "risk genes" has also begun to emerge from the work of Siever.[43]

Although a small percentage (5% to 10%) of borderline patients come from families in which the parents were consistently nurturing, warm, and empathic, most have experienced one or more adverse patterns of child rearing. Parental inability to tolerate the child's quest for independence is one common pattern.[30] Chronic brutalization either by physical violence or verbal abuse is another. Overwhelming early loss, especially the death of the mother in early childhood, contributes heavily toward the development of a borderline condition, particularly in children already vulnerable because of genetic predisposition to a psychosis. The role of incest has been explained in the section on epidemiology. A less dramatic but still important psychosocial factor concerns parental neglect or deprivation. Extreme deprivation may lead to drastic loss of self-esteem and may contribute to the development of a pathologic grandiosity, as a compensatory maneuver. This split in the self-image becomes recognized in adult life as the unintegrated ego and faulty sense of identity characteristic of the borderline level of function. Affect hunger and the propensity to abuse substances are noted typically in deprived persons of this sort.

Differential Diagnosis and Biological Markers

CLINICAL ASPECTS

Some attention has already been paid to differential diagnosis, the details of which are dependent on the diagnostic system employed. Kernberg's borderline structure is, for example, distinguished from neurotic structure by the defective ego-integration of the former and is distinguished from psychotic structure because, in the latter, reality-testing capacity is no longer preserved. Since nuclear schizophrenics show psychotic distortions of various types, such as delusions, hallucinations, and bizarre ego-boundary disturbances, they exhibit a psychotic structure. Kernberg's borderline is thus discriminable from schizophrenia viewed as a clinical category. From a dimensional perspective, however, the situation is less clear: certain attenuated or "spectrum" cases of schizophrenia show adequate reality-testing capacity and operate at the borderline level. These cases are the exception: the majority even of "borderline schizophrenics" ("schizotypal personalities" in *DSM-III*) show poor reality-testing capacity in the interpersonal realm and thus have a psychotic structure.

Similar arguments are relevant for the Gunderson system: borderline personality disorder is discriminable from nuclear schizophrenia because good socialization is lacking in the latter. In some spectrum cases, however, socialization is adequate; if other criteria of borderline personality disorder are met, it will be possible for these schizotypal patients to fit within the Gunderson schema. In fact more "borderline schizophrenics" overlap with the Gunderson borderline personality disorder type than with the Kernberg borderline domain.

Borderline personality as described in the *DSM-III* is a category-based diagnosis discriminable from nuclear schizophrenia for the same reasons mentioned previously. Although some cases of recurrent unipolar depression exhibit enough features of borderline personality to warrant that diagnosis concurrently, the majority do not. Most patients with the recurrent depressive subtype of MDP show only the mood-lowering and vegetative signs of depression but not the irritable or impulsive aspects of borderline personality. Bipolar manic-depressives are easily distinguished in their acute state because of flight of ideas or pushed speech that would not be present in a borderline condition. Some manic-depressives in their interpsychotic phases do not completely return to normal as was once thought[3]; instead, they may manifest a borderline condition.[34]

The diagnosis of *borderline* by any system reviewed here may coexist with any of the other personality types described in the *DSM-III*. One should not get into the habit of labeling sociopathic or alcoholic patients "borderline" where such overlap exists, without assigning first place to the antisocial or substance-abusing disorder, since treatment and prognosis in these cases are shaped more by the personality/habit disorder than by the "borderline" state. The same should be stated of rare syndromes like "multiple personality" and factitious illness or Munchausen syndrome.[44]

BIOLOGICAL MARKERS OF POSSIBLE RELEVANCE

Tests that may aid in the differential diagnosis of borderline conditions consist mainly of biological markers, neurophysiologic procedures, and psychological tests.

Biological markers usually concern biochemical abnormalities that reflect a disturbance in one enzyme system, itself the reflection of one genic error. Many borderline conditions are in the spectra of manic-depression or schizophrenia, but the modes of transmission of these psychoses are probably more polygenic than dependent on a single gene. It is, therefore, less likely that a simple test of one enzyme's activity will suffice to detect either the core condition or its borderline variant. Studies have thus far concentrated on monoamine oxidase (MAO) and plasma cortisol levels. MAO activity has been reported as decreased in some bipolar patients and in some schizophrenics.[43] In a group of volunteers, low platelet MAO levels were found to be associated with sensation-seeking behavior, depression, and suicide in a close relative.[45] Some of the subjects with low MAO levels may be, or become, borderline patients with the affective subtypes. Platelet MAO levels may also be low in some schizotypal borderline patients.[43]

Plasma cortisol levels may return to normal prematurely, following dexamethasone challenge, in patients with endogenous depression but also in a high percentage (25% to 60%) of *DSM-III* borderline patients.[46] There is debate in the literature as to whether borderline patients with concurrent depression of the MDP or endogenous type are more apt to show an abnormal dexamethasone suppression test (DST) (as one might expect, if these cases really were in the MDP spectrum and if the DST were specific for MDP). Since abnormal test results are seen in some anxiety states and schizophrenia cases, it does not appear to be as specific for MDP, let alone for affective borderline states, as one might hope.

The time between onset of sleep and onset of the first rapid eye movement (REM) phase, called REM latency, has been noted to be abnormally brief in both endogenous depressives and in many *DSM-III* borderline patients[39] and may constitute a neurophysiologic marker of some usefulness in this regard. In the area of schizophrenia spectrum conditions, abnormal smooth-pursuit eye movements may be detectable in both core and borderline variants.[43]

Standard psychological tests, although nonspecific for borderline diagnosis, usually show abnormalities of various sorts. Good performance on the structured portions (Weschler Adult Intelligence Scale, Bender Gestalt Test) with poor performance on the unstructured portions (Rorschach Inkblot Test, Thematic Apperception Test) has been emphasized by Gunderson.[28] Differences between Rorschach results in schizotypal versus affective borderline patients have been studied by Carsky and Bloomgarden.[47] Results of the Minnesota Multiphasic Personality Inventory in borderline patients often show an 8–4–2 pattern, noted also, however, in many patients with histrionic personalities and "multiple personality."[48]

Treatment

In a brief survey the complexities and the special features of psychotherapy with borderline patients can only be hinted at. The interested reader should consult any of a number of books devoted to this topic.[49–52] It would be convenient if, to each diagnostic label, there belonged one cause and one optimal treatment. This is rare in psychiatry and is not the case even with the more restrictive definitions for borderline disorders.

THE ROLE OF MEDICATION

The borderline domain, as defined by *DSM-III,* contains depressive patients within the MDP spectrum, many of whom require antidepressant medications episodically for their "vegetative signs" (*viz.,* psychomotor retardation) and despondency; also, it contains characterologically depressive patients, unrelated to the MDP spectrum, who tend not to benefit from antidepressants.[34] Many patients with anorexia/bulimia, especially if hospitalized, are borderline by Kernberg criteria; some, by *DSM-III* criteria; a few, by Gunderson criteria. Some anorexics and "bulimarexics" show significant depressive symptoms plus a family history of MDP. They may benefit from antidepressants or, in the occasional instance where hypomanic traits are also apparent, from lithium. In general, patients with anorexia/bulimia respond better to behavioral modification techniques and supportive psychotherapy than to psychoanalytic therapy. Group therapy in which all the members have eating disorders may prove beneficial with ambulatory borderline anorectics.

Patients with the hysteroid dysphoria syndrome, most examples of which are either Kernberg criteria or *DSM-III* criteria, have been noted to respond specifically to MAO inhibitors,[26] although this proposition is not universally accepted; many such patients do well with tricyclic antidepressant therapy plus psychotherapy or even with psychotherapy alone.[17]

Many borderline women, especially those with prominent depressive symptoms, suffer severe premenstrual irritability or aggravation of depression. Sometimes this "premenstrual syndrome" (PMS) overshadows the other aspects of their condition. The syndrome will generally respond to some form of medication, although this must be discerned empirically: diuretics will suffice in some cases; antidepressants in others; and in a few, irritability and hypomanic features predominate and respond to lithium.[36]

Schizotypal borderlines of the "pure-type" (no admixture of affective symptoms) have, by definition, few of the "target symptoms" (*viz.,* delusions, hallucinations) of classic schizophrenia and respond only in exceptional instances to phenothiazine or other neuroleptic drugs.

Borderline patients who appear to have an organic overlay may show, besides the identity disturbances and other *DSM-III* attributes, fugue states, feelings of uncanniness, micropsia/macropsia, and other strange sensory phenomena, such as odd smells and illusion. Sometimes temporal lobe epilepsy can be documented, but in other cases, despite ample clinical signs, even nasopharyngeal electroencephalographic leads may fail to corroborate the diagnosis. A trial of anticonvulsants, particularly of carbamazepine (Tegretol), may be helpful, if temporal lobe epilepsy is suspected.[40]

PSYCHOTHERAPY: INSIGHT-ORIENTED VERSUS SUPPORTIVE

As the notion of "borderline" cases evolved within the psychoanalytic community, there was a growing awareness that modifications ("parameters") of the classic technique were necessary both to "contain" the more flamboyant symptoms and to allay the intense anxiety to which borderline patients are prone. In these endeavors was born the concept of psychoanalytically oriented psychotherapy. Around this, a rich literature grew up devoted at first to what were thought to be dilute versions of schizophrenia. Now only a fraction of these cases are in the schizophrenia spectrum; most are now considered ''borderline.'' The history[53] and theory[54] of this form of therapy are reviewed elsewhere in this volume.

Only a proportion of borderline patients are ideally suited to insight-oriented psychotherapy. Considerations unrelated to diagnosis are of paramount importance: the degree of motivation, the level of psychological mindedness, and the genuineness of concern about one's illness. If these are of a low order, insight-oriented therapy will not flourish, even if other factors seem favorable. Personality profile has been mentioned earlier as significant also; predominantly depressive or ''infantile''[28] personalities have, on average, a better prognosis than the paranoid or schizoid types. Persistent abuse of drugs (including alcohol) conduce to chaotic life, ''acting-out'' of transference themes, and so on and augur poorly for intensive therapy unless they can be brought under control (*e.g.*, by faithful attendance of Alcoholics Anonymous meetings).

Insight-oriented therapy will include such elements as focus on transference, persistent interpretation of defensive maneuvers, use of confrontation, and particular attention to countertransference issues.[55] Sessions of approximately 45 minutes will usually be scheduled two to three times a week, with therapist and patient face to face, rather than four to five times a week with the patient using the couch, as in classic analysis. Borderline patients tend to ''actualize'' the transference, wishing to make the therapist, to take one common example, into a ''real friend'' rather than to explore the dynamic factors that underlie this wish. In so doing, they often mobilize stronger feelings in their therapists than are evoked by better-integrated patients. Therapists must be careful not to become immersed in these currents of feelings, yet must retain and use awareness of the particular feeling-states active at any given moment. A borderline patient may be too embarrassed to speak of his angry feelings or may be out of touch with them but will deal with the therapist in such a way as to cause him to feel angry (by way of insults, refusing to leave at the end of a session, calling at midnight). It is the therapist's ability to recognize his reaction, to understand the source of the feeling in the patient's own psyche, and to translate this back to the patient. This constitutes one of the most important transactions in the intensive therapy of a borderline patient.

Intensive therapy is indicated for certain hospitalized borderline patients, particularly those who are between the ages of 18 and 35, who, in addition to showing the favorable factors mentioned above, are chronically ill with self-destructive life patterns. When successful, these maladaptive patterns may be given up and replaced by more appropriate modes of interaction, such that the borderline patient is functioning on a level higher than the best premorbid level. In selected cases, long-term hospital treatment of 6 to 20 months is justified, although in others, shorter stays are more effective, especially in patients who tend to lose their motivation in comfortable institutional settings. Intensive therapy works best in hospital units dedicated to work of this kind, where most of the patients are borderline and fairly homogeneous with respect to their potential for recovery, and where the staff has worked together a long time to develop both familiarity with the special problems inherent in this work and good working relationships with each other. When indicated, adjunct pharmacotherapy should be employed. Group therapy will be useful also, especially in dealing with either inhibited patients, whom the group can ''encourage,'' and abrasive patients, whom the group can confront in ways that are less painful than if similar criticism were made by the therapist.

Therapists should be aware that although dramatic improvements can be achieved with selected ambulatory or hospitalized borderline patients using intensive therapy, there will be many failures; many patients may quit abruptly or may persist in undoing the gains of treatment with self-defeating impulsive acts.

Supportive techniques, which will be the mainstays for many borderline patients, must be used in varying degrees and at various times, depending on the presence or absence of ''crisis,'' in all borderline patients. These techniques include clarifications of the here-and-now situation, advice, expressions of concern and sympathy, exhortation, suggestion, and limit-setting. There will be less silence and more spontaneous verbal activity on the part of the therapist than would be the norm for intensive therapy, even though the latter already involves a more active approach than is customary with classic psychoanalysis.

REFERENCES

1. Hughes CH: Moral (affective) insanity: Psycho-sensory insanity. Alienist Neurologist 5:296–315, 1884
2. Rosse IC: Clinical Evidences of Borderland Insanity. J Nerv Ment Dis 17:669–683, 1890
3. Kraepelin E: Manic-Depressive Insanity and Paranoia. Edinburg, E & S Livingstone, 1921
4. Freud S: Instincts and Their Vicissitudes, standard ed, vol 14, pp 111–140, 1915

5. Moore TV: The parataxes: A study and analysis of certain borderline mental states. Psychoanal Rev 8:252–283, 1921

6. Maeder A: Psychologische Untersuchungen an Dementia-praecoxkranken. Jahrb Psychoanal Psychopathol Forschung 2:234–245, 1910

7. Bjerre P: Zur Radikalbehandlung der chronischen Paranoia. Jahrb Psychoanal Psychopathol Forschung 3:759–847, 1912

8. Ekstein R: Vicissitudes of the internal image in the recovery of a borderline schizophrenic adolescent. Bull Menninger Clin 19:86–92, 1955

9. Federn P: Principles of psychotherapy in latent schizophrenia. Am J Psychother 1:129–139, 1947

10. Hoch PH, Polatin P: Pseudoneurotic forms of schizophrenia. Psychiatr Q 23:248–276, 1949

11. Reich W: Der Triebhafte Charakter. Leipzig, Internationale Psychoanalytische, Verlag, 1925

12. Deutsch H: Some forms of emotional disturbance and their relationships to schizophrenia. Psychoanal Q 11:301–321, 1942

13. Frosch J: Psychotic character J Am Psychoanal Assoc 8:544–551, 1960

14. Kasanin J: Acute schizoaffective psychoses. Am J Psychiatry 97:97–120, 1933

15. Stern A: Psychoanalytic investigations and therapy in the borderline group of neuroses. Psychoanal Q 7:467–489, 1938

16. Knight R: Borderline states. Bull Menninger Clin 17:1–12, 1953

17. Stone MH: The Borderline Syndromes: Constitution, Personality and Adaptation. New York, McGraw Hill, 1980

18. Grinker RR, Sr, Werble B, Drye RC: The Borderline Syndrome. New York, Basic Books, 1968

19. Mack JE: Borderline States in Psychiatry. New York, Grune & Stratton, 1975

20. Millon T: Disorders of Personality. New York, John Wiley & Sons, 1981

21. Perry JC, Klerman GL: The borderline patient. Arch Gen Psychiatry 35:141–150, 1978

22. Diagnostic and Statistical Manual of Mental Disorders, 3rd ed. Washington, DC, American Psychiatric Association, 1980

23. Kernberg OF: Borderline personality organization. J Am Psychoanal Assoc 15:641–685, 1967

24. Kernberg OF: The structural diagnosis of borderline personality organization. In Hartocollis P (ed): Borderline Personality Disorders, pp 87–121. New York, International Universities Press, 1977

25. Erikson EH: Growth and crises of the healthy personality. In Senn M: Symposium on the Healthy Personality, pp 91–146. New York, Josiah Macy, Jr, Foundation, 1951

26. Klein DF: Psychopharmacological treatment and delineation of borderline disorders. In Hartocollis P (ed): Borderline Personality Disorders, pp 365–384. New York, International Universities Press, 1977

27. Welner A, Liss JL, Robins E: Undiagnosed psychiatric patients: III. The undiagnosible patients. Br J Psychiatry 123:91–98, 1973

28. Gunderson JG, Singer JT: Defining borderline patients. Am J Psychiatry 132:1–10, 1975

29. Spitzer RL, Endicott J, Gibbon M: Crossing the border into borderline personality and borderline schizophrenia. Arch Gen Psychiatry 36:17–24, 1979

30. Masterson JF: The Narcissistic and Borderline Disorders. New York, Brunner/Mazel, 1981

31. Rinsley DB: Borderline and Other Self Disorders. New York, J Aronson, 1982

32. Kohut H: The Analysis of the Self. New York, International Universities Press, 1971

33. Kety SS, Rosenthal D, Wender PG et al: Mental illness in the biological and adoptive families of adoptive schizophrenics. In Rosenthal D, Kety S (eds): Transmission of Schizophrenia, pp 345–362. Oxford, Pergamon Press, 1968

34. Akiskal HS: Subaffective disorders: Dysthymic, cyclothymic and bipolar-II disorders in the ''borderline'' realm. In Stone MH (ed): Borderline Disorders. Psychol Clin North Am 4:25–46, 1981

35. Sperber MA, Jarvik LF: Psychiatry and Genetics. New York, Basic Books, 1976

36. Stone MH: Premenstrual tension in borderline and related disorders. In Friedman RC (ed): Behavior and the Menstrual Cycle, pp 317–344. New York, Marcel Dekker, 1983

37. Stone MH: Borderline syndromes: A consideration of subtypes. In Stone MH (ed): Borderline Disorders. Psychol Clin North Am 4:3–24, 1981

38. Carpenter WT Jr, Gunderson JG, Strauss JS: Considerations of the borderline syndrome: A longitudinal comparative study of borderline and schizophrenia patients. In Hartocollis P (ed): Borderline Personality Disorders, pp 231–253. New York, International Universities Press, 1977

39. Stone MH: Borderline disorders: Diagnosis, genetics, and personality factors. J Hillside Hosp (in press)

40. Andrulonis PA, Glueck BC, Stroebel CF et al: Organic brain dysfunction and the borderline syndrome. In Stone MH (ed): Borderline Disorders. Psychol Clin North Am 4:47–66, 1981

41. Stone MH: Psychotherapy with schizotypal borderline patients. J Am Acad Psychoanal 11:87–111, 1983

42. Stone MH: Risk factors in suicidal borderlines. J Suicidol (in press)

43. Siever LJ: Genetic factors in borderline personalities. In Grinspoon L (ed): Psychiatry 1982: Annual Review, pp 437–456. Washington, DC, American Psychiatric Association, 1982

44. Stone MH: Factitious illness. Bull Menninger Clin 41:239–254, 1977

45. Buchsbaum MS, Coursey R, Murphy DL: The biochemical high-risk paradigm: Behavioral and family correlates of low platelet monoamine oxidase activity. Science 194:339–341, 1976

46. Carroll BJ, Greden JF, Feinberg M et al: Neuroendocrine evaluation of depression in borderline patients. In Stone MH (ed): Borderline Disorders, Psychol Clin North Am 4:89–99, 1981

47. Carsky M, Bloomgarden JW: Subtyping in the borderline realm by means of Rorschach analysis. In Stone MH (ed): Borderline Disorders. Psychol Clin North Am 4:101–116, 1981

48. Bliss EL: A symptom profile of 47 patients with multiple personalities—with MMPI results (unpublished manuscript)

49. Balint M: The Basic Fault. New York, Brunner/Mazel, 1968

50. Kernberg OF: Borderline Conditions and Pathological Narcissism. New York, J Aronson, 1975

51. Chessick RD: Intensive Psychotherapy of the Borderline Patient. New York, J Aronson, 1977

52. LeBoit J, Capponi A (eds): Advances in Psychotherapy of the Borderline Patient. New York, J Aronson, 1979

53. Stone MH: Treating Schizophrenic Patients. New York, McGraw-Hill, 1983

54. Kernberg OF: The theory of psychoanalytic psychotherapy. In Slipp S (ed): Curative Factors in Dynamic Psychotherapy, pp 21–43. New York, McGraw-Hill, 1982

55. Searles HF: Countertransference and Related Subjects. New York, International Universities Press, 1979

Narcissistic Personality Disorder

The term *narcissism*, first used in a psychiatric sense by Ellis[1] and to describe a sexual perversion by Nacke,[2] entered the psychoanalytic lexicon through Sadger.[3] After mentioning narcissism briefly in various papers, Freud[4] published "On Narcissism: An Introduction," one of his major contributions to psychoanalytic theory. In that essay, Freud refers to narcissism as a form of sexual perversion as well as a characteristic of all perversions; as a stage in libidinal development; as an underlying characteristic of schizophrenia (because of the withdrawal of libido from the external world); and finally with reference to a type of object choice wherein the object is selected because it represents what the subject was, is, or would like to be.

These multiple applications of the word have resulted in considerable confusion about the definition of narcissism. Gradually, however, narcissism as a concept in psychoanalytic theory became distinguished from the clinical use of the term. The latter has come to refer to the preconditions and characteristics of normal and pathological regulation of self-esteem. Descriptions of the narcissistic personality disorder gradually evolved in this second context; the diagnostic category resulted from the observation of a particular constellation of resistances in the psychoanalytic treatment of certain patients—a constellation of resistances that corresponded to a particular type of character pathology also manifest in the ordinary life of these patients.

Jones[5] published the first description of pathologic narcissistic character traits. Abraham[6] was the first to describe the transference resistances of these patients; he pointed to the need for consistent interpretation of their tendencies to look down on the analyst and to use him as an audience for their independent "analytic" work and drew attention to the link between narcissism and envy. Riviere[7] observed that narcissistic resistances were an important source of negative therapeutic reactions: these patients cannot tolerate the idea of improvement because improvement would mean to acknowledge help received from somebody else. Riviere suggested that these patients cannot tolerate receiving something good from the analyst because of their intolerable guilt over their own basic aggression.

Elaborating on Klein's[8] book *Envy and Gratitude*, Rosenfeld[9–12] published in Great Britain the first detailed description of the psychostructural characteristics of narcissistic personalities and their transference developments in the course of psychoanalysis.

Important contributions to the phenomenology and the psychopathology of narcissistic personalities were published in this country by Reich,[13,14] Jacobson,[15] van der Waals,[16] and Tartakoff.[17] On the basis of Jacobson's formulations, and in an effort to integrate the American and British contributions to the diagnosis and treatment of the narcissistic personality within an ego psychology frame of reference, I[18–21] proposed an alternative theoretic and clinical frame to that suggested by Rosenfeld. At the same time, Kohut[22–26] proposed a completely different theoretic frame, clinical explanations, and therapeutic procedure for narcissistic personality disorders.

The proliferation of contributions on narcissism in Great Britain and in this country had a parallel in the contributions of Grunberger.[27] Grunberger, whose work was first published in France in the

1950s and 1960s, focused on the wider clinical and metapsychological aspects of narcissism as observed in the psychoanalytic treatment of a broad range of psychopathology.

Pulver[28] clarified the bewildering expansion of the concept of narcissism within psychoanalytic metapsychology. More recent contributions to the study of the narcissistic personality and the psychoanalytic treatment of these patients have been published by Modell,[29] Volkan,[30,31] and Bach.[32–34] Akhtar and Thomson[35] have provided a broadly based analysis of the narcissistic personality disorder and its relation to the definition of this disorder in the *Diagnostic and Statistical Manual of Mental Disorders (DSM-III)*.

Definition

Given the recent controversies regarding the psychoanalytic theory of narcissism and the influence of differing theoretic formulations on the efforts to clarify the clinical syndrome of the narcissistic personality disorder, it may be helpful to define narcissism at the level of psychoanalytic theory or metapsychology separately from narcissism as a descriptive, phenomenologic, clinical concept. The following definition at the first, metapsychological level will necessarily reflect only one approach to a complex and controversial field. (Other, contrasting, theoretic views are presented in the section on etiology.) At the second, clinical level, there are fewer controversies, and the clinical descriptions arrived at from different theoretic standpoints are reassuringly overlapping. The clinical definitions proposed below should, therefore, prove less controversial than the metapsychological one.

Within traditional psychoanalytic metapsychology, narcissism may be defined as the libidinal investment of the self: "narcissistic libido" is libido invested in the self. The traditional view of "libido" within psychoanalysis as one of the two basic instinctual drives (aggression being the other one) is currently being questioned in many quarters; a discussion of these issues would exceed the frame of this chapter. For practical purposes, the term *libidinal* may also be read as referring to the sum total of affectively positive or rewarding investments, in contrast to affectively negative or aggressive investments. The self is here conceived of as a substructure of the system ego that reflects the integration of all the self-images (or self-representations) that develop throughout experiences of interactions with other humans ("objects" in metapsychologi-

cal language). In contrast, the investment of libido in these objects and in their psychic representations ("object representations") constitutes "object libido." Object libido is in a dynamic relationship with narcissistic libido.

At the clinical level, narcissism may be defined as the normal or pathologic regulation of self-esteem or self-regard. Normally, self-esteem or self-regard fluctuates according to the gratifying or frustrating experiences an individual has in relations with others and according to one's evaluation of the distance between goals and aspirations and one's achievements and success. Clinical experience indicates, however, that the relations between self-esteem, on the one hand, and predominant affects or moods, the extent to which various self-representations are integrated or dissociated, and the vicissitudes of internalized object relations, on the other, are very complicated.

Self-esteem regulation is dependent, among other factors, on the pressures that the superego exerts on the ego: a harsh superego can diminish self-esteem (because of unconscious demands for perfection and infantile prohibitions). Self-esteem regulation may also be affected by lack of gratification of instinctual needs, of both a libidinal and aggressive nature. The regulation of self-esteem depends on the internalization of libidinally invested objects (in the form of libidinally invested object representations), which provide the self with reinforcement of the images of those the individual loves and by whom he feels loved. When excessive conflicts around aggression weaken the libidinal investment of others and, secondarily, of the corresponding object representations, the libidinal investment of the self and self-love also suffer.

For practical purposes, narcissism may be classified into normal adult, normal infantile, and pathologic narcissism. Normal adult narcissism is characterized by normal self-esteem regulation. It is dependent on a normal self-structure related to normally integrated or "total" internalized object representations; an integrated, largely individualized and abstracted superego; and the gratification of instinctual needs within the context of stable object relations and value systems.

Normal infantile narcissism is of importance because fixation at or regression to infantile narcissistic goals (infantile mechanisms of self-esteem regulation) is an important characteristic of all character pathology. Normal infantile narcissism consists in the regulation of self-esteem by age appropriate gratifications that include or imply normal infantile "value systems," demands, and/or prohibitions. A first type of abnormal or pathologic self-esteem regulation, reflecting at the same time the mildest type of narcissistic pathology, coincides with the fixation at or regression to a level of functioning within normal infantile narcissism, represented by the frequent cases of personality or character disorders wherein the regulation of self-esteem seems to be overly dependent on expression of or defenses against childish gratifications that are normally abandoned in adulthood. This is a very frequent and relatively mild disturbance that need not be considered further here.

A second, more severe, but relatively infrequent type of pathologic narcissism was first described by Freud[4] as an illustration of "narcissistic object choice." Here, the patient's self is identified with an object while, at the same time, the representation of the patient's infantile self is projected onto that very object, thus creating a libidinal relation in which the functions of self and object have been interchanged. This is often found among male and female homosexuals: they love another in the way they would have wished to be loved.

A third and very severe type of pathologic narcissism is the narcissistic personality disorder proper, one of the most challenging syndromes met with in clinical psychiatry. The narcissistic personality disorder, which constitutes the focus of the rest of this chapter, is a specific type of character pathology that centers around the presence of a pathologic grandiose self.

Epidemiology

The phenomenologic descriptions and theoretic discussions of the narcissistic personality disorder derive from clinical observations, particularly from the experiences gathered by means of psychoanalytic exploration of character pathology. The relatively recent clinical understanding of this syndrome has not yet led to reliable epidemiologic studies nor, in general, to empiric research leading to reliable diagnostic instruments for such epidemiologic studies. At the same time, in the light of these clinical observations, one gains the impression that narcissistic personalities are a prevalent type of personality disorder, and there exists a widespread though unsubstantiated impression that their incidence may be increasing.

Lasch[36] points to a puzzling convergence between the clinical characteristics of the narcissistic personality as described by Kohut and me and ascending or prevailing patterns of conventional cultural values. I have described the tendency of

groups, particularly large groups, under unstructured or regressive conditions, to select narcissistic personalities for positions of leadership and the surprising facility with which narcissistic personalities assume leadership functions precisely under such circumstances.[37] Beyond such points of contact, between the clinical characteristics of the narcissistic personality and certain cultural and social phenomena, it would seem to be premature to formulate more specific hypotheses regarding the possible social or cultural facilitation of narcissistic personality disorders.

It is possible that, at times of rapid social change and breakdown of traditional social structures, the more severe types of personality disorders emerge because of the loss of the compensating functions of social structure. On the basis of clinical impressions, narcissistic personalities are as prevalent in men as in women and can be found in all socioeconomic and cultural strata.

Clinical Description

The consolidation of the pathologic grandiose self and the appearance of the typical character features of the narcissistic personality disorder probably occurs from childhood on,[38] but most cases in the literature have been late adolescents and adults. The full-fledged picture of the narcissistic personality disorder in adulthood is examined first, and then particular features in special age-groups are presented.

The essential pathologic character traits of these patients center around pathologic self-love, pathologic object love, superego pathology, and a basic characteristic self-state. The *pathologic self-love* of these patients is expressed in excessive self-reference and self-centeredness. They also show grandiosity, reflected in exhibitionistic tendencies, a sense of superiority, recklessness, and a typical discrepancy between inordinate ambitions and limited capabilities or a limiting social reality. Their grandiosity is often expressed in terms of childlike values—physical attractiveness, power, wealth, clothing, manners, and the like. High intelligence may be used as the basis for intellectual pretentiousness. Additional expressions of a pathologic self-love include an overdependency on admiration by others that does not include the capacity for gratitude. Admiration is taken for granted rather than appreciated. Emotional shallowness, reflected in a lack of awareness of depth of human experiences, and dramatic bouts of feelings of insecurity or inferiority convey the impression that these patients feel either superior or totally worthless (and their most terrible fear may be of being "average" or "mediocre"). But of all these indicators of pathologic self-love, grandiosity is the most characteristic.

Regarding the character traits reflecting *pathologic object love,* a key symptom is the excessive, at times overwhelming, manifestation of envy, both conscious and unconscious (the latter reflected in conscious attempts to avoid or deny its presence). Devaluation, largely an expression of defensive efforts directed against potential sources of envy, is another conspicuous characteristic of these patients. Devaluation, consciously manifest as contempt and lack of interest for others' work or productions, also operates at a conscious and unconscious level. Unconscious devaluation shows as a "spoiling" maneuver that consists of incorporating quickly what comes from others and simultaneously devaluating what is incorporated. Exploitativeness, still another manifestation of pathologic object love, constitutes another expression of defenses against envy; these patients are greedy and wish to "steal" or appropriate aggressively what others have; a sense of entitlement often accompanies exploitativeness. Those suffering from narcissistic personality disorder cannot depend on others, another manifestation of pathologic object love. They will temporarily idealize others, but the idealization may quickly shift to devaluation. It is as if these patients were unconsciously experiencing those around them as idols, enemies, and fools. Inability to empathize with others and to make substantive commitments to others are further characteristics of pathologic object love.

Character patterns and affective disturbances indicating the *super ego pathology* of these patients are less decisive in establishing the diagnosis but very important in establishing the prognosis under psychotherapeutic treatment. These characteristics include the incapacity to experience differentiated forms of depression that include remorse, sadness, and self-exploration; the presence of severe mood swings, often initiated by a failure to succeed in grandiose or exhibitionistic efforts, in obtaining admiration from others, or following criticism that shatters their grandiosity; a self-esteem regulated by "shame" rather than "guilt"; and lack of an integrated, internalized value system, reflected in lack of investment in ethical, aesthetic, or intellectual values. These patients have childish values that protect self-esteem and pride; their inordinate dependency on external admiration indirectly reflects their immature superego functioning.

A group of narcissistic patients with particularly severe superego pathology present the syndrome of what I call "malignant narcissism,"[39] characterized by antisocial behavior, ego-syntonic sadism or characterologically anchored aggression, and a paranoid orientation. The antisocial features may range from minor dishonesty to the presence of a full-fledged antisocial personality disorder, illustrating that the antisocial personality may be considered a narcissistic personality with particular additional superego pathology. In clinical practice, the antisocial personality disorder proper can be differentiated from the narcissistic personality disorder as follows: he has no capacity for loyalty to and concern for others or for feeling guilty; he cannot conceive of other people having moral dimensions, nor can he conceive realistically in terms of the future. The ego-syntonic sadism in malignant narcissism may be expressed in a conscious "ideology" of aggressive self-affirmation but also, strangely enough, in chronic, ego-syntonic suicide tendencies. The underlying fantasy is that to be able to take one's life reflects superiority and a triumph over the usual fear of pain and death. To commit suicide is to exercise sadistic control over others. The paranoid orientation reflects the projection onto others of sadistic superego precursors that have not been integrated; it is manifest in an exaggerated experience of others as idols, enemies, or fools. In general, the grandiosity of patients with malignant narcissism is more ego-syntonic than it is for most other narcissistic patients.

Regarding the *basic self-state* in narcissistic personality disorders, these patients typically experience a chronic sense of emptiness, a sense of being alone. They are incapable of learning from others. They have an intense stimulus hunger and a chronic sense of the meaninglessness of life. They characteristically feel bored when their need for admiration and success is not being gratified.

The description of the narcissistic personality disorder in the *DSM-III* is adequate, with the exception of the failure to include these patients' inordinate envy.

Patients with narcissistic personality disorder quite frequently present atypical features. Some of these patients are anxious and tense; instead of the charm and insouciance ordinarily found in narcissistic personality disorder, they are timid and insecure. Their grandiose fantasies and daydreams may take the diagnostician by surprise. Most narcissistic patients are sexually promiscuous but some show sexual inhibition. Such cases are intensely afraid of being rejected and/or ridiculed. This fear, coupled with the inability to establish object relations in depth, may result in their achieving sexual gratification by means of masturbating with narcissistic, grandiose, exhibitionistic fantasies, instead of by promiscuity. Yet another set of atypical characteristics found under this category is general lack of ambition and interest coupled with a primitive hedonistic quality (the person who lives for "TV, beer, and popcorn"), underlying which gross devaluation of most circumstances that otherwise might evoke envy or threaten an unconscious grandiosity renders the quality of daily life empty. One also finds the selfless ideologist, political leader, or social redeemer who couples grandiosity projected onto a world scene with a seeming humility in his daily life. It is not unusual to find guru types who express enormous love for mankind but are totally uninterested and uncommitted to any actual personal relation.

Narcissistic personalities function on a continuum of levels of severity of their pathology, ranging from almost "normal" personalities to functioning that blends with borderline character pathology ("overtly borderline functioning") and with whom a differential diagnosis with psychotic illness may have to be entertained.

At the highest level of functioning are people without neurotic symptoms, who seem to be adaptating and who have very little awareness of emotional illness except for a chronic sense of emptiness or boredom, an inordinate need of approval from others and for personal success, and a remarkable incapacity for intuitive understanding, empathy, and emotional investment in others. Few of these people come to treatment, but over the years they tend to develop complications secondary to their narcissistic pathology.

The middle range of the spectrum of narcissistic personality disorders presents the basic symptoms already mentioned. At the most severe level of the continuum are patients who, in spite of the defensive functions the pathologic grandiose self provides, in social interactions, show overt borderline features (*i.e.,* lack of impulse control and of anxiety tolerance, severe crippling of their sublimatory capacities and a disposition to explosive or chronic rage reactions or severe paranoid distortions).

Adolescent patients with narcissistic personality disorder frequently present a contradictory school record, with ambitiousness and driving efforts on the one hand and almost inexplicable failure and withdrawal from other activities on the other. The explanation lies in the narcissistic adolescents' need either to be the best or to devalue those areas in which they cannot triumph or could achieve their goal only through persistent effort. This pattern is often masked by symptomatic depression related to failure at school. Only a careful evaluation reveals the predominant narcissistic quality of that depression (feelings of defeat and shame over not having triumphed) and the devaluation of what does not come easily or is not immediately rewarding. Difficulty in accepting being a "beginner" is characteristic of (although not exclusive to) narcissistic patients. Adolescent narcissistic patients may also present what one might call an "innocently" charming hedonism, a search for pleasure and enjoyment that often goes with an easy going, superficially friendly nature, a kind of adolescent playboy attitude that can be quite engaging. Such an attitude, combined with talents and high intelligence, may obscure the difficulty these adolescents have in committing themselves to any life goals or to relationships in depth. And on further exploration, warmth and social engagingness reveal a typical poverty of object relations and an absence of long-range investment in value systems and goals other than self-aggrandizement. It is probably only the more severe types of narcissistic personality who come for treatment in adolescence. Therefore, the diagnosis of narcissistic personality disorder in adolescence usually implies that the pathology is severe.

Narcissistic personality disorders frequently undergo a deterioration in middle age.[37] Narcissistic personalities experience throughout the years a worsening of their world of internalized object relations. They unconsciously devalue both their own past (in order not to feel envy of that past) and what others have (in order not to envy others). Hence, these people do not have at their disposal the gratifications that normally accompany memories of past experiences. Pathologic narcissism may thus lead to increasing social isolation and intensify the sense of internal emptiness. In many cases, the vicious circle of devaluation and emptiness becomes insurmountable. Some middle-aged patients with narcissistic personality, however, in spite of, or rather because of worsening of depressive symptoms secondary to their narcissistic personality structure, have a better prognosis for psychotherapeutic treatment than they would have had when they were in their early 20s or 30s. Chronic depressive reactions, a defensive withdrawal from activities, people, and situations that would otherwise evoke envy, and a subsequent increasing sense of loneliness and failure are the most frequent manifestations that bring middle-aged and older narcissistic personality disorders to treatment. Their persistent efforts to deny the passage of time by means of an artificial stress on youthfulness in behavior, attire, activities, and fantasies may lend a somewhat hypomanic (and, at times, pathetic) quality to aging patients with narcissistic personality. Invariably, the key characteristics already described can be found underneath what appears to be a "hypomanic personality."

Etiology

The clinical description of the narcissistic personality disorder derives mostly from the study of these patients in the course of psychoanalytic and psychoanalytically oriented psychotherapeutic treatment. The theories proposed by Rosenfeld, Kohut, and me coincide in pointing to the essentially psychodynamic etiology of these disorders and in focusing on the pathology of self-esteem regulation as the key pathogenic issue. All three approaches also agree in postulating the presence, in these patients, of an abnormal self-structure. The three approaches are in disagreement, however, regarding the origin of this pathologic self-structure, and, as a consequence of their different psychodynamic formulations, they propose significantly different psychotherapeutic techniques within a psychoanalytically based frame of reference.

Rosenfeld, within the theoretic frame of Kleinian psychoanalysis, proposes that narcissistic patients identify themselves with an omnipotently introjected all-good, primitive "part object," thus denying any distinction between self and object. This identification permits the patients to deny any need for dependency on an originally good, external object. Dependency would imply the need for such a loved and potentially also frustrating object who is also intensely hated, with the hatred taking the form of extreme envy.[9] Envy, Rosenfeld assumes, following Klein, is a primary intrapsychic expression of the death instinct, the earliest manifestation of aggression in the realm of object relations. Narcissistic object relations permit the subject to avoid aggressive feelings caused by frustration and any awareness of envy. Rosenfeld[10] also described the complication arising in these personality structures when their self-idealization is contaminated by the idealization of the aggressive parts of the self. The infiltration of the pathologic "mad" self by primitive aggression gives these pa-

tients a quality of violent self-destructiveness. In extreme cases, such patients feel secure and triumphant only when they have destroyed everyone else and particularly when they have frustrated the efforts of those who love them. Rosenfeld[11] thinks this need is responsible for the most severe forms of negative therapeutic reaction. The pathologic grandiose self of these patients reflects a more primitive, severe, and intractable resistance to treatment than the unconscious guilt feelings stemming from a sadistic superego characteristic of milder forms of negative therapeutic reaction.

Kohut[23,25] argued that there exists a group of patients whose psychopathology is intermediate between the psychoses and borderline conditions on the one hand and the psychoneuroses and milder character disorders on the other. This group of narcissistic personality disorders, which he considers analyzable, can in his opinion be differentiated primarily by transference manifestations, not by clinical-descriptive criteria. Kohut diagnoses the narcissistic personality disorder within the psychoanalytic situation by recognizing the development of two types of transference, idealizing and mirroring. The idealizing transference reflects the therapeutic activation of an idealized parent image and derives from an archaic, rudimentary "self-object." Kohut suggested that the intensity of the dependency on these idealized self-objects is due to the patient's wish to substitute them for a missing segment of the psychic structure. The patient's narcissistic equilibrium is safeguarded only through the interest and approval of current replicas of traumatically missing self-objects of the past.

The development of mirror transferences reflects the propensity toward the reactivation of a grandiose self in the psychoanalytic situation. These mirror transferences can be differentiated according to three levels of regression. The most archaic form (a merger transference) represents the revival of an early stage of primary identity of self and object; the alter-ego or twinship transference reflects the patient's assumption that the analyst is either like him or similar to him; through the mirror transference in a narrow sense (the least regressive of the three levels) the patient experiences the analyst as separate but significant only insofar as he is needed by the reactivated grandiose self for its own purpose.

Kohut proposed that these two broad types of transferences—idealizing and mirror—represent the activation in the psychoanalytic situation of an arrested stage of development of an archaic grandiose self. The fragility of that archaic self requires an empathic mother as self-object whose love and ministrations and whose mirroring acceptance of the infant permit the development of that archaic self to more mature forms of self-esteem and self-confidence. At the same time, optimal empathic relations with the mirroring self-object facilitate the development of idealization of the self-object that stands for the original perfection of the grandiose self, now practically preserved in the relationship with such an idealized self-object. This idealization culminates eventually in what Kohut calls the "transmuting internalization" of the idealized self-object into an intrapsychic structure that will originate the ego ideal and provide the idealizing qualities to the superego, thus preserving the now internalized regulation of self-esteem.

Narcissistic psychopathology, in essence, Kohut proposed, derives from the traumatic failure of the mother's empathic function and from the failure of the undisturbed development of idealization processes. These traumatic failures bring about a developmental arrest, a fixation at the level of the archaic infantile grandiose self and an endless search for the idealized self-object needed to complete structure formation, all of which are reflected in the narcissistic transferences already mentioned.

Narcissistic psychopathology, in short, in Kohut's view, reflects the psychopathology of the stage of development that begins with the cohesion of the archaic grandiose self and ends with the transmuting internalization of the ego ideal. This stage centers on the gradual building up of what Kohut has called the "bipolar self." He suggested that one pole, the bulk of nuclear grandiosity of the self, consolidates into nuclear ambitions in early childhood while the other pole, the bulk of nuclear idealized goal structures of the self, is acquired somewhat later. These two polarities of the self derive, respectively, from the mother's mirroring acceptance, which confirms nuclear grandiosity, and her holding and caring, which allow merger experiences with the self-object's idealized omnipotence. Nuclear ambitions and nuclear ideals are linked by an intermediary area of basic talents and skills. Kohut considered these component structures of the bipolar self as reflecting both the origin and the seed of narcissistic psychopathology, in contrast to the drives and conflict-derived psychopathology of the tripartite structure of the mind that characterize the later oedipal period. For Kohut, then, the etiology of the narcissistic personality disorders resides in an arrested stage of development of the normal self.

I have proposed that the specific character features of patients with narcissistic personality disorders reflect a pathologic narcissism that differs from both ordinary adult narcissism and fixation at or regression to normal infantile narcissism.[21,37,39] In contrast to the latter, pathologic narcissism reflects libidinal investment not in a normal integrated self-structure but in a pathologic self-structure. I have redefined the concept of "libido" as the hierarchically supraordinate integration of positive affective investments of self and objects. The pathologic grandiose self, in my view contains real self-representations, ideal self-representations, and ideal object representations. Devalued or aggressively determined self- and object representations are split off or dissociated, repressed, or projected. The psychoanalytic resolution of the grandiose self as part of the systematic analysis of narcissistic character resistances regularly brings to the surface (*i.e.,* activates in the transference) primitive object relations, conflicts, and defensive operations characteristic of developmental stages that predate object constancy. These transferences, however, are always condensed with oedipally derived conflicts, so that they are strikingly similar to those of patients with borderline personality organization.

In my view, the psychic development of the narcissistic personality disorder does not proceed smoothly through the early stages of development described by Jacobson[15] and Mahler,[40,41] whose description of the early stages of infantile autism, symbiosis, separation-individuation, and object constancy underlies my theoretic model. In my view, some time between the ages of 3 and 5 years, the narcissistic personality, instead of integrating positive and negative representations of self and of objects "on the road to object constancy"[42] puts together all the positive representations of both self and objects as well as the idealized representations of self and objects. This results in an extremely unrealistic and idealized idea of himself and a pathologic, grandiose self. Fostering the development of a pathologic grandiose self are parents who are cold, rejecting, yet admiring. The narcissistic personality devaluates the real objects, having incorporated those aspects of the real objects he wants for himself. He dissociates from himself, represses, or projects onto others all the negative aspects of himself and others.

The ideal self- and object representations that would normally become part of the superego are incorporated into the pathologic grandiose self. This leads to a superego containing only the aggressively determined components (the early prohibiting and threatening aspects of the parental images distorted under the impact of the projection onto them of the child's own aggressive impulses). This successfully harsh superego also tends to be dissociated and projected, which leads to further development of "persecutory" external objects and to the loss of the normal functions of the superego in regulating self-esteem, such as monitoring and approval.

The devaluation of others, the emptying out of the internal world of object representations, is a major contributing cause of the narcissistic personality's lack of normal self-esteem and also determines the remarkable inability to empathize with others. The sense of internal void can be compensated for only by endless admiration from others and by efforts to control others to avoid the envy that would otherwise be caused by the autonomous functioning, enjoyment of life, and creativity others enjoy.

Diagnosis and Differential Diagnosis

The narcissistic personality disorder must be differentiated from the antisocial personality disorder. In my view, the *DSM-III* diagnostic criteria for the antisocial personality disorder are problematic. As Frances[43] has pointed out, crucial clinical criteria for the antisocial personality disorder, such as a capacity for loyalty to others, guilt, anticipatory anxiety, and learning from past experiences, are missing. The antisocial personality presents a complete absence of the capacity for concern for others, lacks any capacity to invest in a relation with others that is not of an exploitative, self-serving nature, is incapable of realistic consideration of the future, and cannot understand the moral functions of other persons. Every patient who raises the question of the diagnosis of a narcissistic personality disorder, and who presents antisocial trends (such as a history of chronic lying, stealing, writing false checks, breaking in, association with criminal elements, drug dealing, prostitution, violent assaults, and financial irresponsibility), requires the ruling out of an antisocial personality disorder. This is particularly true for patients presenting the syndrome of malignant narcissism.

The narcissistic personality disorder also must be differentiated from the compulsive personality disorder (the obsessive-compulsive personality), because of the similarity of emotional restriction. The obsessive-compulsive personality, however, presents a capacity for highly differentiated relations with others, for self-awareness and for empa-

thy with others, manifest by the capacity for giving highly differentiated descriptions of significant others in contrast to the narcissistic patients' inability to convey to others an account in depth of persons significant in his life. The obsessive-compulsive patient also has a capacity for commitment in depth to others, for commitment to value systems and, if anything, an excessively rigid set of internalized value systems ("excessive superego pressures") in contrast to the more regressive superego pathology of narcissistic patients.

Another frequent differential diagnosis is with the hysterical and the hysteroid, infantile, or histrionic personality disorders. The *DSM-III*, unfortunately, does not include the hysterical personality disorder proper but only the regressive counterpart to it—the hysteroid or infantile personality, under the headings of histrionic personality disorder and borderline personality disorder. The differential diagnosis with the hysterical personality is necessary particularly with women with narcissistic personality disorder. The sexualized exhibitionism of hysterical patients needs to be differentiated from the cold exhibitionism of the narcissistic personality. The latter is accompanied by a lack of capacity for commitment in depth to a sexual relationship, a tendency toward cold manipulativeness, and a need to control sexual relations. These characteristics are in contrast to the capacity for warmth, commitment, empathy, and highly differentiated relations in the nonsexual sphere of the hysterical personality.

The sexual promiscuity of hysterical and masochistic-depressive personalities needs to be differentiated from the sexual promiscuity of the narcissistic personality disorder. In both sexes, hysterical and masochistic-depressive sexual promiscuity usually represent the acting out of unconscious guilt over sexual intimacy, reflected in the capacity for stable and deep sexual relations with a sadistically experienced object. Narcissistic promiscuity, in contrast, has a detached, coldly exploitative quality or, at least, an indication of a general incapacity for a full relation in depth with others.

The "hypermasculine" demeanor, sexual promiscuity, and histrionic or childlike attitudes or some male narcissistic personalities warrant the differential diagnosis with the hysterical personality disorder in men—what used to be called the "phallic-narcissistic character."[44] The much higher differentiation and quality of object relations in this latter personality disorder, the absence of inordinate envy, grandiosity, and devaluation, and the higher potential for sublimatory channeling, along with mature object relations in the nonsexual realm of the hysterical patient, facilitate this differential diagnosis.

The narcissistic personality disorder at the low level of the continuum described earlier, that is, the narcissistic personality functioning on an overtly borderline level, must be differentiated from the histrionic and/or borderline personality disorder as the *DSM-III* defines it. The most important differentiating feature is the emotional dependency and clingingness of the histrionic, infantile, or hysteroid personality, and the borderline personality disorder, which contrasts to the emotional aloofness of the narcissistic personality disorder.

The social isolation and withdrawal of the schizoid personality disorder can be differentiated from the narcissistic personality disorder by the usually easy and smooth surface social interactions of the narcissistic personality disorder and by the surprisingly subtle and differentiated capacity for evaluating others in depth that is often present in the schizoid personality disorder. Similarly, the atypically timid narcissistic personality does not present the schizoid personality's subtlety and capacity for empathy with others. In all these instances, the combination of several of the chief character features typical for the narcissistic personality disorder usually facilitates the differential diagnosis.

A particularly difficult differential diagnosis is of the narcissistic and the paranoid personality disorders. As already mentioned, some patients with narcissistic personality disorder have marked paranoid features, particularly those functioning at a low or overtly borderline level. There are cases with combined paranoid and narcissistic features and sometimes the decision of which of these two character constellations is dominant must depend on the quality of the prevalent object relations. The typical paranoid personality disorder may be distant, aloof, and suspicious of others, but he does not present the exploitativeness, inordinate envy, devaluation, or childlike grandiosity of the narcissistic personality. The paranoid grandiosity is usually linked with self-righteousness, an ego-syntonic "justified indignation." Ego-syntonic aggression without exploitativeness or inordinate envy speaks for a dominant paranoid structure.

Finally, regarding this same combination of narcissistic and paranoid features, there are patients with atypical paranoid psychoses and patients with paranoid schizophrenia who present grandiose delusions that lend themselves to confusion with narcissistic grandiosity. In all cases of marked, conscious grandiose ideas, it is extremely important to evaluate the patient's reality testing. Loss of reality testing regarding such grandiose ideas indicates a psychotic illness.

Treatment and Prognosis

All three contemporary psychoanalytic approaches to the treatment of narcissistic personalities (Kohut's self-psychology, Rosenfeld's Kleinian approach, and my ego psychology object relations views) agree that psychoanalysis is the treatment of choice for these patients. It needs to be pointed out, however, that Kohut has limited himself to discussing the treatment of analyzable patients with this disorder, whereas Rosenfeld and I have broadened the spectrum of our investigations to include narcissistic personalities with overtly borderline features. Rosenfeld still maintains that this latter group should also be treated by psychoanalysis, but I propose that narcissistic patients with overtly borderline functioning usually have serious contraindications for psychoanalysis proper and should be treated by exploratory or expressive psychotherapy.[39] If psychoanalytic psychotherapy is contraindicated, I propose supportive psychotherapy as the treatment of choice.

Rosenfeld's psychoanalytic technique pretty much coincides with the general technical approach of the Kleinian school of psychoanalysis. It is modified for narcissistic personality disorders only insofar as the specific primitive defenses and object relations of these patients should be explored systematically in the transference. Rosenfeld stresses the importance of interpreting both positive and negative transferences and only modifies his technique with narcissistic patients functioning at the overtly borderline level by exploring very carefully the reality situation that triggers paranoid psychotic transference regressions in order to contain and reduce such regressions.[12]

Kohut stresses the need for permitting the development of the patient's narcissistic idealization of the analyst and avoidance of premature interpretation or reality considerations. This permits the gradual unfolding of mirror transferences. The patient relives the earlier traumatic experiences with a more mature psyche and acquires new psychic structures, with the help of the analyst as self-object, by the process of transmuting internalization. The psychoanalyst must be basically empathic, focusing on understanding the patient's narcissistic needs and frustrations rather than on the drive derivatives and conflicts that emerge at times of narcissistic frustration in the analytic situation. In each of these conditions of narcissistic frustration, the psychoanalyst explores with the patient where and how the analyst has failed in being appropriately empathic and how this relates to past failures of the significant object of the patient's childhood. Kohut insists that this does not require the establishing parameters of technique, that it represents a modification of the standard psychoanalytic technique for non-narcissistic patients only in that it stresses the analyst's empathy in contrast to "objective neutrality" and focuses on the vicissitudes of the self rather than on drives and (not yet existent) interstructural conflicts.

In my view, the most important aspect of the psychoanalytic treatment of narcissistic personalities is the systematic analysis of the pathologic grandiose self as presented in the transference. The activation of the grandiose self can be detected in the psychoanalytic situation by the patient's emotional unavailability, a subtle but persistent absence of the normal or "real" aspects of the relationship between the patient and analyst in which the patient treats the analyst as a specific individual. In contrast, the activation of the patient's pathologic self-idealization alternating with the projection of such self-idealization onto the analyst, conveys the impression that there is only one (ideal, grandiose) person and an admiring yet shadowy complement to it in the room. Frequent role reversals between patient and analyst illustrate this basically stable transference pattern. The analyst has to interpret this transference pattern and the primitive defense mechanisms recruited in its service. This includes the interpretation of the expression of omnipotent control in the transference, of the defensive use of rage reactions, of sudden devaluation of the analyst and his comments, and of negative therapeutic reactions following times when the patient experiences the analyst as helpful. Generally speaking, the primitive defensive operations of omnipotent control, projective identification, primitive idealization, and devaluation are prevalent in the transference of narcissistic patients throughout their treatment and require systematic working through.

Behind the apparently simple activation of narcissistic rage lies the activation of specific primitive unconscious internalized object relations of the past, typically of split-off self- and object representations reflecting condensed oedipal-preoedipal

conflicts. These conflicts may gradually emerge as the pathologic grandiose self is analytically resolved, with a breakthrough of primitive transferences expressing paranoid distrust, direct aggression in the transference, and, eventually, differentiated enactments of internalized object relations in a repetitive alternation or interchange with the analyst of representations of the patient's real and ideal self, ideal objects, and real objects. In the final stages of resolution of the grandiose self, the treatment situation usually resembles that of the psychoanalysis of neurotic patients in that the patient can now establish a real dependence on the analyst, can explore both his oedipal and preoedipal conflicts in a differentiated fashion, and can simultaneously normalize his pathologic object relations and his narcissistic regulatory mechanisms.

The detailed aspects of psychoanalytic technique within any of these competing formulations are beyond the limitations of the present summary. So far, there are no controlled empiric studies available comparing these competing treatment approaches. The discussions regarding their respective merits and problems are based exclusively on the clinical experience of psychoanalysts specializing in this area.

The techniques of psychoanalytic psychotherapy and of supportive psychotherapy with narcissistic personalities functioning on an overt borderline level have been subject even less to systematic validation. I have spelled out both the principles and technique of expressive or exploratory psychotherapy and of supportive psychotherapy for these patients.[39]

In essence, as mentioned earlier, narcissistic personalities functioning on an overt borderline level should be treated with expressive or exploratory psychotherapy rather than psychoanalysis proper. The general psychotherapeutic technique for these cases coincides with that for the borderline spectrum of character pathology ("borderline personality organization"), but with a particular focus on the analysis in the transference of the defensive functions of the pathologic grandiose self and the characteristic defensive operations. Excessive severity of antisocial features, severe and potentially dangerous acting out, severe lack of anxiety tolerance and/or impulse control, and secondary gain of illness are indications for a shift from an expressive to a supportive modality of psychotherapy. Within a supportive psychotherapy, the inappropriate or maladaptive consequences of primitive defensive operations and the pathologic grandiose self may be reduced by stressing reality in tactful and supportive ways and better compromise solutions between character restrictions and environmental adaptive requirements may be worked out.

There are no systematic studies of the prognosis with and without treatment of the narcissistic personality disorder. In my view, the general prognosis for treatment of these patients depends on the extent to which some stability and depth of object relations are still available, and the extent to which antisocial features are present. An additional prognostically crucial dimension is the extent to which aggression has been integrated into the pathologic grandiose self, typical for the syndrome of malignant narcissism. The prognosis here is particularly reserved, and these patients usually have a contraindication for psychoanalysis proper.

Patients with narcissistic personality disorder who do not present significant antisocial features, infiltration of the grandiose self with aggression, or overtly borderline features (that is, patients who can maintain tolerance for anxiety, impulse control, and have a capacity for sublimation) have a favorable prognosis with psychoanalytic treatment. This clinical impression still needs to be empirically validated.

REFERENCES

1. Ellis H: Auto-erotism: A psychological study. Alienist Neurolgist 19:260–299, 1982
2. Nacke P: Die sexuellen Perversitaten in der Irrenanstalt. Psychiatrische en Neurologische Bladen 3, 1899
3. Sadger J: Fragment der Psychoanalyse eines Homosexuellen. Jahrbuch fur Sexuelle Zwischenstufen 9:339–424, 1908
4. Freud S: On narcissism: An introduction. In Strachey J (ed): The Standard Edition of the Complete Works of Sigmund Freud, Vol 14, pp 69–102. London, Hogarth Press, 1914
5. Jones E: The God complex. In Essays in Applied Psycho-Analysis, vol 2, pp 244–265. London, Hogarth Press, 1951
6. Abraham K: A particular form of neurotic resistance against the psychoanalytic method. In Selected Papers of Karl Abraham. London, Hogarth Press, 1949
7. Riviere J: A contribution to the analysis of the negative therapeutic reaction. Int J Psychoanal 17:304–320, 1936
8. Klein M: Envy and Gratitude. New York, Basic Books, 1957
9. Rosenfeld H: On the psychopathology of narcissism: A clinical approach. Int J Psychoanal 45:332–337, 1964
10. Rosenfeld H: A clinical approach to the psychoanalytic theory of the life and death instincts: An investigation into the aggressive aspects of narcissism. Int J Psychoanal 52:169–178, 1971
11. Rosenfeld H: Negative therapeutic reaction. In Giovacchini PL (ed): Tactics and Techniques in Psychoanalytic Therapy, Vol II, Countertransference, pp 217–228. New York, Jason Aronson, 1975
12. Rosenfeld H: Notes on the psychopathology and psychoanalytic treatment of some borderline patients. Int J Psychoanal 59:215–221, 1978
13. Reich A: Narcissistic object choice in women. J Am Psychoanal Assoc 1:22–44, 1953
14. Reich A: Pathologic forms of self-esteem regulation. Psychoanal Study Child 15:215–232, 1960
15. Jacobson E: The Self and the Object World. New York, International Universities Press, 1964
16. van der Waals H: Problems of narcissism. Bull Menninger Clin 29:293–311, 1965
17. Tartakoff H: The normal personality in our culture and the Nobel prize complex. In Loewenstein RM, Newman LM, Schur M, Solnit AJ (eds): Psychoanalysis: A General Psychology. New York, International Universities Press, 1966
18. Kernberg O: Borderline personality organization. J Am Psychoanal Assoc 15:641–685, 1967
19. Kernberg O: Factors in the treatment of narcissistic personalities. J Am Psychoanal Assoc 18:51–85, 1970
20. Kernberg O: Further contributions to the treatment of narcissistic personalities. Int J Psychoanal 55:215–240, 1974
21. Kernberg O: Borderline Conditions and Pathological Narcissism. New York, Jason Aronson, 1975
22. Kohut H: The psychoanalytic treatment of narcissistic personality disorders. Psychoanal Study Child 23:86–113, 1968
23. Kohut H: The Analysis of the Self. New York, International Universities Press, 1971
24. Kohut H: Thoughts on narcissism and narcissistic rage. Psychoanal Study Child 27:360–400, 1972
25. Kohut H: The Restoration of the Self. New York, International Universities Press, 1977
26. Kohut H: Two analyses of Mr Z. Int J Psychoanal 60:3–27, 1979
27. Grunberger B: Narcissism: Psychoanalytic Essays. New York, International Universities Press, 1979
28. Pulver S: Narcissism: The term and the concept. J Am Psychoanal Assoc 18:319–341, 1970
29. Modell A: The holding environment and the therapeutic action of psychoanalysis. J Am Psychoanal Assoc 24:255–307, 1976
30. Volkan V: Transitional fantasies in the analysis of a narcissistic personality. J Am Psychoanal Assoc 21:351–376, 1973
31. Volkan V: The "glass bubble" of the narcissistic patient. In Leboit J, Capponi A (eds): Advances in Psychotherapy of the Borderline Patient. New York, Jason Aronson, 1979
32. Bach S: Narcissism, continuity and the uncanny. Int J Psychoanal 56:77–86, 1975
33. Bach S: On narcissistic fantasies. Int Rev Psychoanal 4:281–293, 1977
34. Bach S: On the narcissistic state of consciousness. Int J Psychoanal 58:209–233, 1977
35. Akhtar S, Thomson JA Jr: Overview: Narcissistic personality disorder. Am J Psychiatry 139:12–20, 1982
36. Lasch C: The Culture of Narcissism: American Life in an Age of Diminishing Expectations. New York, WW Norton, 1978

37. Kernberg O: Internal World and External Reality. New York, Jason Aronson, 1980

38. Egan J, Kernberg P: Pathological narcissism in childhood. J Am Psychoanal Assoc 32:39–62, 1984

39. Kernberg O: Severe Personality Disorders: Psychotherapeutic Strategies. New Haven, Yale University Press, 1984

40. Mahler M, Furer M: On Human Symbiosis and the Vicissitudes of Individuation. New York, International Universities Press, 1968

41. Mahler M, Pine F, Bergman A: The Psychological Birth of the Human Infant. New York, Basic Books, 1975

42. Mahler M: Selected Papers of Margaret S. Mahler. New York, Jason Aronson, 1979

43. Frances A: The DSM-III personality disorders section: A commentary. Am J Psychiatry 137:1050–1054, 1980

44. Reich W: Character Analysis. New York, Farrar, Strauss & Giroux, 1933

Hysterical and Histrionic Personality Disorders

Definitions

Two related personality disorders are described in this chapter. First is the hysterical personality disorder, characterized by an essentially intact sense of identity; the capacity for stable, discriminating, emotionally rich and empathic, internal and interpersonal relations with others, including the capacity to tolerate ambivalence and complexity; and a predominance of defense mechanisms centering on repression. The hysterical personality disorder as here defined is not listed in the *Diagnostic and Statistical Manual of Mental Disorders (DSM-III)*.

The second is the histrionic personality disorder, which is included as here defined under that heading in the *DSM-III*. The histrionic personality disorder corresponds to what others have called the "infantile," the "hysteroid," the "hysteroid dysphoric," the "emotionally unstable," and the Zetzel[1] type 3 and 4 hysterics (patients whose manifest hysterical symptoms disguise deeper pathology). The histrionic personality disorder belongs to a group of severe regressive personality disorders characterized by "borderline personality organization," that is, these patients present the syndrome of identity diffusion (or lack of identity integration), severe pathology of object relations, and a predominance of primitive defensive operations centering around the mechanism of splitting. Identity diffusion, the central feature of borderline personality organization, is characterized by a lack of integration of the self-concept and concepts of significant others, reflected in an inability to differentiate relationships with other people and to evaluate others in depth, and the consequently inappropriate selection of sexual and marital partners.

Both the hysterical and histrionic personality disorders present different characteristics in men and women that warrant separate descriptions for them. The features of both personality disorders common to both genders should become apparent in these descriptions.

Controversial Issues

Confusing and overlapping terminology plague this area of the personality disorders, as well as shifting clinical and theoretic frames of reference that deal with psychopathology formerly brought together under the heading of "hysteria."

A number of empiric studies carried out during the past 30 years here and abroad (comprehensively summarized by Mersky,[2] the contributors to Roy's volume on *Hysteria*,[3] and Cavenar and Walker[4]) have provided some clarification of these questions, while pointing to areas in which lack of aggreement and information persists.

First, there exists an emerging agreement that the more severe the patient's personality disorder within the hysterical spectrum, the more likely it is that severe and multiple somatic symptoms corresponding to "conversion hysteria" will be present. By the same token, patients with the severe type of "dissociative reactions" or even psychotic reactions who in the past might have been classified as "hysterical psychoses" are also patients who present the more severe type of personality disturbances within the broad spectrum called "hysterical" in the past. However, these severe personality disturbances appear to overlap with the personality disturbances now classified under the "borderline" spectrum.

To the contrary, the more typical the personality disorder corresponds to the "hysterical personality" of the psychoanalytic literature (*i.e.*, personality disturbances close to the better functioning or "neurotic" end of the "hysterical" personality spectrum), the weaker are the connections between conversion symptoms, dissociative reactions, and the hysterical personality disorder proper. In short, the paradoxic impression conveyed by the literature on hysteria of the past 30 years is that the relation between personality disorder, conversion reaction, and dissociative reaction is strongest when the personality disturbances are most severe and merge with other severe personality types and that this relationship is weakest when the hysterical personality appears with its most distinctive characteristics.

The recent tendency to make a sharper distinction between the conversion syndrome, the dissociative syndrome, and the personality disorder seems, therefore, a reasonable first approach to clarifying this entire area of psychopathology.

Turning to the hysterical personality proper, the chief problem that has been debated in the literature over the years[5-17] is whether the hysterical personality should be considered in terms of severity of pathologic character traits ranging from a high or "neurotic" level to a low or "borderline" level, or whether a distinction should be made between two restricted, circumscribed specific disorders. The first would be the "hysterical personality disorder" functioning within the "neurotic" range and corresponding to the classic psychoanalytic descriptions formulated by Abraham,[18] Wittels,[19] Reich,[20] and Fenichel.[21] The second would be the personality disorder that corresponds to the more regressive, "borderline" level of personality organization, referred to in the literature as the "hysteroid,"[7] "Zetzel type 3 and 4,"[1] or "infantile" personality.[22]

A careful exploration of the *DSM-III* definition of the histrionic personality disorder places this personality disorder clearly within this second, more severely disturbed type. It could be argued that the *DSM-III* has opted for designating the entire spectrum of the hysterical personality disorder under the heading histrionic personality disorder, rather than adopting the restrictive, two-type solution referred to here. The clinical description of this disorder in the *DSM-III*, however, negates such an as-

sumption: the description corresponds only to the regressive end of the spectrum and leaves out what might be called the "hysterical personality."

In short, the problem of the spectrum of hysterical personality disorders merges, at the pole of severest conditions, with that of the description of the borderline patient. Regardless of where one stands in terms of the conceptual, clinical, and research issues that may influence one's view regarding this area of psychopathology, the following conclusions are suggested as a reasonable approach to clarifying at least the semantic issues involved:

The classic hysterical personality includes a broad spectrum of related pathologic character traits ranging from the hysterical personality disorder proper at the "higher" level to the "histrionic" (in the sense of *DSM-III*), or hysteroid, or infantile, or Zetzel type 3 and 4 personality disorder at the lower level.

This "lower level" personality disorder also corresponds to what *DSM-III* and the empiric researchers working in this area have designated the "borderline personality disorder." The psychostructural concept of Stone[23] and Kernberg[24] considers the infantile personality (or borderline personality disorder in the *DSM-III* sense) as one personality type within the broader spectrum of "borderline personality organization," characterized by identity diffusion, a predominance of primitive defensive operations, and good reality testing.

For heuristic reasons, in what follows the term *hysterical personality disorder* will be used to describe the higher level of this continuum and will be described separately from the "histrionic personality disorder," which corresponds to the lower level of this spectrum and coincides with the infantile personality, the Zetzel type 3 and 4 personality, and the histrionic personality disorder in the *DSM-III*. Actually, however, the clinician will find patients that present intermediate levels of psychopathology, so that these "pure," "polar" types may either be considered as extreme types of a continuum or discrete personality types with intermediate forms.

Epidemiology

Studies of the prevalence of the hysterical and the histrionic personality disorders have been affected by the conceptual and semantic confusions troubling this area of personality disorders. A few general agreements seem to be emerging, but even these are subject to question. For example, are the hysterical and the histrionic personality disorders found much more frequently in women than in men because the description of these personality disorders has been in terms related mostly to the psychology of women? It is possible that the development of diagnostic approaches focusing on the psychopathology of women have produced an artificially high female-to-male sex ratio for these disorders.[6,25]

Clinical experience gives the impression that both the hysterical and the histrionic personality disorders are frequently found in outpatient populations and only the histrionic personality disorder is a frequent diagnosis on psychiatric inpatient services. There are, however, so far no reliable epidemiologic studies of the overall prevalence of these personality disorders and of their relationship to socioeconomic and cultural factors. Many hypotheses formulated in this area still require validation. Comprehensive summaries of current epidemiologic hypotheses and findings regarding the hysterical and the histrionic personality disorders may be found in the work of Temoshok and Attkisson[26] and in Cavenar and Walker's overview.[4]

Clinical Descriptions

HYSTERICAL PERSONALITY IN WOMEN

A dominant characteristic in women with hysterical personality is their emotional lability. They relate easily to others and are capable of warm and sustained emotional involvements—with the important exception of an inhibition in their sexual responsiveness. They are usually dramatic and even histrionic, but their display of affects is controlled and has socially adaptive qualities. The way they dramatize their emotional experiences may give the impression that their emotions are superficial, but exploration reveals otherwise: their emotional experiences are authentic. These women may be emotionally labile, but they are not inconsistent or unpredictable in their emotional reactions. They lose emotional control only selectively, vis-à-vis a few closely related persons concerning whom they have intense conflicts, especially of a sexual and competitive nature.

With these particular people, hysterical women are prone to develop emotional crises, but they al-

ways have the capacity to ''snap out'' of such crises and evaluate them realistically afterward. They may cry easily and tend toward sentimentality and romanticism, but their cognitive capacities are intact and their understanding of complex human reactions is in sharp contrast to the apparent immaturity of their emotional display. The difference between their generally appropriate social interactions and the specific object relations that have sexual implications represents a general tendency to show infantile, regressive behavior only in circumstances that are either actually or symbolically sexual or that are concerned with persons they experience as having parental functions. These women's impulsiveness is restricted to such specific interactions or to occasional temper tantrums.

Hysterical patients tend to be essentially extraverted, outgoing, and involved with others. This extraversion shows in easy social contacts and blends with a tendency to exhibitionism and excessive dependence on others. Hysterical personalities want to be loved, to be the center of attention and attraction, particularly in circumstances with sexual implications. Their dependence on other persons' judgment and evaluation of them is balanced by a clear sense of what socially realistic requirements they must meet to obtain such love and approval, and their childlike, clinging dependency is confined to sexual contexts. In fact, the childlike attitudes in intimate relations and generally mature attitudes in ordinary social interactions are key characteristics of the hysterical personality.

Some hysterical women may seem shy or timid but nonetheless subtly convey a provocative, sexual seductiveness that may even be accentuated by this timidity.

Women with hysterical personality typically show a pseudo hypersexuality in combination with sexual inhibition; they are both sexually provocative and frigid. Their sexual involvements have ''triangular qualities'' in that they are with unavailable men or men involved with other women. Their provocative behavior may induce sexual responses from men, which these women may then experience as intrusive or shocking and to which they react with fear, indignation, and rejection.

The hysterical woman is competitive both with men and with other women for men. The competitiveness with men contains implicit fears and conflicts having to do with a consciously or unconsciously assumed inferiority to them. Subtypes of a submissive or competitive hysterical personality reflect charcterologic fixations of these submissive (often masochistic) and competitive patterns. Psychoanalytic exploration typically reveals that regressive infantile behavior is being used defensively against the guilt aroused by the adult aspects of sexual involvement. Some women tend to submit to men whom they experience as sadistic in expiation of guilt feelings and as a price to be paid for sexual gratification. Intense competitiveness with men compensates for fantasied inferiority to them, or, to the contrary, self-defeating behaviors in competitive situations with men are an expression of deep-seated fantasies of inferiority to them. What is of great interest is the difference between the nature of the competitiveness with men and with women in these patients, in contrast to the more regressively undifferentiated patterns of pathologic reactions toward men and women in patients with histrionic personality disorder. Some additional aspects of the hysterical personality described in the early literature have recently been questioned. For instance, it had earlier been assumed that hysterical patients were highly suggestible. Recent observations point to the idea that suggestibility may emerge only in the context of idealized, romanticized, and clingingly dependent relations and that it may easily change to suspiciousness, distrust, pouting, or stubbornness under conditions of intense competitiveness with men or women. Another characteristic classically attributed to the hysterical personality is excessive dependency. However, as mentioned before, inappropriate, infantile, clinging dependency only characterizes a few, very intense relations. A third assumed characteristic of hysterical patients was that of "egocentricity," a self-centered, self-indulgent, vain quality conveyed by the exhibitionistic, attention-seeking behavior of these patients and their excessive sensitivity to other people's reaction. But such a characteristic does not correspond to their actual capacity for deep involvements with others, their stability in engagements, their loyalty, and their commitment. By the same token, other characteristics that imply lack of capacity for emotional investment coupled with deficiency in moral functioning are definitely not part of this personality disorder. Thus, for example, the early literature mentioned emotional shallowness, fraudulent affects, mendacity, and pseudologia fantastica: all these are characteristics that may be found in the histrionic personality disorder but are definitely not part of the hysterical personality disorder, which, to the contrary, usually displays a solid and well-integrated superego structure reflected in normal moral functioning, absence of antisocial features and, as mentioned before, the capacity for object relations in depth.

Shapiro[27] and Horowitz[28] have described a cognitive style of hysterical patients characterized by their tendency toward global (in contrast to detailed) perception, selective inattention, and impressionistic rather than accurate representations. These characteristics may reflect a generally repressive organization of defensive functions, which, together with inhibition of competitiveness (because of an unconscious sense of inferiority as a woman), may contribute to intellectual inhibition.

HYSTERICAL PERSONALITY IN MEN

Blacker and Tupin[14] have summarized the characteristics of male patients with hysterical and histrionic personality disorders (their descriptions used a model of continuity of character pathology ranging in severity under the global heading of "hysterical structures"). Men with hysterical personality reveal the same tendency toward emotional dramatization and affective lability seen in hysterical women. They also present emotional outbursts or temper tantrums and impulsive and infantile behavior under conditions of intimate emotional involvements, while maintaining the capacity for differentiated behavior under ordinary social circumstances.

Several patterns of disturbances in their sexual adaptation characterize men with hysterical personality. One pattern is characterized by a pseudo hypermasculine quality, a histrionic accentuation of culturally accepted masculine patterns, usually a stress on independence, and an attitude of dominance and superiority over women, combined with childlike sulkiness when such aspirations cannot be fulfilled. A related, though superficially an apparently contrasting pattern is that of a seductive, subtly effeminate, infantile sexual behavior that combines flirtatiousness and heterosexual promiscuity with a dependent, childlike attitude toward women. Or there is a type of childlike Don Juan who combines a stress on masculine attires and manners with a subtly dependent and childlike behavior, prone to engage in dependent though transitory relations with dominant women. Both the effeminate and hypermasculine types reveal in treatment underlying conscious or unconscious guilt over sexual relations in depth with women, a surprising inability to identify with an adult male sexual role in approaching women that is in sharp contrast to their surface behavior. These characteristics, particularly as presented by the pseudo hypermasculine type correspond to what used to be called the "phalic-narcissistic character."[20] These cases need to be differentiated from the more severe, histrionic personality disorder in men and from sexual promiscuity as a symptom of the narcissistic personality disorder in men with the corresponding severe pathology of object relations.

HISTRIONIC PERSONALITY IN WOMEN

These patients' self-centered, self-indulgent behavior may still be accompanied by the capacity for and need of intense dependency on others, but their general clinging dependency needs do not show the mutuality of the relationships of the hysterical personality disorder. At the same time, histrionic patients still do have a higher capacity for emotional involvements than the emotionally aloof and distant narcissistic personality disorder. Their very clingingness and the stability of their highly immature involvements contrast to the absence of this feature in the narcissistic personality.

In contrast to the hysterical personality disorder, histrionic personalities present diffuse emotional lability, undifferentiated relations with significant others, and immature, self-centered emotional investments. In contrast to the socially appropriate extraversion of the hysterical personality, the histrionic personality overidentifies with others and projects unrealistic, fantasied intentions onto them. Here the dramatization of affects, the emotionally volatile and labile behavior, the general excitability, and the inconsistency of reactions convey an underlying emotional shallowness and lack of the capacity for differentiated object relations. Histrionic personalities have difficulty understanding others, as well as themselves, in depth, and the childlike, clinging nature of all their object relationships contrasts to the differentiated capabilities of the hysterical personality in this respect. Their selection of marital and/or sexual partners is usually highly inappropriate.

Dependent and exhibitionistic traits are less sexualized in the histrionic personality disorder than in the hysterical personality disorder, in the sense that the histrionic personality seeks a childlike dependency in itself rather than as a defense against more mature sexual commitments. The histrionic personality may use sexualized behavior crudely and inappropriately to express exhibitionistic and dependent needs. The histrionic personality tends to have fewer sexual inhibitions and is more frequently promiscuous than the hysterical personality. There are fewer repressive features in the histrionic personality's sexual life and more generalized dissociative features, such as the alternation of contradictory sexual fantasies and engagements (expressed in polymorphous infantile sexual behavior). In the pathology of interpersonal relations, the

degree of disturbance in any particular interpersonal relationship is in proportion to the intensity of involvement or intimacy with the other person.

The histrionic personality disorder may present masochistic tendencies, but these are less closely linked to sexual behaviors. Histrionic personalities have diffuse impulsive tendencies, which make for an unpredictability that reinforces the unstable and intense relations with others, and they show inappropriate, intense anger or lack of control of anger and severe mood swings. They are prone to suicide gestures and attempts and to use authentic suicide fantasies and wishes to attract attention and reassurance. Manipulative suicide threats are only one aspect of generally manipulative interpersonal relations, and these patients frequently lie and manifest antisocial behavior and pseudologia fantastica. These latter cases require differentiating from the antisocial and narcissistic personality disorders: the prognosis, with or without treatment, is much poorer for the antisocial personality.

Histrionic patients are prone to develop feelings of depersonalization and, under extreme stress, transitory psychotic symptoms of insufficient severity or duration to warrant an additional diagnosis. These characteristics, in addition to their identity disturbances and the general characteristics already described, also correspond to these listed for the borderline personality disorder in the *DSM-III*. With these reservations, the diagnostic criteria for the histrionic personality disorder outlined in the *DSM-III* adequately cover the crucial characteristics of female patients with this personality disorder.

HISTRIONIC PERSONALITY IN MEN

These patients also present the characteristics of identity diffusion, severe disturbances in object relations, and lack of impulse control. Histrionic personalities in men usually present severely promiscuous, often bisexual and polymorphous perverse sexual behavior, antisocial tendencies, and, with surprising frequency, conscious or unconscious exploitation of organically determined or psychogenically determined physical symptoms. Male patients with "compensation neurosis" and/or hypochondriasis often present the generalized emotional immaturity, dramatization, affective shallowness, and impulsiveness characteristic of the histrionic personality disorder, together with antisocial features and exploitative tendencies in their relation to the helping professions. These so-called chaotic or impulse-ridden personality disorders of earlier descriptions that did not correspond to the antisocial personality proper reflected what today would be diagnosed as histrionic and narcissistic personality disorders functioning on an overt borderline level. In fact, in all cases of male patients with histrionic features, the differential diagnosis with the narcissistic personality and the antisocial personality disorders is important for its prognostic and therapeutic implications.

HYSTERICAL AND HISTRIONIC PERSONALITY DISORDERS IN CHILDREN AND ADOLESCENTS

Hysterical and histrionic personality disorders in children have received increasing attention in recent years.[29-31] Both the hysterical and the histrionic or infantile personality disorders may be observed in girls from the ages of 6 to 8 years on, thus contributing clinical evidence in this area that is accumulating for other personality disorders as well, namely, that at least some of them may be diagnosed and treated in the later years of childhood. These observations are as yet too limited, however, to warrant a systematic description of these personality disorders in childhood.

The hysterical personality disorder is diagnosed quite frequently from late adolescence on and may first become apparent in the context of sexual inhibition, heterosexual conflicts, and work or study inhibitions. Similarly, the histrionic personality disorder also becomes evident during adolescence, and the more severe the personality disorder, the earlier it may disrupt an adolescent's life. The firm social structuring of an early adolescent's life may compensate for milder types of personality disorder, but the deep emotional turmoil, the difficulty in establishing object relations in depth, and the failure at school and work bring patients with histrionic personality disorder to the attention of the helping profession.

Clinical Course and Prognosis

Although there are no empiric studies as yet providing solid evidence regarding the prognosis for the hysterical and the histrionic personality disorders, women with hysterical personality disorder have been observed to improve their functioning in later adulthood and old age, raising the question to what extent the good ego strength of these patients,

their capacity for engagement with others, in work and professions, and the gradual compensation of sexual inhibitions and conflicts throughout life may combine in facilitating a better social and intrapsychic adaptation in later years. The histrionic personality disorder, in contrast, appears to decompensate in later adulthood and old age. The cumulative effects of the incapacity to pursue personal, professional, cultural, and social values, the frequent disruption of and failure in intimate relations, and the identity diffusion typical of these patients' personality may interfere with ordinary social learning and create a circular reaction that worsens their functioning with the years.

The hysterical personality disorder has an excellent prognosis with psychoanalytic treatment. The histrionic personality disorder has only a moderately favorable prognosis within modified psychoanalytic treatment but a better prognosis with psychoanalytic or exploratory psychotherapy, with varying degrees of parameters of technique. The development of psychoanalytic psychotherapy for the borderline spectrum of personality disorders in recent years has improved the prognosis for these patients. The psychotherapy research project of the Menninger Foundation[32] is the first and only empiric study of the outcome of long-term psychotherapy with these cases.

Etiology

GENETIC STUDIES

The persisting failure to differentiate the hysterical from the histrionic personality disorders in empiric studies and the confusing tendency in some epidemiologic studies to lump the interpersonal disturbances of a hysterical or histrionic kind with the antisocial personality seriously weaken the currently available contributions to the genetics of these personality disorders. In my view, there is as yet no evidence for genetic predisposition to the personality disorders within the hysterical-histrionic spectrum.

PSYCHOANALYTIC CONTRIBUTIONS

The hysterical personality disorder was the principal type of psychopathology that Freud[33-37] explored in both developing and applying the psychoanalytic theory of the neuroses. The Dora case[33] continues as a basic illustration of the unconscious impulses and defenses described in the psychoanalytic theory of these disorders and the transference manifestations of these unconscious conflicts in psychoanalytic treatment.

Krohn[15] offers a masterful summary of Freud's basic contributions to the psychoanalytic understanding of the hysterical personality. Krohn states:

(1) hysteria involves an infantile conflict at the phallic-oedipal stage; (2) the hysterical ego resorts primarily to repression, dissociation, amnesia and, less important, to reaction formation as defenses; (3) the hysterical symptom commonly shows itself as a conversion reaction, hysterical attack, or phobia, and carries with it secondary advantages; (4) the hysteric's superego tends to be relatively pliable, less severe than that of the obsessional; (5) the hysterical symptom becomes synthesized with the ego and may itself secondarily become recruited to gratify the unconscious needs that it was used to fend off; (6) the hysteric tends to fend off internal conflict by internally blocking perception of or physically withdrawing from external stimuli that promised to spark unconscious needs or their derivatives; and (7) unconscious fantasy is an essential intermediary step in the formation of the hysterical symptom.

Freud stressed the essential nature of the infantile genital stage of development and of the Oedipus complex in hysteria. Abraham[18] complemented these dynamics with his study of the female castration complex, specifically, the development of a "wish-fulfillment type" and a "revenge type" of hysterical personality in women. He elaborated on aspects of penis envy as an unconscious conflict in relation to descriptive aspects of the hysterical personality. Wittels,[19] Reich,[20] and Fenichel[21] further developed an understanding of the relation of unconscious intrapsychic conflicts to the phenomenologic characteristics of the hysterical personality. They all stressed the predominance of the Oedipus complex and of castration anxiety and penis envy as dynamic features of the hysterical personality and proposed that pregenital conflicts, particularly oral fantasies and character traits, represented a defensive regression against dominant oedipal features. They all stressed the prevalence of repression and related defenses, such as displacement, affect storms, reversal of affects, and hystrical types of identification and pointed to the manifestations of instinctual conflicts and defenses in the transference neurosis of hysterical patients.

Marmor,[5] in sharp contrast to these authors, proposed that oral fixations are of basic importance in the hysterical character, that they give the subsequent Oedipus complex of these patients a strong pregenital cast, and that the greater frequency of hysteria in women as compared with men might reflect in part the cultural facilitation of "oral aggressivity, dependency, and passivity" as feminine traits, making them more acceptable in women than in men. Subsequent discussions in the psychoanalytic literature stimulated by Marmor's paper gradually led to the realization that there were indeed patients with predominently oral conflicts centering around pathologic dependency, passivity, and above all, evidence of severe disturbances in preoedipal mother–infant relations, but that these cases corresponded to what we are now calling the histrionic, infantile, or hysteroid personality disorder, whereas the psychodynamics of castration anxiety and the Oedipus complex correspond to the hysterical personality proper as now defined. Easser and Lesser,[7,8] Zetzel,[1] and Kernberg[22] focused on the relation between levels of severity within the hysterical spectrum and corresponding differences in prevalent unconscious conflicts, defensive operations, ego structure, and transference characteristics. According to these authors, the predominant conflicts of the hysterical personality proper are oedipal and relate to the genital phase of psychosexual development. The ego structure of these patients is organized around repression and is characterized by solid ego identity, as reflected in the typical manifestations of neurotic transference developments. Oral regressions in these patients are temporary defensive regressions that may be interpretively resolved, thus leading to the central oedipal conflicts. Histrionic, infantile, hysteroid, or Zetzel "type 3 and 4" personality disorders, in contrast, typically present a condensation of preoedipal and oedipal features under the predominance of preoedipal (especially oral) aggression, an ego organization centering around primitive dissociation or splitting and related defensive mechanisms, and are expressed in the treatment in the primitive "part object" transferences typical for borderline patients.

FAMILY DYNAMICS AND CULTURAL FACTORS

Although most information in this area stems from the review of patients' records and psychoanalytic exploration of individual patients' past experiences, this literature conveys a growing consensus that women with hysterical personality disorder come from rather stable families with the following characteristics. Their fathers are described as seductive, often combining sexually seductive and overstimulating behavior toward their daughters with abrupt and authoritarian and at times sexually puritanical attitudes toward them: seductiveness during childhood typically shifts into prohibition against sexual and romantic involvements in adolescence. These patients' mothers are described as domineering and controlling of their daughter's life in subtle and pervasive fashions, often conveying the impression that they were attempting to realize their unfulfilled aspirations through their daughters. At the same time, these mothers were effective and responsible at home and in their community functions.

There is less information available regarding the family background of the histrionic personality disorder. In general, it appears that these patients come from more disturbed families, with profound and chronic conflicts involving the mother–child relations and severe personality disturbances in the mothers.

A consensus seems to be growing among students of the psychodynamics of the hysterical and the histrionic personality disorders that cultural factors may play a fundamental role in determining the organization of pathologic character traits that mediate the relationships between unconscious intrapsychic conflict and social adaptation. Cultural stereotypes regarding gender roles, the power relation between the sexes, and the boundaries of encouraged and permitted (in contrast to censored, denied, or suppressed) sexual behavior are considered of crucial importance in the dynamic organization of pathologic character traits. Although the literature in this area is still mostly speculative, perhaps empiric studies will contribute to clarifying these issues beyond the temptation to decide them on the basis of theoretic bias or ideologic commitments.

Diagnosis and Differential Diagnosis

The most important differential diagnosis of the hysterical and histrionic personality disorders is, first of all, from each other. Only secondarily need they be differentiated from other personality disorders. The importance of this differential diagnosis lies in the prognosis and treatment, which are significantly different for each. The clinical description presented earlier should permit making this differential diagnosis.

Regarding the differential diagnosis with other personality disorders, the hysterical personality needs to be differentiated, first of all, from the narcissistic personality disorder with which it tends to be confused. The chief difference is in the capacity for object relations. Narcissistic personalities characteristically show a lack of capacity for investment in depth in others and for empathy; they are unstable in their sexual involvements and show a coldness that contrasts to the warmth and commitment of the hysterical personality, even if both are attention-seeking and exhibitionistic.

In women with high intelligence and a rich cultural background, the hysterical personality disorder tends to be confused with the obsessive-compulsive personality (the "Compulsive Personality Disorder" in the *DSM-III*). These women's competitiveness with men and women may take predominantly intellectual forms, giving a pseudo-obsessive quality to their rationalizations and use of intellectualization.

In hysterical women with strong masochistic features reflecting unconscious prohibitions against sexual freedom and enjoyment, the differential diagnosis with the depressive-masochistic personality disorder is of interest. This category, omitted from the *DSM-III*, has been described by Laughlin,[38] who classifies the character traits of the depressive-masochistic personality disorder as traits reflecting excessively harsh superego functioning; those reflecting overdependency on support, love, and acceptance from others; and those reflecting difficulties in the expression of aggression. In many ways, all three categories have the faulty "metabolism" of dependency needs as a predominant issue. These patients feel guilty because of intense ambivalence toward loved and needed objects, and they are easily frustrated if their dependent longings are not gratified. In contrast to the hysterical personality disorder, however, sexual conflicts and, specifically, sexual inhibition are much less dominant in their psychopathology.

The symptom of sexual promiscuity, present in the hysterical, histrionic, and narcissistic personality disorders, often leads to the exploration of the differential diagnosis of these conditions. Sexual promiscuity in the depressive-masochistic and hysterical personality disorders stems from unconscious guilt. These patients typically give evidence of stability only in sexual relations that have a masochistic quality. The hysterical personality in particular may tolerate a satisfactory sexual experience only when it is carried out under conditions of objective or symbolic suffering. These patients' capacity to understand, differentiate, and empathize with their love objects is remarkably high, in contrast to the corresponding incapacity on the part of the narcissistic personality disorder. Sexual promiscuity in the narcissistic personality disorder goes hand in hand with severe pathology of object relations. In addition, narcissistic personality disorders present the characteristic dominance of the defense mechanisms of grandiosity and omnipotence, projective identification, idealization, and devaluation, while the hysterical personality disorder presents predominantly repression, reaction formation, higher levels of projection, and rationalization. The sexual promiscuity of the histrionic personality disorder is part of a generally polymorphous perverse quality of their sexual life, with much less repression of sexual fantasy and uninhibited, often chaotic sexual behavior.

All personality disorders may present depression as a prevalent symptom. The depressive masochistic, hysterical, histrionic, and narcissistic personality disorders frequently present acute or chronic depressive reactions, jointly constituting the so-called "characterological depression." The term *hysteroid dysphoria*[39] refers precisely to histrionic patients with such chronic dispositions to depression, and the question has been raised as to what extent some of these patients may have a genetic predisposition to major affective illness that colors or codetermines their character pathology. The mechanisms by which depression is triggered in all these cases vary.

Regarding the differential diagnosis of the histrionic personality disorder and the borderline personality disorder (although on the surface the *DSM-III* stresses the exhibitionistic and histrionic qualities of the histrionic, in contrast to the borderline personality disorder), a careful comparison reveals that the *DSM-III* describes the borderline personality disorder as presenting traits similar to those presented by the histrionic personality disorder. Both are described as impulsive or unpredictable, with patterns of unstable and intense interpersonal relations, showing inappropriate, intense anger or lack of control of anger and affective instability, prone to suicide gestures and attempts, and presenting incessant efforts to attract attention and reassurance. Although the *DSM-III* explicitly describes the borderline personality disorder as presenting an identity disturbance, the characteristic histrionic personality equally manifests identity disturbance. And both histrionic and borderline personality disorders are described as prone to developing brief psychotic episodes. In practice, therefore, the histrionic and the borderline personality disorder of the *DSM-III* are largely overlapping or coincidental and this area of the *DSM-III* would seem to need a revision.

Treatment

The treatment of the hysterical personality disorder is essentially psychotherapeutic, with psychoanalysis typically the treatment of choice. It needs to be underlined, however, that the hysterical personality disorder, like the obsessive-compulsive and the depressive-masochistic personality disorders, has an excellent prognosis for the entire spectrum of psychoanalytically oriented psychotherapies, although psychoanalysis appears to be the treatment with broadest psychotherapeutic results.[32] In practice, patients who consult for relatively mild or minor neurotic symptoms that complicate a hysterical personality disorder may not require more than the treatment of their symptoms. For example, milder forms of psychosexual dysfunctions (such as inhibited female orgasm) may respond satisfactorily to sex therapy. To what extent the hysterical personality disorder is of sufficient severity to warrant treatment beyond the symptomatic resolution is thus still open to question. Many patients consulting a psychiatrist for relatively time-limited interpersonal conflicts linked to conversion symptoms, phobic reactions, or dissociative experiences may benefit from expressive or exploratory psychotherapy. When the patient complains only about minor symptoms, however, and the diagnostician sees that the hysterical personality disorder might have serious effects on the patient's marriage, work, or profession, a major psychotherapeutic intervention such as psychoanalysis may be warranted.

The specific technical difficulties in the psychoanalytic treatment of the hysterical personality disorder include early, intense transference developments with pseudoerotic defenses against aggressive impulses, regressive transference developments as a defense against the activation of more directly expressed oedipal conflicts, development of affect storms as a form of acting out, and dissociation of affects from their unconscious meanings. These patients may give the therapist trouble in detecting negative transference elements because of their eroticized transferences.

The treatment for the histrionic personality disorder is not psychoanalysis but is essentially psychotherapeutic, with expressive or exploratory psychoanalytic psychotherapy usually the treatment of choice. Supportive psychotherapy is indicated when the patient presents contraindications for exploratory psychotherapy. These contraindications include the presence of marked antisocial features, an unusually severe pathology of object relations, and severe acting out that offers the patient secondary gain. Histrionic personality disorders with secondary depressive symptoms or characterologically determined depression may respond to monoamine oxidase inhibitors or tricyclic or tetracyclic antidepressants. In my experience, however, medication should be reserved only for patients with severe depression and discontinued if no clear and definite improvement of the depression occurs within a few months.

All cases of histrionic personality disorder should be treated psychotherapeutically and as early as possible after the diagnosis is made. Whereas the hysterical personality disorder may gradually improve in internal and interpersonal adjustment over the years, the usual course of the untreated patient with histrionic personality disorder is precarious at best, with a danger of gradual worsening as life opportunities are missed or destroyed.

If the patient falls into the intermediate range between the hysterical and the histrionic personality (Zetzel types 2 and 3), a difficult therapeutic problem ensues. In my view, patients with such intermediate cases should tentatively be treated with psychoanalysis and only shifted into psychoanalytic psychotherapy if psychoanalysis is contraindicated for individual reasons. Such reasons include high secondary gain of illness, lack of motivation, and/or conspicuous inability for emotional introspection. There exists a growing tendency in the literature, however, to recommend starting out with exploratory or psychoanalytic psychotherapy in cases with dubious indication for psychoanalysis and to transform such psychotherapy into psychoanalysis later on.

The principal difficulties in the psychotherapeutic treatment of histrionic personality disorders are the patient's tendency toward massive acting out, secondary gain of the treatment situation itself as a refuge from life, development of apparently "chaotic" treatment situations as an expression of primitive transferences, and severe regression in the communicative process in the treatment so that nonverbal behaviors dominate over verbal communication. These difficulties coincide to all intents and purposes with the general technical problems in the psychotherapy of the borderline spectrum of personality disorders and will not be explored further here. As already mentioned, the growing understanding of the technical difficulties in the treatment of borderline patients and their management

has improved the prognosis for the histrionic personality disorder in an adequate, long-term psychoanalytically oriented psychotherapy. With the exception of the Menninger Psychotherapy Research Project,[32] however, empiric research in this area is still badly lacking.

REFERENCES

1. Zetzel E: The so-called good hysteric. Int J Psychoanal 49:256–260, 1968
2. Mersky H: The Analysis of Hysteria. London, Baillière-Tindall, 1979
3. Roy A (ed): Hysteria. New York, John Wiley & Sons, 1982
4. Cavenar JO Jr, Walker JI: Hysteria and hysterical personality. In Cavenar JO Jr, Brodie HF (eds): Signs and Symptoms in Psychiatry, vol 4, pp 59–74. Philadelphia, JB Lippincott, 1983
5. Marmor J: Orality in the hysterical personality. J Am Psychoanal Assoc 1:656–671, 1953
6. Chodoff P, Lyons H: Hysteria, the hysterical personality, and "hysterical" conversion. Am J Psychiatry 14:734–740, 1958
7. Easser BR, Lesser SR: Hysterical personality: A reevaluation. Psychoanal Q 34:390–415, 1965
8. Easser BR, Lesser SR: Transference resistance in hysterical character neurosis: Technical considerations. In Goldman G, Shapiro D (eds): Developments in Psychoanalysis, pp 69–80. New York, Hafner, 1966
9. Lazare A, Klerman GL, Armor DJ: Oral, obsessive, and hysterical personality patterns: An investigation of psychoanalytic concepts by means of factor analysis. Arch Gen Psychiatry 14:624–630, 1966
10. Lazare A, Klerman GL, Armor DJ: Oral, obsessive, and hysterical personality patterns. J Psychiatr Res 7:275–290, 1969–1970
11. Lazare A: The hysterical character in psychoanalytic theory. Arch Gen Psychiatry 25:131–137, 1971
12. Luisada PV, Peele R, Pittard EA: The hysterical personality in men. Am J Psychiatry 131:518–521, 1974
13. Chodoff P: The diagnosis of hysteria: An overview. Am J Psychiatry 131:1073–1078, 1974
14. Blacker KH, Tupin JP: Hysteria and hysterical structures: Developmental and social theories. In Horowitz MJ (ed): Hysterical Personality, vol 2, pp 97–140. New York, Jason Aronson, 1977
15. Krohn A: Hysteria: The Elusive Neurosis. New York, International Universities Press, 1978
16. Millon T: Disorders of Personality. New York, John Wiley & Sons, 1981
17. Tupin JP: Histrionic personality. In Lion JR (ed): Disorders: Diagnosis and Management, pp 85–96. Baltimore, Williams & Wilkins, 1981
18. Abraham K: Manifestations of the female castration complex. In Selected Papers of Karl Abraham. London, Hogarth Press, 1949
19. Wittels F: Der hysterische Charakter. Psychoanal Bewegung 3:138–165, 1931
20. Reich W: Character Analysis. New York, Farrar, Straus & Giroux, 1972

21. Fenichel O: The Psychoanalytic Theory of Neuroses. New York, WW Norton, 1945

22. Kernberg O: Borderline Conditions and Pathological Narcissism. New York, Jason Aronson, 1975

23. Stone MH: The Borderline Syndromes. New York, McGraw-Hill, 1980

24. Kernberg O: Severe Personality Disorders: Psychotherapeutic Strategies. New Haven, Yale University Press, 1984

25. Lerner HE: The hysterical personality: A woman's disease. Compr Psychiatry 15:157–164, 1974

26. Temoshok L, Attkisson CC: Epidemiology of hysterical phenomena: Evidence for a psychosocial theory. In Horowitz M (ed): Hysterical Personality, pp 145–222. New York, Jason Aronson, 1977

27. Shapiro D: Hysterical Styles. Neurotic Styles. New York, Basic Books, 1965

28. Horowitz MJ: Structure and the Process of Change. In Horowitz MJ (ed): Hysterical Personality, pp 331–399. New York, Jason Aronson, 1977

29. Metcalf A: Childhood: From process to structure. In Horowitz MJ (ed): Hysterical Personality, pp 225–281. New York, Jason Aronson, 1977

30. Kernberg P: Hysterical personality in child and adolescent analysis. In Anthony EJ, Gilpin D (eds): Three Further Clinical Faces of Childhood, pp 27–58. New York, FP Medical and Scientific Books, 1981

31. Anthony EJ: Hysteria in childhood. In Roy A (ed): Hysteria, pp 145–162. New York, John Wiley & Sons, 1982

32. Kernberg O, Burstein E, Coyne L et al: Psychotherapy and psychoanalysis: Final report of the Menninger Foundation's psychotherapy research project. Bull Menninger Clin 36:1–275, 1972

33. Freud S: Fragment of an analysis of a case of hysteria. In Strachey J (ed): The Standard Edition of the Complete Works of Sigmund Freud, Vol 7, pp 3–122. London, Hogarth Press, 1905

34. Freud S: Hysterical phantasies and their relation to bisexuality. In Strachey J (ed): The Standard Edition of the Complete Works of Sigmund Freud, Vol 9, pp 157–166. London, Hogarth Press, 1908

35. Freud S: Some general remarks on hysterical attacks. In Strachey J (ed): The Standard Edition of the Complete Works of Sigmund Freud, Vol 9, pp 229–234. London, Hogarth Press, 1909

36. Freud S: Introductory lectures on psycho-analysis. In Strachey J (ed): The Standard Edition of the Complete Works of Sigmund Freud, Vol 15, London, Hogarth Press, 1915–16

37. Freud S: Inhibitions, symptoms and anxiety. In Strachey J (ed): The Standard Edition of the Complete Works of Sigmund Freud, Vol 20, pp 77–174. London, Hogarth Press, 1926

38. Laughlin HP: The Neuroses. New York, Appleton-Century-Crofts, 1967

39. Liebowitz MR, Klein DF: Interrelationship of hysteroid dysphoria and borderline personality disorder. Psychiatr North Am Clin 4:67–88, 1981

Compulsive Personality Disorder

Certainly since Freud's description in 1908[1] of the anal character, typified by the traits of orderliness, parsimoniousness, and obstinacy, the general notion of a compulsive personality type has been one of the most consistent and enduring categories of personality disorders in clinical literature. In his well known 1921 essay entitled "Contributions to the Theory of the Anal Character," Abraham elaborated on Freud's formulations, sustaining Freud's view that such disorders stem from difficulties encountered in the anal erotic stage of psychosexual development.[2] In 1945 Wilhelm Reich presented a similar dynamic understanding of the origins of this disorder, extending the clinical description to include other features such as ruminative thinking, indecision, and affect-block; however, he preferred the term "compulsive character."[3]

Although concepts of the dynamics and etiology of this disorder have broadened because of the influences of Rado, Erikson, Salzman, Shapiro, and others, the basic view remains intact, that is, a psychopathologic condition called *compulsive personality disorder* does exist, which clinicians can fairly readily identify. *Diagnostic and Statistical Manual of Mental Disorders,* 3rd ed (*DSM-III*) cites the first essential feature of this disorder as "restricted ability to express warm and tender emotions;" this feature and the four additional *DSM-III* criteria for this disorder closely resemble the descriptions of, presumably, the same disorder in the early clinical literature. Although in 1980 Vaillant and Perry suggested that "of all the personality disorders, compulsiveness is the most occupationally adaptive, and . . . it is the personality disorder least often confused with misbehavior," compulsive personality disorder can be a cause of significant distress or impairment in functioning.[4]

Research studies are needed to test the clinical wisdom that supports this diagnosis. In the *DSM-III* Field Trials, the interrater reliabilities for the specific personality disorders were reported to be quite low (kappas ranging from 0.26 to 0.75); figures were not reported for individual disorders. These preliminary results were disappointing, in contrast to the quite good interrater reliability of most Axis I conditions. One possible source of this discrepancy, because many patients may have had both Axis I and Axis II diagnoses, could be the distorting effect that Axis I syndromes may have on Axis II conditions, as discussed by Frances in 1980,[5] Hirschfeld and co-workers in 1983,[6] and Akiskal and co-workers in 1983.[7] A second source of low Axis II reliability, as Frances suggested in 1980, may be the lack of clear boundaries between personality disorders and normal personality traits, along with indistinct boundaries between some of the personality disorders themselves. Recent developments of semi-structured research interviews to survey *DSM-III* personality disorders will minimize interview variability, providing some promise that more extensive and useful reliability data will be forthcoming. Subsequent prevalence studies, family studies, and genetic studies should shed further light on the question.

Definition

The following features are currently considered the most important ones for diagnosis of this disorder; four of them must be present to establish a *DSM-III* diagnosis of compulsive personality disorder:

1. Restricted ability to express warm and tender emotions
2. Perfectionism that interferes with the ability to grasp "the big picture"
3. Insistence that others submit to his or her way of doing things, and lack of awareness of the feelings elicited by this behavior
4. Excessive devotion to work and productivity to the exclusion of pleasure and the value of interpersonal relationships
5. Indecisiveness

The triad of traits typifying the compulsive character in the early psychoanalytic literature has remained intact in this current definition of the disorder. Thus, orderliness roughly corresponds with criterion #2, parsimoniousness is reflected as a tendency to be stingy, associated with criterion #1, and obstinacy corresponds with criterion #3. In 1982 Emmelkamp summarized the results of several factor analytic studies, concluding that they clearly demonstrate a relationship among orderliness, parsimony, and obstinacy as originally predicted from psychoanalytic theory, in contrast to less consistent results for certain other personality disorders.[8] As reflected in the *DSM-III* criteria, current views of compulsive personality disorder, although clearly including these three features, also emphasize lack of emotionality, indecisiveness, and excessive devotion to work.

In the pre-*DSM-III* clinical literature, patients with this disorder were referred to using terms like compulsive character,[3] obsessive style,[9,10] obsessive behavior,[11] or rigid character.[12,13] In a recent detailed work on personality disorders in 1981, Millon, one of the members of the initial Task Force established by the American Psychiatric Association for developing *DSM-III*, indicated his preference to describe this disorder as a compliant or conforming pattern of behavior.[14] As he put it, "The *DSM-III* employs the label 'compulsive personality' to characterize this syndrome. The author considers this designation to be inappropriate since the great majority of these patients exhibit neither compulsions nor obsessions. Moreover, there is an 'obsessive-compulsive' anxiety syndrome with which the personality diagnosis may readily be confused." Gunderson (in Frosch, 1983) expressed similar objections, although he preferred that the disorder continue to be called obsessive-compulsive personality.[15] However, the term compulsive personality disorder was selected for this *DSM-III* Axis II condition in contrast to the Axis I syndrome referred to as obsessive-compulsive disorder.

Epidemiology

Data are not available to establish the epidemiology of compulsive personality disorder. Although the clinical descriptions in the literature of this disorder have much in common, the reliability with which the diagnosis can be made has not been established. In particular, the discrimination between those persons with compulsive personality traits and those with the disorder itself is often obscure. Recently, *DSM-III* criteria have been used to establish the diagnosis of obsessive compulsive disorder in clinical research studies on this Axis I condition, which has been reported to be "many times more prevalent than is commonly believed."[16] However, few comparable studies have yet appeared of the Axis II compulsive personality disorder. Newly developed semistructured interviews covering all 11 *DSM-III* disorders may pave the way for large scale epidemiologic studies of the personality disorders.

Cross cultural studies have suggested that if a country is isolated and homogeneous, it may have what has been referred to as a national character, yet most larger nations are quite diverse in their populations. Cultures that place a high premium on work, punctuality, and orderliness may well have a higher incidence of obsessional traits among their populations, but whether or not a correspondingly high incidence of compulsive personality disorder occurs as well is not known.

It is traditionally reported in the clinical literature that compulsive personality disorder is more common in men than in women, occurs more often in the oldest child in a family, and is more frequently encountered in professions or occupations that require perseverance, methodical attention to detail, or expertise with facts, figures, classification, and categories. It seems likely that the reported greater prevalence of this disorder among men may represent a reflection of traditional sociocultural patterns and that the percentage of women with this disorder could increase as a result of the influence of cultural and occupational changes and of changes in parents' expectations for their daughters.

Clinical Description

HISTORICAL REVIEW

Freud's short essay in 1908 on the anal character, in which he described the traits of orderliness, parsimoniousness, and obstinacy, was subsequently enriched and extended by other psychoanalysts interested in character formation, including Jones, Abraham, and Reich.[1] In 1918 Jones described some aspects of typical behavior that he referred to as anal-erotic character traits.[17] He stressed that two opposing psychological forces—keeping back and giving out—led to two sets of, sometimes contradictory, character traits. Thus, procrastination and hoarding miserliness may be present, yet also a passion for thoroughness and completeness along with organized determination and persistence. Jones emphasized that such character-disordered persons are often preoccupied with time, money, and cleanliness, all of which Jones viewed as derivatives of early childhood anal-stage preoccupations.

Although Abraham's 1921 paper is also couched in the framework of early psychoanalytic theory, it remains a rich source of clinical material, which is remarkably congruent with contemporary descriptions of compulsive personality disorder.[2] Abraham emphasized the compulsive person's pleasure in indexing, classifying, and compiling lists, his tendency to arrange things symmetrically and to divide things with minute exactness, and his ambivalence toward order or cleanliness betrayed by fastidiousness on the surface but disarray or lack of cleanliness underneath. He also noted the compulsive person's pleasure in possession, often resulting in an inability to throw away worn out or worthless objects. The compulsive's penchant to postpone every action is combined with an often unproductive perseverance and a preoccupation with preserving correct social appearances. Yet, in close personal relationships, the compulsive refuses to accommodate himself to others, expects compliance, has an exaggerated criticism of others, and insists on controlling interactions with others. Finally, Abraham noted the generally morose or surly attitude of the compulsive, reflecting a state of constant tension.

Many of these characteristics were stressed not only in the psychoanalytic literature, but also by early pioneers of psychopathologic classification. As reviewed by Millon in 1981, two such nosologists, Kretschmer and Schneider, described person-

ality types probably similar to compulsives.[14] In 1918 Kretschmer described sensitive types who had ruminative, action-inhibited, and indecisive characteristics. In 1923 Schneider described an insecure personality type which he suggested be called anankastic personality. He emphasized that an exaggerated concern to behave correctly and a compulsion to control concealed an extreme inner insecurity.

Wilhelm Reich was especially interested in character pathology, again from a psychoanalytic perspective, and in 1945 he stressed several important additional features of the compulsive character.[3] He noted that the compulsive person's mental processes are typified by indecision, doubt, and distrust, and although he often feels guilty, he is "just as ill-disposed toward affects as he is acutely inaccessible to them," leading at times to a complete affect-block. Perhaps Reich's most succinct description of compulsive persons was to refer to them as living machines.

In 1974 Rado referred to the obsessive person as the ultimate perfectionist, yet as one who specializes in trifles and "is always in danger of missing the essentials."[11] He added that "the obsessive patient is almost never completely free from tension and irritability." In 1974 Monroe described the person with an obsessive personality as ideal for middle management, and he strikingly contrasted the description the obsessive's employer might give of him—a conservative hard worker with integrity—with the description that the obsessive's wife might give of her husband—a pedantis, inefficient, stubborn, self-centered, inflexible hair-splitter.[18]

In a 1968 clinical study of the obsessive personality, as well as in a more recent report (1980), Salzman viewed obsessional behavior on a spectrum, from normal obsessional behavior to obsessional personality to symptomatic obsessional neurosis.[9,10] He emphasized in all obsessionals the need to be in control, and that "the consistent theme in all obsessionals is the presence of anxieties about being in danger because of an incapacity to fulfill the requirements of others and to feel certain of one's acceptance." In addition to the typical features of the compulsive that have been mentioned, Salzman added emphasis on an internal sense of omnipotence, a hesitancy to form deep commitments to others, and a sexual reticence.

David Shapiro, first in 1965 and more recently in 1981, wrote about what he calls the obsessive-compulsive style or the rigid character.[12,13] His extensive clinical descriptions focused and elaborated on many of the characteristics described by others, and he added detailed case material. Shapiro emphasized the excessive devotion to work characteristic of compulsive patients, "These people may be enormously productive in socially recognized ways, or they may not; however that may be, they are, typically, intensely and more or less continuously active at some kind of work." He pointed out that even leisure time is approached as if it were a job, "The compulsive person tries just as effortfully to 'enjoy' himself at play as he does to accomplish or produce at work." The "single most characteristic thought-content of obsessive-compulsive people," according to Shapiro, is "'I should.'" This trait he later described as a special kind of conscientiousness, producing obsessive-compulsive rigidity as a behavior pattern, and concealing obsessional doubt, worry, and rumination.

In Millon's recent review of personality disorders, he too, emphasized the compulsive patient's fear of disapproval of others, notably his superiors or persons invested with authority, as a major determinant of his behavior.[14]

In summary, compulsive people have been described as anhedonic, driven people, who often work inefficiently, torn by a struggle between dread of rules and deadlines and resentful or anxious procrastination. They lack warmth, and they tend to be stubborn and insensitive to others; yet they are indecisive in the context of perfectionistically seeking to follow rules, avoid mistakes, and maintain a picture of dedicated hard work.

CLINICAL EXAMPLE

A 29-year-old physicist sought treatment for lifelong feelings of insecurity and lack of confidence. The oldest child of four siblings, he remembered his father as a stranger and his mother as distant and demanding. Warmth and closeness were lacking, and he learned to seek approval by excelling at school, although he felt little satisfaction with the honors he earned. After years of stalling, beset with doubts, he married for fear of losing his fiancee. He was neither affectionate nor demonstrative; the marriage failed as his wife despaired that she could never be sure that he loved her. Indecisiveness, doubt, and inhibitions haunted him; he was a poor judge of other people, leading to new disappointments; and he spent most of his time on a joyless treadmill of work and worry. He could experience affection or aggression when alone, yet these feelings always evaporated in the presence of the person toward whom he had the feeling. As he put it,

"It's difficult for me to say 'I don't understand, I need help.' I have difficulty being aggressive. You don't always get help. My natural inclination is to say 'yes yes' to people and thank them, when it's no help. . . . When I was a student I simply could not ask a question in class. It was a tremendous effort to do it. It

was contrived. Because the whole focus . . . I had to work myself up so to ask the question that I couldn't listen to the answer. To pursue asking questions forces me to reveal part of myself. I hit it off in technical areas and math. Those were to some extent deliberate choices to protect myself, to avoid seminars—participation where I had to write papers or express real opinions about things. So, in college I missed out on a lot. I work too hard. I always have. I work a lot of the time. I'll go home and read. I don't know why I do it. I feel a real need to have to be working, to be striving for something. I don't know why that is. If I'm not working then I don't know what to fill the time with. It's always been the case. It was a problem for me in college. I'd read everything about everything. I remember a guy—I envied him. I'd talk to him and his eyes would light up. He was interested in what he was doing—excited. This guy would walk into the library and say 'wow look at all the exciting things;' I'd walk into the library and say 'how depressing—look at all I have to know and don't.' I cannot make a committment. I know it's self-defeating. I end up heading off in all directions."

COURSE AND PROGNOSIS

As with all personality disorders, compulsive personality disorder represents an enduring constellation of characteristics which, although entailing subjective distress or significant impairment in functioning, generally is thought to remain stable over time. Many individuals with this disorder may not seek treatment, because their immersion in work can maintain them in financially secure circumstances as well as in habitual contact with others. They often resist change, and treatment itself is frequently seen as a threat to their regular routines and sense of self-control. As a result of these circumstances, combined with the lack of epidemiologic studies using current diagnostic criteria, little is known with certainty about the course or prognosis of compulsive personality disorder.

Clinicians have traditionally described that when under stress, compulsive patients are prone to develop paranoid or depressive conditions. Paranoid projective mechanisms have been suggested as a second line of defense beyond emotional isolation, to externalize the compulsive patient's unacceptable impulses. Relatedly, the strict controlling superego of the compulsive patient has been thought to make him more vulnerable to certain pathologic grief reactions, perhaps particularly late-onset major depression with melancholia. Whether the compulsive patient's presumed susceptibility to paranoia or depression also reflects a genetic predisposition is not known, nor is it known how frequently these developments occur. The question of covariance of other disorders with compulsive personality disorder is reviewed further in the discussion of differential diagnosis below.

Etiology

GENETIC CONSTITUTIONAL COMPULSIVE PERSONALITY DISORDER

In a recent study on the genetics of neurosis, Torgerson stated that "any conclusion from twin studies, as to the relative contribution of heredity and environment in the development of neurosis, will depend upon sampling," and he demonstrated different findings depending on sex, severity of illness, and type of illness.[19] Such variables apply for personality disorders as well, which, in addition to the diagnostic imprecision in past studies, make it difficult to interpret the role of heredity in the etiology of personality disorders.

In 1967 Eysenck reviewed the earlier literature on hereditary and personality, concluding mainly that the role played by heredity is likely to be significant in many cases.[20] In 1978 Carey and co-workers reported that, in spite of major methodologic problems in genetic studies, the personality dimension of introversion was the most heavily influenced by genetic factors; this conclusion was consistent with that of previous work by Gottesman, one of the co-authors of this study.[21] Clearly, however, introversion could apply to many personality types, although possibly including some compulsive patients. Family studies have been contradictory and inconclusive, and adoption studies have focused mostly on Axis I conditions. Siever recently reviewed the evidence for a role played by genetic factors in personality disorders.[15] Although more convincing data exist pointing to a genetic factor in the Axis I obsessive compulsive disorder, some studies suggest that a genetic factor may be a predisposition for the development of obsessional traits. Future research studies are needed to extend our knowledge of the likely role played by genetics in compulsive personality disorders itself.

Outside of the area of experimental research, many clinicians have proposed that constitutional factors play a crucial etiologic role in the development of compulsive personality disorder. Freud clearly felt that the anal character derived his character traits as direct expressions of, alterations of, or reactions against constitutionally derived anal-erotic instincts. Psychoanalysts subscribing to Freud's libido theory or its revision, the structural theory, generally maintained similar views. For example, in 1974 Rado said, "Presumably, the acquired predisposition to obsessive behavior is based on a genetic predisposition in which the over-strength of rage may be linked with the pleasure deficiency of the sexual orgasm."[11]

Most recently, clinicians have speculated that constitutional factors affect temperament and, as a result, contribute to the etiology of personality disorders. In the case of compulsive personality disorder, Millon speculated that a constitutionally-based anhedonic temperament may be involved.[14]

PSYCHODYNAMIC COMPULSIVE PERSONALITY DISORDER

Early psychoanalytic theorists believed that compulsive behavior derived from unconscious guilt related to infantile anal-erotic libidinal impulses, compounded by the child's perception of his parents' disapproval during the toilet training process. As Freud put it, "We can at any rate lay down a formula for the way in which character in its final shape is formed out of the constituent instincts: the permanent character-traits are either unchanged prolongations of the original instincts, or sublimations of those instincts, or reaction-formations against them."[1] This view, of the central role of anal-erotic impulses in the etiology of this disorder, is no longer widely accepted, and, as well, the specific importance of the toilet training experience itself has been discounted.[8] Rado suggested that compulsive patients had constitutionally excessive amounts of rage, inducing power struggles with others from an early age.[11] Although such a hypothesis remains plausible, it has not been established. MacKinnon and Michels viewed the obsessive patient as "involved in a conflict between obedience and defiance . . . (leading) to a continuing alternation between the emotions of fear and rage."[22] They added that such a patient "must keep his conflicting emotions and indeed all emotion, as secret as possible . . . ," leading to defense mechanisms of emotional isolation and intellectualization. In their view, the conflict originated in childhood experiences and retains a childish quality in the adult patient.

Vaillant and Perry preferred Erikson's developmental model of the stage of autonomy versus shame as explanatory in this disorder, emphasizing the importance of the child's interactions with his parents and their responses to him.[4] This vantage point implies that, because Erikson was describing a normal developmental stage, the future compulsive patient, as a child, either was inherently excessively autonomous, or that the parents doled out inordinant reproof and control. Indeed, variations of the latter formulation seem to be the most frequently proposed psychodynamics of this disorder in the current clinical literature. Salzman emphasized the obsessional patient's need to maintain an illusion of perfection and infallibility to defend against feelings of insecurity brought about by overbearing parents.[9,10] Shapiro stressed that the compulsive patient's personality is structured around a need for approval.[12,13] Ingram[23] suggested that the compulsive patient's need to control represents identification with authoritarian parents, while Millon saw it as a need to keep impulses, mainly hostile ones, at bay due to overcontrolling parents.[14]

In viewing the child in the context of the family, Lidz stated, "it has become increasingly evident that major determinants of the type of psychopathology from which a patient suffers are to be found in the continuing family transactions, which include the influence of the child's inherent makeup, and presence upon the other family members and their interactions with one another, as well as the effects of the family milieu and style."[24] He added, "One might surmise, for example, that the parents of obsessional patients tend to be obsessional themselves, unable to tolerate expressions of instinctual drives and autonomy in themselves or in the children and actually teach the use of isolation, undoing, and reaction formation as a means of handling aggression and sexuality, both by their own behavior and by what they approve and disapprove in the children. These obsessional parents would be apt to use rigid bowel training and would almost certainly seek to limit the young child's autonomy, and thereby foster ambivalence, stubbornness, shame, and undoing defenses in many ways other than through bowel training."

How much each of these dimensions of the early family experiences of the compulsive character contributes to the disorder's etiology remains unclear, but it seems likely that these early interactional patterns may be at least partially etiologically significant. Carefully controlled studies of the families of compulsive patients should add to our knowledge in this crucial area.

Diagnosis and Differential Diagnosis

The diagnosis of compulsive personality disorder is complicated by the difficulty of distinguishing between the disorder itself and normal obsessional behavior. Especially in the case of the compulsive patient, whose pathology may be ego-syntonic, the clinician must decide if there is significant impairment in social or occupational functioning to warrant making the diagnosis. As Frances pointed out, such a judgment may be highly subjective and variable among clinicians, and he prefers a dimensional system of diagnosis for the personality disorders.[5] Similarly, Gunderson felt that "it would be valuable to attempt to better integrate the personality diagnoses with the studies of personality traits derived from healthier populations."[15]

To date, there are no known laboratory examinations to assist in the diagnosis of compulsive personality disorder. Projective psychological tests may be helpful by providing corroboration of compulsive traits such as rigidity, orderliness, indecisiveness, and emotional isolation.

The discrimination between compulsive personality disorder and obsessive compulsive disorder is relatively straightforward because the diagnosis of the Axis I disorder is based on the presence of ego-alien symptoms. Still, the presence of obsessive compulsive disorder or other Axis I disorders may well significantly diminish the validity with which the Axis II disorder can be diagnosed concurrently.[5,7]

There is considerable disagreement regarding the frequency with which the obsessive-compulsive Axis I "state disturbance" may occur in persons who already have the Axis II compulsive trait disturbance. Redlich and Freedman went so far as to say, "all patients with obsessive symptoms show an obsessive character structure;"[25] other clinicians would not put it so categorically. Goodwin and Guze reported that "many individuals with obsessional neurosis have obsessional personalities antedating the illness," but they added that the frequency of this pattern was unknown.[26] In contrast, Nemiah stated that "there is no necessary connection between obsessional character traits and obsessive-compulsive symptoms,"[27] and, similarly, Weintraub said, "Most compulsive characters do not develop neurotic symptoms and many compulsive neurotics do not have compulsive character traits."[28]

Emmelkamp, in an attempt to clarify this controversial question, reviewed the experimental evidence in the literature, and he concluded that "taken together, these data indicate that there is a strong relationship between premorbid obsessional personality traits and the development of obsessional neurosis."[8] He noted, however, that it is not a one-to-one relationship. In virtually all of these studies, as well as the anecdotal opinions of clinicians, the focus is usually on the premorbid personality or character structure of patients who develop obsessive compulsive disorder. The percentage of those patients identified as premorbidly obsessional who would be diagnosed as having compulsive personality disorder is not known.

Millon summarized what he felt to be the most frequent Axis I disorders that covary with compulsive personality disorder.[14] In his opinion, the most common Axis I conditions which covary, in addition to obsessive compulsive disorder, are phobic disorders, anxiety disorders, affective disorders, and, less frequently, somatoform disorders, dissociative disorder, brief reactive psychosis, and schizophreniform disorder.

Clinicians have frequently felt that depression in particular is prone to occur in obsessional patients. Akiskal and co-workers reviewed this question in careful detail; although they emphasized caution due to methodologic shortcomings in many clinical and retrospective studies, they concluded that the literature supports a link between bipolar affective psychoses, as well as some unipolar depressions, and "a driven work-oriented obsessoid quality" in the pre-existing temperaments of such patients.[7]

The frequency with which other personality disorders coexist with compulsive personality disorder is not known. Weintraub considered compulsive and paranoid personalities together, as two diseases of the intellect, and in his opinion "compulsive and paranoid traits or symptoms may coexist in the same individual."[28] Millon concurred with this view, and he cited dependent personality disorder as a second Axis II condition that may covary with compulsive personality disorder.[14] Whether such multiple Axis II diagnoses accurately reflect discrete coexisting disorders, or whether a dimensional approach to Axis II is preferable, remains to be established.

Treatment and Prevention

The compulsive patient who seeks treatment usually does so only after his equilibrium has been threatened. Either he has been left by an exasperated spouse, has failed at his job, or has encountered unexpected stress. Occasionally, the subjective wear and tear of the disorder on the patient himself brings him for help, as he becomes increasingly dissatisfied with his unfulfilling life full of repetitive routine and lacklustre friendships.

Compulsive personality disorder is often treated by psychoanalysis or psychoanalytically oriented psychotherapy. Auchincloss and Michels suggested that the primary indication for psychoanalysis today is a character disorder, and that "psychoanalysis (as a technique) and character analysis have become synonymous."[15] Particularly with compulsive patients, clinicians have reported their belief that only by such intensive insight-oriented efforts can the all-too-durable defenses of the patient be altered, leading to greater awareness, tolerance, and understanding of his intense inner affective life, as well as of the origins of these affects and the defenses that kept them hidden.

Salzman emphasized the need for the therapist to take an active role in treatment of compulsives, focussing on the here and now, to deal with the patient's emotional isolation and his need to control.[9,10] The ego-syntonicity of much of the compulsive patient's character pathology also dictates an active therapeutic technique, and such an approach is not inconsistent with modern character analysis. As Auchincloss and Michels described it, "if the patient presents ego-syntonic character pathology, the analyst spends a great deal of time trying to weaken the patient's unquestioning acceptance of these character patterns . . . The attempt is to make character ego-alien, at least to the extent that the patient can observe it and analyze it, whether or not he ultimately reclaims it as his own."[15] Outcome studies of these forms of treatment for this disorder are not available.

In some ways, there may be certain similarities between aspects of traditional psychoanalytic anxiety-provoking treatment and the response prevention and deliberate exposure behavioral techniques recently reported as promising for treatment of obsessive-compulsive disorder.[29] Especially since, as described before, there may be a strong relationship between premorbid compulsivity and the Axis I obsessive-compulsive disorder, it is possible that these behavioral techniques might be beneficial for some patients with compulsive personality disorder as well. Similarly, recent reports indicate significant improvement in obsessive-compulsive patients treated with newer psychopharmacologic agents;[30] the possibility that these and other psychopharmacologic agents could be helpful to patients with compulsive personality disorder should be explored.

Summary

Although the title has changed, the category of compulsive personality disorder has remained a distinctly described type of character pathology in the clinical literature since Freud's brief report on the anal character in 1908.[1] Consisting of, usually ego-syntonic traits, such as (1) restricted emotional warmth (parsimoniousness), (2) perfectionism (orderliness), and (3) insistent, insensitive control of others (obstinacy), along with (4) a "workaholic" pattern, and (5) indecisiveness, the Axis II condition can be differentiated from Axis I obsessive compulsive disorder by the absence of ego-alien symptomatic obsessions and compulsions. It is more difficult to distinguish the personality disorder from normal obsessional behavior, a commonly found type of adaptive functioning. The prevalence of compulsive personality disorder is not known. A genetic component may be involved in the etiology of this disorder, although further study of this possibility is needed. Clinicians, having generally moved away from the original psychodynamic formulations of this disorder, currently see it as largely the product of family influences on the patient during his formative developmental years. Psychoanalysis or psychoanalytically-oriented psychotherapy are the generally recommended treatments for this disorder, involving active techniques on the part of the therapist.

REFERENCES

1. Freud S: Character and Anal Erotism (1908). London, The Hogarth Press, 1968
2. Abraham K: Contributions to the theory of the anal character (1921). In Abraham K: On Character and Libido Development. New York, Basic Books, Inc., 1966
3. Reich W: Character Analysis. New York, Simon and Schuster, 1945
4. Vaillant GE, Perry JC: Personality disorders. In Kaplan HI, Freedman AM, Sadock BJ: Comprehensive Textbook of Psychiatry, 3rd ed. Baltimore, Williams & Wilkins, 1980
5. Frances A: The DSM-III personality disorders section: A commentary. Am J Psychiatry 137:1050–1054, 1980
6. Hirschfeld RMA, Klerman GL, Clayton PJ et al: Assessing personality: Effects of the depressive state on trait measurement. Am J Psychiatry 140:695–699, 1983
7. Akiskal HS, Hirschfeld RMA, Yerevanian BI: The relationship of personality to affective disorders. Arch Gen Psychiatry 40:801–810, 1983
8. Emmelkamp PMG: Phobic and Obsessive-Compulsive Disorders. New York, Plenum Press, 1982
9. Salzman L: The Obsessive Personality. New York, Science House, 1968
10. Salzman L: Treatment of the Obsessive Personality. New York, Jason Aronson, 1980
11. Rado S: Obsessive behavior. In Arieti S (ed): American Handbook of Psychiatry, 2nd ed. New York, Basic Books, Inc., 1974
12. Shapiro D: Neurotic Styles. New York, Basic Books, Inc., 1965
13. Shapiro D: Autonomy and Rigid Character. New York, Basic Books, Inc., 1981
14. Millon T: Disorders of Personality. New York, John Wiley & Sons, 1981
15. Frosch JP: Personality Disorders. Washington, DC, American Psychiatric Association Press, Inc., 1983
16. Runck B: Research is changing views on obsessive-compulsive disorder. Hosp Community Psychiatry 34:597–598, 1983
17. Jones E: Anal-erotic character traits. In Jones E: Papers on Psychoanalysis, Baltimore, Williams & Wilkins, 1949
18. Monroe RR: Obsessive behavior: Integration of psychoanalytic and other approaches. In Arieti S (ed): American Handbook of Psychiatry, 2nd ed. New York, Basic Books, Inc., 1974
19. Torgersen S: Genetics of neurosis. Br J Psychiatry 142:126–132, 1983
20. Eysenck HJ: The Biologic Basis of Personality. London, Routledge and Kegan Paul, 1967
21. Carey G, Goldsmith HH, Tellegen A et al: Genetics and personality inventories: The limits of replication with twin data. Behav Genet 8:299–313, 1978
22. MacKinnon RA, Michels R: The Psychiatric Interview in Clinical Practice. Philadelphia, WB Saunders, 1971
23. Ingram DH: Compulsive personality disorder. Am J Psychoanal 42:189–198, 1982
24. Lidz T: Family studies and changing concepts of personality development. Can J Psychiatry 24:621–631, 1979
25. Redlich FC, Freedman DX: The Theory and Practice of Psychiatry. New York, Basic Books, Inc., 1966
26. Goodwin DW, Guze SB: Psychiatric Diagnosis. New York, Oxford University Press, 1979
27. Nemiah JC: Psychoneurotic disorders. II: Obsessive-compulsive and neurotic depressive reactions. In Freedman AM, Kaplan HI: Comprehensive Textbook of Psychiatry. Baltimore, Williams & Wilkins, 1967
28. Weintraub W: Compulsive and paranoid personalities. In Lion JR (ed): Personality Disorders, Baltimore, Williams & Wilkins, 1981
29. Steketee G, Foa EB, Grayson JB: Recent advances in the behavioral treatment of obsessive-compulsives. Arch Gen Psychiatry 39:1365–1371, 1982
30. Insel TR, Murphy DL, Cohen RM, et al: Obsessive-compulsive disorder. Arch Gen Psychiatry 40:605–612, 1983

Antisocial Personality

Antisocial personality is a clinical diagnosis which mixes social and moral concepts with those of clinical psychiatry. The clinician who takes seriously the effect of the mind on life-style and behavior, and the effects of genetics and environment on the development of the mind, must consider antisocial personality (and its somewhat dated synonyms "psychopathy" and "sociopathy") within the disease model of psychiatric disorders rather than in a primarily environmental or behavioral context. The chapter that follows presents some of the evidence for such a conclusion, and discusses clinical correlates, treatment, and social and legal issues.

History

Pinel recognized as early as the eighteenth century that some forms of antisocial behavior were associated with, and perhaps the result of, mental illness. His clinical concept of *manie sans délire* was different from the legal concepts, present since prebiblical times, of mental illness's potential interference with responsibility for one's acts.[1] In the early nineteenth century, Prichard described "moral insanity," which bore considerable resemblance to later descriptions of sociopathy, in *A Treatise on Insanity*.[2]

Nineteenth century efforts to define antisocial syndromes had mixed effects. Koch's "medicalization" of the concept of psychopathy by naming it "constitutional psychopathic inferiority," provided a semblance of clinical accuracy.[3] Kraeplin's theoretical psychodynamic explanations of the disorder—developmental inhibitions that predisposed the patient to infantile characteristics—were clinically elegant but lacked evidence of their validity.[4] Franz Alexander felt there was a strong neurotic component within most chronic antisocial behavior. His "neurotic characters" were persons whose primary conflicts led to alloplastic activity rather than to classic neurotic symptoms.[5] Karpman's analytic work a few years later bore out Alexander's prediction of the existence of purely psychopathic individuals, without guilt or self-destructive symptoms. Karpman named these people "anethopaths."[6]

An association of antisocial personality with criminality has persisted since the beginning of the concept. Between the late 1930s and about 1975, almost all research and clinical writing on the subject stressed criminal behavior or delinquency. In addition, pessimism with respect to treatment or change became well established by the work and publications of Cleckley, the McCords, and others.[7,8] Unfortunately, this preoccupation with illegal, sometimes aggressive pursuits, often limited rather than clarified understanding of those with antisocial personality, because they were confused with many other kinds of criminals and because nonaggressive symptoms of the disorder were ignored by many clinicians and the lay public.

On the other hand, that period was one in which longitudinal and analytic studies gave rise to most of our understanding of the psychodynamic aspects of psychopathy. Cleckley is the person most associated with such in-depth understanding. His ideas, which are summarized in *The Mask of Sanity*, have survived relatively unchanged for almost 40 years.[7]

During the mid-twentieth century there was

again a movement toward scientific definition and understanding of antisocial personality. Efforts to establish physiologic parameters of the disorder focused primarily on electroencephalography at first, then on physiologic characteristics associated with anxiety (such as cardiovascular and electrodermal responses). The former never led to any significant correlates with sociopathy, although group data appeared to suggest some nonspecific similarities among antisocial subjects.[9] Psychophysiologic studies were similarly nonproductive, at least in any practical sense, except perhaps for certain findings that the recovery limbs of conditioned electrodermal response curves are significantly altered in some antisocial subjects.[10] Like much social and clinical research of the same era, the results suffer from a lack of adequate definition of the antisocial disorders studied, as well as from difficulties in replicating data and making use of them.

Diagnosis

There are at least three viewpoints from which to consider antisocial personality, each of which should be kept in mind throughout this chapter. First, antisocial personality is a specifically-defined disorder that fits best into a disease model of understanding, and which is not defined by any single kind of outward behavior.

Second, so many people still confuse antisocial behavior with antisocial personality that it is necessary to discuss syndromes, especially chronic ones, which do not fit the diagnostic criteria for psychopathy but which are commonly cited in clinical situations in which aggression or illegal activity predominate. Finally, in spite of the apparent specificity of the official diagnostic criteria in use in the United States (the American Psychiatric Association's *Diagnostic and Statistical Manual,* 3rd ed [*DSM-III*], those criteria establish definition, not clinical fact.[11] The author recommends that attention be given to a subgroup of those who meet *DSM-III* criteria and in addition convey an impression of emptiness and affectionlessness, much as described by Karpman during the 1940s[6] and more recently by Reid.[12,13]

Until 1980, most definitions of antisocial personality were based in large part upon Cleckley's original sixteen diagnostic points, all of which he felt to be part of the personality of the psychopath.[7] These include superficial charm, unreliability, poverty of affective reactions, lack of remorse or shame, poor judgement, and "egocentricity and in-

capacity for love." Cleckley noted a conspicuous absence of psychotic or psychoneurotic symptoms.

DSM-III places antisocial personality in a cluster that contains histrionic, narcissistic, and borderline personalities.[11] The essential features of the *DSM-III* diagnosis (301.7) are a clear continuum of antisocial behavior from childhood well into adulthood; continuously antisocial or inadequate behavior, without major interruptions, in which others' rights are violated; and failure to sustain competence in vocation or life's work over several years. This chronic condition and behavior must not be the result of mental retardation, schizophrenia, or affective illness. Mental retardation may coexist in some unusual cases. It may be pointed out that violation of the rights of others does not always imply criminality. This is further discussed below.

The *DSM-III* criteria are consistent with those of the *International Classification of Diseases,* 9th ed (*ICD-9*). They provide for far more reliable diagnosis than was possible in the past, and thus allow more consistent statistical comparison of this diagnosis with others. Unfortunately, the validity of the criteria is not as secure as the reliability. Furthermore, *DSM-III* criteria for the other personality disorders are far less refined or specific than those for antisocial personality.

Classification can be the beginning of differentiation. Since the publication of the *DSM-III* criteria, more and more studies have separated patients with antisocial personality from antisocial persons who more properly deserve some other (or no) diagnosis. Jail and prison populations, adolescent delinquent groups, and other populations are seen to be composed of a broad variety of individuals, a fact that has profound implications for treatment planning, prognosis, and sentencing of persons who have come to trial.

It is especially important that children and adolescents not receive a diagnosis of antisocial personality. Aggressive or delinquent behavior of some youths continues into adulthood, at which time a diagnosis of psychopathy may be made provided other criteria are present. Many teenagers, however, do not develop the complete antisocial syndrome; adolescent behavior, or behavior induced by particular family or personal stresses of childhood, can take many forms. The label of "psychopath" must not be applied lightly. In addition, the author feels that young adults, especially those experiencing an extended adolescence because, for example, of continued schooling, should be allowed several years of signs and symptoms before the diagnosis is made.

Although considered subjective by modern diagnostic standards, Cleckley's concepts have a great deal of value to today's clinical psychiatry. Many of them remind one of the *intrapsychic* nature of this disorder; this is a disease of the psyche, not basically one of socialization. One example of the importance of the psychodynamic aspects of the disorder has to do with the overriding importance of the quality of the patient's interpersonal relationships to the making of the diagnosis, or to the establishment of its severity. An absolute paucity of close relationships bespeaks a core personality defect involving basic trust or the ability to internalize important parts of the infant environment.[14] This in turn may form the basis for a diagnosis of a more severe "true" antisocial or "anethopathic" personality.

DIFFERENTIAL DIAGNOSIS

As implied above, "All that glitters is not gold," and all that is antisocial, asocial, hedonistic, narcissistic, frustrating, or refractory to treatment is not antisocial personality.[13] Chronic criminal behavior, for example, is not by any means pathognomonic of psychopathy. People become and remain criminals for many reasons—cultural, religious, financial, and neurotic. Socialized or consistently purposeful aggression or criminality should not be confused with antisocial personality (although a person with antisocial personality may be found in, or drift to, such activity).

The clinician must differentiate antisocial personality from other major psychiatric disorders. Careful attention to the *DSM-III* criteria should prevent confusion of the personality disorder with antisocial manifestations of psychoses, affective disorders, subtle organic central nervous system deficits, substance abuse, or other conditions. The treatments of these are quite different from that of primary antisocial personality, as are their prognoses.[15]

Differentiating the many personality disorders that may predispose the patient to antisocial behavior requires even more care. Borderline and narcissistic disorders contain features in common with antisocial personality. The former implies little affective stability, however, and a propensity to decompensate under only moderate loss or other stress. Problems with self-image are much closer to the surface in both of these disorders than in antisocial personality, and seemingly antisocial behavior may have a transparent self-destructive theme. The borderline patient's difficulty with relationships has a plaintive and intolerant quality that is seen in the psychopath by only the very empathic therapist.

The person with paranoid personality characteristically lacks the chronicity of antisocial behavior—and the child-to-adult continuum—found in the psychopath. His acts are more consistent with projection and paranoia, without the stimulating quality usually seen in antisocial personality. Passive-aggressive personality may predispose one to resistive-resistant features, substance abuse, and the like, but rarely provides the entire spectrum of criteria for antisocial personality. Histrionic personality deserves special mention not because of its diagnostic confusion with antisocial personality, but because of its possible genetic, or at least familial, relationship with the disorder (see below).

A number of non-*DSM-III* personality disorders have been proposed to clarify specific syndromes described in the clinical or social literature. *Inadequate personality* is a term used by Cameron and others that seems to describe a condition similar to that of the nineteenth century "constitutionally inferior" individual.[16] "Dyssocial" and "asocial" character traits or styles should be differentiated from antisocial personality. The former has more to do with society than with the psyche (*cf.*, this author's frequent use of the term "psychopath") and does not imply the same difficulty with interpersonal relationships as is found in antisocial personality.[17] The latter usually describes persons unable to tolerate socialization, often because of severe narcissism.

The phrase "emotionally unstable" has been used to describe a particular personality or character by a number of authors and clinicians. If such a personality disorder does exist, it has not been accepted as such by any major group or text. Rifkin and co-workers attempted to separate a subset of patients with chronic maladaptive behaviors and short bipolar swings from other affectively disordered patients and place them in such a category.[18] The syndrome is probably not closely related to antisocial personality.

"Impulse-ridden" or "impulsive" personality is a diagnosis seen in some older texts. It seems similar in manifestations to the "disorders of impulsive control" found in more recent nomenclature (such as the *DSM-III*), in which one finds pathologic gambling, kleptomania, explosive disorders, and the like. Patients with these disorders appear to behave with some purpose (*e.g.*, in the case of pyromania or kleptomania), within which there is a sort of driven quality. Other such patients exhibit subtle neurologic signs, verbal or other triggers for behavior, or unusual sensitivity to drugs or alcohol (especially in the case of explosive disorders). The full syndrome of antisocial personality is not present.

Finally, ordinary aggressive or antisocial behavior must be differentiated from antisocial personality. *DSM-III* accomplishes this well, allowing alternative, behavioral diagnoses (*e.g.*, adjustment disorder with disturbance of conduct), or nonpathologic "V-codes" (*e.g.*, adult antisocial behavior). These differences must be kept in mind when working with, for example, criminals or delinquent youth, and when reviewing the literature on understanding and treating antisocial syndromes, because diagnostic methods are frequently poorly documented (especially in papers published before 1980).

Clinical Correlates

ORGANIC

Although the psychopath's brain appears to function normally, emotional defects are obvious on closer observation; physical defects may be present as well. The search for neurologic correlates with, or causes of, antisocial personality continues. Some antisocial or aggressive behaviors are clearly associated with specific or diffuse lesions. However, these tend not to be directly related to antisocial personality. Elliott and others have described anatomic neurologic sources of antisocial behavior, such as those secondary to trauma, infection, neoplasm, or deterioration.[19]

Neurologic correlates with personality disorders themselves, including antisocial personality, are much more difficult to define. The most diligent search has been for electroencephalographic correlates. Conventional techniques do not differentiate groups of patients with antisocial personality from other groups, in spite of some early papers that reported nonspecific changes (*e.g.*, bilateral slowing similar to that found in physically immature brains) associated with chronic antisocial behavior.[9,20] Elliott reported frequent electroencephalographic (EEG) abnormalities in aggressive patients and their families, but these findings have more relevance to the general topic of antisocial behavior, and to issues of familial influence on antisocial syndromes, than to antisocial personality itself. Activating procedures, such as chemical (*e.g.*, bemegride) or photic stimulation, increase positive findings in many syndromes, including antisocial personality, but are inconsistent and have not been well studied since clarification of diagnostic criteria in the late 1970s.[9,19]

Psychophysiologic research has provided a more convincing case for central nervous system deficit in antisocial personality, in part because this kind of work measures neurologic function—at least small, highly specific parts thereof—much more directly than does electroencephalography. The most reliable data stress autonomic characteristics that indicate lowered levels of baseline anxiety, lessened autonomic reaction to some forms of stress, and changes in speed of autonomic recovery from such stress. Some researchers infer from these findings a relationship between autonomic defect and conditioned responses to fear or anxiety, such as those implicated in early development of the ability to learn from experience.[9,21] Results should be seen as inconclusive at this time.

A few authors have recently attempted to link possible neurologic deficit in antisocial personality with apparently similar signs in childhood attention deficit disorder (ADD).[22] Longitudinal studies of children with behavioral disorders, including ADD, show a clear statistical relationship to adult behavioral problems.[23,24] This has some implications for the treatment of a few antisocial adults, for example with methylphenidate; however, when one examines these data more closely, it seems likely that the so-called hyperactive adult is part of a discrete subgroup of those with antisocial syndromes.

BIOCHEMICAL FINDINGS

Correlations between biochemical findings and antisocial personality are unproved to date. Unreplicated studies of serum cholesterol, phenylethylamine production, and some other parameters provide some of the very little evidence that psychopaths are biologically different from other persons. Preliminary measurements of urinary 3-methoxy-4-hydroxyphenolglycol (MHPG), serum dopamine-β-hydroxylase (DBH), and platelet monoamine oxidase have thus far shown no reliable differences from nonantisocial groups.[13,25,26]

EMOTIONAL DEVELOPMENT AND PSYCHODYNAMIC CORRELATES

No early developmental experience, or set of experiences, is highly predictive of later sociopathy.

Many authors cite maternal deprivation, chaotic mother–child relationships, and lack of parental bonds of affection.[27-36] The presence of the father in the home has been given importance by some; however, the most important single issue with respect to fathers appears to be whether or not they are "sociopathic."[31] Antisocial fathers have been consistently associated with antisocial or criminal behavior in offspring in a statistical sense, although there are not data to indicate that this is a predictor of true antisocial personality.

Many authors have written about the early development of narcissistic persons and antisocial adolescents, usually describing immature parents who, rather than providing consistent and unselfish parenting, tended to be overly stimulating or needed to be gratified by the child.[30,32-36] Because this is a rather broad concept, the reader is referred particularly to the work of Leaff for a more comprehensive discussion of this topic.[28]

The psychodynamics of the adult reveal pathology that is more severe than that of most other character disorders. This has been described as "semantic aphasia";[7] severe disturbance of the ego, superego, and instinctual integration;[28] and in other ways, but most authors agree that there is a basic integrity of self-object relations in the true psychopath.

Several authors refer to self-destructive aspects of the psychopath's character and behavior. Lindner's *Rebel Without a Cause* is an example of a famous case.[37] Halleck, Menninger, Stürup, and others discuss the resilient defenses that the patient with antisocial personality has against feelings of helplessness and dependency.[3,38,39] These are sometimes seen as stimulation, but almost always they lead to suffering by the psychopath as well as by those around him.

It is instructive to examine the Jungian viewpoint of the psychodynamics of antisocial personality. Talley observes the puerile characteristics found in virtually all of these patients.[40] Guggenbühl-Craig describes a similar immaturity and sadness in these highly disabled individuals.[41] Reid and Ellis have discussed the Jungian concept of initiation and passage with respect to the psychopath. They note that the adult who has successfully gone through at least a symbolic passage from adolescence feels competent and worthwhile. Such a person understands that mature people do not "cheat." In contrast, the person who believes, rightly or wrongly, that he has not completed the requirements for this passage may view himself as a "trickster," not deserving of the rights, privileges,

and label of the adult, and may behave accordingly.[42]

The above Jungian view is consistent with some work of Hott in which antisocial patients were found to have idealized images of behavior, which they should exercise.[17] These "shoulds" of unconscious morals and guilt are, in Hott's view, externalized, felt as social pressures from others, and then overthrown through ruthless or guiltless activity. This concept of the aggression that is often seen with antisocial personality is similar to this author's view of the psychopath as one who may not be particularly aggressive *per se*, but may instead be defending himself against the fantasied onslaught of others.[12] Leaff describes that kind of aggression as existing within a severely narcissistic personality structure. He feels that the psychopath may need to attack potential providers to prove to himself that they, and the things they symbolize, cannot be trusted.[28] This implies that there is a foundation for the formation of object relationships in those with antisocial personality, albeit an immature, self-directed one. One might thus expect the formation of a transference similar to that seen in severely narcissistic patients in psychotherapy with these individuals.

GENETICS

Schulsinger, Crowe, and others have carried out careful adoption studies using strict diagnostic criteria for antisocial syndromes.[43,44] Their work suggests that there are familial, and perhaps genetic, factors in the etiology of antisocial personality.

Indirect evidence supporting hypotheses of genetic influence (as opposed to the more general "familial" influence) comes from the finding of what some term antisocial "equivalents" in the pedigrees of carefully diagnosed psychopaths. These include hysterical syndromes in women, alcohol abuse syndromes,[45,46] and some slight evidence for genetic relationships between psychopathy and psychotic disorders.[47]

The relationship between antisocial personality and hysteria has been studied by a number of people, notably Tupin and Horowitz.[48,49] Although the author feels that the true incidence of antisocial personality is probably about the same for men and women, the incidence of culturally recognized antisocial behavior is about five times as great in males.[31] There is some evidence that the psychodynamics, and perhaps the genetics as well, of histrionic personality are similar—a sort of "mirror image"—to those of antisocial personality.[48,50]

A few years ago there was considerable interest in the relationship between certain rare genotypes involving the sexual chromosomes and criminal or aggressive behavior. The most commonly implicated genotype was the XYY. It is now felt to be doubtful that genotype alone is consistently correlated with criminal behavior.[51,52,53] Hook in particular has pointed out at least three ways in which these unusual XYY individuals might come to the attention of society and be used erroneously as evidence for the genotypic aberrance hypothesis.[53]

SOCIAL CORRELATES

Psychopathy and Criminality

Many individuals convicted of felonies fulfill criteria for a diagnosis of antisocial personality. This number is statistically significant when compared to samples from virtually any other population, and applies to both men and women (although the women usually have associated diagnoses such as alcoholism, substance dependence, or hysteria).[54] A few studies find that fewer than one fourth of all convicted criminals qualify for a diagnosis of antisocial personality,[55,56,57] and one places this number at only 7% (although diagnostic criteria for this study were vague).[56] The studies that yield these figures often do not include petty criminals, those not sent to prisons, or those who are never caught.

Associating criminality with psychopathy is not the same as associating psychopathy with criminality. The two sets of individuals certainly overlap; however, it is likely that the subset of psychopaths who are criminals by American legal standards occupies no more than 50% of the entire group of those with antisocial personality. This figure may of course be considerably less; there are no studies that provide reliable data on this subject.

Psychopathy and Charisma

At one time it was fashionable to speak of some severely antisocial individuals as "successful" or "creative." One view held that when the antisocial individual's sources of gratification were in concert with the wishes or needs of a particular social group, the result was someone who emerged as a hero or otherwise respected person. Harrington held that even highly symptomatic psychopaths represent a sort of social evolutionary breakthrough that allows the individual and those around him to transcend their compulsive, morally restricted day-to-day lives.[58]

This author disagrees. The person with antisocial personality is one with an emotional deficit. This

deficit limits his quality of life and prevents the attainment of truly close relationships, productivity, or true pleasure. The psychopath is best seen by the clinician as a victim of his disturbance rather than the happy bearer of it.

COURSE AND PROGNOSIS

Antisocial personality is a chronic disorder. Its characteristics may change with time, but there is little evidence that adequately diagnosed psychopathy will remit of its own accord before the individual reaches the middle years of life.

Authors differ in their descriptions of antisocial personality after this time. There is a common perception that some such individuals "burn themselves out" as the physical strength and emotional stamina needed to continue the stimulating, hustling life become too much. The aging psychopath has difficulty competing with younger ones, and with his own drive for relief, stimulation, and defense against his inner self. This "burning out," if it does occur naturally, should not be confused with the burn-out syndrome described in some drug abusers. The latter seems more clearly related to social competition and physical strength, as well as to bodily deterioration from the effects of drugs, illness, or malnutrition. The aging psychopath, rather, is often seen as one who is still antisocial, but has become less successful at it. He is described as a criminal who commits lesser crimes or who is now permanently incarcerated, as a "skid row" person, or as someone whose efforts at stimulation and defense have turned from outwardly antisocial activity to more passive pursuits such as drug abuse or alcoholism.

The author has spoken of another view of the course of true psychopathy—a paradigm represented by deterioration into severe depression.[12] This view arises from observation of severely antisocial persons who are, through no direct wish of their own, rendered incapable of stimulating themselves, and from the case reports of analysts and therapists, including the author, who describe the experiences of carefully diagnosed psychopaths within intensive psychotherapy or psychoanalysis.[6] In the first instance, severe illness or injury, for example, may cause a sudden, enormous barrier of reality between the individual and his defensive system. In the latter, a few therapists consistently report their antisocial patients' first experiences with affect (usually depression) during treatment, extraordinary fear of it, support by the therapist, and subsequent development of depressive syndromes. In both situations, there is a lasting despair—and anxiety about that despair—which supplants the symptoms of antisocial personality as if it had come from beneath those symptoms. The patient can and should then be treated as a depressed individual, not a psychopathic one.

Treatment

PSYCHOTHERAPY

Insight-oriented treatment, particularly that of sufficient intensity to eventually penetrate the psychopathic defensive structure, requires extraordinary dedication of the patient and the therapist. The former is likely to be unwilling to take on this task; the latter may not wish to spend his or her time treating an antisocial patient instead of one with some other disturbance. It is thus unusual to find cases in which therapists and patients work together in this way, but this rarity in itself does not alter the quality or principles of psychotherapeutic treatment when it is possible.

Countertransference issues are extremely important in psychotherapy with severely antisocial patients.[59] The therapist experiences powerful feelings of both seduction and revulsion within the treatment, and may encounter therapeutic dilemmas unique to his or her experience (particularly in the case of young therapists). Consultation or supervision is highly recommended.

Briefer psychotherapy, ordinary group therapy, and other traditional approaches are usually unsuccessful. The danger here is that the inexperienced therapist encounters a patient who appears to be bright and motivated, but later is disappointing or, at worst, devastating to the therapist's image of himself as a competent professional. When considering beginning treatment with patients with antisocial personality or related syndromes, the therapist should carefully weigh the potential benefits and detriments to all concerned, and should try to ascertain his or her true reasons for either accepting or not accepting the patient.

MENTAL HEALTH SYSTEMS

Special Hospitals

There are very few institutions that devote part or all of their resources to the treatment of antisocial persons who have no other mental illness. Setting aside hospitals and psychiatric units for mentally disordered sex offenders and those who are "criminally insane," there are fewer than one half dozen large mental health facilities in the world that focus on changing psychodynamic or personality characteristics of antisocial persons.

The most successful institutional approach to lasting changes in social and interpersonal behavior and in patients' intrapsychic functioning is that which devotes great time and energy to providing a therapeutic milieu that is inescapable. The patient ordinarily enters at the lowest point in a several-level hierarchy. In most such systems he knows that the only alternative to progress is prison, and there is only one way to progress—by convincing highly experienced staff, and often peers, that one is changing.

Treatment methods in such hospitals are different from those of traditional mental health facilities. Medications are rarely used. Great emphasis is placed on the individual's responsibility for himself and others in the program. Whether stated or implied, some of the major goals of group and individual therapy are to increase the individual's ability to feel affect, to fantasize, to trust, and to develop empathy. The very basic fragility of these persons' self-images is recognized, in spite of their tough exteriors. Consistent support, short of coddling, is extremely important, taking the form of stable relationships with staff, work toward both long- and short-term goals, and considerations such as private rooms or cells where the patient can reflect on new experiences and express affects without exposing himself to others (although sharing of feelings with others is important later in the treatment program).

Staff members in such institutions often have the dual role of therapist and jailer. Even the correctional staff should be chosen for sensitivity and lack of sadistic characteristics. There must be excellent communication among staff for mutual support and consistent treatment approaches. Many institutions use the same staff for both inpatient and outpatient treatment, carefully attending to the crucial period of transition between the hospital and the community.

The demise of indeterminate sentencing in the United States has caused some to doubt whether special institutions such as those described above can be effective, since they no longer fully dictate the patient's release date. Preliminary data indicate that by accepting only patients who have several years left on their sentences, and often by remaining influential within the parole system. Success rates of the above programs, measured in rates of rearrest, return to prison, future employment status, and so on, tend to be good compared to those of ordinary correctional institutions. The situation is far from one of panacea, however, and criticisms of such facilities are common. In this author's opinion, those criticisms not only reflect realistic appraisals of therapeutic results, but often show some of society's prejudice against the concept of treating those who have callously hurt us.

Community Programs

The Probationed Offenders Rehabilitation and Treatment (P.O.R.T.) program designed by F. A. Tyce, MD in Rochester, Minnesota, provided a paradigm for modern, successful community treatment programs for nonmentally-ill offenders. These programs share some characteristics with the longer, more intensive residential approaches just described (*e.g.,* hierarchical structure) but are briefer, less physically restrictive, and far less reliant on a therapy model. In general, the most successful ones follow most of the principles outlined below.

Offenders are referred to community treatment programs by sentencing judges, often because they are young, first offenders, or have an attorney who is aware that such a program exists. Thus, the treatment population is one that tends to be more highly selected for persons who are young, have committed lesser felonies, and are not felt by the sentencing judge to be a potential danger to the community (although several programs accept fairly violent individuals).

Once in the program, the offender is expected to become employed or start full-time schooling immediately. He then passes through several stages toward more physical freedom. From the beginning he is expected to be responsible not only for his behavior but for that of his peers in the program. Restitution to victims and payment to the program itself are common requirements. This may be arranged in a number of ways; offenders are rarely refused because of lack of ability to pay.

The physical pressures in community programs such as these are few. The doors are not locked. If one fails in the program, the immediate result is return to other sentencing alternatives (usually jail or prison). Many antisocial individuals find the always-present pressure to be responsible, feel affect, and grow away from criminal life to be highly stressful. In some programs up to 50% drop out and return to incarceration. Escapes are quite unusual and crimes while in the programs are rare.

The results of these programs are promising. Such programs are very cost-effective ways to deal with the offenders who are referred to them. *Per diem* costs are quite low, in the range of $35 to $45. This is often made even lower by reimbursement from the offenders' own work and returns to the community in the form of taxes and commerce.

Rearrest rates tend to be significantly lower than those for similar ex-convicts or persons in other kinds of transition facilities (such as halfway houses), provided the client completes the entire program successfully. These findings extend across many kinds of criminals, but are worse for counterfeiters and other "con-men" than for other groups.[60] Substance abusers often have lower rates of success. Those programs that accept both juveniles and adults report fewer successes with the juvenile groups.

Wilderness Programs

Another useful program for many kinds of offenders is the wilderness experience. Such programs are short-term (2–4 weeks) and do not follow medical or psychological models of treatment. The experiences are sometimes compared to those of the well-known "outward bound" programs, although there are clear differences in goals and process.

Those wilderness programs with which the author is familiar accept offenders at stages of court diversion, sentencing alternative, and prerelease evaluation. Referrals usually consist of first- or second-offenders who have commited minor felonies. Offenders are usually accepted without regard to crime committed, unless the judge feels that an individual is intractably violent. Mentally ill offenders, including schizophrenics in remission and mildly retarded persons, have completed strenuous wilderness programs and have benefited considerably. Most authors in this area feel that modifying the experience in order to make it easier for either handicapped or normal patients has a deleterious effect on its efficacy. Success may depend on one's going through a difficult but conquerable passage.

Wilderness programs usually consist of three phases. In the first phase, a few days are spent teaching the offenders something about camping, the country in which they are to have the experience, and the need for cooperation among all members of the expedition if it is to survive. Survival is indeed an important concept here, as in later stages there will be situations in which participants could be seriously injured or even killed (although to this author's knowledge very few such tragedies have occurred). At this introductory point a small percentage of participants drop out, but most go on to an 8- to 14-day wilderness trip that consists of several offenders and a few wilderness-trained counselors working together to achieve some complex physical goal. Finally, the offenders are prepared for an expedition alone, during which time the counselors watch from a distance.

The dropout rate for wilderness programs is far lower than that for community or institutional rehabilitation. After completing the program, clients are released into their communities and followed up with careful efforts to support their vocational, educational, and interpersonal successes therein. Recidivism rates for both juveniles and adults are far lower than those for similar individuals who have been incarcerated, or for offenders who have experienced an "easy" wilderness program, such as a simple camping trip.

In addition to simple rearrest rates, persons involved in some wilderness programs (especially those headed by Will Matthews, MD in the New Mexico forensic treatment system) have undergone broad social and psychological testing before, after, and long after their experience. Results are unusually positive, showing shifts toward normality on many scales of objective and subjective tests.[61]

OTHER TREATMENT METHODS

There are a number of other treatment methods that are designed for certain kinds of antisocial, often criminal behavior. These are only briefly mentioned here, because they do not specifically address antisocial personality or generically antisocial individuals. For example, depot injections of medroxyprogesterone or cyproterone acetate have been shown to consistently and safely supress testosterone levels in sexually aggressive or predatory males. Psychosurgery is sometimes indicated in situations in which rare seizure foci or, for example, basal ganglionic syndromes produce intractable violence in individuals of otherwise normal personalities. These and other approaches to particular, often organically-based syndromes, are discussed elsewhere, particularly in work by Elliott, Reid and Gutnik, Cavanaugh and co-workers, Tupin, and others.[19,62–64]

ANTISOCIAL PERSONALITY AND THE GENERAL PSYCHIATRIC HOSPITAL

Most persons with antisocial personality, when they do find their way to inpatient psychiatric care,

end up in ordinary mental hospitals, where they are placed on treatment units with patients of other types. In some cases the patient is hospitalized for only a short time, for example, long enough for the personality disorder to be diagnosed and a decision to discharge the patient implemented. In other instances the psychopath may need extended evaluation (perhaps while awaiting trial) or the hospital may have a disposition problem when it tries to discharge him. Experienced clinicians know that antisocial patients can wreak havoc in ordinary treatment programs and may exploit or abuse both patients and staff. Although this author's purpose is not to have those with antisocial personality treated unfairly, the good of others and of the therapeutic milieu may require that few psychopathic patients be admitted to some units, that their behavior be discussed openly among staff and patients in order to prevent confusion and exploitation, and that a firm "stick-to-the-rules" approach be taken whenever possible. These patients often complain and almost always try to rationalize their behavior. Patients must be treated according to their needs, not according to a strict democracy. If such a patient is caught directly hurting others, such as by bringing drugs onto the ward or extorting patients or staff, this author recommends legal action and removal from the unit. Nevertheless, the clinician must be aware of the sometimes subtle line between discharge and abandonment of the patient.

Antisocial Personality and the Family

The family of the psychopath deserves the understanding and support of the clinician. Family members are often wracked with guilt about what they may have done wrong in bringing up the individual. They may wonder whether their younger children are destined for the same fate. They may try over and over again to get the "antisocial offspring" to return their love and finally to grow out of it.

The clinician can help by supporting family members, pointing out the needlessness of their guilt, and encouraging them to separate from the individual who is draining them. It is difficult to convince parents or spouses that their antisocial kin will never begin paying back his debt to them, or that bailing him out of jail is really more harmful than helpful. This author recommends focussing on lessening the damage to the family and attempting to have family members realize that the entire family need not deteriorate with the affected member.

Antisocial Personality and Dangerousness

To some, the terms psychopathic and dangerous are almost interchangeable. Because of the way psychopaths often present to mental health professionals, and because of sensational media portrayals of "psychopaths" who really do not deserve the label, most laymen and many psychiatrists view these people as dangerous, even sadistic, by definition.

This view is erroneous. The dangerousness associated with psychopathy is more accurately linked to the indirect victims of his need to stimulate and defend himself. While this may make the victims feel no less pain, it should be clearly understood that most of those hurt by persons with antisocial personality are by-products of his activity (*e.g.*, people who trust him and then suffer a loss when he breaks his word, or victims of an accident caused by his reckless driving). It is unusual for the psychopath to begin some activity with the sole intent of hurting others; rather, he begins his activity without considering its effect on others. As noted above, empathy, the fantasy of another's pain, and the lasting thought that one "shouldn't" do something are not within his planning ability, much as attention to detail or self-destructive possibilities elude his predictions.

There is one form of danger related to the social phenomenon of psychopathy that this author believes is quite significant. That is the danger that in our efforts to contain antisocial behavior within our society, we will injure the very structure of our democratic way of life. The person with antisocial personality not only lacks feelings of concern or justice, he does not perceive them in others. At least, when he does see them, they become objects of curiosity (or perhaps envy) for him, which can be used to his advantage rather than our own. The more society creates stringent laws and encourages a harsh judicial system, the more it limits every segment of society except the antisocial one it wishes to address. The population as a whole thus falls victim to its own efforts to contain the antisocial behaviors it fears so much, while the person who engenders this fear goes about his business as he sees fit.

REFERENCES

1. Pinel P: Abhandlung über Geisteverirrungen oder Manie. Wien, Carl Schaumburg, 1801

2. Prichard JC: A Treatise on Insanity. London, Sherwood, Gilbert and Piper, 1835

3. Halleck SL: Psychiatry and the Dilemmas of Crime. New York, Hoeber Medical Division/Harper & Row, 1967

4. Kraeplin E: Psychiatrie, 8th ed. Leipzig, Barth, 1915

5. Alexander F: The neurotic character. Int J Psychoanal 11:292, 1930

6. Karpman B: On the need for separating psychopathy into two distinct types: The symptomatic and the idiopathic. J Crim Psychopathol 3:112, 1941

7. Cleckley HM: The Mask of Sanity. St. Louis, CV Mosby, 1941

8. McCord W, McCord J: Psychopathy and Delinquency. New York, Grune & Stratton, 1956

9. Hare RD: Psychopathy: Theory and Research. New York, John Wiley & Sons, 1970

10. Venables PH: Progress in psychophysiology: Some applications in a field of abnormal psychology. In Venables PH, Christie M (eds): Research in Psychophysiology. New York, John Wiley & Sons, 1975

11. American Psychiatric Association: Diagnostic and Statistical Manual III. Washington DC, American Psychiatric Press, 1980

12. Reid WH: The sadness of the psychopath. Am J Psychother 32(4):496, 1978

13. Reid WH: Antisocial personality and related syndromes. In Lion JR (ed): Personality Disorders: Diagnosis and Management, 2nd ed. Baltimore, Williams & Wilkins, 1981

14. Reid WH: Diagnosis of antisocial syndromes. In Reid WH (ed): The Psychopath: A Comprehensive Study of Antisocial Disorders and Behaviors. New York, Brunner/Mazel, 1978

15. Reid WH: Treatment of the DSM-III Psychiatric Disorders. New York, Brunner/Mazel, 1983

16. Cameron FL: Personality Development and Psychopathology. Boston, Houghton Mifflin, 1963

17. Hott LR: The antisocial character. Am J Psychoanal 39(3):235, 1979

18. Rifkin A, Quitkin F, Carillo C et al: Lithium carbonate in emotionally unstable character disorder. Arch Gen Psychiatry 27:519, 1972

19. Elliott FA: Neurological aspects of antisocial behavior. In Reid WH (ed): The Psychopath: A Comprehensive Study of Antisocial Behaviors. New York, Brunner/Mazel, 1978

20. Knott JR, Platt EB, Ashby MC: A familial evaluation of the electroencephalograms of patients with primary behavior disorder the psychopathic personality. Electroencephalogr Clin Neurophysiol 5:363, 1953

21. Hare RD, Cox DN: Psychophysiological research on psychopathy. In Reid WH (ed): The Psychopath: A Comprehensive Study of Antisocial Disorders and Behaviors. New York, Brunner/Mazel, 1978

22. Stringer AY, Josef NC: Methylphenidate in the treatment of aggression in two patients with antisocial personality disorder. Am J Psychiatry 140(10):1365, 1983

23. Menkes MH, Rowe JS, Menkes JH: A 25-year follow-up study on the hyperkinetic child with MBD. Pediatrics 39:393, 1967

24. Morrison JR, Minkoff K: Explosive personality as a sequel to the hyperactive child syndrome. Compr Psychiatry 16:343, 1975

25. Sandler M, Ruthven CRJ, Goodwin BL et al: Phenyl-

ethylamine overproduction in aggressive psychopaths. Lancet 8103:1269, 1978

26. Virkkunen M: Serum cholesterol in antisocial personality. Neuropsychobiology 5:27, 1979

27. Bowlby J: Forty-four juvenile thieves. Int J Psychoanal 25:19, 1944

28. Leaff LA: The antisocial personality: Psychodynamic implications. In Reid WH (ed): The Psychopath: A Comprehensive Study of Antisocial Disorders and Behaviors. New York, Brunner/Mazel, 1978

29. McCord W, McCord J: The Psychopath: An Essay on the Criminal Mind. Princeton NJ, Van Nostrand, 1964

30. Hare RD: Psychopathy and laterality of cerebral function. J Abnorm Psychol 88:605, 1979

31. Robins L: Deviant Children Grown Up. Baltimore, Williams & Wilkins, 1966

32. Mahler MD, Pine F, Bergman A: The Psychological Birth of the Human Infant. New York, Basic Books, 1975

33. Stubblefield RL: Antisocial personality in children and adolescents. In Freedman AM, Kaplan HI, Sadock BJ (eds): Comprehensive Textbook of Psychiatry, 2nd ed. Baltimore, Williams & Wilkins, 1975

34. Rexford EN: A developmental concept of the problems of acting out. J Am Acad Child Psychiatry 2:6, 1963

35. Reich W: Character Analysis. New York, Noonday Press Division of Farrar, Straus, and Giroux, 1949

36. Glueck S, Glueck E: Towards a Typology of Juvenile Offenders. New York, Grune & Stratton, 1970

37. Lindner RM: Rebel Without a Cause: The Hypoanalysis of a Criminal Psychopath. New York, Grune & Stratton, 1944

38. Menninger K: Man Against Himself. New York, Harcourt, Brace, 1938

39. Stürup GK: Treating the "Untreatable:" Chronic Criminals at Herstedvester. Baltimore, The Johns Hopkins University Press, 1968

40. Talley JE: A Jungian viewpoint. In Reid WH (ed): The Psychopath: A Comprehensive Study of Antisocial Disorders and Behaviors. New York, Brunner/Mazel, 1978

41. Guggenbühl-Craig A: Eros on Crutches. Irving, TX, Spring Publications, University of Texas, 1980

42. Reid WH, Ellis M: Psychodynamics of successful treatment programs: A Jungian view. Unpublished data

43. Schulsinger F: Psychopathy: Heredity and environment. International Journal of Mental Health 1:190, 1972

44. Crowe RR: An adoption study of antisocial personality. Arch Gen Psychiatry 31:785, 1974

45. Rada RT: Sociopathy and alcohol abuse. In Reid WH (ed): The Psychopath: A Comprehensive Study of Antisocial Disorders and Behaviors. New York, Brunner/Mazel, 1978

46. Rada RT: Sociopathy and alcoholism: Diagnostic treatment and implications. In Reid WH (ed): The Treatment of Antisocial Syndromes. New York, Van Nostrand Reinhold, 1981

47. Eysenck HJ, Eysenck SBG: Psychopathy, personality and genetics. In Hare RD, Shalling D (eds): Psychopathic Behavior: Approaches to Research. London, John Wiley & Sons, 1978

48. Tupin JP: Histrionic personality. In Lion JR (ed): Personality Disorders: Diagnosis and Management, 2nd ed. Baltimore, Williams & Wilkins, 1981

49. Horowitz MJ: Hysterical Personality. New York, Jason Aronson, 1977

50. Guze SB, Woodruff RA Jr, Clayton PJ: Hysteria and antisocial behavior: Further evidence of an association. Am J Psychiatry 127(7):957, 1971

51. Baker D: Chromosome errors and antisocial behavior. CRC Crit Rev Clin Lab Sci 3:41, 1972

52. Reid WH, Bottlinger J: Genetic aspects of antisocial disorders. Hillside Journal of Clinical Psychiatry 1(1):87, 1979

53. Hook EB: Behavioral implications of the human XYY genotype. Science 179:139, 1973

54. Guze SB: Criminality and Psychiatric Disorders. New York, Oxford University Press, 1976

55. Glueck BA: A study of 608 admissions to Sing Sing prison. Mental Hygiene 2:85, 1918

56. Bromberg W, Thompson CB: The relation of psychosis, mental defect and personality types to crime. Journal of Criminal Law Criminol 28:70, 1937

57. Oltman JE, Friedman S: A psychiatric study of one hundred criminals. J Nerv Ment Dis 93:16, 1941

58. Harrington A: The coming of the psychopath. Playboy 18(12):203, 1971

59. Lion JR: Countertransference and other psychotherapy issues. In Reid WH (ed): The Treatment of Antisocial Syndromes. New York, Van Nostrand Reinhold, 1981

60. Reid WH, Solomon GF: Community-based offender programs. In Reid WH (ed): The Treatment of Antisocial Syndromes. New York, Van Nostrand Reinhold, 1981

61. Reid WH, Matthews WM: A wilderness experience treatment program for antisocial offenders. International Journal of Offender Therapy and Comparative Criminology 24(2):171, 1980

62. Reid WH, Gutnik BD: Organic treatment of chronically violent patients. Psychiatric Annals 12(5):526, 1982

63. Cavanaugh JL, Rogers R, Wasyliw OE: Mental illness and antisocial behavior. In Reid WH (ed): The Treatment of Antisocial Syndromes. New York, Van Nostrand Reinhold, 1981

64. Tupin J: Treatment of impulsive aggression. In Reid WH (ed): The Treatment of Antisocial Syndromes. New York, Van Nostrand Reinhold, 1981

The Avoidant Personality

Avoidant personality is a new term in the official psychiatric nomenclature, having been coined by Millon as a descriptive designation for patients characterized by a long-standing, pervasive, and active withdrawal from social relationships.[1] Although derived initially in a theoretical manner, the clinical features hypothesized as characteristic of the avoidant personality accurately portray cases well known to practitioners and correspond in most details to descriptively similar, though conceptually and metapsychologically diverse, entities reported for decades in the nosologic literature. Features of a cast similar to the avoidant personality have been described most frequently in conjunction with conceptions of the schizoid personality and in portrayals of phobic character traits. Although this literature is modest in scope, an attempt is made to identify these major historic parallels. Before doing so, it may be useful to note that the mistrustful interpersonal style of the avoidant and the characteristic developmental history of parental deprecation represent features that have been ascribed, notably by analytic theorists, to a broad range of other personality disorders, for example, to the schizoid character by Fairbairn[2] and, more recently, to the narcissistic personality by Kohut.[3] This chapter, however, is concerned with authors whose conceptions of both the phenomenology and etiology of the personality types they have studied are clear forerunners of the *Diagnostic and Statistical Manual of Mental Disorders,* 3rd ed (*DSM-III*) avoidant pattern, described as follows in the official manual.[4]

The essential feature is a Personality Disorder in which there are hypersensitivity to potential rejection, humiliation, or shame; an unwillingness to enter into relationships unless given unusually strong guarantees of uncritical acceptance; social withdrawal in spite of a desire for affection and acceptance; and low self-esteem (p 323).

Historical Forerunners

This presentation of the historical and theoretical precursors of the avoidant personality is subdivided into three groups—those investigations that have been guided by a constitutional viewpoint, clinicians oriented by psychoanalytic formulations, and more recent theorists of a biosocial-learning persuasion.

CONSTITUTIONAL THEORIES

Having coined the term schizophrenia, Bleuler was also the first to employ the label *schizoid.*[5] However, the view that the symptoms of "dementia praecox" were dramatic accentuations of preexisting traits was recorded earlier in the clinical literature by Kahlbaum,[6] Binet,[7] and Hoch.[8] For example, in describing his "shut-in" type, Hoch wrote, "what is, after all, the deterioration in dementia praecox if not the expression of the constitutional tendencies to their extreme form."[8]

Kraepelin also wrote of a prodromal form of dementia praecox, describing it as "certain abnormal personalities with mild defect states . . . a product of dementia praecox experienced in earliest childhood, and then brought to a standstill."[9] He elaborated this view in later texts, speaking of these patients as "autistic personalities," characterizing them as inclined to "narrow or reduce their external interests and contacts and their preoccupation with inward ruminations."[10]

Bleuler coined the term *schizoidie* to present a cluster of prepsychotic traits akin to Hoch's "shut-in" and Kraepelin's "autistic" types.[11,12] He described them as "people who are shut in, suspicious, incapable of discussion, people who are comfortably dull at the same time sensitive.[13]

It was not until Ernst Kretschmer that the constitutional view reached its clearest formulation.[14] More important perhaps was his recognition that the schizoid character may arise from a combination of two, diametrically opposite levels of sensitivity. The seeming contradiction in Bleuler's quote in the previous paragraph—"comfortably dull at the same time sensitive"—was explained by Kretschmer in his distinction between hyperaesthetic and the anaesthetic constitutional proclivities. Although most individuals exhibit a mix of these temperament extremes, clear-cut clinical entities are seen among those who fall at one or the other polarity of the continuum. This distinction of Kretschmer's is the prime forerunner of the differentiation that has been made between the DSM-III schizoid and the DSM-III avoidant personalities. Those at the anaesthetic pole, similar to the DSM-III schizoid, are characterized by Kretschmer as indifferent, affectively insensitive, flavorless, boring, unfeeling, emotionally empty, cold, and soulless. In contrast, those at the hyperaesthetic pole are clinical types that clearly anticipate the features of the DSM-III avoidant personality. Kretschmer describes them as abnormally tender, constantly wounded, sensitively susceptible, feeling all the harsh, strong colors and tones of life, wishing to deaden all outside stimulation; beneath the "cover of a sulky silence" is an inner tension which "gets heaped up" and which "cannot be spoken out."

PSYCHOANALYTIC CONCEPTIONS

There have been a number of analytic descriptions and explanatory schemas that clearly correspond to the characteristics and etiology of the avoidant personality; these formulations have invariably been associated with the "schizoid character." Now that the traditional schizoid concept has been subdivided into several DSM-III personality types—schizoid, avoidant, and schizotypal—it is necessary that we reassess the earlier literature on the schizoid and identify those propositions that are most relevant and applicable to modern formulations of the avoidant and schizotypal syndromes. What follows is a summary of analytic proposals that were initially addressed to the schizoid character, but which appear today to be more pertinent to the avoidant personality; a detailed historical review and comparison of this literature may be found in Millon.[15]

The essential theme of analytic theorists is that the schizoid character evolves as a defensive consequence of early parental rebuff or indifference. This defense and disillusion model of development seems most applicable in the background of avoidants; by contrast, the defect and deficit model appears relevant to the history of schizoids. To the English analyst Fairbairn, these character types have experienced an "unsatisfactory emotional relationship with their parents and particularly with their mothers."[2] As a consequence, they are incapable of either giving love or being loved, having learned to depersonalize and "de-emotionalize" object relationships. Deutsch's proposal of an "as if" type is similar to that presented by Fairbairn.[16] However, "as if" personalities seem intrinsically lacking in affect, that is, devoid of empathic and emotional sensitivity. Because they exhibit no social apprehension, nor an awareness of their social insensitivity, this type appears to be more properly a forerunner of the DSM-III schizoid, rather than the avoidant character. Closer to the avoidant concept is Winnicott's proposal of a "false self" personality.[17] These seemingly unfeeling and detached individuals protect their deeper sensitivities or "true self" by interposing a false self between it and the outer world. This front hides and protects the true self from the pains and failures of life, shielding it with a false ego-strength, so to speak, so that it can be preserved in an unaffected state. Guntrip and Laing have elaborated the proposals of Fairbairn and Winnicott.[18,19] Both provide sensitive portrayals of the inner feelings and defensive struggles that typify the avoidant personality, although the label they append to their writings is that of the schizoid.

Similar analytic formulations have been offered by Horney, Arieti, and Burnham.[20,21,22] Horney characterizes her "detached" type as one who has learned to "move away" from people. She speaks of him as experiencing an "intolerable strain in associating with people, and solitude becomes primarily a means of avoiding it." There is a need to put distance between self and others, and to follow a set of negative goals in life, such as not to be involved, not to need anyone, and not to let anyone intrude or be influential. According to Arieti, the lack of involvement and overt insensitivity of these patients is a defense against their profound vulnerability to personal and social pain. What distinguishes Arieti's view is his contention that this vulnerability is repressed so successfully that there is no awareness of personal needs, nor is there any pain or longing for social affection. Burnham, following an object-relations framework, attributes the syndrome to a so-called need–fear dilemma. To him, this patient's "very psychological existence depends on his maintaining contact with objects," but the excessiveness of his need makes others inordinately dangerous because they "can destroy him through abandonment." His only recourse to alleviate the pain of his dilemma is "object avoidance."[22]

Another line of psychoanalytic thought, originated largely in the writings of Fenichel, has generated the concept of a "phobic character," described as a person who actively seeks to avoid situations and persons originally wished for.[23] Similarly, Rado has formulated a parallel syndrome which he terms "overreactive disorders," noted by their use of phobic avoidance as a precautionary mechanism.[24] Although this adaptation strengthens the individual's defensive safeguards against anxiety, it spreads as in a vicious circle from situation to situation, leading almost inevitably to a pervasive avoidance style. More recently, Mackinnon and Michels have described patients who exhibit "phobic character traits."[25] Aptly conceived in a manner that foreshadows the avoidant personality, these character types appear overly preoccupied with security, fear threats to it, and constantly imagine themselves in situations of danger.

BIOSOCIAL LEARNING THEORY

A recent deductive system proposed by Millon seeks to generate and coordinate all of the major personality syndromes.[15,26,27] Drawing on three polarities of psychological functioning that were posited by European theorists early in the century,[28,29,30] Millon combined the dimensions of active–passive, subject–object, and pleasure–pain to construct a full-range personality typology. Freud, for example, claimed that "our mental life as

a whole is governed by three polarities, namely the following antitheses:[28]

Subject (ego)—Object (external world)
Pleasure—Pain
Active—Passive

By manipulating the elements comprising these polarities, it is possible to deduce a wide range of personality orientations that "govern" the psychological life of patients. To illustrate this, individuals who are (quite normally) motivated both by the evasion of pain and the seeking of pleasure, but have learned that it is best to wait (passive) for others (objects) to arrange these aims for them, might be spoken of as possessing a passive-dependent pattern, a governing style that corresponds to the *DSM-III* portrayal of the dependent personality. Among other combinations of the three-fold polarity elements are those characterized by a paucity of pleasurable life experiences, a concurrent excess of painful ones at the hands of both oneself (ego) and others (object), and a vigorous drive (active) to evade the latter; this combination exhibits what Millon terms an active-detached pattern, an orientation that corresponds to the *DSM-III* avoidant personality, the subject of this chapter.

Definition and Criteria

The following clinical features and diagnostic criteria were presented by the author in 1975 as the initial working draft of the avoidant syndrome for the personality subcommittee of the DSM-III Task Force.

This pattern is typified by an apprehensive and fearful mistrust of others. There is a depreciation of self-worth, a marked social awkwardness, and a general distancing from interpersonal closeness. Desires for affection may be strong, but they are self-protectively denied or restrained. Recurrent anxieties and a pervasive mood disharmony characterize the emotional life. Thought is periodically distracted and confused, and there is an overalertness to potential social derogation that is intensified by tendencies to distort events in line with anticipated rejection.

Since adolescence or early adulthood at least three of the following have been present to a notably greater degree than in most people and were not limited to discrete periods nor necessarily prompted by stressful life events.

Affective dysphoria (*e.g.*, notes a constant and confusing undercurrent of tension, sadness, and anger; exhibits vacillation between desire for affection, fear, and numbness of feeling)

Mild cognitive interference (*e.g.*, relates being bothered and distracted by disruptive inner thoughts; irrelevant and digressive ideation upsets effective social communication)

Alienated self-image (*e.g.*, describes life as one of social isolation and rejection; devalues self and reports periodic feelings of emptiness and depersonalization)

Aversive interpersonal behavior (*e.g.*, tells of social pan-anxiety and distrust; protectively seeks privacy to avoid anticipated social derogation)

Perceptual hypersensitivity (*e.g.*, vigilant scanning for potential threats to self; overinterprets innocuous behaviors as signs of ridicule and humiliation)

Epidemiology

Little systematic data concerning prevalence, incidence, as well as a host of useful demographic indices have been gathered on this newly labeled syndrome. Nevertheless, preliminary information on these variables has begun to show up in the literature. For the present, they are limited to prevalence and sex ratio research. For example, recently Kass, Spitzer, and Williams have reported that approximately 6% of all personality disorders are diagnosed as avoidant types.[31] Of these, two fifths are males and three fifths are females. The results of a more recent and ongoing study, reported here for the first time, includes data from a substantially larger population than reported by Kass and co-workers. Based on a national sample of both inpatient and outpatient settings, and employing the results of the *DSM-III* correlated psychological test, the Millon Clinical Multiaxial Inventory (MCMI),[23] approximately 11% of all personality diagnoses were of the avoidant disorder. Notable here is the fact that male and female prevalence rates are almost identical. Table 1 summarizes MCMI prevalence percents and sex ratio diagnoses for all eleven *DSM-III* Axis II personality disorders.

Clinical Description

The *DSM-III* considers the essential features of avoidants to be hypersensitivity to potential rejection, humiliation, and shame. They exhibit an unwillingness to enter into social relationships unless there is assurance that they will be uncritically accepted. Particularly significant is the fact that they withdraw socially, despite strong desires for affection and acceptance. Devastated by disapproval, they distance from others for fear that they will be denigrated and rejected.

Avoidants feel their loneliness deeply, experience being out of things, and have a strong, though often repressed, desire to be accepted. Despite their longing to relate and participate actively in social life, they fear placing their welfare in the hands of others, or trusting and confiding in them. Thus, the social detachment of avoidants does not stem from deficit drives and sensibilities, as in the schizoid personality, but from an active and self-protective restraint. Although they experience a pervasive estrangement, they do not expose themselves to the defeat and humiliation that they anticipate.

Because their affective longings cannot be expressed overtly, they cumulate and are vented in an inner world of rich fantasy and imagination. Their need for contact and relatedness may pour forth in poetry, be sublimated in intellectual pursuits or a delicate taste for food and clothing, or be expressed in finely detailed and expressive artistic activities.

Isolation and protective withdrawal result in a variety of secondary consequences that compound the avoidant's difficulties. Avoidants' apparently tense and fearful demeanor often pulls ridicule and deprecation from others, that is, leaves them open to persons who gain satisfaction in taunting and belittling those who dare not retaliate. To most observers who have but superficial contact with them, avoidant personalities appear timid and withdrawn or perhaps cold and strange—not unlike the image conveyed by the schizoid personality. However, those who relate to them more closely recognize that they are anxious, hypersensitive, evasive, and mistrustful.

Avoidant personalities are alert to the most subtle feelings and intentions of others. Although this vigilance serves to protect them against potential danger, it floods them with excessive stimuli and distracts them from attending to the ordinary features of their environment. In the course of a typical day, avoidants may be so attuned to matters that bear on how others feel toward them that they can attend to little other than the routine aspects of their daily life. Cognitive processes of avoidants are not only interfered with by this flooding or irrelevant environmental details, but also are compli-

TABLE 1. Sex Ratios of Axis II Personality Diagnoses in Adult Patients

Diagnoses	Males	Females	Sex Ratio (M/F)	N or Percent of Total
Cases with at least one personality diagnosis	1574	1611	.98	3185 (.80)
Cases with two or more personality diagnoses*	1008	1128	.89	2136 (.54)
Paranoid	192	95	2.02	5.4
Schizoid	166	48	3.46	4.0
Schizotypal	229	186	1.23	7.8
Histrionic	72	421	.17	9.3
Narcissistic	209	91	2.30	5.6
Antisocial	230	52	4.42	5.3
Borderline	242	397	.61	12.0
Avoidant	284	281	1.01	10.6
Dependent	225	497	.45	13.6
Compulsive	311	265	1.17	10.8
Passive-Aggressive	254	248	1.02	9.4
Mixed/Atypical	168	158	1.06	6.1
Total	2582	2739	.94	5321

N = 3967 (M = 1874; F = 2093)
* Only the two most prominent personality diagnoses have been included in this table.

cated further by an inner emotional disharmony. These feelings upset their cognitive processes and diminish their capacity to cope effectively with many of the tasks of ordinary life. This cognitive interference, a cardinal feature of the avoidant personality, is especially pronounced in social settings. It is here that they must protect themselves from anticipated humiliation and rejection.

Avoidants describe themselves typically as ill-at-ease, anxious, and sad. Feelings of loneliness and of being unwanted and isolated are often expressed, as are fear and distrust of others. People are seen as critical, betraying, and humiliating. With so trouble-laden an outlook, we can well understand why their social behavior is characterized by interpersonal aversiveness.

Disharmonious emotions and feelings of emptiness and depersonalization are especially noteworthy. Avoidant personalities tend to be excessively introspective and self-conscious, often perceiving themselves as different from others, and they are unsure of their identity and self-worth. The alienation they feel with others is paralleled, then, by a feeling of alienation from themselves. They voice futility with regard to the life they lead, have a deflated self-image, and frequently refer to themselves with an attitude of contempt and derision more severe then they hear from others.

Avoidant personalities are beset by several notable conflicts. The struggle between affection and mistrust is central. They desire to be close, show affection, and be warm with others, but they cannot shake themselves of the belief that such actions will result in pain and disillusion. They have strong doubts concerning their competence and, hence, have grave concerns about venturing into the more competitive aspects of our society. This lack of confidence curtails their initiative and leads to the fear that their efforts at autonomy and independence will only fail and result in humiliation. Every route toward gratification seems blocked with conflicts. They are unable to act on their own because of marked self-doubt; on the other hand, they cannot depend on others because they mistrust them. Security and rewards can be obtained neither from themselves nor from others; both provide only pain and discomfort. They are trapped in the worst of both worlds, seeking to avoid both the distress that surrounds them and the emptiness and wounds that inhere within them.

The avoidant's prime intrapsychic recourse is to break up, destroy, or repress these painful thoughts and the emotions they unleash. These personalities struggle to prevent self-preoccupations and seek to intrude irrelevancies by blocking and making their normal thoughts and communications take on different and less significant meanings. In effect, and through various intrapsychic ploys, they attempt to interfere actively with their own cognitions. Similarly, the anxieties, desires, and impulses that surge within them must be also restrained, denied, turned about, transformed, and distorted. Thus, they seek to muddle their emotions also, making their affective life even more discordant and disharmonious than it is typically. To avoidants it is better to experience diffuse disharmony than the sharp pain and anguish of being themselves. Despite their efforts at inner control, painful and threatening thoughts and feelings periodically break through, disrupting more stable cognitive processes and upsetting whatever emotional equanimity they are able to muster. Fantasies occasionally serve as an outlet for venting frustrating impulses, but they too prove distressing in the long run because they point up the contrast between desire and objective reality. Repression of all feelings is often the only recourse, hence accounting for the avoidant's initial appearance of being flat, unemotional, and indifferent, an appearance that belies the inner turmoil and intense affect these persons truly experience.

Etiology

For pedagogical purposes, it is often necessary to separate biogenic factors from psychogenic factors as influences in personality development. This bifurcation does not exist in reality. Biological and experiential determinants combine and interact in a reciprocal interplay throughout life. This sequence of biogenic-psychogenic interaction evolves through a never-ending spiral. Each step in the interplay builds on prior interactions and creates, in turn, new potentialities for future reactivity and experience. Etiology in psychopathology must be viewed, further, as a developmental process in which intraorganismic and environmental forces display not only a reciprocity and circularity

of influence but also an orderly and sequential continuity throughout the life of the individual.

With the foregoing as a precis, let us outline a number of biological and psychosocial factors that are believed to interact to shape the avoidant personality pattern.

HEREDITY

Genetic predispositions to avoidant behavior must not be overlooked, despite the lack of empirical data. Many physiologic processes comprise the physical substrate for complex psychological functions. It would be naive to assume that these substrates do not vary from person to person. Studies that demonstrate a high correspondence within family groups in social apprehensiveness and withdrawal behavior can be attributed in large measure to learning, but there is reason to believe, at least in some cases, that this correspondence may partially be assigned to a common pool of genotypic dispositions within families.

FEARFUL INFANTILE PATTERN

Infants who display hyperirritability, crankiness, and withdrawal behaviors from the first days of postnatal life may not only possess a constitutional disposition toward an avoidant pattern but may prompt rejecting and hostile attitudes from their parents. Such tense infants typically induce parental dismay, an attitude that may create a stereotype of a difficult-to-manage child. In these cases, an initial tendency toward anxiety may be aggravated further by parental rejection.

PARENTAL REJECTION AND DEPRECATION

Even attractive and healthy infants may encounter parental devaluation and rejection. Reared in a family setting in which they are belittled and censured, youngsters have their robustness and optimism crushed, and acquire in its stead attitudes of self-deprecation and feelings of social alienation. We can well imagine the impact of these experiences on a child who was not especially robust to start with.

The consequences of parental rejection and humiliation are many and diverse. The opportunity for creating the basis for tension and insecurity through mismanagement is greatest at the earliest stages of life. Infants of cold, rejecting parents acquire a diffuse sense that the world is harsh and unwelcoming. They learn, in their primitive way, to avoid attaching themselves to others. They acquire a sense of mistrust of their human surroundings and, as a result, feel helpless and alone. Parents who scorn their offspring's first stumbling efforts markedly diminish feelings of self-competence and the growth of confidence. Although normal language and motor skills may develop, the youngster often uses these aptitudes in a hesitant and self-doubting manner. He may internalize his parents' criticisms and begin to turn against himself. The roots of self-deprecation begun earlier in life may take firm hold over time. The image of being a weak, unlovable, and unworthy person may take on a strong cognitive base. The future avoidant may become increasingly aware of himself as unattractive, a pitiful person, and one who deserves to be scoffed at and ridiculed. Little effort may be expended to alter this image because nothing he attempts can succeed, given the deficits and inadequacies he sees within himself.

PEER GROUP ALIENATION

The give and take of friendship, school, athletic competitions, and heterosexual dating make demands that the healthy youngster is prepared to meet. Other youngsters who are less fortunate, approach this era of life convinced of their inadequacies. The feeling is conveyed to peers and in turn is reinforced by them. Peer group interactions can be devastating for the future avoidant. Many such youngsters feel shattered by constant humiliation as they expose their scholastic, athletic, physical, or social inadequacies. Unable to prove themselves, they are not only derided and isolated by others, but become sharply critical of themselves for their lack of worthiness and esteem. Feelings of loneliness and rejection are now compounded by severe self-judgments of personal inferiority and unattractiveness. They are unable now to turn either to others for solace and gratification or to themselves.

RESTRICTED SOCIAL EXPERIENCES

Avoidants assume that the atypical experiences to which they were exposed in early life will continue to be their lot forever. In defense, they narrow the range of activities in which they participate. By circumscribing their life, however, they preclude the possibility of corrective experiences, experiences which may show them that "all is not lost," that there are kindly and friendly persons who will not disparage and humiliate them. By detaching themselves from others they are left to be preoccupied with their own thoughts and impulses. Limited to these stimuli, they can only reflect about past events, with all the discomforts they bring forth. Since experience is restricted largely to their past, life becomes a series of duplications. They relive the painful events of earlier times rather than experience new events that might alter their attitudes and feelings.

Differential Diagnosis

Because the syndrome is new to mental health practitioners, and because several of its features are similar to those of other disorders, the avoidant personality diagnosis requires greater differential clarification than usual. Especially problematic may be distinctions that need to be drawn among avoidant, schizoid, and schizotypal personality diagnoses; to a lesser extent, difficulties might occasionally arise in differentiating among avoidant, dependent, and borderline designations.

AVOIDANT-SCHIZOID DISTINCTION

Schizoids differ from the similarly appearing avoidant personalities in that they possess a defect or deficit in their capacity to relate socially and empathically. By contrast, avoidants are excessively sensitive to social feelings and defensively withdraw from interpersonal relationships for fear of experiencing humiliation and rebuff. Unfortunately, many clinicians, especially those of an analytic persuasion, consider an overt lack of affect or social blandness to signify a protective emotional blunting and isolation due to repressed childhood disappointments, conflicts, and anxieties. The notion that affect and social insensitivity signifies an adaptive defensiveness does not apply to the DSM-III conception of the schizoid personality, but it does apply to the avoidant personality. Although the DSM-III avoids specifying etiologies for its syndromes, the schizoid category was formulated to represent asocial and affectless individuals who are neither conflicted nor suffer social anxieties or the desire for interpersonal warmth or closeness; their detached and unemotional characteristics derive from inherent deficits in personal sensitivity and empathy. Clinicians who correctly ascribe their patients' bland exteriors to defensive actions consequent to conflict or disillusion should employ the new avoidant personality designation to represent their views. These patients are emotionally sensitive and, despite their restraint and withdrawal, do desire interpersonal warmth and social acceptance. On first examination, avoidants may appear to be cooly detached; their warmth and neediness will be exhibited on closer contact. Schizoids, however, continue to be distantly connected and emotionally disengaged.

Avoidants may be spoken of as being actively detached.[1,15] They are oversensitive to social stimuli and hyperreactive to the moods and feelings of others, especially those which portend rejection or humiliation. By contrast, schizoids are best considered passively detached. They are underaroused, undermotivated, and insensitive. As a consequence of their deficits they simply fail or are unable to respond to the incentives that activate interpersonal behaviors and stimulate relevant and mutually rewarding social relationships.

AVOIDANT–SCHIZOTYPAL DISTINCTION

In general, the behaviors, perceptions, and thought processes of the schizotypal suggest that he possesses a more severe form of pathology in personality organization than is found in the avoidant.[1,15] More specifically, schizotypals exhibit obvious eccentricities such as odd speech, ideas of reference, magical thinking, and recurrent illusions—essentially, features that often typify schizophrenia without the characteristic delusions and hallucinations. Avoidants exhibit fewer dramatic peculiarities and bizarre behaviors, expressing instead an anxious anticipation of humiliation, a fear of interpersonal rejection, low self-esteem, and an unrequited desire for social acceptance.

According to Millon, the schizotypal personality may be best understood as a more severe or decompensated variant of the avoidant and schizoid personalities.[15] Endowed with a less advantageous constitutional makeup, or subjected to more deleterious life experiences, the schizotypal pattern may gradually and insidiously unfold through earlier and milder avoidant or schizoid phases.

AVOIDANT–DEPENDENT DISTINCTION

Dependents are trusting souls; they seek out intimate and affectional relationships in both the hope and the assumption that they will be secured. In contrast, avoidants are rarely trusting; they anticipate social rejection and, hence, fail to seek warmth and maintain distance from personal closeness. They withdraw from affection and intimacy, whereas dependents are at their most comfortable and secure when experiencing a bond and a sharing with another. Should a dependent sense that he may be abandoned or rejected by a significant other, he will do anything to regain his favored place, increasing his compliance and submitting to whatever the other wishes, throwing all caution to the winds and exposing himself to even further deprecation. Not only does the avoidant rarely chance a bond that may result in rejection or humiliation, but should such signs become evident in a formerly secure affiliation, he will neither submit nor demean himself to regain favor, but quickly and protectively withdraw, repressing his pain and closing off all avenues that might reactivate it.

AVOIDANT-BORDERLINE DISTINCTION

As with the schizotypal personality, the borderline syndrome signifies a pathologic level of personality organization that is usually more severe and dysfunctional than that observed among avoidants. The affective instability, repetitive impulsivity, and pervasively erratic relationships of the borderline signify a long-standing and weak level of social and personal adaptation. Although borderlines occasionally exhibit a loneliness and an anticipation of social failure that is akin to that seen in the avoidant, these signs are transient symptoms rather than persistent traits, a minor and passing facet of a larger spectrum of unregulated emotions and conflict-filled relationships. The criteria of the borderline designation clearly aligns the syndrome within the affective disorders spectrum. It represents a moderately severe affective personality pattern in the same sense as the schizotypal syndrome represents a moderately severe personality within the schizophrenic spectrum.

Concomitant Disorders

Avoidant types are among the most vulnerable of the personality patterns to Axis I symptom disorders; they not only exhibit more of them but experience them more frequently and more intensely than all other types—with the possible exception of the borderline personality, in whom these symptoms often achieve the characterologic quality of chronicity. Because the avoidant designation is among the newest of the personality syndromes, it may be useful to elaborate on their associated clinical syndromes.

ANXIETY DISORDERS

The most common of the avoidant's symptoms is the generalized anxiety disorder, typically seen for prolonged periods and consisting of moderately intense and widely exhibited apprehensions. The interpersonal abilities of avoidants are barely adequate to the social strains and challenges they must handle. As such, they characteristically seem on edge, unable to relax, easily startled, tense, worrisome, irritable, preoccupied with calamities, and prone to nightmares; and they have poor appetites and suffer fatigue and intangible physical ailments.

PHOBIC DISORDERS

Social phobias, of course, are so deeply ingrained and pervasive a part of the avoidant that it is difficult to say where the personality trait ends and where the phobic symptom begins. Avoidants try to keep their specific or focal phobias to themselves. For them, the phobic symptom does not serve to solicit attention, as it does in dependents or histrionics, since they are convinced that such attentions will bring forth only ridicule and abuse. As with anxiety, phobias are an expression, albeit a symbolic one, of feeling encroached upon or of being pressured by excessive social demands. Crystallized in phobic form, these patients have an identifiable and circumscribed anxiety source that they can then actively avoid.

DISSOCIATIVE DISORDERS

As noted repeatedly, avoidant personalities experience frequent and varied forms of dissociative disorder. Feelings of estrangement may arise as a protective maneuver to diminish the impact of excessive stimulation or the pain of social humiliation. These symptoms may also reflect the patient's devalued sense of self. Thus, without an esteemed and integrated inner core to which experience can be anchored, events often seem disconnected, ephemeral, and unreal. Self-estrangement may also be traced to the avoidant's characteristic coping maneuver of cognitive interference, which not only serves to disconnect normally associated events but deprives these persons of meaningful contact with their own feelings and thoughts.

AFFECTIVE DISORDERS

Given their "detached" style, one might think that avoidants would not be among those who display affective disorders. This belief would be consistent with their characteristic effort to flatten emotions and suppress or otherwise interfere with feelings. Despite their efforts in this regard, these patients do sense a deep sadness, emptiness, and loneliness. Added to this melancholic tone is the contempt these patients feel for themselves and the self-deprecation they experience for their unlovability, weaknesses, and ineffectuality. Though hesitant to display this self-contempt before others, lest it invite a chorus of further derision, tactful probing will readily elicit both the self-deprecatory comments and the genuinely felt moods of futility and dejection. Repetitive affective disorders, particularly of a depressive nature, are therefore among their more notable Axis I symptoms.

SCHIZOPHRENIC DISORDERS

Among the more severe or psychotic disorders, disorganized schizophrenic episodes signify a surrendering by the avoidant of all coping efforts. Although every pathologic pattern may exhibit this disorder, it is an active coping maneuver in some personality types, thereby increasing the likelihood of its occurrence. Moreover, some personalities are more disposed than others to surrender their controls and thus to collapse into a fragmented state. Avoidant personalities are among those especially inclined to this disorder, not only because they are easily overwhelmed by external and internal pressures but because disorganization is an extension of their characteristic protective maneuver of interfering with their cognitive clarity. By blocking the flow of thoughts and memories, they effectively distract themselves and dilute the impact of painful feelings and recollections. Disorganized (hebephrenic) schizophrenia may arise, then, as a direct product of either intolerable pressures or self-made confusions, or both. The upshot is a clinical picture of forced absurdity and incoherence, and a concerted effort to disrupt cognitive logic and emotional stability.

Avoidant features often develop in other personality patterns as they begin to withdraw socially and experience critical and unsupportive responses from others. Whether initially dependent, passive-aggressive, compulsive, or whatever, the troublesome moods and actions that these patients exhibit often provoke both the rejection and the humiliating experiences that characterize the background of the avoidant from the start. In addition to these insidiously developing similarities, there are personality syndromes that naturally combine with the avoidant pattern. Research using the MCMI,[23] the *DSM-III* correlated self-report inventory, shows that profiles including the avoidant pattern are shared most often with dependent, passive-aggressive, borderline, and schizotypal personalities.

Treatment

Not only are the habits and attitudes of avoidants pervasive and ingrained, as are all personality patterns, but most find themselves trapped in an environment that provides them with few of the supports and encouragements they need to reverse their lifestyle. Moreover, because of their mistrust of others, they are not likely to be motivated to seek or to sustain a therapeutic relationship. Involved in treatment, it is probable that they will engage in maneuvers to test the sincerity and genuineness of the therapist's feelings and motives. Most terminate treatment long before remedial improvement occurs. This tendency to withdraw from therapy stems not only from doubts and suspicions regarding the therapist's integrity, but also from an unwillingness to face the humiliation and anguish involved in confronting their painful memories and feelings. They intuitively sense that their defenses

are weak and that facing their feelings of unworthiness, no less their repressed frustrations and impulses, will simply overwhelm them, driving them into unbearable anxieties and even to (as they fear it) "insanity."

To add to these fears, the potential gains of therapy may not only fail to motivate the avoidant but may actually serve as a deterrent. It may reawaken what these personalities view as false hopes. That is, it may remind them of the dangers and humiliations they experienced when they tendered their affections to others but received rejection in return. Now that they may have found a modest level of comfort by detaching themselves from others, they would rather leave matters stand, keep to the level of adjustment to which they are accustomed, and not "rock the boat" they have so tenuously learned to sail.

Therapists must take great pains not to push matters too hard or too fast because avoidants often feel they have a fragile hold on reality. Therapists should seek, gently and carefully, to build a sense of genuine trust. Gradually, attention may be turned to the patient's positive attributes, addressing these as a means of building confidence and enhancing feelings of self-worth. This is likely to be a slow and arduous process, requiring the reworking of long-standing anxieties and resentments, bringing to consciousness the deep roots of mistrust, and, in time, enabling the patient to reappraise these feelings more objectively.

In approaching therapy as a formal technique, note that a first approach would be to assist the patient in arranging for a rewarding environment and facilitating the discovery of opportunities that would enhance self-worth. Supportive therapeutic approaches may be all such patients can tolerate until they are capable of dealing comfortably with their more painful feelings. Psychopharmacologic treatment may be used to diminish or control anxieties. Behavior modification may prove useful as a way to learn less fearful reactions to formerly threatening situations. As avoidants progress to trust and feel secure with their therapists, they may be amenable to methods of cognitive reorientation designed to alter erroneous self-attitudes and distorted social expectancies. The deeper and more searching procedures of psychoanalysis can be useful in reconstructing unconscious anxieties and mechanisms that pervade all aspects of these patients' behavior. Family techniques can be usefully employed to moderate destructive patterns of communication that contribute to or intensify the avoidant's problems. Last, group therapy may assist these patients in learning new attitudes and skills in a more benign and accepting social setting than they normally encounter.

REFERENCES

1. Millon T: Modern Psychopathology: A Biosocial Approach to Maladaptive Learning and Functioning. Philadelphia, WB Saunders, 1969

2. Fairbairn WRD: Schizoid factors in the personality. In Psychoanalytic Studies of the Personality. Tavistock, London, 1952

3. Kohut H: The Analysis of Self. New York, International Universities Press, 1971

4. American Psychiatric Association. Diagnostic and Statistical Manual of Mental Disorders (DSM-III). American Psychiatric Association, Washington, DC 1980

5. Bleuler E: Dementia Praecox oder Gruppe der Schizophrenien. Deuticke, Leipzig, 1911. English translation: Dementia Praecox. New York, International Universities Press, 1950

6. Kahlbaum KH: Heboidophrenia. Allgemeine Zeitshrift Psychiatrie 46:461–482, 1890

7. Binet A: Double consciousness in health. Mind 15:46–57, 1890

8. Hoch A: Constitutional factors in the dementia praecox group. Neurol Psychiatr 8:463–475, 1910

9. Kraepelin E: Psychiatrie: Ein Lehrbuch, 8th ed, Vol 3. Leipzig, Barth, 1913

10. Kraepelin E: Dementia Praecox and Paraphrenia. Livingstone, Edinburgh, 1919

11. Bleuler E: Die probleme der schizoidie und der syntonie. Zeitschrift Gesamte Neurol Psychiatrie, 78:373–388, 1922

12. Bleuler E: Syntonie-schizoidie-schizophrenie. Fortschütte der Neurologie und Psychopathologie 38:47–64, 1929

13. Bleuler E: Textbook of Psychiatry. English Translation. New York, MacMillan, 1924

14. Kretschmer E: Korperbau und Charakter. Berlin, Springer–Verlag, 1925. English translation. Physique and Character. London, Kegan Paul, 1926

15. Millon T: Disorders of Personality: DSM III: Axis II. New York, John Wiley & Sons, 1981

16. Deutsch H: Some forms of emotional disturbance and their relationship to schizophrenia. Psychoanal Q 11:301–321, 1942

17. Winnicott DW: Primitive emotional development. In Collected Papers. London, Tavistock, 1958

18. Guntrip H: A study of Fairbairn's theory of schizoid reactions. Br J Med Psychol 25:86–104, 1952

19. Laing RD: The Divided Self. Chicago, Quadrangle, 1960

20. Horney K: Our Inner Conflicts. New York, Norton, 1945

21. Arieti S: Interpretation of Schizophrenia. New York, Brunner, 1955

22. Burnham DL, Gladstone AI, Gibson RW: Schizophrenia and the Need–Fear Dilemma. New York, International Universities Press, 1969

23. Fenichel O: The Psychoanalytic Theory of the Neuroses. New York, Norton, 1945

24. Rado S: Adaptational Psychodynamics. New York, Science House, 1969

25. MacKinnon RA, Michels R: The Psychiatric Interview in Clinical Practice. Philadelphia, WB Saunders, 1971

26. Millon T: Millon Clinical Multiaxial Inventory. Minneapolis, National Computer Systems, 1977

27. Millon T, Millon R: Abnormal Behavior and Personality. Philadelphia, WB Saunders, 1974

28. Freud S: The instincts and their vicissitudes. In Collected Papers, English translation, Vol 4. London, Hogarth, 1925

29. Heymans G, Wiersma E: Beitrage zur speziellen Psychologie auf grund einer massenuntersuchung. Z Psychol 42, 46, 49, 51:1906–1909

30. Kollarits J: Charakter und Nervositat. Budapest, Knoedler, 1912

31. Kass F, Spitzer RL, Williams JBW: An empirical study of the issue of sex bias in the diagnostic criteria of DSM III Axis II personality disorders. Am Psychol 38 799–801, 1983

William A. Frosch, James P. Frosch, and John Frosch

The Impulse Disorders

Some degree of impulsivity is part of the human condition. As Oscar Wilde said, "I can resist everything but temptation." As a symptom it appears in many syndromes; as an aspect of typical modes of behavior, it appears in a number of personality disorders. Impulsivity may also be the defining feature of specific monosymptomatic syndromes or the characteristic feature distinguishing a particular personality style.

Dictionary definitions of *impulsive* tend to stress suddenness, explosiveness, and driven movement to action. Within psychiatry, *impulse* is similarly defined as a generally unpremeditated emergence of a drive to an action; it is hasty, impetuous, and lacks deliberation; it is apparently irresistible and accompanied by tension. An impulse may be sudden in onset and transitory, or tension may crescendo to an explosive expression of the impulse, at times resulting in violence without regard for self or others. What makes such an impulse pathologic is an inability to resist it and its expression in an unsuitable and non-phase-related setting.

Both the impulse and the act to which it leads are experienced by the individual as consonant with the conscious ego state and aims of the psyche; they are ego-syntonic at the moment of expression. They are also often directly understandable by others in the sense that an aggressive impulse is likely to result in an aggressive act consonant with the accompanying affect and ego state: anger results in aggressive assault; sexual wishes lead to sexual acts. Although impulsive behavior is often used as a defense, the degree of distortion of the original impulse is not as great as, for example, in the neuroses, and, at the moment of expression, the original impulse is identifiable in the act (*e.g.*,

stealing in kleptomania). This is in contrast to the often bizarre, meaningless, ego-alien character of a compulsion, in which, for example, the aggressive wish may be expressed in the forced ritual of touching and erasing, of doing and undoing. There is also a primary pleasurable component: in contrast to compulsive patients, who do not primarily enjoy their rituals despite the often accompanying lessening of anxiety and tension, individuals with an impulse disorder enjoy the act at the moment of action, although they may later be horrified by their wish and their enjoyment of it.

Impulsive behavior is often incorrectly referred to as *acting out*. However, not all action meets the meaning of that technical term, which originally referred to fantasies about the therapist or treatment enacted in some disguised manner outside the treatment instead of being talked about within the treatment. The fantasy was "acted out" of the transference situation and the original wish remained hidden. This concept has been considerably broadened but is probably best restricted to behaviors clearly based on the enactment of unconscious mental content, on a fantasy or repressed memory, and not extended to all inappropriate or antisocial activity.

Developmental Issues

To experience an impulse is ubiquitous; to permit its expression on occasion is human. However, to have an impulse disorder requires a continuing or recurrent imbalance between the pressure of the impulse and the strength of the mechanisms for its control that results in impairment of function. The usual biopsychosocial mechanisms have been suggested. There is now ample evidence for neonatal individual variations in motility patterns and in the modes of coping with frustration.[1,2] These differing givens are acted on as development proceeds. As the brain matures, cortical control is imposed on drives and subcortically generated impulses. The role of normal control can be seen clearly in the frequency of difficulties in impulse control in patients with a variety of brain diseases or toxicity. Fever, trauma, and encephalitis have all been noted to be precipitants, along with more diffuse cerebral dysfunction, such as is found in patients with attention deficit disorder. Alcohol and other drugs are often used in order to permit expression of impulse but are also known to lessen controls and permit the surfacing of impulses.

Constitutional, developmental, or traumatic deficits in the ability to delay are central in disorders of impulse control. Neural development is essential to the potential for delay that is inherent in the development from presumed hallucination to percept, thought, speech, and evaluative judgment. However, early experiences with "good-enough mothering" that foster phase-related delay, development of the potential for anticipation, and imitation and identification with the mother are important. Both too much and too little frustration and both undergratification and overgratification interfere with the development of the ability to anticipate and delay. There is a failure, on the one hand, to incorporate the parents' nurturing and protective functions and, on the other, to experience parental permission for controlled, graduated, phase-related initiative, exploration, and risk taking.[3] Later in life, circumstance and specific physiologic and psychologic stresses may modulate both impulse and control. Social forces can also have powerful effects on these aspects of behavior. Marcus[4] has focused on the way a particular culture or subculture can reinforce the development of socio-syntonic and ego-syntonic impulsivity. "What Engels has seen is that the counterpart of the deprivations, instabilities, degradations and depression of the working-class life he knows, is its tendency to be impulse-ridden. This has always been the classical diagnosis of the culture of poverty; it remains so today. It consists of behavior and attitudes that are generally regarded as "nonadaptive." In addition to drunkenness, Engels discusses the other classical components of this syndrome; impulsive and promiscuous sexuality, general improvidence, lack of foresight, inability to plan for the future,

insufficient internalization of disciplines, regularities and normative controls and adaptive inflexibilities . . . The behavior in question is short-term and consummatory, and Engels includes among it certain kinds of theft and even suicide . . ."

Classification

The impulse disorders have been ignored[5,6] or variously categorized. Some years ago it was suggested that the symptom impulse disorders be separated from those character disorders in which impulsivity is pathognomonic, pervades the character structure, and is not limited to a particular kind of impulsive act.[7,8] Among the symptom disorders included were the simple impulsive act, aggressive or sexual; the impulsive neuroses such as kleptomania, pyromania, and some addictions; perversions such as exhibitionism, voyeurism, sadism, and masochism; the catathymic crisis, an isolated, non-repetitive explosive act; and intermittent explosive behavior.

In the *Diagnostic and Statistical Manual of Mental Disorders (DSM-III),*[9] of the symptom impulse disorders described previously, the simple impulsive act does not qualify for a diagnosis, and the addictions and perversions are classified under other headings, such as substance use disorder and paraphilia. The impulsive character is to be found either in attention deficit disorder, residual, or other personality disorders (the text does mention impulsive personality disorder but without specifying criteria). The *DSM-III* includes a diagnostic class of disorders of impulse control not elsewhere classified whose essential features include failure to resist an impulse harmful to self or others; increasing tension prior to the act; and ego-syntonicity and accompanying pleasure, gratification, or release at the moment of the act. The act may be premeditated or not; resisted or not; or followed by regret, self-reproach, or guilt or not. The class contains five specific categories: (1) pathologic gambling, (2) kleptomania, (3) pyromania, (4) intermittent explosive disorder, and (5) isolated explosive disorder; there is also a residual category, atypical impulse control disorder.

PATHOLOGIC GAMBLING

Gambling exists in every culture, and it is a rare individual who goes through life without ever making a wager. Greenberg,[10] in his comprehensive review of the psychology of gambling, suggested that the appeal of ordinary gambling derives from the fact that gambling allows risk taking in a controlled setting and it permits the gambler to entertain the momentary illusion of unlimited personal power with omnipotent control over fate. For the normal gambler, these illusions do not seriously interfere with the ability realistically to assess the situation, and he generally limits losses or quits while ahead. For the compulsive gambler, the act of gambling becomes an addiction; the "game" takes over life and disrupts personal, family, or occupational pursuits. This disruption, and the experience of the typical build up and release of tension characteristic of all the impulse disorders, define pathologic gambling in the *DSM-III:*[9]

> The essential features are a chronic and progressive failure to resist impulses to gamble and gambling behavior that compromises, disrupts, or damages personal, family, or vocational pursuits.

This must be distinguished from gambling secondary to a manic phase of bipolar affective illness, from social gambling, and from gambling in the antisocial personality. Although the compulsive gambler may commit various antisocial acts, this is usually done only in order to enable continued gambling, with later feelings of guilt and regret.

Custer[11] and Lesieur[12] have studied the broadest spectrum of gamblers and have provided a vivid picture of the natural history of the disorder. It generally begins in adolescence, and, over the course of several years, the preoccupation with gambling increases, until "the chase" becomes irresistible. An occasional big win reinforces the possibility of recouping losses with one throw of the dice, and eventually the gambler uses any available option to obtain more money to remain in the betting. When not gambling, there is a sense of boredom and deadness; during the game, one feels excited and full of life. As with the drug addict, eventually the gambler's existence is dominated by repeated cycles of financial collapse, bail out, and then continued gambling to the point of ruin. No matter how ruinous the circumstances, the gambler denies them and hopes to outwit fate.

Pathologic gambling is more common in men than in women. Predisposing factors in childhood are said to be a parent or other significant older person who gambled; parental alcoholism; loss of a parent before age 15 by death, separation, or divorce; and inconsistent or inappropriately harsh parental discipline.

There is an extensive literature about the psychodynamics of gambling. Freud,[13] in his essay on Dostoyevsky, suggested that gambling arose from a need for self-punishment to appease unconscious guilt about patricidal wishes. He noted that after a big loss Dostoyevsky experienced freedom from creative inhibitions and did his best writing. Bergler[14] also believed the gambler was motivated by a powerful unconscious wish to lose because of guilt about his hatred of parents who "deprived" him of his infantile sense of omnipotence. Greenson[15] believed that gambling behavior served to gratify multiple oedipal and pre-oedipal wishes. He viewed the gambler as reenacting a family drama in which fate at times represented the tyrannical father whom the gambler wished to defeat and at other times the mother he wished to woo and whose bounty he longed to receive.

Custer takes the view that gamblers are prone to depression and use gambling as an antidepressant. He does agree with the psychoanalytic writers that the gambler seeks to recapture the atmosphere of early childhood in which, in the mind of the child, time, death, and limitation of control do not exist. The gambler is engaged in a duel against the odds that constrain us all.

With the exception of Bergler,[14] most psychoanalytic writers have been pessimistic about the efficacy of psychotherapy for gamblers. The gamut of other modalities has been used, including behavior therapy.[16,17] The most successful treatment has been Gamblers Anonymous, either alone or in conjunction with psychotherapy. This group is built on the same principles as Alcoholics Anonymous and uses the empathic confrontation of peers who struggle with the same impulses. For most gamblers, psychotherapy is not likely to be successful unless coupled with such a group.

KLEPTOMANIA

Kleptomania was described by a number of English and European psychiatrists in the 19th century, notably Marc and Esquirol, who reported several such individuals, including two kings, who were compulsive thieves. In order to satisfy the *DSM-III* criteria for kleptomania, the following features must be present: recurrent failure to resist impulses to steal objects that are not for immediate use or monetary gain; increasing the sense of tension before committing the act; experience of either pleasure or release at the time of committing the theft; stealing is done without long-term planning and assistance from others; and stealing is not due to conduct disorder or antisocial personality. Thus kleptomania must be distinguished from ordinary stealing and from stealing secondary to another major disorder, such as schizophrenia or an organic syndrome.

Most shoplifters are not kleptomaniacs. Bradford and Balmaceda[18] reported on 50 shoplifters apprehended in Ottowa, Canada, and found kleptomania in only two of these cases. Other studies reviewed by these authors suggested a range of 3.8% to 8% of shoplifters. The disorder is believed to be more common in women, and, according to Bradford and Balmaceda, the typical shoplifter is a middle-aged, married, professional woman suffering from mild depression who steals an item of insignificant value to herself.

A young woman was seen by one of us because she repeatedly stole watches from her fellow students. After the theft she would give away the watches on a nearby street. She resented her peers, who she believed were superior: the theft was an act of revenge and an attempt to obtain what she felt both entitled to and deprived of. In this patient, as with many reported in the literature, there was a feeling of injustice, of having been deprived, and the theft was an attempt to take something to make up for the deprivation. Both the object stolen and the nature of the act may have special symbolic significance for the person. It may unconsciously represent milk, penis, child, or any valued and desired object. In more disturbed patients, the symptom may be a means of establishing identity and self-cohesion. One such patient kept the stolen objects, frequently fondling them while savoring her power and triumph. She panicked at the thought of stopping the stealing, saying that without it she would not feel alive or real. In other patients the act of stealing may represent an unconscious wish to be punished.[19]

Since true kleptomania is rare, little is known about treatment. Psychoanalytically oriented therapy has been successful in some cases, and behavior therapy has also been used.[20]

Pyromania

Fire has always been irresistibly fascinating to humans. It both maintains life and threatens it. Its many forms and functions can evoke different feelings and can become symbolic of a variety of activities. At times it symbolized warmth, security, safety, or sustenance; at other times it stands for sexual passion; and at yet other times, for hate and destruction. Arson, defined as "the willful or malicious burning, with or without intent to defraud, a dwelling house, public building, motor vehicle, aircraft, or personal property of another,"[21] is probably as old as our ability to light a fire. Arson is now commonplace. Conservative estimates suggest that in 1975 arson resulted in a death toll of over 1,000, with 10,000 persons injured and property damage over $1.4 billion.

The delineation of a psychiatric syndrome in which pathologic firesetting is the major feature dates from 1833, when Marc coined the term *monomanie incendiarie,* a condition he believed was linked to the frustration of sexual satisfaction.[22] Ray, in 1871, described patients who were not psychotic, and who experienced an "irresistible impulse to burn" with no other motive in setting fires.[22] For a time pyromania was not considered a discrete clinical entity but a symptom found in various mental disorders. However, in the *DSM-III* it is once again regarded as a specific mental disorder.

In the DSM-III, pyromania is defined as follows:

> The recurrent failure to resist impulses to set fires, intense fascination with the setting of fires, and seeing fires burn. Prior to setting the fire, there is a build up of tension. Once the fire is under way, the individual experiences intense pleasure or release. . . . The diagnosis is not made when fire setting is associated with conduct disorder, antisocial personality disorder, schizophrenia or organic mental disorder.

Although it shares the characteristic features of other impulse disorders (*i.e.,* ego-syntonicity, minimal distortion of the original impulse, and pleasurable component), the original sexual or aggressive impulse is somewhat more distorted than in the simple impulsive act.

Pyromania must be differentiated from other forms of arson, especially since the other forms are far more common. In his excellent review, Blumberg[23] identified five distinct groups of firesetters: (1) nonpsychologically motivated firesetters, such as those who set fires for profit; (2) juvenile and adolescent firesetters; (3) pyromaniacs; (4) psychotic firesetters; and (5) female firesetters. Estimates vary on the proportion of firesetters who are pyromaniacs: although some have suggested it may be as high as 40%, recently investigators believe it to be a rare condition. Kosen and Dvoskin[24] studied 26 consecutive pretrial arsonists referred to Bridgewater State Hospital and failed to find a single patient who satisfied the current criteria for pyromania. Lewis and Yarnell's[22] study of 1,584 firesetters remains the broadest survey of this population in the literature. Of the entire sample, which were mostly adult men, only 50 could be diagnosed as having true pyromania. The others, who were often psychotic or retarded, were not motivated by an irresistible impulse but set fires for other reasons, most often to obtain revenge for a narcissistic injury.

Pyromaniacs have an intense fascination in both the fire and in the efforts to extinguish it. The build up of tension preceding the act may at times be sexual and at times is accompanied by orgasm. After setting the fire, they will frequently sound the alarm and join in attempts to put it out, or they may stand apart, enjoying the secret knowledge of how the fire started. One patient, the employee of a hospital, asked to be transferred to the fire watch component of the housekeeping department. He would start a fire, then turn in the alarm, and rush to join the attempts to extinguish it. During these episodes he experienced intense sexual pleasure, often culminating in orgasm. He reported lighting matches to piles of paper as a child, masturbating as he did so.

There have been numerous psychodynamic formulations about the motives of pyromaniacs. In a classic paper in 1932, Freud[25] speculated that the "shape and movements of a flame suggest a phallus in activity," and that in order to tame fire primitive man had to relinquish the homosexual wish to urinate on the fire. Subsequent contributions noted the importance of sadism and pre-oedipal conflicts in firesetting. Vandersall and Wiener[26] and Boling and Brotman[27] both note that more recent dynamic thinking has shifted from an exclusive focus on sexual drive to include aggression and the overall state of the ego.

In their description of firesetters, Lewis and Yarnell[22] noted that these patients identified with the power of firemen who extinguish the fire and that firesetting frequently stemmed from the wish to avenge a narcissistic insult. Physical deformities, low intelligence, poor occupational and marital adjustment, and alcoholism were thought to be associated or contributory features. The younger pyromaniacs were frequently from broken homes.

Macht and Mack[28] studied four adolescent firesetters. All of these patients had fathers whose work was involved with fire, and firesetting served to reestablish a lost and longed-for connection with the father. Many other associated factors and causal mechanisms have been suggested. The link between urethral preoccupation and fascination with fire noted by Freud has been documented in some subsequent work. Wax and Haddox[29] believed that the triad of enuresis, firesetting, and cruelty to animals in adolescent males was predictive of future assaultive behavior. It appears that many factors contribute to the choice of firesetting as a primary symptom, and no one formulation will explain its occurrence in every affected individual.

Very little has been written about the treatment of pyromaniacs. Movromatis and Lion[30] noted that the denial and resistance to treatment of these patients make therapy difficult. With children who set fires, the symptom must be considered in the context of the family and family therapy may be indicated. However, there is nothing thus far in the literature to suggest the efficacy of specific strategies with pyromaniacs, and psychotherapeutic technique should derive from an assessment of various factors, including the patient's level of ego development, motivation, capacity for insight, and ability to establish a therapeutic alliance. Those on the primitive end of the spectrum will require a therapy that is structured and makes use of limit setting, confrontation, and assistance in evaluating the consequences of action. With those who have some capacity for delay and who can use fantasy as trial action, conventional exploratory techniques may be utilized.

INTERMITTENT EXPLOSIVE DISORDER AND ISOLATED EXPLOSIVE DISORDER

The diagnostic criteria for intermittent explosive disorder in the *DSM-III*[9] include the following: (1) several discrete seriously assaultive or destructive aggressive episodes; they are out of proportion to any precipitant or stress; they occur in the absence of interepisode impulsivity or aggressiveness; and they do not appear as a symptom of schizophrenia, antisocial personality disorder, or conduct disorder. The criteria for isolated explosive disorder are identical except that it is a single episode. This has been referred to as a "catathymic crisis" by Wertham.[31] In a review of these rare syndromes, Rickler[32] concludes the following:

> The penchant for tight classifications has exceeded current capability. The disorder appears to be a spectrum of behavior and should be termed episodic dyscontrol syndromes, rather than suggest a single entity. The exploration of explosive behavior will be more productive if the concepts involved are recognized to be evolving rather than final truths.

This caution is well taken; most reports are clinical anecdotes, and there has been little formal data collection.

Characteristically, in the absence of prior thought or conscious intent, although at times preceded by increasing tension or accompanied by subtle changes in sensorium, there is a sudden, at times paroxysmal, assault or other destructive behavior. The patients may be surprised or startled by their behavior, feel as though they are impelled beyond their control despite awareness of responsibility for their actions, and feel genuine regret and self-reproach at its consequences. Monroe[33] has noted a number of so-called soft neurologic signs as associated features, including hyperacusis, photophobia, minor motor asymmetries or awkwardness, as well as nonspecific electroencephalographic abnormalities. The latter are most likely to be uncovered through the use of activation techniques, such as hyperventilation or sleep induction, or by using nasopharyngeal leads. Attention deficit disorder may be antecedent to intermittent explosive disorder. Onset is most commonly in the second or third decade or may follow brain trauma or infection. It is apparently more common in men than women, with the former often finding their way to correctional institutions and the latter to mental health facilities. Some have linked this syndrome to sensitivity to alcohol idiosyncratic intoxication. Explosive disorders need to be distinguished from episodes or outbursts of aggressiveness that occur in other disorders, in antisocial personalities, or in patients with mania, paranoia, or schizophrenia.

Although many patients show some evidence of brain dysfunction (perhaps primarily limbic), it is clear that early life experience and learning also are important determinants of explosive behavior. Early deprivation and increased aggressivity within the family are associated with violent behavior and perhaps with this disorder. A wide variety of psychodynamics have all been suggested as contributing mechanisms. Both Elliott[34] and Ervin and Mark[35] have noted the role of particular significant others in eliciting violence.

The complexity of the syndromes included in this category demands thorough neurologic and psychosocial evaluation for both diagnosis and treatment planning. Anecdotal case reports suggest the usefulness of anticonvulsants in some patients even in the absence of clear-cut seizure activity. Studies, some done in correctional institutions, support the use of lithium in helping patients maintain control of violent impulses.[36,37] Propranolol has been reported to reduce violent behavior associated with chronic brain syndromes.[38] Despite the lack of evidence, and the reluctance of many psychiatrists to become involved with such patients, psychotherapy is often recommended and may be useful for some.

Impulsive Personality Disorder

The impulse-ridden character is permeated by a diffuse impulse disturbance not limited to a specific kind of impulse.[8] Impulsivity itself is the pathognomonic feature. Patients are usually infantile, immature, and intolerant of tension or anxiety. They may act instead of thinking, unable to postpone action. A wish is experienced as an immediate need. Such impulsivity may manifest itself in many spheres and lead to a restless running from one activity to another. These patients are rarely able to be by themselves or to maintain concentration. Explosive behavior may be followed by self-reproach, self-castigation, depression, and at times suicidal impulses. Although not accepted by the *DSM-III* task force, the following criteria have been suggested:

> This disorder is characterized by a diffuse impulse disturbance permeating the personality without attaching itself to one kind of impulse. The clinical manifestations are ego-syntonic and may consist of aggressive or sexual acts characterized by lack of deliberation and impetuosity. The impulse is apparently irresistible and impelling and occurs in a setting of tension. There is minimal distortion of the original impulse, and the expression is accompanied by a directly pleasurable component.

ASSOCIATED FEATURES. Patients in this group are usually infantile, immature, and intolerant of tension or anxiety. Their frustration tolerance is low, and they tend to react explosively in the face of deprivation. The patient may recognize this and berate himself for his impulsive behavior, and he frequently becomes depressed by his actions, at times to the point of attempts at self-destruction.

AGE AT ONSET. Onset is typically in childhood or adolescence. It may occur later in life as a complication of brain disease or damage.

IMPAIRMENT. Severe impulse dyscontrol may result in serious difficulties both at home and at work. This may range from slight disturbance of social or occupational functioning to relatively total inability to maintain a job or social relations.

COMPLICATIONS. Both sexual and aggressive impulses when uncontrolled may expose the individual to a variety of diseases, accidents, and damage. For example, an impulsive patient may get angry when somebody cuts him off on the highway and may accelerate abruptly and crash into the offending car.

PREDISPOSING FACTORS. There is suggestive evidence that at least some individuals with impulsive personalities also suffer from minimal brain dysfunction, have an early history of encephalitis, or have nonspecific abnormal electroencephalographic patterns. In addition, early experiences of deprivation may also be predisposing.

PREVALENCE. The prevalence of this disorder is unknown.

SEX RATIO. Impulsive personality is apparently more common among men.

FAMILIAL PATTERN. The familial pattern is unknown.

DIFFERENTIAL DIAGNOSIS. This disorder needs to be separated from other immature personalities and the behaviors carefully distinguished from more structured symbolically significant forms of acting out that occur in the neuroses.

Many of those patients with a clear history of early onset will meet the criteria of attention deficit disorder. Others with diagnosed organic brain disease are appropriately diagnosed as having organic personality syndrome. The differential diagnosis also includes mania, paranoia, and a variety of personality disorders, which may, as one of their features, show impulsivity. In both mania and paranoia other symptoms are also prominent, and the impulsivity is apt to be intermittent rather than pervasive and characteristic. Similar distinctions can be made between the impulsive and other personality disorders.

It has been suggested that real psychologic or physiologic trauma at critical stages of development may play an important role in reinforcing the leap from impulse to action. The earlier the trauma, the greater the interference in the development of the capacity to tolerate delay and the greater the likelihood of problems with impulse control. Greenacre[39] postulates that trauma early in development, when body motion and activity are the major communications, may inhibit speech development and alter the later balance between acting and speaking, with acting continuing as communi-

cation and discharge. The specifics of the experience, the nature of the trauma, and the stage of psychic development will determine the specific coloring of the impulsivity, for example, the focus on aggression or sexuality.

Few patients present with pure syndromes. In most patients with personality disorders the impulsivity lies along a spectrum from defect to defense, from action to acting out, from a relatively contentless discharge of biologically driven need to the enactment of a complex fantasy or reenactment of early life experience. However, when the problems are primarily defect, we may try to patch, repair, or replace; we cannot usefully interpret. Defects in the capacity for delay contribute to impairments in the evaluation of reality and in reality testing. The therapist may have to act as auxiliary ego once a working relationship and therapeutic alliance have been established. It then becomes possible to point out the consequences of behavior, to impose limits, to help strengthen the patient's own resources in the service of control, and to teach the patient to recognize the prodromata. These patients live from crisis to crisis; the therapist's accessibility is important to counter their loneliness and fear of abandonment. Particularly in those patients with either attention deficit disorder or diagnosed organic brain disease, medication is often useful.

When defense is most important or when the impulsive behavior reflects structured fantasy, as it does in acting out, then exploration, clarification, confrontation, and interpretation are appropriate. Often treatment starts supportively even when the goal is to undo early damage by exploratory therapy and the understanding of fantasy.

REFERENCES

1. Fries M, Woolf PJ: Some hypotheses on the role of the congenital activity type in personality development. Psychoanal Study Child 8:48–62, 1953
2. Thomas A, Chess S, Birch H et al: Behavioral Individuality in Early Childhood. New York, New York University Press, 1963
3. Khantzian EJ, Mack JE: Self-preservation and the care of the self: Ego instincts reconsidered. Psychoanal Study Child 38:209–232, 1983
4. Marcus S: Engels, Manchester and the Working Class. New York, Random House, 1974
5. Diagnostic and Statistical Manual of Mental Disorders. Washington, DC, American Psychiatric Association, 1952
6. Diagnostic and Statistical Manual of Mental Disorders, 2nd ed. Washington, DC, American Psychiatric Association, 1968
7. Frosch, J, Wortis SB: A contribution to the nosology of the impulse disorders. Am J Psychiatry 111:132–138, 1954

8. Frosch J: The relation between acting out and disorders of impulse control. Psychiatry 40:295–314, 1977

9. Diagnostic and Statistical Manual of Mental Disorders, 3rd ed. Washington, DC, American Psychiatric Association, 1980

10. Greenberg H: The psychology of gambling. In Freedman AM, Kaplan HI, Sadock BJ (eds): Comprehensive Textbook of Psychiatry. Baltimore, Williams & Wilkins, 1980

11. Custer R (in press)

12. Lesieur HR: The Chase: Career of the Compulsive Gambler. Garden City, NY, Anchor Books, 1977

13. Freud S: Dostoyevsky and patricide. In Strachey J (ed): The Standard Edition of the Complete Works of Sigmund Freud, vol 21, p 177. London, Hogarth Press, 1961

14. Bergler E: The gambler, a misunderstood neurotic. J Crim Psychopath 4:379, 1943

15. Greenson R: On gambling. Am Imago 4:61, 1947

16. Barker JC, Miller MB: Aversion therapy for compulsive gambling. J Nerv Ment Dis 146:4, 1968

17. Greenberg D, Rankin H: Compulsive gamblers in treatment. Br J Psychiatry 140:364–366, 1982

18. Bradford J, Balmaceda R: Shoplifting: Is there a specific psychiatric syndrome? Can J Psychiatry 28:248, 1983

19. Alexander F: The neurotic character. Int J Psychiatry 6, 1930

20. Robertson J, Meyer U: Treatment of kleptomania: A case report. Scand J Behav Ther 5:87, 1976

21. Boudreau J, Kwan Q, Faragher W et al: Arson and arson investigators survey and assessment (1977). Presented before the National Institute of Law Enforcement and Criminal Justice, October 1977

22. Lewis N, Yarnell H: Pathological Firesetting. New York, Nervous and Mental Disease Monographs, 1951

23. Blumberg NH: Arson update: A review of the literature on firesetting. Am Acad Psychiatry Law Bull 9(4), 1981

24. Kosen D, Dvoskin J: Arson: A diagnostic study. Bull Am Acad Psychiatry Law 10(No. 1), 1982

25. Freud S: The acquisition and control of fire. In Strachey J (ed): Standard Edition of the Complete Works of Sigmund Freud, vol 22, p 185. London, Hogarth Press, 1964

26. Vandersall TA, Wiener JM: Children who set fires. Arch Gen Psychiatry 22:63, 1970

27. Boling L, Brotman C: A firesetting epidemic in a state mental health center. Am J Psychiatry 132:946, 1975

28. Macht LB, Mack JE: The firesetter syndrome. Psychiatry 31:277, 1968

29. Wax DE, Haddox UG: Enuresis, firesetting and animal cruelty: A useful danger signal in predicting vulnerability of adolescent males to assaultive behavior. Child Psychiatry Hum Dev 4:151–156, 1974

30. Mavromatis M, Lion J: A primer on pyromania. Dis Nerv System 38:954, 1977

31. Wertham F: The catathymic crisis: A clinical entity. Arch Neurol Psychiatry 37:974–978, 1937

32. Rickler KC: Episodic dyscontrol. In Benson DF, Blumer D (eds): Psychiatric Aspects of Neurological Disease, vol 2, pp 49–73. New York, Grune & Stratton, 1982

33. Monroe RR: Episodic Behavioral Disorders. Cambridge, MA, Harvard University Press, 1970

34. Elliott FA: Neurological factors in violent behavior (the dyscontrol syndrome). In Sadoff RL (ed): Violence and Responsibility. New York, Spectrum, 1978

35. Ervin FR, Mark VH: Violence and the Brain. New York, Harper & Row, 1970

36. Sheard MH, Marini JL, Bridges CI et al: The effect of lithium on impulsive aggressive behavior in man. Am J Psychiatry 133:1409–1413, 1976

37. Tupin JP, Smith DB, Classon TL et al: Long term use of lithium in aggressive prisoners. Compr Psychiatry 14:311–317, 1973

38. Yudofsky SC, Stevens L, Silver J et al: Propranolol in the treatment of rage and violent behavior associated with Korsakoff's psychosis. Am J Psychiatry 141:114–115, 1984

39. Greenacre P: General problems of acting out. Psychoanal Q 19:455–467, 1950

Dependent and Passive-Aggressive Personality Disorders

The two disorders to be considered in this chapter reveal the heterogeneity of the personality disorder concept. Unlike those that reflect a major problem in personality organization, or those that appear, at least from a psychodynamic point of view, to represent a complex but stable system of compromise formations, the terms *dependent* and *passive-aggressive* personality disorders denote characteristic, fixed modes of relating to other people in otherwise relatively well-integrated personality structures. Indeed, in many individuals, such patterns of relating will operate with reasonable adaptive success. In such cases we refer to character or personality patterns or types, rather than disorders. It is only when these modes of relating are so fixed and inflexible, so intense and importunate, that they lead to maladaptive consequences that we refer to them as disorders.

Dependent Personality Disorder

The historical background of the notion of an overly dependent personality type has been admirably sketched by Millon.[1] Although frequently observed and described in varying and often pejorative terms, such individuals did not, as Millon points out, achieve a diagnostic home in most early classification systems. In the writings of 19th century psychiatrists, emphasis was placed on moral considerations with such descriptions as "shiftless" (Kraepelin) and "weak-willed" (Schneider); the

analogue in the *Diagnostic and Statistical Manual of Mental Disorders*, 2nd ed (*DSM-II*) was "inadequate." The passivity, ineffectuality, and excessive docility of these patients were seen as failures in moral development or (in the terminology that Freud sought constantly to refute) "degeneracy."

It was in the context of psychoanalytic character theory that efforts were first made to deal with such conditions outside the realm of moral or constitutional judgments. In his efforts to apply Freud's concepts of psychosexual stage development to the study of character, Abraham[2] spoke of the "oral" character types who are "dominated by the belief that there will always be some kind of person—a representative of the mother, of course—to care for them and give them everything they need. This optimistic belief condemns them to inactivity." Furthermore, he wrote of others who are "burdened throughout their whole lives with the aftereffects of an unsatisfied sucking period . . . These people always seem to be asking for something. One might almost say that they 'cling like leeches'. . . They particularly dislike being alone, even for a short time." Thus, Abraham clearly related excessive and maladaptive dependency to either overindulgence or deprivation in the oral-sucking stage of development. Levy,[3] in his now classic study of "maternal overprotection," found that although most children who experienced this distortion of development tended to show behavior disorders with manipulative tendencies, many had overdependent traits as well; they were demanding, lacked initiative, and insisted that others do for them things they professed inability to do for themselves.

DEFINITION

As defined in the *DSM-III,* the salient characteristics for the diagnosis of dependent personality disorders are as follows:

1. Gets others to assume responsibility for major areas of one's life (*e.g.,* getting others to make important decisions or to initiate actions)
2. Subordinates own needs to those of supporting persons in order to avoid any possibility of having to rely on self (*e.g.,* tolerates abusive spouse)
3. Lacks self-confidence (*e.g.,* sees self as helpless, stupid)
4. Suffers intense discomfort when alone for more than brief periods

Such individuals experience themselves as desperately needy and devote extraordinary efforts to the pursuit of an external agent or "magical helper" who will meet all their needs, make all their life decisions, rescue them from helplessness, and provide them with the love and nurturance without which they cannot, they believe, live. (Horney[4] referred to this pattern as "the neurotic need for affection.") In some cases, this position may represent a regressive expression of unsatisfied phallic longings; unconsciously, the patient may hope that through her dependent attachment she may extort from the "magic helper" a penis that, she believes, is necessary for self-esteem. These persons often tolerate severe physical and/or mental abuse and humiliation in order to retain, if only in fantasy, an attachment to such an idealized, aggrandized object. For the dependent personality, abandonment is experienced as the supreme danger, to be defended against at virtually any cost. Since the attachment is often tenuous and precariously maintained, anxiety is a common feature in the face of the omnipresent threat of disappointment and desertion and, should such an eventuality occur, depression, accompanied by feelings of helplessness, may supervene. Hypochondriacal complaints are frequent, serving to accent the patient's neediness and helplessness. An example of a typical case study follows:

> A 45-year-old Hispanic woman came to the clinic because she felt depressed. Tearfully, she complained that her husband does not take her seriously when she tells him of her concern about pains in her neck. She has had 14 children: 10 live at home and 2 have cerebral palsy. Her life has been devoted to her home and family; she rarely goes out, has few friends, and has little social life. Her only excursions outside the home are to church and to various doctors for care of mild asthma, pains in her neck, and feelings of "depression."
>
> She has been crying daily since her local doctor dismissed her neck pains and advised her to take aspirin for them. She has, however, slept soundly, had no loss of energy, has been maintaining her family effectively, and has experienced no loss of concentration. She has had no loss of sexual interest, no guilt feelings, and no suicidal ideation. Her principal focus of concern is her husband's indifference to her somatic complaints and his tendency to laugh them off. Apart from her sad, somewhat anxious demeanor, her mental state is unremarkable. She urgently requests medication for her symptoms, but it is to be noted that during a previous visit 4 months earlier with similar complaints she failed to take medication that was prescribed for her.

It is noteworthy that this patient's preoccupation is less with her symptoms than with her husband's lack of attention to them. It seems evident that her physical complaints are primarily a vehicle for communication with him and her "depression" is an expression of her resentment and feelings of helplessness at what she regards as his inadequate response.

EPIDEMIOLOGY AND ETIOLOGY

The incidence of dependent personality disorder is not known. It would seem that it has never been systematically studied. Clinical impression suggests, however, that it is not uncommon. It appears to occur predominantly in women, at least they more frequently receive the diagnosis than do men. It is not clear whether there exists some biological basis for this disproportion, but there are strong suggestions of both sociogenic and cognitive factors. Most cultures, and particularly Western industrialized societies, have stressed as normative a dominant aggressive role for males and a submissive "passive" role for women. Furthermore, Gilligan[5] has proposed that there exist two fundamental ways in which people think about and experience human relationships: (1) a hierarchical, power-oriented mode and (2) a mutually dependent, interactive mode. In her studies, males tended to emphasize the former, while women tended to see relationships primarily in the latter manner, with emphasis on dependence, nurturance, and care as crucial elements. This pattern could form the cognitive foundation for what, in exaggerated, even caricatured form, becomes the dependent personality disorder.

No known biological factors can be associated with this syndrome, but it is possible that certain innate temperamental variants may predispose to its development. One could speculate that, for instance, a child who demonstrates, in the terms of Thomas and Chess,[6] a low activity level and a low persistence level might elicit parental responses that would tend to promote a pattern of reduced initiative and excessive reliance on others. It is such early interaction patterns that appear to be of primary etiologic importance. Their own presumed temperamental characteristics, combined with particular parental needs, have stifled the development of individuation in these persons and of the formation of a stable sense of personal autonomy.[7] In the terms of Mahler's schema,[8] the practicing subphase of the separation-individuation process has been stunted, leading to a diminished sense of self-confidence and persistent reliance on the parent viewed as an omnipotent figure (or, in Kohut's[9] terms, "idealized parent-imago"). Such children then fail, Mahler suggests, to resolve the "rapprochment crisis" of the second year, experiencing intense separation anxiety and maintaining, therefore, a clinging attachment to the mother that interferes with the normal evolution of differentiated self and object representations. As a consequence, progression toward object constancy, or the ability to maintain stable images of both the self and the absent love object, is impaired, as reflected in the intolerance of such patients for being alone and their constant terror of abandonment.

Significant in this process is the role of *ambivalence*. The usual description of the overdependent person stresses his intense, often erotic attachments. Less often specified is the prominence of latent and unconscious aggression and hostility in his relations to the primary figures in his life. Inevitable disappointments in the idealized self-object evoke intense reactions of narcissistic rage. Through dependent clinging the patient is often able to exert a significant measure of control over the object; furthermore, his demands often mask unspoken reproach. His cloying sweetness and submissiveness can often be understood as a *reaction formation,* an unconscious defense against the expression of hostile feelings that, in his view, could threaten the maintenance of the relationship that seems to him to be vital to his very existence.

DIAGNOSIS AND DIFFERENTIAL DIAGNOSIS

The diagnosis of dependent personality disorder rests on the criteria set forth in *DSM-III* and cited previously. It should be noted, however, that as an Axis II diagnosis it may be consistent with a number of Axis I diagnoses with which it may coexist and from which it may be difficult to differentiate. These may include the following:

1. Agoraphobia without panic attacks. Here the intense dependence on another person, the anxiety about being alone, and the predominant occurrence in women may generate confusion. In fact, as Millon points out, "dependents are especially vulnerable to agoraphobia attacks."
2. Affective disorders. When confronted with the loss of a significant figure, particularly the "magic helper," the dependent person is likely to experience feelings of helplessness and/or hopelessness and progress to clinically significant depressive symptoms. This may be facilitated by the tendency of such patients to repress the rage they experience in response to object loss and to direct it against themselves, thus intensifying their usual self-depreciation and at the same time issuing implicit demands for care and reassurance to those around them.

In addition, differentiation from the following Axis II diagnoses will sometimes present problems:

1. Borderline personality disorder. In the intensity of attachments, the severity of their reactions to separation or loss, and their fear of being alone, patients with dependent personality disorders show resemblances to patients with borderline personality disorders. Usually they are less labile, less likely to engage in substance abuse, and more likely to have satisfactory work histories, but the lines between them may be thin indeed; a patient with a decompensating dependent personality disorder may show many of the features of a borderline personality disorder, such as affective lability and impulsive suicidal gestures.
2. Masochistic personality disorder. Although not represented in *DSM-III*, this diagnosis has a long-standing place in psychiatric nomenclature that is favored by many, particularly those who are psychoanalytically oriented. The willingness of patients with dependent personality disorder to submit to abuse and humiliation and to abase themselves is, by such observers, taken to suggest an unconscious gratification from pain, or at least a willingness to accept pain and degradation as the price of gratification. This willingness is considered to be the hallmark of "moral masochism."[10] Many dependent personality disorder patients will, however, succeed in maintaining a dependent attachment

without this necessity; in these cases, this diagnostic confusion will not arise.

3. Schizoid personality disorder. The passivity, low self-esteem, and lack of initiative of schizoid patients may at times appear comparable to that of dependent personality disorder patients, but their social isolation and affective aloofness are distinguishing characteristics.

Psychological testing, particularly projective tests, such as the Rorschach Inkblot Test and Thematic Apperception Test, which address questions of object relatedness, fantasies about interpersonal relationships, and self-image, can be of assistance in clarifying diagnosis. Of greatest value, however, is a carefully taken history that emphasizes premorbid patterns of adaptation as well as current relationships.

TREATMENT AND PREVENTION

It should be noted at the outset that patients with dependent personality disorder are difficult to treat. Not only are their maladaptive patterns chronic and deeply entrenched, but they also provide, when they work, substantial secondary gains in the form of attention, nurturance, and relief from life's responsibilities. One is often in the position of treating the consequences of failure of the basic dependent modes of relating in the form of anxiety, depression, or phobic symptoms; once these have been relieved, the patient may be indifferent to further therapeutic efforts. Alternatively, he may establish an intensely dependent relationship on the therapist, seeking the same gratification he customarily derives from other important figures in his life. In the latter case, long-term psychotherapy aimed at encouraging and supporting the patient's efforts at achieving autonomy and gaining self-esteem through active pursuits will often be of value. Countertransference reactions can be intense and require careful monitoring; these may range from feelings of anger and frustration to oversolicitude and inappropriate reassurance and support. No medication is useful in treating the basic personality disorder, but antidepressants and anxiolytics may be employed for short-term management of acute symptoms that may occur when the characteristic defenses and coping mechanisms fail to function.

Since no etiology is known, preventive efforts can only be addressed to those developmental factors believed to be causally relevant, if not necessary and sufficient. Parent education directed toward encouraging developmentally appropriate initiative and self-reliance and early (preferably preschool) educational programs promoting optimal development of the ego resources would seem likely to be helpful in reducing the incidence of this disorder.

Passive-Aggressive Personality Disorder

Of the various diagnostic entities defined in *DSM-III*, passive-aggressive personality disorder is one of the more controversial and, perhaps, the least clearly delineated. A specific interpersonal mechanism is constituted here as the determining criterion for and dynamic basis of a personality or character type and its maladaptive form. This notion has, apparently, demonstrated some clinical use in the past, since the term, in one or another variant, has appeared in each *DSM* edition. As Millon[11] points out, however, in his skeptical review of the syndrome, little attention has been paid to it in the literature over the years. The 19th century European systematizers (Kraepelin, Bleuler, Schneider) spoke of patients who were "ill-tempered," "querulous," and "pessimistic," presumably on a constitutional basis.

It was, again, primarily Abraham[12] who formulated, within the framework of Freud's psychosexual theories, a developmental hypothesis about the origins and dynamic functions of this pattern. After citing Sadger's description of persons who showed "great perseverance side by side with a tendency to put off doing everything to the last moment," he went on to describe oppositional tendencies in children, primarily around issues of defecation, and the tendency "in anal characters of postponing every action." The anal character, he says, "tends to procrastination and hesitation" and may also manifest a "melancholic nervousness which passes over into marked pessimism." This is not, however, "directly of anal origin, but goes back to a disappointment of oral desires in the earliest years." Thus to Abraham these tendencies toward pessimism, surliness, procrastination, and avoidance of action had their roots in pregenital conflict, both oral and anal, which generate intense unresolvable ambivalence. As Millon points out, Reich's[13] description of the "masochistic character" strongly resembles the present syndrome, with its provocative defiance, covert sadism rationalized as masochistic suffering, and the reliance on externalization as a major defense. This similarity represents, in fact, one of the major difficulties surrounding the diagnosis of passive-aggressive personality disorder.

DEFINITION

The defining characteristics of passive-aggressive personality disorder, according to *DSM-III*, are as follows:

1. Resistance to demands of adequate performance in both occupational and social functioning
2. Resistance expressed indirectly by at least two of the following: a) procrastination, b) dawdling, c) stubbornness, d) intentional inefficiency, e) forgetfulness
3. As a consequence of (1) and (2), pervasive and long-standing social and occupational ineffectiveness (including roles of housewife or student), such as intentional inefficiency that has prevented job promotion
4. Persistence of the behavior pattern even under circumstances in which more self-assertive and effective behavior is possible

The name of this disorder is based on the psychodynamic assumption that the observed passive behavior is a mask for covert aggression. Indeed, in some cases, the hostility and resentment toward authoritative figures may be conscious and expressed overtly. At the same time, these persons show little or no awareness that the occupational and social failures from which they suffer are the consequence of their dilatory or resistant behavior; blame is ascribed to those who make "unreasonable" demands, and a generally misanthropic and pessimistic attitude is pervasive. Indeed, at times this dysphoria may lead to overt depression and/or efforts to ward it off by means of alcohol or other chemical substances. Relations with others are characterized by truculence and irritability; compliance is grudging and experienced as submission, which is, in turn, felt to be threatening. This characteristic poses significant difficulty in treatment.

EPIDEMIOLOGY AND ETIOLOGY

No precise knowledge of the incidence of this disorder exists, but the pattern of passive-aggressive behavior is seen frequently and may occur in the context of a wide variety of psychiatric conditions.

According to Millon, diagnostic agreement on this syndrome was relatively poor in *DSM-III* field trials; this would make epidemiologic study difficult and unlikely to yield reliable results.

Small and co-workers[14] reported that of patients in public mental hospitals in 1966, 3.1% carried this diagnosis (*DSM-II*) while 1% of those in private mental hospitals and 9% of patients in outpatient clinics were so diagnosed. In his own study, 3% of admitted patients met *DSM-II* criteria for passive-aggressive personality disorder. On the other hand, of 408 consecutive admissions to the Payne Whitney Psychiatric Clinic of New York Hospital in 1982–1983, this term was employed as a primary or secondary diagnosis in only two cases (dependent personality disorder, in contrast, was used 28 times). Similarly, of 1000 consecutive outpatient cases, only two received a primary diagnosis of passive-aggressive personality disorder; subsequent retrospective review suggests that in neither case was this diagnosis the correct one. At the very least, such discrepant data suggests the difficulty in establishing the incidence or the definability of this condition.

There are no known biological foundations for this disorder. As noted above, early theorists, including Freud and Abraham, postulated undefined "constitutional" bases for the intense ambivalence and "libidinal fixations" that were thought to predispose to such characterologic deviations. It is possible, although it has not been demonstrated, that certain innate temperamental patterns, such as that characterized by Thomas and colleagues[15] as that of the "difficult infant"—negative responses to new stimuli, slow adaptability to change, frequent negative mood—may generate the kind of parent–child relationship that many believe contributes to the development of this disorder, and to the "oppositional disorder of childhood" (*DSM-III*) that often precedes it.

The passive-aggressive personality pattern appears to emerge out of parent–child interactions characterized by inconsistency of demands that are poorly and unstably internalized and by inconsistency of gratification that generates marked ambivalence that is never resolved. The aggressive component of this ambivalence is, however, not expressed directly. The passive-aggressive individual is, characteristically, not openly defiant or manifestly hostile; he does not overtly refuse to do what he is asked or in all cases even protest against it. He simply does not do it or delays interminably or does it wrong or forgets about it. He subverts his conscious intention and the demands of others, while disclaiming responsibility or blame for doing so; indeed, he characteristically attributes the blame to others. Unlike the obsessive-compulsive personality, whose exaggerated compliance and meticulousness are a caricature of introjected parental demands, the passive-aggressive personality disorder patient neither submits nor openly defies: he maintains an ambivalent inconsistent posture that generates hostility in others. This evoked hostility serves to confirm his sense of injustice, to justify his feeling of injured innocence, and thus to generate a pattern that closely resembles, if it is not identical to, that of a "masochistic character" (cf. Bergler's[16] concept of the "injustice collector").

DIAGNOSIS AND DIFFERENTIAL DIAGNOSIS

The diagnosis of passive-aggressive personality disorder is based on the criteria set forth in the *DSM-III* cited previously. As noted, however, there is considerable overlap between this diagnosis and that of other personality disorders; the passive-aggressive mechanism can be seen in a wide range of personality types, and many passive-aggressive patients show features of other disorders. Dependency features are prominent, however, and may lead to confusion with dependent personality disorder. The masochistic features described above may also create differential diagnostic problems, particularly for those who regard this as a distinct diagnostic type.

Small and co-workers[14] offered a number of factors that, in their view, serve to define and discriminate the syndrome. Characteristically, their index patients had developed emotional disturbances in adolescence, on a background of significant familial alcoholism. There was no gender differential. Their life histories were marked by serious interpersonal strife, verbal but not physical aggressiveness, impulsivity, and manipulativeness. Disturbances of affect were frequent, with impulsive rages and outbursts of tearfulness. Somatic complaints were frequent.

Of their 100 cases, 30 had signs and symptoms of depressive illness, while 18 met *DSM-II* criteria for the diagnosis of alcoholism. All the rest (52) had signs and symptoms of "significant psychiatric disorder" but did not meet specific diagnostic criteria. Their findings confirmed the impression that passive-aggressive personality disorder is, in *DSM-III* terms, primarily an Axis II diagnosis compatible with a wide range of Axis I disorders and lends support to Millon's reservations about its discreteness and usefulness as a diagnostic category.

TREATMENT AND PREVENTION

As indicated earlier, patients with strong passive-aggressive mechanisms are not easy to treat. Since they resist what they construe to be demands imposed on them by others, they are likely to respond similarly to the therapist's "demands" for change. Treatment is generally initiated by a decompensation of their characteristic coping devices, with the emergence of anxiety or depression, usually seen by the patient as purely situational. Initial treatment will involve, then, measures addressed to this acute symptomatology; these may be psychotherapeutic or psychopharmacologic or both. Once relieved of such urgent distress, many of these patients will lose interest in treatment. Vigorous confrontation is likely to increase their resistance; yet capitulation to their withdrawal will be seen as a lack of interest and concern. The therapist must walk a fine line between these positions. He must be alert to the countertransference rage that he is likely to experience in response to these patients' stubborn provocativeness.

Since repeated confrontation is necessary to assist such patients in developing interest in and capacity for self-observation, family and group therapies, where such confrontations are offered by peers and familiar persons rather than the therapist, may be particularly helpful. In any case, treatment, where it can be sustained, is likely to be prolonged. No drug therapy has been found helpful in dealing with the basic personality disorder.

In their follow-up study, Small and co-workers[14] found that only 9 of their 100 patients "recovered" from the condition diagnosed 7 to 15 years earlier. Although depressive symptoms and somatic complaints tended to increase over time, psychotherapy appeared to have helped those who received it.

In the absence of specific etiology, preventive measures will be difficult to specify. When feasible, parent education programs that stress consistency and clarity in the communication of parental expectations and that promote an understanding of children's developmental needs and capacities may be helpful.

REFERENCES

1. Millon T: Dependent personality: The submissive pattern. In Millon T: Disorders of Personality: DSM-III, Axis II, p 107. New York, John Wiley & Sons, 1981
2. Abraham K: The influence of oral erotism on character for-

mation (1924). In Abraham K: Selected Papers on Psychoanalysis, p 393. London, Hogarth Press, 1968

3. Levy D: Maternal Overprotection. New York, WW Norton & Co, 1966

4. Horney K: The Neurotic Personality of Our Time. New York, WW Norton & Co, 1937

5. Gilligan C: In a Different Voice: Psychological Theory and Women's Development. Cambridge, MA, Harvard University Press, 1982

6. Thomas A, Chess S: Temperament and Development. New York, Brunner/Mazel, 1977

7. Erikson EH: The problem of ego identity. In Erikson EH: Identity and the Life Cycle. New York, International Universities Press, 1959

8. Mahler M: On the first three subphases of the separation-individuation process. Int J Psychoanal 53:333, 1972

9. Kohut H: Forms and transformations of narcissism. J Am Psychoanal Assoc 14:243, 1966

10. Berliner B: The role of object relations in moral masochism. Psychoanal Q 27:38, 1958

11. Millon T: Passive-aggressive personality disorder: The negativistic pattern. In Millon T: Disorders of Personality: DSM-III, Axis II, p 244. New York, John Wiley & Sons, 1981

12. Abraham K: Contributions to the theory of anal character (1921). In Abraham K: Selected Papers on Psychoanalysis, p 370. London, Hogarth Press, 1968

13. Reich W: The masochistic character. In Reich W: Character Analysis, p 208. New York, Orgone Institute Press, 1949

14. Small I, Small J, Alig V et al: Passive-aggressive personality disorder: A search for a syndrome. Am J Psychiatry 126:973, 1970

15. Thomas A, Chess S, Birch H: Temperament and Behavior Disorder in Children. New York, International Universities Press, 1968

16. Bergler E: The Basic Neurosis: Oral Regression and Psychic Masochism. New York, Grune & Stratton, 1949

The Masochistic Personality

The term masochism is often used interchangeably but incorrectly with the perversions and the masochistic personality disorders. These are two separate and distinct entities, but confusion between the two has been longstanding. The *Diagnostic Statistical Manual III* (*DSM-III*) has compounded the problem by omitting masochistic personality from the classification of personality disorders, while specifically including the masochistic perversions under the sexual perversions. The authors apparently intended to subsume the personality disorder under the narcissistic and passive-aggressive disorders. However, these categories are inadequate to encompass the very special features of the masochistic personality.

It is probable that the ambiguity between the perversion and the personality disorder began with Krafft-Ebing's original description in 1895 of what is essentially sexual masochism.[1] He created the term *masochism* from the name Leopold von Sacher-Masoch. This was a 19th century author who had written several romances dealing with certain men whose sexual gratifications lay in being painfully treated by a special kind of woman (*e.g., Venus in Furs*).

Definition

DSM-III does attempt a brief definition of the masochistic personality disorder but without providing a special category for it. In a one sentence statement, the manual notes that the personality traits "such as the need to be disappointed or humiliated are distinguished from sexual masochism by the fact that they are not associated with sexual excitement."[2]

Krafft-Ebing himself did not insist that actual physical pain is part of the symptom complex. "The common element in all these cases is the fact that the sexual instinct is directed to ideas of subjugation and abuse by the opposite sex."[1] Many of the attempts to refine Krafft-Ebing's definitions tend to get lost in the morass of trying to explain such a willingness to tolerate, and even to seek out, suffering. The distinction between the perversion, which requires pain for sexual gratification, and the personality disorder, with its more remote sexual aims, frequently appears blurred.

Lion still maintains that self-mutilation is a common aspect of the masochistic personality.[3] He states that the tensions of primitive sexual and aggressive feelings are relieved by these acts of self-mutilations. Sack and Miller define the personality in behavioristic terms, as "behavior in which ordinarily painful or unpleasant experiences do not produce the expected responses. . . In short, the individual's reactions to ordinarily aversive events is anomolous."[4]

Psychoanalysis emphasizes the dynamic elements in addition to the phenomenology. In his pioneering study of character, Reich says ". . . love and affection are sought but result in pain; by making themselves unlovable, masochists avoid pain but, as a consequence, prevent themselves from achieving the love they desire."[5]

The personality disorder can probably be most fully defined as a life-long pattern of unconsciously arranged difficulties or failures in multiple areas of functioning. Brenner adds the psychoanalytic dictum that such seeking after discomfort is in the service of obtaining sexual pleasure and "that either the seeking or the pleasure or both may often be unconscious rather than conscious."[6] Today many analysts would no longer agree with this statement.

Epidemiology

No statistics are available as to either the general or gender incidence of masochistic personality disorders. The impression of most psychiatrists is that it is a common phenomenon with equal distribution among men and women. Certainly, some elements of masochism seem pervasive in our culture. By contrast, the perversion seems to be much more limited in the population, although here, too, no specific statistics are available. Again, by contrast, what is known but not well explained is that the perversion occurs almost exclusively in men with few, if any women, reported in the literature. Even in the small number of women in whom the perversion does seem to appear, its main incentive seems to reflect a need to maintain a relationship with a man who requires these acts. The woman who acts out a masochistic perversion apparently does so with the aim of holding onto a relationship with a sadistic man. The sexual element itself is not the prominent aspect in the woman's masochistic perversion as it is with men. Women's involvement in masochistic perversions is much more attenuated and lacks the ecstatic and intense lust of masochistic sexual experiences.

Clinical Description

The masochistic personality demonstrates a need to be unnecessarily encumbered, or even to fail, in most endeavors. He displays an inability to succeed fully, if at all, in whichever goal he may choose. The category includes those who are the "losers" of our society, the ones who succeed in wresting failure out of the teeth of success. This is usually consistent in all areas of functioning—school, work, love relationships—although in varying degress. Endowment with innate talent or high intelligence can counterbalance the need to fail to some degree, but most success is achieved at a great emotional expense and at a level far below what should be ex-

pected. Unable to appreciate his/her own role in thwarting success, the masochist tends to perceive failure as a defeat by an external agency, usually fate.

Unlike with the perversion, another person is not necessary as the punitive figure. Just as they cannot recognize their own role in their frustrations and failures, masochists need to see their difficulties as arising from the world outside themselves. "Fate, a late and impersonal father substitute, has replaced the humiliating and beating partner."[7]

The personality style is frequently presented in an exhibitionistic manner. He often has a need to exhibit to the world the "slings and arrows of outrageous fortune" that are defeating him. But it is also in this exhibiting quality that the aggressiveness of the masochist is experienced. His constant overt or covert complaints frustrate or stimulate guilt in their object relationships. This creates major difficulties in therapy.

Submission is a prominent aspect of the masochistic personality. Its aim includes the need to arouse guilt in the other person (for what he or the original loved one did in the past) and helps to explain certain typical masochistic object relations that would otherwise be perplexing. These are instances in which a clearly destructive relationship is continued, with the masochist persisting in thrusting himself into closeness with a hurtful partner who is incapable of guilt feelings. In contrast, the normal adult, when he or she experiences rejection in a love affair, hates in return and gives up the object. The masochist blindly and repeatedly and progressively humiliates himself in submission to the denigrating partner, always hoping that by his increasingly flagrant and humiliating submissions, he will succeed in provoking guilt. The movie "The Blue Angel" is a powerful story of just such a painful relationship in which a highly successful, highly principled and moral man submits to an unprincipled woman—lower class in ethics, morality, and life values. She uses him, exploits him, and eventually destroys him. The almost literally fatal fascination that such a self-indulgent, amoral woman has for this previously highly self-controlled, respected, and honored man, is confounding to the observer, unless one appreciates the desperate need of the masochist to arouse the guilt feelings that seem absent in the exploiting and cruel partner. The attraction this woman has lies in her hedonistic, guiltless abandon, which the moral man envies but also attempts to bring down, because he requires himself to forgo such hedonistic gratifications and because she is very likely a representation of a hated, earlier person. His continued failure to elicit such guilt escalates to ever-greater shameful humiliations, until he is destroyed. The unconscious fantasy seems to be, "Look what you've done to me, my destruction will show them what an evil destructive person you are; you *must* feel guilty about this." An additional important determinant is the element, "You *will* love me because I degrade myself and suffer. I know that this is what you require in order for me to be loved by you." It is a clinical example that illustrates Frued's pithy comment, "The true masochist always holds out his cheek whenever he sees the chance of receiving a blow."[8]

An interesting but relatively unexplored phenomenon is the ability of certain masochists to contaminate and then arouse similar masochistic actions in their objects. Fowles' *The French Lieutenant's Woman* illustrates just such a relationship. In the novel (and the movie) a woman with a shadowy past is reputedly dominated by feelings of rejection by a deceitful lover. She maintains a mysterious, distant but enticing stance in her community, until she ensnares a young man. The man, at the zenith of his fortunes, is seduced by her air of sadness and desolation at her years-ago desertion. After a brief inner struggle, he succumbs to her and renounces all his successes—career, wealth, reputation and a loving fiancee—all in a kind of masochistic orgy. He is then, in turn, inevitably deserted by the woman. This is a familiar pattern and one that can be explained by analytic concepts. It probably represents a revitalization of an earlier libidinal tie to an internalized sadistic object, one that had been unstably repressed, as will be discussed further.

Although one can usually find evidences of the masochistic personality all along the individual's life course, its intensity does vary considerably. It is often difficult to anticipate the varying intensity of the need to suffer or fail, but there is a pattern of increasing self-thwarting behavior whenever a greatly desired situation presents itself. Related to those characters Freud described, who have a tendency to be "wrecked by success," whose achievements, or approaching achievements, are "too rich for my blood" (as one patient sardonically muttered) the disorder is stimulated by the smell of success.[9] The masochistic need seems less marked, however, when fate has independently presented one with a severe affliction or personal loss. Whether facilitated long in advance by the personality disorder itself, or through an unfortunate exigency of life, such actual sufferings usurp the masochistic need to arrange for them and the personality disorder may become less intense, although usually only for the period of suffering.

Personality structures permeated with a marked masochistic proclivity frequently function quite well in other areas. These individuals tend to have a high level of personality organization. As a group, they are dependable, hard-working people. If they have some talent, their achievement can be quite impressive to others, although they remain dissatisfied and self-critical. On the whole, their more superficial associations with people are quite good but the severity of the demands they place on themselves, and often onto others, can eventually become unpleasant and even unwelcome burdens in more significant and intimate relationships.

Masochistic behavior patterns usually begin to become manifest in middle to late adolescence and tend to become more fixed and distinctive as life progresses. Without treatment the course is usually inexorable, sometimes advancing to severe depression and even suicide later in life. Since masochism is a personality style that is fed by internal needs, environmental changes rarely relieve the pathology. There are two possible exceptions. In some cases a life partner is found who has complementary needs and a long-lasting, balanced, and gratifying relationship may ensue. In other situations, the postponing of gratifications and the expectation that their sacrifices, hard work, and turning the other cheek, will eventually be appreciated and the long-awaited reward be forthcoming, is suddenly recognized as no longer realistic. These are the perfectionistic men and women who have driven themselves all their lives until they reach their 40s and 50s, and younger people are now being promoted over them.

In other cases their families are being dispersed and they find themselves clutching at empty air, rather than receiving the kudos and embracing love for which they have been paying in advance all their lifes by martyrdom. These are the individuals whose personality disorders now fail whatever adaptive or maladaptive functions they have served. Their pathology begins to slide into depressions or alcoholism or other substance abuse. Depending on the degree to which their previous life achievements may continue to serve as supports, they may fade away into withdrawn, passive, depressive, misogynist, querulous personalities, inwardly (sometimes outwardly) railing against the unfairness of life. It is unusual for the masochistic personality to compromise with their inner demands and to settle into a comfortable, satisfied way of life.

Etiology

Despite the multiplicity of explanations that have been suggested, the etiology of masochistic personalities is basically unknown. A discussion from two view points, the possible biological origins and the psychodynamic explanations, should help organize the current theories.

BIOLOGY AND ETHOLOGY OF MASOCHISM

In the psychiatry of the 19th and early 20th century, genetic influences were always given great weight in psychopathology, and this was also true for masochistic behavior. This belief then shifted to a tendency to deemphasize heredity and to emphasize rather early conditioning and the dynamic influences of early family life. Masochism is usually considered an exclusively human propensity. The more complicated social development of humans, the long period of helplessness during infancy with dependence on the parents for care and love, the high capacity for symbolization and the complexities of human interactions have supported this belief that masochism is a purely human vicissitude of life. Beginning with Freud's 1923 claim that "masochism was a derivative of an inborn death instinct," part of the inevitable direction towards entropy of all living organisms, reemphasized the sometimes overriding importance of constitutional endowment.[10] Long before DNA was understood, he stated that "each ego is endowed from the first with individual dispositions and trends . . . even before the ego has come into existence the lines of development, trends, and reactions that it will later exhibit are already laid down for it."[11] Recently renewed interest in tracing phylogenetic patterns of masochistic or submissive behavior has appeared. Evidence accumulated by some experimental psychologists, and especially the animal ethologists Lorenz and Tinbergen, are influencing clinicians and theorists to reexamine the role of genetics in the area of masochistic precursors.[12]

Some of the work with imprinting phenomena in chicks has shown that painful stimuli presented during the critical first 18 hours of life establish a more rapid and more firmly entrenched attach-ment to the parent object than occurs in controls.[13] This is suggestive of the dynamics of some forms of human masochism, where the subject is willing to endure suffering or deprivation if it believes that an important love object will become more loving. A chick imprinted with an associated electric shock will "follow the parent object significantly more than a group of control animals which had not received shock. This . . . is not unreasonable from the survival value of such behavior because the animal in a painful situation at that moment when it depends on the parent to a tremendous degree to survive, seeks to get even closer to the parent object."[14] Punishment does facilitate behavior, at least experimentally. Sack and Miller have collected a number of similar aversive experiments with animals that seem to support these findings.[4] Jay Weiss, of Rockefeller University, has been studying the varying behavior of rats who have different amounts of alpha II receptors for norepinephrine in their locus ceruleus.[15] This is clearly a genetic disparity that Weiss believes influences the sociology of the rat colony, the dominance hierarchy, or the pecking order. Those rats with fewer alpha II receptors allowed themselves to submit to and be dominated by the rats with a greater number of the receptors.

Wilson, a sociobiologist, is a major advocate of the role of genetics in masochism. Extrapolating from his observations of the social insects, such as bees and ants, and their altruistic self-sacrifice for the preservation of the family group, he suggests that these primitive activities may be phylogenetic precursors of masochism; that ". . . the emotions we feel, which in exceptional individuals may climax in total self-sacrifice [perhaps] stem ultimately from hereditary units that were implanted by the favoring of relatives during a period of hundreds or thousands of generations."[16]

Lorenz claims that intra-species aggression is the basis of "bonding."[12] By this thesis, aggression, with its components of dominance and submission, is integral to the formation of a closely knit social group. Bonding, then, including its implied masochistic submission, may be a significant requirement for communal life. Since some form of submission is a frequent concomitant of masochism, it seems worthwhile to explore such patterns of yielding and deference. Lorenz makes the intriguing inference that "good manners" are social forms that are attenuated derivates of early dominance–submission conflicts. Each social group has its own group of conforming characteristics. These are culturally ritualized exaggerations of submissive gestures, usually derived from phylogenetically ritualized motor patterning. The rather outmoded social convention of bowing, and the more contemporary nodding of one's head, are such signs of submission. Tipping one's hat is derived from opening one's helmet vizor to indicate nonbelligerence; while the social etiquette of shaking hands evolved from the need to show that one is empty handed (*i.e.*, that weapons have been put aside).

Lorenz describes how different phyla of animals have different forms of submission. In a fight, dogs and wolves signify surrender by suddenly adopting a submissive attitude and presenting their vulnerable neck with the unprotected jugular vein to the dominant animal. This could be the origin of the term, a ''hang dog'' look, used to describe people who give up and submit masochistically. Although such patterns of inhibiting aggression or forming a bond are usually not described in humans, they are part of the sequence of actions that lead to the ''group cohesion'' described by sociologists. In effect, they point to the significance and useful role that some form of masochism plays in human relations.

In another area, isolated clusters of self-destructive phenomena that are known to be genetically determined have been observed in humans. One of the more bizarre phenomena is the hereditary Lesch–Nyham disorder that stimulates the afflicted young children (usually males) to compulsive self-mutilation (even to the extent of biting off their fingers). In a 1979 panel on masochism, Cooper made reference to Lesch–Nyham disease stating, ''it seems clear that this syndrome is physiological in origin, but this extraordinary behavior may indeed reveal something of the biological matrix for self-inflicted aggression.''[17]

Psychodynamic Explanations

Krafft-Ebing believed that states of subjugation and passivity could be more important to certain masochists then the experience of physical pain.[1] He considered this as a mental mechanism, ''ideeler masochismus.'' Freud went much further in explicating and delineating this nonsexual masochism which he later labeled ''moral masochism.'' His earlier theory had claimed that sadism was a primary instinct.

Analytic theory holds that the individual feels as responsible for unconscious forbidden wishes as for the act itself (as long as a wish remains unconscious it is claimed that it cannot be distinguished from the deed itself). Freud maintained that such guilt, from unconscious but still active remnants of infantile oedipal wishes, led to masochism. This was sadism turned against the self as a punishment. Freud explained this as a wish for punishment which he attributed to the development of a group of internalized goals and restrictions classified under the rubric of the superego. Punishment is wished for, usually unconsciously, as a penance or expiation for forbidden thoughts or impulses. As a result, it is understandable that masochistic tendencies occur to some extent in the normal character also.

By 1920, Freud introduced an additional concept. Influenced by his knowledge of the ''laws of entropy,'' which he presumed were common to all living matter, he now theorized that each living cell contained a drive towards dissolution and death.[10] His concept of a ''death instinct'' (essentially a part of his philosophy rather than derived from clinical observation) was now considered by him to be beyond the pleasure principle, which was the earlier Freudian principle of mental functioning. He now advanced masochism as a primary instinct by itself. The analytic community never fully accepted the role of a death instinct in the development of masochism, and the theory is rarely used today. However, Freud's term ''moral masochism'' is a widely held analytic concept, essentially synonymous with masochistic personality.

Freud's theory included the additional idea that masochism is an integral part of female psychology. He believed that feminine masochism arose out of women's normal development, since suffering and pain associated with childbirth, menstruation, and defloration, are integral parts of their normal biological functions. Helene Deutsch went much further and elaborated this thesis into a dissertation on ''The Psychology of Women.''[18] In recent years analysts have placed less significance on female masochism, because the importance of societal influences in its genesis has minimized the need to see female masochism as exclusively determined by biology.

Analytic theory has attempted to explain the two main characteristics of the masochistic personality that contrast with the perversion—that it is not associated with any manifest sexual pleasure, and that an obvious partner is not always required.

The punishing and restricting figure, derived from an important relationship early in development (usually a parent) is often experienced as an internal part of one's self, or disguised by displacement and then abstracted into fate, destiny, or God. The ''moral'' part of the term is unfortunately often misunderstood as referring to society's morals. It does not signify submission to an external sadistic figure. It refers rather to the masochist's personal conflict within himself between various aspects of his own personality that require him to fail and to restrict his gratification. It is postulated that early relationships become part of the character structure during development and are often reexperienced as different parts of the self. One's goals, one's self-restrictions, one's ideals, and one's moralities, are to a great extent determined by the identifications that had been made with early important people, usually parents. Some individuals never fully separate from these early significant figures who remain as important internal arbiters of what is vulnerable or bad. They remain more or less intact, as flies trapped in amber, as internalized objects. With regression, these internal clusters of ideals and rules that are titled superego, become more pronounced and the individual feels driven to please and be loved by them even more intensely. The masochist experiences severe guilt and remorse because he then usually feels he has violated the rules and standards of these internalized objects at some time (normally in childhood). This is the basis of a large portion of his need to suffer and pay penance. He needs to fail to undo his "sadistic" gratification in success, since success to him means the triumphant destruction of the conquered rival. In the masochist, the internal relationships with parts of his own psychic structure are often more important than relationships with external objects. Although the moral masochist frequently involves external objects or situations in his suffering, these are often being used to satisfy the primitive requirements of the puritanical internal object relationship. Clinically, what the observer sees, are the various phenomena that result from these internal conflicts being bounced off the object world manifested as fate neuroses, as manifested by negative therapeutic reactions, in repeated failures in love relationships, failures at work, and sometimes in suicide. In each instance, however, careful listening usually reveals that the patient is reacting as if an internal structure is looking on approvingly, as if these constructs of psychic structures have been personified and actually exist, and as if someone inside is watching, judging, and approving. Psychoanalysis labels these structures as either the critical or ideal aspects of the superego, and claims that the masochistic phenomena we see clinically are fabricated by the hypertrophy and skewing of these internal imagos. Whatever in their development slanted their lifestyle in this way, at some time a special ego pattern had been established ruling that only by suffering does one get love or approval.

This role in life of failure or of limited gratification is a caricature of the Protestant ethic; the praiseworthy goal has become one that demands deprivation and work foremost, with pleasure in the real world coming only secondarily, if at all. Just as the good Calvinist is favored by God if he chooses the life of discipline, hard work, and eschews pleasure, the "need to suffer" of the moral masochist similarly seems to reflect strivings to be loved in the special style that has been learned, an ideal epitomized by the suffering martyr.

Berliner followed similar ideas in describing masochism as a disturbance of interpersonal relations, a pathological way of loving.[19] Normally, one rejects an unloving person. The masochist, by contrast, is attracted by the sadism of the loved one. He has a need to be loved by a hating or rejecting person. A child who is mistreated by a parent does not love this suffering, but because he loves the person who is responsible for it, the ill-treatment becomes a significant and even required part of the relationship. It helps explain the confounding attachment even a severely battered child usually has for the battering parent. The masochist insists on being loved by the punishing person because it may be the only kind of intimacy he has known. (Actually, it is uncommon to find a history of severely punitive parents in the childhood of the moral masochist, although not uncommon in the early life of the masochistic perversion).

In the masochistic perversions, the relationship is to a superego element that has been externalized, and so is more easily recognized because the chosen partner is required to act out the role. By contrast, the moral masochist's internal conflict remains internal and can only be inferred. Freud's "criminals out of the sense of guilt"[9] similarly try to force an outside object to play the role of punisher.[9] This type of criminal usually commits antisocial acts in order to be punished, to alleviate guilt over unconscious infantile aggressive impulses toward the parent. However, one often can also discern the additional aim of coercing the object into a sado-masochistic relationship.

An extreme example of this dynamic can be discovered in many suicides, the ultimate masochistic act. The suicide often has the fantasy that he is passively experiencing the act, that it is being carried out by the loved person, the "hidden executioner,"[20] (usually the one to whom the suicide note is addressed). In the classical suicide style of Russian roulette, or overdosing with pills, the defiant demand is framed, "you, (fate, the lover, the therapist) must protect me from the loaded chamber of the gun, must rescue me before the overdose takes lethal effect." In fantasy, the love object is forced to be the executioner, enslaved by the act and bound tightly to the suicide. In the masochist's suffering lies the hidden fantasy of two incompletely separated personae, now acting and experiencing the suicide in concert. This fantasied cooperation is remarkably similar to the "bonding" Lorenz had described in certain animal species.

Diagnosis and Differential Diagnosis

The diagnosis of the masochistic personality disorder should be limited to a life-long pattern of failures in multiple areas of functioning. Even if attainment of life goals does approach achievement, these individuals find their path complicated by undue obstacles and difficulties they somehow arrange. Their lives are characteristically burdened and unhappy, not because of fortuitous events, but rather as a result of self-defeating complications to which they have unwittingly exposed themselves.

Masochism is often used interchangeably, but incorrectly, with masochistic sexual perversions and the masochistic personality disorders. The masochistic perversions encompass a wide variety of physically painful practices, including whippings and mutilations, to which the subject responds with sexual excitement and pleasure. Masochistic personality disorder is usually distinct from the perversion in at least two aspects—(1.) unlike the perversion it is not associated with a sexual act or sexual gratification, (2.) physical pain is not consciously sought out or arranged.

There is a group of phenomena that are sometimes considered as masochistic behaviors, but which are neither sexual perversions nor aspects of a masochistic character structure. Familiar examples are the initiation rites and related forms of submission and minor mutilation that are found in almost all societies, such as the community's requirement for such rituals of circumcision or scarification, which dynamically signify a *pars pro toto* castration, or the knighting of the young squire by the king's merely touching the youth's shoulder with a sword. These rituals obliged the powerful authority to grant to the supplicant the rights of an adult, (including sexuality) and to provide protection and favor. Specific cultural rituals should not be considered as part of a masochistic personality.

The masochistic character does share features with several of the personality disorders and other categories described in *DSM III*—the passive-aggressive and the narcissistic personality disorders. Dysthymic depression and the obsessional character also have similar features. However, the masochistic character has too many distinctive features to be subsumed by any one of these.

The main area of convergence with these clinical entities lies in their characteristic difficulty in expressing aggression overtly, with some exceptions, in their interpersonal relationships. But while thinly disguised oppositional interpersonal relations are familiar enough in the passive-aggressive and obsessional characters, they almost never exhibit the self-defeating and self-punishing styles of the moral masochist. One recognizes, usually by inference, a greater degree of intra-psychic distress over interpersonal conflict in the masochist, although this is also characteristic of the depressive. In truth, there are sufficient similarities with the depressive character structure to support those psychopathology taxonomists who suggest that masochism is intimately related to the affective disorders. There are many masochistic personalities who do manifest depression at various times, and some may even progress to a clinical depression later in life. Conversely, some dysthymic disorders and even major depressions may merge into a masochistic life-style when the affective disorder is in remission. There is a close dynamic relationship between the two groups, especially since each suffers from an overly severe self-critical, demanding conscience. However, the depressed mood, vegetative signs, and withdrawal from social contacts that are typical of the depressive, are distinguishing elements, as is the life history with its proclivity to facilitate difficulties and failures of the pure masochistic personality. Nor is there as yet any strong evidence for a similar biological etiology in the two categories, either in family history or in response to pharmacologic intervention.

The compulsive is more isolated than the masochist, and has less of a need for a loving response in relationships. The compulsive is constantly struggling to control his sadistic impulses and thoughts through a variety of rituals and obsessions. He protects his objects by a tendency to remain intellectually aloof from affective relationships. This is reflected in their stubborn treatment problems, manifested by their usually great reluctance and difficulty in establishing a transference.

Treatment

Although the treatment of all personality disorders is difficult, masochism is especially so. Because the narcissistically significant aspects of their self-esteem regulation is mainly an internal affair, they deemphasize the value of changing disappointing relationships or even of modifying their environment to improve their sense of well-being. As a result, their destructive patterns tend to continue. In working with such patients, the hostile element is felt soon enough in their determination to have the therapist see their misfortunes and helplessness with fate. These are poorly disguised reproaches to the world, to the significant others, of their failures with treatment, of their lack of love. Paranoid elements often contaminate the relationship as the patient struggles with his need to fail, to thwart the therapist, and to arouse guilt in him. A curious but large element of pride over the control the patient achieves over the people who would help him is frequently prominent.

One young man succeeded in stalling his career for several years, despite his extraordinary brilliance and ability, because he wanted to "do it on my own." Whichever interpretations were made would be responded to as debating points and with great skill and gleeful pride he would destroy their usefulness. When it was pointed out that his opposition to therapeutic interventions seemed strange because his life was falling apart all around him and he obviously wanted to continue treatment and get help, he would smugly reply that it was more important that he not allow himself to be forced to submit (presumably to the therapist's interpretations). As is true of most masochistic personalities, he was rarely aware of how aggressive and belittling his attacks were, and specially, unaware of the obstacles he was constantly placing in the path of what would otherwise be certain success in his career.

These are probably the most frustrating patients a therapist has to treat. They are the most prone to manifesting negative therapeutic reactions, that is, their response to a correct interpretation or environmental manipulation is often to negate its effect, or to become even more symptomatic.[23] Successful treatment is unconsciously forbidden and is similar to Freud's category of those individuals who are wrecked by success. Their internal value system abjures success.

At present there is no pharmacologic treatment for masochism (although the depressions to which these patients are prone can and should be treated somatically). Behavior modification has been only questionably successful, as is true for most personality disorders. However, psychotherapy, although difficult and trying, can be successful in many cases.

The resistance to improvement, the overt and covert provoking of the therapist, and the patient's paradoxic pride in his pathology are often insurmountable obstacles in therapy. The therapist is provoked by the patient's twin aims, to make treatment fail, and to evoke a critical response. This second aspect arises from the need to make transference fantasy real, to convert the therapist into the cruel and disappointing person of his early relationships. Until the patient's pride in suffering and thwarting treatment is brought into awareness and helped to become ego-dystonic, little successful work can be done. To achieve this awareness usually requires helping the patient recognize his fantasy that someone approves of his suffering and privations in treatment. One patient hid for a long time that he was imagining his dead mother hovering over him during his sessions, sternly approving of his successes in denigrating the therapist's efforts. The uncovering of this fantasy helped explain the cryptic half-smile that flitted over his face whenever he would dismiss an interpretation (usually a correct one) that would have helped ease his difficult life situation. Only after this fantasy was dealt with could therapy progress.

The continuing attempts to provoke a negative response must be repeatedly dissected into their component parts. The therapeutic alliance needs to be maintained, constantly inviting the patient to examine with the therapist his ego ideal which is the "secret ally" that applauds the patient for both his suffering and for his "victory" over the therapist. A cool, distant stance is antitherapeutic because it confirms the transference fantasy of a rejecting parent.

Although the sadistic aspects of his masochism must eventually be recognized by the patient, this should be postponed until treatment is well along. Instead, persistent and sympathetic pointing out of his need to be victimized is necessary. Therapy should repeatedly and carefully demonstrate how the people he accuses are actually people he covertly loves.

A sympathetic, understanding therapist who does not respond to the patient's provocative onslaughts with the expected criticisms, rejections, and punishments is required to provide a more benign internal representation. Much of the therapeutic aim with such patients is to work through and modify their early destructive identifications. Although the therapist should not be primarily a deliberate role model, such a role may be useful with masochistic patients (as is often true also in working with depressives and in negative therapeutic reactions). In these clinical conditions, it can be a valid technique to allow the benign therapeutic stance to be available for identification, as a replacement for the cruel superego. It is a modified corrective emotional experience. This is a narrow line, but a careful therapist can achieve this function without falling into the role of the omnipotent and omniscient early transference object.

Finally, because of the usual course of a drawn-out treatment with the draining negative counter-transference that needs to be constantly understood and guarded against, it is probably unwise to treat more than one such patient at a time. On the other hand, when advances are made in treatment, and especially if treatment is even moderately successful, it is extremely rewarding for the therapist. One learns an enormous amount about human psychology from such patients.

REFERENCES

1. von Krafft-Ebing RF: Psychopathia Sexualis. London, FA Davis Co, 1895
2. Diagnostic Statistical Manual of Mental Disorders III, 3 ed. p 274. American Psychiatric Association, 1980
3. Lion JR: Personality Disorders. Baltimore, Williams and Wilkins, 1981
4. Sack LS, Miller W: Masochism: A clinical and theoretical overview. Psychiatry, 38:244, 1975
5. Reich W: Character Analysis. New York, Orgone Institute Press, 1933
6. Brenner C: The masochistic character: Genesis and treatment. J Am Psychoanal Assoc 7:197, 1959
7. Reik T: Masochism in Modern Man. New York, Strauss and Co, 1941
8. Freud S: The Economic Problem of Masochism. S.E.19:157. London, Hogarth Press, 1924
9. Freud S: Some Character Types Met With in Psychoanalytic Work. S.E.14:311. London, Hogarth Press, 1916
10. Freud S: Beyond the Pleasure Principle. S.E.18:3. London, Hogarth Press, 1920
11. Freud S: Analysis Terminable and Interminable. S.E.23:209. London, Hogarth Press, 1937
12. Lorenz K: On Aggression. New York, Harcourt, Brace and World, 1966
13. Hess EH: Imprinting. Science 130:133, 1959
14. Mitchell WM: Observations on animal behavior and its relationship to masochism. Diseases of the Nervous System 30:124, 1969
15. Weiss JM, Bailey WM, Goodman PA et al: Model for neurochemical study of depression. In Spiegelstein MY, Levy A (eds): Behavioral Models and the Analysis of Drug Action, p 195. Amsterdam, Elsevier Publishing Co, 1982
16. Wilson EO: On Human Nature. Cambridge, MA, Harvard University Press, 1978
17. Fischer N: Masochism: Current concepts, Panel Discussion. J Am Psychoanal Assoc 29:673, 1981
18. Deutsch H: The Psychology of Women. New York, Grune and Stratton, 1944
19. Berliner B: The role of object relations in moral masochism. Psychoanal Q 27:38, 1958
20. Asch SS: Suicide and the hidden executioner. Int Rev Psychoanal 7:51, 1980
21. Fenichel O: The Psychoanalytic Theory of the Neuroses. New York, WW Norton, 1945
22. Bak RC: The phallic woman. Psychoanal Study Child. New York, International Universities Press 23:15, 1968
23. Asch SS: Varieties of negative therapeutic reactions and problems of technique. J Am Psychoanal Assoc 24:383, 1976

SUGGESTED READING

Bergler E: The Basic Neurosis: Oral Regression and Psychic Masochism. New York, Grune and Stratton, 1977

Brennan M: On being teased and the problem of moral masochism. Psychoanal Study of Child. New York, International University Press 7:264, 1952

Herman I: Clinging—going in search. Psychoanal Q 45:5, 1976

Speigel L: Moral masochism. Psychoanal Q 47:209, 1978

Stolorow R: The narcissistic function of masochism (and sadism). Int J Psychoanal 56:441, 1975

David Bear, Roy Freeman, and Mark Greenberg

Changes in Personality Associated With Neurologic Disease

If personality is an "enduring style of relating to the environment,"[1] there can be little doubt that structural or physiologic pathology within the nervous system may profoundly alter it. In the presence of gross evidence of neurologic malfunction such as memory loss, aphasia, or severe dementia, one is readily led to identify an "organic brain syndrome" and seek its physical cause. However, neurologic lesions may selectively affect areas of the human brain highly specialized for emotional functions, producing patterns of emotional and behavioral change without gross motor, sensory, or elementary cognitive deficits.

A dramatic example of such an organic alteration in personality was provided by the case of Phineas Gage, which was reported in 1878.[2] Gage was a conscientious railroad worker whose frontal lobes were pierced by a crowbar following a dynamite explosion. The resulting lesion was well documented by a physician, who digitally probed the trajectory of the crowbar from its entry point above the eyes to its exit through the anterior dorsum of the skull; by postmortem observations of extensive laceration of prefrontal cortex; and by the dramatically deformed Gage skull, which is still on display next to the "surgical" iron crowbar.

Despite his dramatic injury, Gage was able to walk away from the accident, answering questions, speaking normally, and retaining memory of daily activities and friends. Gage's frontal lobe personality changes only became apparent over a longer period of time: his polite, quiet comportment was replaced by facetious jocularity, deterioration in grooming, lapsing social graces, irreverence in church, and loss of interest in events beyond the moment that terminated his working life.

In keeping with a pattern that has frequently characterized the study of the functions of cognition and emotion, initial clinical identification of personality changes in humans following frontal lobe injury prompted studies of behavior in lesioned animals; most notable was the work of John Fulton and associates at Yale University.[3] However, the behavioral consequences of frontal lesions in animals, even in the higher primates such as the rhesus monkey or chimpanzee, proved more subtle yet less complex than those in humans. This perhaps led to a premature transfer of oversimplified laboratory observations back to clinical medicine in the form of the therapeutic frontal lobotomy. For an unfortunate period of time, physicians became the prime producers of an organic personality disorder![3]

Other examples of cross-fertilization between the animal laboratory and the study of human emotional functions were less problematic. Kluver and Bucy codified behavioral changes following bilateral temporal lobectomy in the rhesus monkey, observing dramatic alterations in aggression, sexual behavior, exploration of the environment, and feeding.[4] This pattern of behavioral change has subsequently been described in humans and may appear as a personality change in early stages of some cortical dementias.[5] Alterations in emotions and behavior observed during the interictal period in temporal lobe epilepsy had been noted by many clinicians, including Kraepelin, during the previous century. These have been conceptualized as the converse of Kluver and Bucy's alterations, reflecting overactivation rather than destruction of temporal limbic structures.[6] The importance of the hypothalamus in modulation of aggression, sexuality, and feeding, which has been extensively elucidated by experimentation with animals, has also been documented in humans[7] and may account for organic behavioral changes associated with concussion, encephalitis, or currently obscure states such as the Kleine-Levin syndrome and some forms of anorexia nervosa.

The study of organic alterations in personality is important to the general psychiatrist for several reasons. Most commonly cited is the need to identify those patterns of behavioral change that herald organic illness, lest the psychiatrist confirm the darkest mutterings of his medical and neurologic colleagues by, for example, providing psychotherapy to a patient experiencing personality alterations due to a brain tumor. Such concerns would certainly justify the knowledge of characteristic patterns of organic behavioral change. However, it is well to remember that differential diagnosis is a double-edged sword. Thus, insecurity regarding the organic personality disorders is as likely to lead to a vague overdiagnosis of the organic disorder as to the much-feared failure to detect physical pathology. Either form of error is tragic when a treatable condition that might have been diagnosed by knowledge of relevant organic personality syndromes is assigned to the wrong side of the functional-organic border. This is as true of pseudoseizures in the setting of character disorder or late-life depression mimicking structural dementia as of operable subfrontal meningiomas or normal pressure hydrocephalus.

Additional benefits accrue from the study of organic personality disorders. Following the medical or neurologic identification of such conditions as frontal lobe injury, temporal lobe epilepsy, infarction of the right cerebral hemisphere, or Huntington's disease, physicians are faced with multidimensional problems of management. Alterations in the patient's behavior, which may powerfully affect family dynamics, are often the most incapacitating aspects of these neurologic illnesses, and psychiatric intervention (pharmacologic, behavioral, sociodynamic, and psychotherapeutic) is strongly indicated. In these common and perplexing situations, an understanding of the nature of the underlying organic behavioral alterations is the keystone of effective psychiatric management.

Finally, we believe that organic personality alterations are of great theoretic interest to psychiatrists. In many of these syndromes, a biologically defined "independent" variable in the form of a neuroanatomically localized lesion has produced distinctive alterations in emotions and behavior, which may thus be studied as "dependent" variables. These are model conditions, rarely duplicated in the investigation of idiopathic psychiatric illness, and they provide unique opportunities for structure–function correlations. Such observations of altered structure and function provide the basis for a "neurology of emotion," a nascent understanding of the mechanisms of affective processing in the human nervous system. This additional perspective on emotional functions promises to enrich the neurochemical, psychodynamic, behavioral, and even sociodynamic models of behavior.[8]

Definition

In defining changes in personality associated with neurologic disease, we are aware that many idiopathic behavioral syndromes, such as schizophrenia, may eventually be related to organic abnormalities. However, in this chapter, we restrict our consideration to structural or electrical alterations of the central nervous system detectable by current methodology that are regularly correlated with specific changes in emotions and behavior.

Furthermore, we have focused on alterations in emotion and behavior in the absence of gross disruption of cognition, following the tradition of the *Diagnostic and Statistical Manual of Mental Disorders* (*DSM-III*),[1] of separating "organic personality syndrome" from "organic brain syndrome." However, there are possible misunderstandings of the commonly used rubric "organic personality disorder."

First, it will become clear that there is a plurality of patterns of organically induced personality changes that are strikingly different from one another. For example, the deep and persistent emotions that may be associated with temporal lobe epilepsy are readily differentiated from the flattened, transient affects seen with frontal lobe disorder. The concept of a single "organic personality disorder" characterized by a bewildering potpourri of pathologic emotional and behavioral reactions is an unfortunate legacy from the past and a continuing source of error.

A second potential source of confusion in the definition of organic behavioral alterations is the assumption that these are necessarily "disorders" of personality. This presumes a clear concept of normal or "ordered" personality, which at best would reflect a collective social judgment of what constitutes appropriate behavior under many complex circumstances. In general, personality "disorders" are characterized by grossly dissocial aggressive or sexual behavior, aberrant social relationships, or disordered thoughts. However, it must be stressed that organic processes may produce subtle rather than gross alterations in behavior and that characteristic features of particular organic syndromes such as a heightened interest in religion or a tendency to write at length need not be socially dysfunctional or attract psychiatric attention.

A related misunderstanding could result from the attempt of the *DSM-III* to differentiate "organic affective" or "organic psychotic" from "organic personality syndromes."[1] Among the patterns of organic personality change that we will review, some alteration of affective intensity, appropriateness, or range is a fundamental feature. Depending on the neuroanatomic location of dysfunction, some syndromes will include disruption in flow of thought or failure to modify behavior appropriately with regard to the environment (disturbed reality testing) that could be termed *psychotic*. Thus it would be erroneous to exclude these psychiatric features from the organic personality syndromes.

On the other hand, behavioral changes produced by organic lesions, when examined closely, rarely reproduce or precisely copy idiopathic psychiatric syndromes such as depression, mania, or schizophrenia. Rather, we suggest that the organic behavioral syndromes are better understood as phenomena in their own right, reflecting alterations at specific stages in the neurologic processing of affect. The advantages of objective behavioral description over premature application of psychiatric labels are both practical and theoretic. Such an approach facilitates the identification of features that differentiate organic syndromes from their functional "phenocopies," and it may provide a neutral base for correlating function with neuroanatomic structure, eventuating in novel neurologic models from which to redefine the idiopathic psychiatric syndromes.[8]

Finally, we offer several clarifications regarding the interaction of organic and functional factors in our definition of organic personality alterations. First, there are cogent reasons to believe that the organic personality syndromes presented below do not represent "secondary" or psychodynamic reactions to deficit or illness. For example, syndromic behavioral changes associated with temporal lobe epilepsy or frontal lobe injury are not seen in response to such medical illnesses as myocardial infarction, rheumatoid arthritis, or life-threatening neurologic disease.[3,9,10] The indifference reaction associated with infarction of the right parietal lobe, which often includes minimization of illness, will

be seen to differ extensively from the psychological denial observed in cardiac disease.[11] In the organic personality syndromes, one does not generally encounter an intensification of prior personality patterns or coping styles, as might be expected in response to illness outside the nervous system.[3] Rather, the direct involvement of emotion-mediating circuits in the brain tends to modify underlying personality, often dramatically, producing recognizable patterns of behavioral alteration that are more the result of the anatomic location of the lesion than the prior personality of the patient.

Furthermore, it should not categorically be assumed that remnants of prior personality or psychodynamic factors will inevitably interact with the organic process to produce a "holistic" behavior picture. It is essential to appreciate the nature and especially the localization of the organic impairment in order to determine whether prior learning, environmental interaction including psychotherapy, or even pharmacotherapy are likely to alter the aberrant behavior.

Prevalence and Etiology

Organic alterations in personality are not rare or esoteric curiosities but are common psychiatric occurrences. It has been estimated that 30% of first admissions to psychiatric hospitals have an organic basis.[12] Since the more obvious cognitive deterioration characterizing delirium and dementia lead readily to neurologic and medical referral, it is probable that many of these patients were admitted for personality changes only subsequently linked to organic pathology.

A wide range of conditions such as traumatic, infectious, vascular, degenerative, demyelinating, or neoplastic processes may affect emotion-controlling structures within the nervous system. However, some etiologies are especially prevalent causes of organic personality syndromes in particular periods of life.

Among young adults, head trauma is an unfortunately frequent cause of organic personality change. Many different syndromes may develop, such as postconcussion changes, perhaps reflecting diencephalic and caudal brainstem dysfunction; personality alterations secondary to contusion especially of the temporal poles or orbital frontal cortex; behavior change with posttraumatic limbic epilepsy; or frontal-subcortical changes secondary to late developing hydrocephalus.[13]

Temporal lobe epilepsy is an important cause of behavior change in adolescence and middle adulthood. Representing the most common of the adult epilepsies, with a prevalence of approximately 3 per 1000, temporal lobe epilepsy may be associated with hypothalamic dysfunction or, of the greatest importance to psychiatrists, with a syndrome of interictal alteration in behavior.[3,6,9] Temporal lobe epileptic foci can, of course, signal the presence of other etiologies such as neoplasm or encephalitis, in which cases the behavioral changes may result from structural or epileptogenic processes within the limbic system.

Among other important etiologies of organic personality change in this age-group are demyelinating disorders such as multiple sclerosis, in which plaques may concentrate in the white matter of the frontal lobes, and collagen vascular diseases, such as systemic lupus erythematosus, in which the pathologic alterations may include multifocal vasculitis within the central nervous system.[14]

Although comparatively rare, such conditions as Huntington's disease or Wilson's disease may present as organic personality alterations in early adulthood, frequently years before the development of overt movement disorder or dementia. Their importance stems not from high prevalence but from the need of early diagnosis for treatment and effective genetic counseling.[15]

In middle life, neoplasia and cerebrovascular accidents are prominent etiologies. Tumors affecting the prefrontal cortex are especially likely to produce personality alterations in the absence of conspicuous elementary neurologic deficits. Although metastatic lesions are more prevalent than primary brain tumors, slow-growing intrinsic meningeal tumors (such as olfactory groove or parasagittal meningiomas) may present an initial picture of organic personality change. These lesions are benign, but they may eventually produce irreversible mass effects on surrounding brain tissue.[3,15]

Cerebrovascular accidents (ischemic or hemorrhagic) are prevalent illnesses that often produce prominent behavioral changes.[14] Although distinctive syndromes are associated with damage in various locations, the special psychiatric significance of infarction in the distribution of the right middle cerebral artery requires emphasis. The initial presentation of this type of stroke may be agitation or confusion without clear motor, sensory, or language deficit.[16] When the structural lesion includes dorsal aspects of the right hemisphere, particularly the parietal association cortex, a pervasive alteration in personality characterized by indifference to

illness and disrupted emotional priorities frequently results.[11,15]

Profound alterations in personality, frequently combining features of temporal limbic and medial frontal degeneration, can also be the initial presentation of malignancy outside the central nervous system. The behavioral changes associated with the syndrome of "limbic encephalitis" may be seen in association with bronchial and other neoplasms.[17]

In later mid life and among the elderly, dementing illnesses become the most prominent cause, by far, of organic personality changes. Recent estimates suggest that between 4.5% and 8% of persons over 65 may develop some form of dementia.[5]

Personality alterations may develop prior to clear cognitive deterioration, especially in the pathologic entity of Pick's disease. In this illness, neuronal degeneration is concentrated in the rostral temporal poles and prefrontal cortex; personality changes may include aspects of the Kluver-Bucy syndrome.[3,5]

Personality alteration frequently accompanies Alzheimer's disease, the most common structural dementia.[5] Although the later clinical pictures of Alzheimer's disease and Pick's disease are similar, the pathologic process in Alzheimer's disease often begins more posteriorly, in the association cortex of the parietal lobes, the hippocampal gyrus, and the hippocampus. As a result, anomic aphasia, spatial disorientation, and memory loss often precede conspicuous personality deterioration. The later involvement of the prefrontal cortex typically produces organic personality change.

Profound alterations in personality with rapid onset of dementia and myoclonic movements are characteristic of Jakob-Creutzfeldt disease. Degenerative changes involve temporal and frontal lobes as well as the basal ganglia. The etiology may be slow virus infection. Personality changes that accompany a stepwise, progressive loss of intellectual functions, often in the setting of hypertension, may be the consequence of cumulative frontal-subcortical lesions in the syndrome of "multi-infarct dementia."[18]

Anatomic Overview of Organic Personality Alterations

Neurologic alterations in personality are frequent and may result from a host of etiologies. Clearly, no single picture of "the organic personality" can do justice to the variety of altered emotions and behavior that the clinician may confront.

However it would be an error to overlook the important similarities and systematic relationships among organic personality disorders produced by diverse etiologies. It is the disturbance of specific, neuroanatomically localized functions that accounts for the emergence of several characteristic patterns of altered behavior. Familiarity with these recurrent behavioral patterns is essential to fundamental understanding of the organic personality disorders and offers a unique insight into the neurology of "normal" emotional processing.

Many aspects of behavior traditionally categorized as "emotional" involve the biological drives such as aggression, reproduction, or self-protection. Neurologic regulation of these drives involves a hierarchical organization of structure and function (Fig. 1).

Within the brainstem, the hypothalamus represents a crucial pathway for activation of consummatory drive behaviors, such as attack or copulation, which are often accompanied by characteristic autonomic and neuroendocrine responses. In general, sensory information projected directly to the hypothalamus is focused on the internal milieu—chemoreception and visceroception. The hypothalamus thus plays a vital role in homeostatic adjustments and the mediation of drive responses. However, in the primate brain, the hypothalamus is essentially ignorant of the external world; it does not have direct access, for example, to cortical visual areas involved in the discrimination of particular "stimulus" objects.[6]

Thus disturbances at the hypothalamic level of drive control tend to be quantitative (*e.g.,* too much or too little hunger, anger, or sex), independent of the objects normally eliciting these emo-

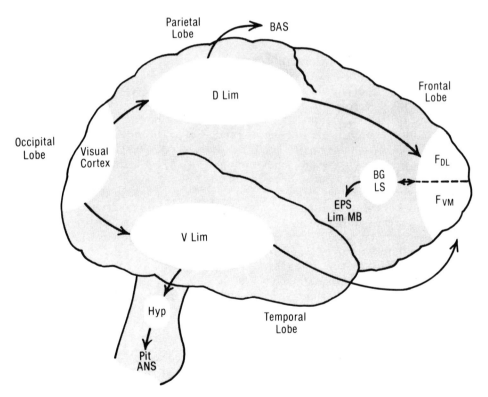

FIG. 1. Neuroanatomic systems associated with specific emotional functions in the human brain. (*Hyp,* hypothalamus; *Pit,* pituitary axis; *ANS,* autonomic nervous system; *V Lim,* ventral limbic system including amygdala, hippocampus, and associated cortex of the temporal lobe; *D Lim,* dorsal limbic system, including cingulate and associated cortex of the parietal lobe; *BAS,* brainstem arousal systems, including midbrain reticular formation, median raphe, locus ceruleus; F_{DL}, association cortex of dorsolateral convexity of frontal lobe; F_{VM}, association cortex of ventromedial region of the frontal lobe; *BGLS,* basal ganglia [*e.g.,* caudate nucleus] and adjacent limbic striatum [*e.g.,* nucleus accumbens septi]; *EPS,* extrapyramidal motor system; *Lim MB,* limbic midbrain [*e.g.,* ventral tegmental area])

tional responses. Other predictable signs of hypothalamic and adjacent brainstem involvement are disrupted homeostasis (*e.g.,* defects in thermoregulation, endocrine dysfunction, autonomic irregularities, and alteration of sleep–wake cycles).[6,7,19]

Converging evidence suggests that limbic structures within the temporal lobe, especially the amygdala, play a role in linking the hypothalamus with neocortical sensory systems, such as vision. In order to associate a particular object, such as a sexual partner, with the appropriate drive response, a pathway from the primary visual cortex through visual association areas in the occipital lobe, inferotemporal visual cortex, amygdala, and hypothalamus is presumably activated. The ventral limbic structures (amygdala, hippocampus, and adjacent temporal cortex) appear to be necessary for both the initial visual-emotional association and its subsequent storage or memory.[6,20]

Two forms of ventral limbic dysfunction may be contrasted. Structural lesions might be expected to "disconnect" sensory areas from drive centers, resulting in inappropriate sexual, aggressive, or appetite responses to visually discriminated objects— the proposed basis of the Kluver-Bucy syndrome of personality alteration.[21] Alternatively, irritative processes, like epileptic foci that activate limbic structures, might result in the formation of fortuitous sensory-emotional connections, which is the suggested mechanism of excessive emotional association in the interictal behavior syndrome of temporal lobe epilepsy.[6] Thus, processes impinging on the ventral limbic structures affect the qualitative association of object with drive rather than the quantitative intensity of drives.

Although the ventral limbic structures mediate associations between perceptions and drive responses, a dorsal sensory-limbic processing system involving parietal association cortex, the cingulate, and dorsolateral convexity of the frontal lobe appears to perform a complementary function. Whereas the ventral system receives highly analyzed information from central vision suitable for object recognition, the dorsal system receives projections from all visual sectors, with emphasis on the periphery of space. Laboratory and clinical investigations suggest that this system is involved in surveillance of the environment for detection and spatial placement of drive-relevant stimuli. On their detection, projections to brainstem arousal centers affect general activation and attentional shifts, while pathways to frontal eyefields and motor systems allow for visual or tactile orientation to the object.[11]

As a consequence of the hemispheric specialization that underlie language development, this emotional "early warning system" appears to be lateralized to the nondominant hemisphere in humans. A disturbance of emotional surveillance functions may account for the "indifference" reaction and disruption of affective priorities associated with parietal-frontal lesions of the right hemisphere.[11,15]

The extensive granular cortex anterior to the motor strip in the frontal lobe is the phylogenetically newest of the areas specialized for emotion. In essence, it performs executive decision-making functions, based on integration of hypothalamic input concerning the internal milieu, highly processed sensory information regarding the external environment, and signals from limbic systems regarding stimuli of affective significance.[11,22] Before initiating motor behaviors, the prefrontal cortex makes a complex "judgment," assigning priorities among the biological drives or, more typically in human society, modifying drive responses in accordance with acquired social rules.[3,11]

This complex process may be localized to two subsystems that stand in hierarchical relation to the dorsal and ventral limbic systems, respectively. The dorsolateral convexity of the frontal lobe appears to energize or initiate behavioral responses, perhaps when "notified" of an arousing stimulus by the dorsal limbic system. Lesions in this region of the frontal lobe result in reduced behavioral activity: flattened affects, apathy, and abulia.[3,11,15] By contrast, the medial and orbital undersurface of the frontal lobe, which receives "focal" information about a specific drive stimulus from ventral limbic structures, appears crucial for determining social appropriateness before engaging in a drive response. Destruction of this region characteristically produces impulsive, socially inappropriate, sexual, eliminative, or aggressive responses. The personality becomes childlike, reminiscent of the situation before social rules were acquired.[3,11,15] On the other hand, epileptic activation of this region has been reported to produce embarrassment, the typical affective response to social opprobrium.[23]

The basal ganglia, especially the caudate nucleus, bear a close anatomic and functional relationship to the prefrontal cortex. In the higher primates a point-to-point mapping of frontal cortex onto the caudate has been demonstrated. Caudate lesions may reproduce behavioral deficits associated with frontal lesions.[15] The extrapyramidal motor system is a major efferent pathway of the limbic system, mediating emotional expression through facial movements, posture, and vocal modulation. A set of structures adjacent to motor components of the striatum also uses dopamine as a major neurotransmitter. These areas, such as the nucleus accumbens septi, have been labeled "limbic striatum," suggesting their involvement in affective processing.[15,24]

These relationships may account for the combination of movement disorder and emotional alteration in conditions affecting the basal ganglia. For example, the reduction of dopaminergic transmission in parkinsonism is associated with masked facies, hypophonia, and other deficits in emotional expression.[15] Structural lesions in the basal ganglia or the right hemisphere have resulted in loss of emotional intonation or prosody in speech.[25] In Huntington's disease, degeneration beginning in the caudate nucleus is associated with some of the personality changes of the frontal lobe syndromes, accompanied by choreic movement disorder.[26]

Clinical Presentation

The preceding section presented an overview of neuroanatomic areas known to mediate distinctive emotional functions in the human brain. We shall now review important clinical syndromes that result from lesions in these regions. In this section, we shall present detailed behavior descriptions of the evolution of behavioral symptoms followed by a consideration of superficially similar psychiatric conditions from which they must be distinguished and by approaches to behavioral management.

HYPOTHALAMIC SYNDROMES

Hypothalamic lesions have resulted in specific behavioral changes.[7,27,28] Characteristic features include irritability, outbursts of rage, changes in eating patterns, mood changes, apathy, somnolence, confusion, hallucinations, and inappropriate behavior. Disruption of endocrine, autonomic, and other vegetative functions are commonly associated with the behavioral changes. Such disturbances include diabetes insipidus, pituitary insufficiency, galactorrhea, circadian rhythm disturbances, obesity or weight loss, and loss of temperature regulation.[19,29,30] The clinical descriptions confirm the extensive experimental literature (with precise interspecies and intraspecies, clinicoanatomic correlation) elucidating the role of the hypothalamus in the integration of autonomic, endocrine, visceral, and somatic responses.[9,29,30] Documented causes have included congenital malformations, infections and other inflammatory conditions, trauma, vascular events, metabolic abnormalities, and tumors.[29]

Although pathologically verified lesions confined to the hypothalamus are rare, behavioral alterations reflecting hypothalamic dysfunction may underlie a variety of clinical conditions. For example, personality changes such as irritability, apathy, and sleep–wake cycle disturbance have been described as a postconcussive syndrome.[3] The Kleine-Levin syndrome is a periodic disorder, typically occurring in young men and characterized by hypersomnolence, hyperphagia, and hypersexuality.[31] Anorexia nervosa, a disorder in many ways the antithesis to the Kleine-Levin syndrome, occurs in adolescent females and includes weight loss due to decreased food intake, hyperactivity, hyposexuality, amenorrhea, and hypothermia.[31] Hypothalamic dysfunction may be implicated in all of these disorders.[31]

TEMPORAL LOBE SYNDROMES

A distinctive cluster of cognitive, emotional, and behavioral traits has been recognized in a significant proportion of patients with temporal lobe epilepsy.[3,9]

Heightened emotional reactivity often dominates the clinical picture and is variously manifested as anxiety states, phobic reactions, episodic dysphoria, frank paranoia, ecstatic experiences, and smoldering anger. Other characteristic features include intense philosophic and religious interests, diminished or altered libido, a tendency to write copiously, and obsessive circumstantial thinking. These traits are stable, enduring personality characteristics and not episodic, ictal events. These alterations have been collectively termed an *interictal behavior syndrome* of temporal lobe epilepsy. Less frequent behavioral features include episodes of destructive violence, multiple suicide attempts, sexual paraphilias, dissociative reactions, and florid psychoses.[32]

The patient with the typical interictal behavior syndrome appears as a warm, engaging, intense individual who tends to take both himself and the world seriously ("humorless sobriety"). Clinicians often remark on the instant intimacy and extraordinary candor revealed in the initial sessions. This warmth and social adhesiveness have been termed *viscosity*. Such patients are insensitive to social cues that regulate and terminate conversation. Even punctual therapists find themselves running over the time alloted for sessions. History taking can be frustrated by the patient's verbose recitation of endless peripheral detail and circumstantial associations. Such patients have difficulty in giving "straight answers" even to direct questions. They feel obliged to preface their answers, qualify and hedge substantive statements, and cavil over semantics. The temporal lobe epileptic often presents his doctors with voluminous materials: letters to doctors, editors, politicians; diaries of seizure frequency; lists of medications and side-effects; poetic, literary, and graphic offerings; as well as overly detailed autobiographical accounts.

Many such patients have documented complex partial seizures ("psychomotor epilepsy"), which may include olfactory auras, déja vu, fear, depression, derealization, auditory and/or visual hallucinations, speech arrest, epigastric pain, and automatic movements. These may be followed by generalized tonic-clonic seizures and postictal confusion. However, often the seizures are subtle, infrequent, or nocturnal and the patient may not initially be identified as epileptic. Therefore, the presence of multiple interictal behavioral traits should alert the clinician to the possibility of temporal lobe epilepsy. The subsequent evaluation should include comprehensive history taking with emphasis on possible ictal events, birth status, history of head trauma, family history of neurologic disease; a neurologic examination; objective mental status testing; electroencephalography and computed tomography when indicated. However, normal findings on examination, electroencephalography, or computed tomography do not exclude the presence of a medially situated epileptic focus. Carbamazepine (Tegretol) has become the drug of choice for seizure control in limbic epilepsy; however, its efficacy in ameliorating the symptoms of the interictal behavior syndrome has not been established. Medications aimed at reducing the intensity of interictal affect may be effective in some patients, but controlled clinical trials are needed.

Differential diagnosis can be difficult, because patients manifest multiple psychiatric symptoms that are common to a wide range of psychiatric disorders. Periods of dysphoria mimic depressive episodes; religious and philosophical preoccupations suggest paranoia; extreme verbosity parallels the cognitive style of neurosis; excessive warmth and emotionality resemble the hysterical personality; tangential mentation suggests a schizophrenic thought disorder; the history of violence and suicide attempts suggest the borderline personality. It is the *syndromic* quality of the clinical picture (the tendency of these disparate traits to occur in the same patient) that raises the diagnostic suspicion of temporal lobe epilepsy. Furthermore, certain qualitative features in the behavior of the temporal lobe epileptic may aid in the differential diagnosis. For example, in patients with poorly controlled aggressive outbursts, the presence of remorse or despair over their actions helps to rule out the diagnosis of idiopathic sociopathy. In the patient with long-standing temporal lobe epilepsy who develops the florid symptoms of psychosis ("schizophreniform" psychosis of epilepsy[33]) interpersonal warmth is often preserved and the clinician's sense of estrangement (the "praecox feeling") is distinctly absent.

A common mechanism may underlie the various manifestations of the interictal behavior syndrome, namely, impairment in the process of assigning emotional significance to external stimuli.[6] The interictal behavior syndrome can be conceptualized as a dysfunction of cathexis, with some ideas and objects hypercathected and others hypocathected. This hypothesis is consistent with current understanding of the limbic system: limbic structures such as the amygdala may act as a bridge between neocortical representation of the external world and diencephalic control of the internal milieu. Thus, the interictal behavior syndrome can be viewed as a result of an irritative limbic focus that forges fortuitous or inappropriate "sensory-limbic hyperconnections."

It is of great theoretic as well as clinical interest that destructive lesions of the temporal lobe tend to produce a converse clinical picture. In the monkey these changes were defined by Kluver and Bucy.[4] Following bilateral temporal lobe ablation, animals became placid, tame, hypersexual, and socially withdrawn. Additional features included a tendency to explore the environment relentlessly and a proclivity to mouth objects ("hyperorality"). Fortunately in humans, vascular, neoplastic, and traumatic diseases of the nervous system rarely destroy limbic structures bilaterally. However, infectious and degenerative diseases with a predilection for the temporal lobe may produce features of the Kluver-Bucy syndrome. In Pick's disease, late-stage Alzheimer's disease, herpes simplex encephalitis, and limbic encephalitis, patients can undergo dramatic personality change, including indifference to family and friends, passivity, sexual disinhibition, and a compulsion to mouth nonfood objects.

RIGHT HEMISPHERE SYNDROMES

The association between right hemisphere damage and the lack of concern over illness has been repeatedly confirmed since 1914, when Babinski coined the term *anosognosia,* describing the denial of disability in two patients with left hemiplegia.[34,35]

In its extreme form, patients with severe, incapacitating sensory or motor impairments claim to be in good health and demonstrate in word and deed a marked unconcern with their predicament. In a variant known as autopagnosia, the patient actually denies the existence of an affected body part, typically a paralyzed limb. Sometimes the patient dissociates the body part from the self by naming it "my dummy" or "this stupid thing." These extreme forms of denial are usually accompanied by hemi-neglect of extracorporeal space. A less extreme form (often emerging later in the course of recovery) consists of minimization of illness. The patient describes a hemiparetic limb as "a bit slow" and his general state of health as "not 100%." When confronted with the realities of hospitalization, confinement to a wheelchair, or inability to carry out skilled movements with one side of his body, the anosognosic patient will typically confabulate and rationalize. For example, a patient was asked to raise a glass of water with her weak left hand. She refused and commented, "I'm just not thirsty."

The parietal lobe is the most frequent site of pathology in anosognosia. Heilman and Valenstein maintain that neglect syndromes can also result from damage to the frontal lobe and cingulate gyrus.[36] (These areas comprise the dorsal limbic system schematized in Figure 1.) Lesions of the nondominant (usually right) parietal lobe are most likely to produce these syndromes; in the study of Nathanson and associates, there was a 2 : 1 ratio of right-to-left hemisphere lesions in patients with anosognosia.[37] Right-sided lesions also result in a greater severity and duration of the syndrome.

Explicit denial of illness and dissociation of body parts are dramatic features of a more subtle, global cognitive and emotional style encountered in patients with right parietal damage. This right parietal lobe syndrome includes chronic, euphoric unconcern for nonmedical issues, such as pressing family matters, financial obligations, problems in the world at large, and other situations that typically elicit worry and concern. Sometimes this chronic alteration in personality is the only remnant of neurologic insult after recovery of sensory and motor functions. This incapacity to experience distress can be punctuated with brief bouts of paranoid ideation and affectively laden false beliefs. Both reactions present formidable obstacles to establishing and maintaining a therapeutic alliance. The carefree, unconcerned patient is unmotivated to engage in psychotherapy, and often must be coerced into initiating treatment by concerned family members. The clinician is often frustrated by the patient's inability to identify a focus for therapy or a target symptom. Further strain is placed on the therapeutic relationship during episodes of misdirected, inappropriate affect. An extreme example of how unconcern can sabotage recovery is provided by a patient with mild residual motor weakness who refused to use a cane and subsequently fell down a flight of stairs, sustaining severe injury. Following right hemisphere damage, a second patient failed to observe many signs of a deteriorating marriage. Attempts by the therapist to draw her attention to the situation elicited frank delusions about a covert relationship between the therapist and her husband, creating an impasse in treatment. The standard psychotherapeutic techniques designed to counter the psychological defenses of denial and resistance may have little or no impact on the patient with organic denial syndrome. Rather, we suggest that the clinician accept the denial of illness as a given and focus on spared areas of insight to mitigate the dysfunctional intrapsychic and interpersonal effects of excessive unconcern.

There is converging evidence that the right hemisphere syndrome reflects unopposed emotional tendencies of the intact left hemisphere. Sackeim and co-workers reviewed 14 cases of total adult right hemispherectomy.[38] Twelve patients became euphoric and unconcerned following surgery, a reaction presumably mediated by the isolated left hemisphere. Evidence from unilateral lesions[39] and unilateral pharmacologic inactivation (Wada test[40]) support the hypothesis that the isolated left hemisphere is biased toward euphoria and that the right hemisphere patient has lost the capacity for subjective anxiety and dysphoria. It is important to emphasize that failure to exhibit distress can coexist with the vegetative features of depression and/or paranoid ideation, symptoms that are associated with intense psychological distress in the intact brain.

Several authors have described the aprosodias, a class of deficits in paralinguistic communication associated with right hemisphere damage.[25,41] Such patients may have impairments in perceiving or expressing emotional intonation in speech. For example, a monotonous drone can belie the patient's internal affective state. A related deficit in the visual modality is seen in the patient who has difficulty interpreting emotion from facial expression. For example, such a patient may be unable to discriminate among the expressions of fear, disgust, surprise, and anger, crippling interpersonal communication.[42]

In summary, following right hemisphere damage, the usual mechanisms for the perception, experience, and expression of emotion can be disrupted. Therefore, the clinician must be cautious in making inferences about the subjective-affective world of the patient.

FRONTAL LOBE SYNDROMES

Lesions in the frontal lobes may produce characteristic and dramatic alterations in personality, with only subtle impairment of overall intellectual functioning.[43,44] The hallmarks of frontal involvement include deficits in self-regulation (difficulties in planning and executing a course of action), deficits in judgment (lack of foresight, inability to profit from experience, and disregard for social conventions), and disturbances of affect (diminished and/or enhanced emotionality). These changes are most obvious when the patient is in an unstructured environment where external cues to guide and direct behavior are minimal.

Two clinical variants of the frontal lobe changes have been identified, each with a distinct neuroanatomic substrate. These have been termed the *dorsolateral* and *ventromedial frontal lobe syndromes*. The ventromedial syndrome is associated with damage to the orbital frontal regions. Characteristically, such patients tend to be highly impulsive, acting first and thinking later. They do not deliberate over action, fail to anticipate consequences of their behavior, and have difficulty delaying gratification. Impulsive speech and behavior is noted during the interview, and an impulsive response style is evident on tests of cognitive function. Such patients are prone to affective overreactions in response to environmental cues. External stimuli provoke intense paroxysmal bursts of emotional behavior that quickly subside. The evanescent nature of these responses has led to the term *shallowness of affect*. Furthermore, discourse with orbital frontal patients is characterized by joking, punning, and silliness ("Witzelsucht").[45] Such patients cannot resist making light of situations, seem to be immune to embarrassment, and are undeterred by social censure.

These traits can be charming and captivating in the right circumstance but usually cause consternation among those spending time with the patient. Collectively, these three features can be conceptualized as evidence for behavioral "hyperreflexia" or stimulus boundness. It is as if the "pull" of environmental stimuli overrides the modulating effects of social convention. This clinical picture bears superficial similarity to both mania and sociopathy. However, the periodic outbursts of the patient with frontal lobe disease are not sustained mood changes; the talkative facetiousness is not true elation and the patient rarely succeeds in carrying through an elaborate course of action. Although a typical sociopath also behaves impulsively and fails to profit from experience, his antisocial behavior is deliberate and calculated and his selective disregard of social rules is in contrast to the loss of social judgment by the patient with frontal lobe disease. However, the life-style of many sociopaths places them at high risk for frontal lobe damage from head trauma, potentially complicating this differential diagnosis.

If the orbital frontal lobe syndrome is characterized by behavioral "hyperreflexia," the patient with dorsolateral frontal damage typically exhibits behavioral "hyporeflexia"—underresponsiveness to environmental stimuli. A profound anhedonia and apathy can emerge. These patients lack initiative and are unmotivated and uninterested in directing the course of their life. Marked reduction of behavioral output has been termed *abulia*. Their lack of reactivity to environmental stimuli is accompanied by a slowing of cognitive and motor function and by impairments in attention. In extreme cases the patient fails to engage in basic self-care. Perseveration in thought and action is manifest. There is difficulty "switching mental sets." Flashes of irritability, sadness, or elation are common but are short-lived. To family members the patient appears to be like "a bump on the log." The clinical presentation of the dorsolateral frontal syndrome can be distinguished from a retarded depression by the lack of a ruminative sadness or guilt. Vegetative changes in sleep or appetite are not typical. In addition, incontinence, a frequent accompaniment of the dorsolateral frontal syndrome, is extremely rare in depression.

For purposes of exposition, we have distinguished between dorsolateral and ventromedial frontal lobe syndromes. However, many lesions will involve both anatomic regions, producing an admixture of clinical profiles. The resulting personality has been described as "irritable, euphoric apathy."[46]

Common causes of the frontal lobe syndromes are head trauma, neoplasia, degenerative diseases (especially Pick's disease and Alzheimer's disease), multiple sclerosis, and hydrocephalus.

Behavioral Syndromes With Disease of the Basal Ganglia

Disease of the basal ganglia may result in fundamental alterations of emotional expression or behavior, typically in association with characteristic disorders of movement. These disorders may be broadly classified by reference to the nature of the movement abnormality: Parkinson's disease, progressive supranuclear palsy, Wilson's disease, and the multiple system atrophies are examples of the akinetic-rigid forms of basal ganglia disease; Huntington's disease and Sydenham's chorea are choreoathetotic forms.[47] Parkinson's disease and Huntington's disease will be discussed as prototypes of basal ganglia disorders.

PARKINSON'S DISEASE

A resting tremor, motor rigidity, and bradykinesia are cardinal features of Parkinson's disease. These are frequently associated with paucity of facial expression, stooped posture, hypophonic dysarthria, and a festinating gait. Such clinical features are frequently misdiagnosed as depression, especially early in the disease. Later in the course of the illness characteristic features of a depressive syndrome, including dysphoria, may develop.[48] It has been shown that depression occurs more commonly in Parkinson's disease than in other equally disabling conditions, suggesting that the mood change is not merely an appropriate reaction to illness.[48,49] This association has raised the possibility of a direct disturbance of mood based on underlying alterations in catecholamine function. The depressive syndrome may be responsive to tricyclic antidepressants.

Subtle changes in personality occur early in Parkinson's disease and include decreasing spontaneity, lack of imagination, forgetfulness, lethargy, and difficulties in sustaining a conversation.[50] With further progression of the disease, memory impairment, slowness of thought, apathy, and difficulty

with manipulation of acquired knowledge appear. Several workers have drawn attention to the absence of aphasia, apraxia, and agnosia, which would be characteristic of the cortical dementias.[51] Late in the disease an extensive loss of cognitive functions may develop. This late dementia has been correlated with neurofibrillary tangles, senile plaques, and neuronal loss in the basal forebrain nuclei.[52–54]

Dramatic changes in personality may also appear as a complication in the treatment of Parkinson's disease. Both L-dopa and dopamine agonists such as bromocriptine may precipitate an overt psychosis. Psychoses occurring on the initiation of treatment are often associated with a prior underlying thought disorder. However, psychotic symptoms may develop following a prolonged course with dopamine agonists, usually in conjunction with vivid dreams and hallucinations.[55] This perhaps reflects overstimulation of dopaminergic receptors in mesolimbic and mesocortical regions.[56]

HUNTINGTON'S DISEASE

Huntington's disease is an autosomal dominant disorder with complete penetrance. It thus occurs in every generation, affecting 50% of the progeny. The illness is characterized by personality changes occurring in conjunction with a movement disorder, which most frequently is choreic. However, alterations in personality, affect, and thought processes frequently precede the movement disorder by several years.[18]

Subtle personality changes such as distractibility, mental fatigue, inefficiency, and loss of interest occur as early features. At a later stage, poor insight, judgment, and impulse control with sexual promiscuity and social deviance may occur.[57] Inability to appreciate humor, irritability, and even frank aggression are not infrequent manifestations. Depression with rumination, guilt, self-deprecation, and delusions may be presenting features of Huntington's disease. This perhaps accounts for the striking incidence of suicide. The depressive symptoms may be responsive to tricyclic agents or electroconvulsive therapy. Manic and hypomanic behavior with elation, pressured speech, flight of ideas, and grandiosity are also seen in Huntington's disease and has been successfully treated with neuroleptics and lithium carbonate.[58]

A thought disorder described as ''delusionary-hallucinatory'' or schizophrenialike has also been reported. The psychosis typically has a paranoid quality and is often accompanied by auditory and tactile hallucinations; paranoid schizophrenia is among the common misdiagnoses of Huntington's disease.[59]

As noted, behavioral features may occur before the appearance of an obvious movement disorder. However, the astute observer may search for subtle "piano-playing" finger movements appearing while walking, occasional pursing of the lips and swallowing movements, bobbing head and neck movements, and slow saccadic eye movements.[60]

Dopamine antagonists, such as tetrabenazine, and the neuroleptic agents may temporarily alleviate both chorea and psychotic thought disturbances. Experimental therapies aimed at increasing available gamma-aminobenzoic acid and acetylcholine have yielded disappointing results.

REFERENCES

1. Diagnostic and Statistical Manual of Mental Disorders, 3rd ed. Washington, DC, American Psychiatric Association, 1980

2. Harlow JM: Recovery from the passage of an iron bar through the head. Publications Mass Med Soc 2:329–346, 1868

3. Blumer D, Benson DF: Personality changes with frontal and temporal lobe lesions. In Benson DF, Blumer D (eds): Psychiatric Aspects of Neurologic Disease, vol 1. New York, Grune & Stratton, 1975

4. Kluver H, Bucy PC: Preliminary analysis of functions of the temporal lobes in man. Arch Neurol Psychiatry 42:979–1000, 1939

5. Cummins J: Cortical dementias. In Benson DF, Blumer D (eds): Psychiatric Aspects of Neurologic Disease, vol 2. New York, Grune & Stratton, 1982

6. Bear D: Temporal lobe epilepsy: A syndrome of sensory-limbic hyperconnection. Cortex 15:357–384, 1979

7. Reeves AG, Plum F: Hyperphagia, rage and dementia accompanying a ventromedial hypothalamic neoplasm. Arch Neurol 20:617–624, 1969

8. Bear DM: An approach to the study of organic behavioral changes. In Gazzaniga M (ed): Handbook of Behavioral Neurobiology. London, Plenum Press, 1979

9. Bear DM, Fedio P: Quantitative analysis of interictal behavior in temporal lobe epilepsy: Arch Neurol 34:454–467, 1977

10. Wilson H, Olson WH, Gascon GG et al: Personality characteristics in multiple sclerosis. Psychol Rep 51:791–806, 1982

11. Bear D: Hemispheric specialization in the neurology of emotion. Arch Neurol 40:195–202, 1983

12. Malzberg B: Important statistical data about mental illness. In Arieti S (ed): American Handbook of Psychiatry, vol 1. New York, Basic Books, 1959

13. Alexander MP: Traumatic brain injury. In Benson DF, Blumer D (eds): Psychiatric Aspects of Neurologic Disease, vol 2. New York, Grune & Stratton, 1982

14. Benson DF: The treatable dementias. In Benson DF, Blumer D (eds): Psychiatric Aspects of Neurologic Disease, vol 2. Grune & Stratton, 1982

15. Bear DM, Arana G: Neurologic syndromes affecting emotions and behavior. In Guggenheim F, Nadelson C (eds): Major Psychiatric Disorders. New York, Elsevier Press, 1982

16. Mesulam MM, Waxman SG, Geschwind N et al: Acute confusional states with right middle cerebral artery infarction. J Neurol Neurosurg Psychiatry 39:84–89, 1976

17. Corsellis J, Goldberg GJ, Norton AR: Limbic encephalitis and its association with carcinoma. Brain 91:481–498, 1968

18. Adams RD, Victor M: Degenerative diseases of the nervous system. In Principles of Neurology. New York, McGraw-Hill, 1977

19. Plum F, VanUtert R: Neuroendocrine diseases and disorders of the hypothalamus. In Reichlin S, Baldesserini RJ, Martin JB (eds): The Hypothalamus. New York, Raven Press, 1978

20. Jones B, Mishkin M: Limbic lesions and the problem of stimulus-reinforcement associations. Exp Neurol 36:362–377, 1972

21. Geschwind N: Disconnexion syndromes in animals and man. Brain 88:237–294, 1965

22. Nauta W: The problem of the frontal lobe: A reinterpretation. J Psychiatry Res 8:167–187, 1971

23. Devinsky O, Hafler D, Victor J: Embarrassment as the aura of a complex partial seizure. Neurology 32:1284–1285, 1982

24. Stevens JR: An anatomy of schizophrenia? Arch Gen Psychiatry 29:177–189, 1973

25. Ross ED, Mesulam MM: Dominant language functions of the right hemisphere? Arch Neurol 36:144–148, 1979

26. Folstein SE, Folstein MF, McHugh PR: Psychiatric syndromes in Huntington's disease. In Chase T, Wexler N, Barbeau A (eds): Advances in Neurology, vol 23. New York, Raven Press, 1979

27. Haugh RM, Marksbery WR: Hypothalamic astrocytoma: Syndrome of hyperphagia, obesity and disturbances of behavior and endocrine and autonomic function. Arch Neurol 40:560–563, 1983

28. Beal MF, Kleinman GM, Ojemann RG et al: Gangliocytoma of the third ventricle: Hyperphagia, somnolence and dementia. Neurology 31:1224–1228, 1981

29. Martin JB: Neurological manifestations of hypothalamic disease. In Martin JP, Reichlin S, Brown GM (eds): Clinical Neuroendocrinology, pp 247–273. Philadelphia, FA Davis, 1977

30. Moore-Ede MC, Czeisler CA, Richardson GS: Circadian time keeping in health and disease. N Engl J Med 301:469–476, 1983

31. Young JK: A possible neuroendocrine basis for two clinical syndromes: Anorexia nervosa and the Kleine-Levin syndrome. Physiol Psychol 3:233–330, 1979

32. Bear DM, Freeman RL, Greenberg MS: Interictal behavioral alterations in temporal lobe epilepsy. In Blumer D (ed): Psychiatric Aspects of Temporal Lobe Epilepsy. Washington, DC, American Psychiatric Association Press, 1983

33. Slater E, Beard AW: Schizophrenia-like psychoses of epilepsy. Br J Psychiatry 109:95–150, 1963

34. Babinski J: Contribution a l'étude des troubles mentaux dans l'hemiplegic organique cérébrale (anosognosie). Rev Neurol 22:845–848, 1914

35. Critchley M: The Parietal Lobes. New York, Henner Publishing, 1966

36. Heilman KM, Valenstein E (eds): Clinical Neuropsychology. New York, Oxford University Press, 1979

37. Nathanson M, Bergman PS, Gordon GG: Denial of illness. Arch Neurol Psychiatry 68:380–397, 1952

38. Sackeim HS, Greenberg MS, Weiman AL et al: Hemispheric asymmetry in the expression of positive and negative emotions: Neurologic evidence. Arch Neurol 39:210–218, 1982

39. Gainotti G: Emotional behavior and hemispheric side of the lesion. Cortex 8:41–55, 1972

40. Terzian H: Behavioral and EEG effects of intracarotid sodium amytal injection. Acta Neurochir 12:230–239, 1964

41. Heilman KM, Scholes R, Watson RJ: Auditory affective agnosia: Disturbed comprehension of affective speech. J Neurol Neurosurg Psychiatry 24:323–325, 1971

42. Benowitz LI, Bear DM, Rosenthal R et al: Hemispheric specialization in nonverbal communication. Cortex 19:5–11, 1983

43. Teuber HL: The riddle of frontal lobe function in man. In Warren JM, Akert K (eds): The Frontal Granular Cortex and Behavior. New York, McGraw-Hill, 1964

44. Luria AR: The frontal lobe syndrome. In Vinton PJ, Bruyn GW (eds): The Handbook of Clinical Neurology, vol 2. Amsterdam, North-Holland, 1969

45. Hecaen H, Albert M: Disorders of mental functioning related to frontal lobe pathology. In Benson DF, Blumer D (eds): Psychiatric Aspects of Neurologic Disease, vol 1. New York, Grune & Stratton, 1975

46. Geschwind N: Personal communications, 1983

47. Marsden CD: Basal ganglia disease. Lancet 182:1141–1147, 1982

48. Mayeux R, Stern Y, Rosen J et al: Depression, intellectual impairment and Parkinson's disease. Neurology 31:645–649, 1981

49. Hall S: Some psychological factors in parkinsonism. Neurol Neurosurg Psychiatry 37:27–31, 1974

50. Leif AJ, Smith E: Cognitive deficits in the early stages of Parkinson's disease. Brain 106:257–270, 1983

51. Albert ML: Subcortical dementia. In Katzman R, Terry RD, Bick KL (eds): Alzheimer's Disease: Senile Dementia and Related Disorders, pp 173–179. New York, Raven Press, 1978

52. Whitehouse PJ, Hedreen JC, White CL et al: Basal forebrain neurons in the dementia of Parkinson's disease. Ann Neurol 13:243–248, 1983

53. Hakim AM, Mathieson G: Dementia in Parkinson's disease: A neuropathologic study. Neurology 29:1209–1214, 1979

54. Boller F, Mizutani R, Roessman U et al: Parkinson's disease, dementia and Alzheimer's disease: Clinicopathological correlations. Ann Neurol 7:329–335, 1980

55. Klawins HL: Parkinsonism. In Textbook of Neuropharmacology. New York, Raven Press, 1981

56. Javoy-Heid F, Agid Y: Is the mesocortical dopaminergic system involved in Parkinson's disease? Neurology 30:1326–1330, 1980

57. Bruyn GW: Huntington's chorea—History, clinical and laboratory synopsis. In Vinken PJ, Bruyn GW (eds): Handbook of Clinical Neurology, vol 6, pp 298–378. Amsterdam, North-Holland, 1968

58. Bear DM: Emotional and behavioral changes in Huntington's disease. In Report of the Commission for the Control of Huntington's Disease, vol 3, part 1. Washington, DC, Department of Health, Education and Welfare, 1977

59. McHugh PE, Folstein MF: Psychiatric syndromes in Huntington's disease. In Benson E, Blumer D (eds): Psychiatric Aspects of Neurologic Disease, pp 267–285. New York, Grune & Stratton, 1975

60. Paulson GW: Diagnosis of Huntington's disease. In Chase TN, Wexler NS, Barbeau A (eds): Advances in Neurology, vol 23, pp 177–184. New York, Raven Press, 1979

SUGGESTED READING

Benson DF, Blumer D (eds): Psychiatric Aspects of Neurologic Disease, vols 1 and 2. New York, Grune & Stratton, 1975, 1982

Heilman KM, Valenstein E: Clinical Neuropsychology. New York, Oxford University Press, 1979

Lishman A: Organic Psychiatry. Oxford, Blackwell Scientific Publications, 1978

The authors wish to acknowledge the generous support of the Delbert Coleman Foundation in the preparation of this chapter.

Introduction to the Neuroses

It was no surprise, but in the view of many a mistake, that when the third edition of the *Diagnostic and Statistical Manual of Mental Disorders* (*DSM-III*) was published the concept of neurosis as a category of classification was abandoned from the official American classification nomenclature. The writers of the *DSM-III*, who were primarily representatives of phenomenologic and biological schools of psychiatry, regarded the term to be without descriptive use and believed it referred to a specific etiologic theory based on the psychoanalytic model of mental functioning. In an effort to develop a criterion-based nomenclature that was free of etiologic assumptions, the neuroses were discarded as a nosologic class and the conditions previously included in it were redistributed into newly established categories characterized by the dominant symptom. Depressive neurosis was placed in the affective disorders; phobic, anxiety, and obsessive-compulsive neuroses were placed in a new category, anxiety disorders; and hysterical neurosis was divided into two conditions, somatoform disorders and dissociative states (Table 1).

Both biologically and psychodynamically oriented psychiatrists, here and abroad, have argued that the *DSM-III* Task Force underestimated the descriptive usefulness of the term *neurosis,* as well as the advantages of maintaining an historically familiar and internationally accepted category in the absence of any superior alternative. Psycho-dynamic psychiatrists questioned the narrowness and superficiality of the Task Force's definition of the phenomenology that could be assessed reliably. These dynamic psychiatrists maintained that some psychodynamic observations, including those relating to the "dynamic unconscious" and defense mechanisms, were no more inferential than many of the descriptive observations found in the *DSM-III*.[1]

The use of the term *neurosis* was chosen in organizing this section, despite the Task Force's rejection of it. This introduction will review the major issues associated with the concept of neurosis and present the basis for the decision to retain it.

Definitions

In the final stages of its work, the *DSM-III* Task Force began to appreciate that their view of neurotic disorder as exclusively an etiologic psychodynamic concept was misguided and that there was a long tradition of the neuroses as a descriptive nosologic category. As a result, they made the useful distinction between *neurosis* as a descriptive term for a disorder and neurosis as an etiologic process. The following definitions are from the *DSM-III* glossary[2]:

1. *Neurotic Disorder.* A mental disorder in which the predominant disturbance is a symptom or group of symptoms that is distressing to the individual and is recognized by him or her as unacceptable and alien (ego-dystonic); reality testing is grossly intact. Behavior does not actively violate gross social norms (though it may be quite disabling). The disturbance is relatively enduring or recurrent without treatment, and is not limited to a transitory reaction to stressors. There is no demonstrable organic etiology or factor.

2. *Neurotic Process.* A specific etiological process involving the following sequence: (1) unconscious conflicts between opposing desires or between desires and prohibitions, which cause (2) unconscious perception of anticipated danger or dysphoria, which leads to (3) use of defense mechanisms that result in (4) either symptoms, personality disturbance, or both.

These definitions require amplification in many aspects. Is there a specific relationship between neurotic disorder and neurotic process? Does the sequence of unconscious conflict, danger, defense mechanisms, and symptom formation occur only in the neurosis and if so, in what sense, if any, is it etiologic? It leaves uncertain the relationship of neurosis to personality disorders and intermediate states. For example, what of pathologic symptoms that are experienced as distressing but are believed to be an integral part of the personality (*e.g.,* an oppositionalism to superiors, severe procrastination, or a repetitive tendency to fall in love with individuals who are unable to reciprocate)?

Historical Perspective

It is a common error to assume that the study of the neurotic disorders begins with Freud. Ackerknecht

TABLE 1. Comparison of the Classification of Neuroses in the *DSM-II* and the *DSM-III*

DSM-II Neurosis		DSM-III Equivalent	
300.0	Anxiety Neurosis	Anxiety Disorders	
		300.01	Panic disorder
		300.02	Generalized anxiety disorder
300.1	Hysterical Neurosis	No equivalent	
300.13	Hysterical Neurosis, Conversion Type	Somatoform Disorders	
		300.11	Conversion disorder
		307.80	Psychogenic pain disorder
300.14	Hysterical Neurosis, Dissociative Type	Dissociative Disorders	
		300.2	Psychogenic amnesia
		300.13	Psychogenic fugue
		300.14	Multiple personality
300.2	Phobic Neurosis	Anxiety Disorders	
		300.21	Agoraphobia with panic attacks
		300.22	Agoraphobia without panic attacks
		300.23	Social phobia
		300.29	Simple phobia
300.3	Obsessive-compulsive neurosis	Anxiety Disorders	
		300.30	Obsessive-compulsive disorder
300.4	Depressive Neurosis	Major Depression	
		296.22	Single episode, without melancholia
		296.32	Recurrent, without melancholia
		300.40	Dysthymic disorder
		Adjustment Disorder	
		309.00	Adjusted disorder with depressed mood
300.5	Neurosthenic Neurosis	No equivalent	
300.6	Depersonalization Neurosis	Dissociative Disorder	
		300.60	Depersonalization disorder
300.7	Hypochondriacal Neurosis	Somatoform Disorder	
		300.70	Hypochondriasis

dates the serious study of this group of diseases to the 17th century. Although interest in hysteria dates to antiquity, he cites the conviction of Thomas Sydenham (1621–1698) that half of his nonfebrile patients were hysterical. Another English physician, George Cheyne (1671–1749), believed that a third of his patients were "nervous," and in 1733 he published the *English Disease,* which claimed that the English were particularly prone to this illness.[3]

The word *neurosis* was first used to refer to a class of diseases in 1769 by an Edinburgh physician, William Cullen, as a neologism referring to their neural etiology; the neuroses were "affections of the nervous system." Among the diseases that Cullen included in his widely translated nomenclature were chorea, apoplexy, paralysis, hypochondria, tetanus, epilepsy, palpitations, asthma, whooping cough, diarrhea, diabetes, hysteria, melancholia, and mania. After Cullen it was no longer scientifically acceptable or fashionable to attribute illness to vapors or humors. People now suffered from "nerves" or diseases of the nervous system.[4,5]

Over the next 150 years the scope of neurosis as an umbrella or "wastepaper basket" diagnosis narrowed. Pathologic anatomy revolutionized medicine in the 19th century. Structural lesions were found for many of the "neuroses" so that diseases such as chorea and tetanus were set apart from the neurotic rubric. What remained, for example, were hypochondriasis, hysteria, and cataplexy, which were the morbid states described as nervous disorders before Cullen broadened the concept. These neurotic disorders failed to yield a structural lesion. The major psychoses might be equally unyielding, but confidence in their basically organic etiology remained. The neuroses were "diseases without lesions."[6]

Not only were the neuroses a negative category of classification with regard to pathologic anatomy, but they were also negatively defined with regard to psychopathology. The psychoses could be defined by hallucinations, delusions, or other florid evidence of defective reasoning or impaired reality testing that required institutionalization. The neuroses showed no comparable defects. Janet, in a paper delivered at the centennial celebration of the psychiatric division of New York Hospital in 1921, summarized the state of affairs as follows: "But above all, one preserved the conviction that these queer disorders (the neuroses) were very different to the mental disorders of lunacy (the psychoses). These peculiar individuals had, it was said, all their reason; they remained capable of understanding their fellow creatures and of being understood by

them; they were not to be expelled from society like the poor lunatics."[6]

Two approaches to this dilemma of the neuroses as a "negative category" appeared. The first was to relegate the neuroses to a minor status and to turn one's attention to the psychoses, which with the growth of the asylum in the 19th century became the dominant focus of psychiatry during that period and resulted in the major contributions of Kretschmer, Kraepelin, and Bleuler. Another solution was to investigate the pathophysiology of the disease. Pinel had regarded the neuroses as "moral disorders." Neurotic patients suffered from "mental alienation," a psychological concept implying the deleterious impact on behavior of faulty education and noxious environmental conditions.[3] The major studies on the pathophysiology of the neuroses were conducted by Charcot, Jane, and Freud.

Jean Martin Charcot (1835–1893) reestablished the importance of the neuroses toward the end of the century. After establishing a reputation as the great neuropathologist of his age, he shifted his investigations to the neuroses, especially hysteria. The "Napoleon of the Neuroses" used hypnosis to evaluate the pathophysiology of hysterical paralysis and seizures. Although many of his descriptions of the mechanisms of hysteria have proved incorrect (he proposed the existence of specific hysterogenic zones on the body that when stimulated produced the symptoms) he is credited by Ellenberger with the development of the concept of unconscious ideas as the nuclei for certain diseases.[7]

Pierre Janet (1859–1947) is cited by historians and by Freud for developing a systematic dynamic psychopathology of the neuroses that proposed the existence of "subconscious fixed ideas" that could be split off in the personality of the hysteric, lead an autonomous life and development, and at some point produce symptoms.[7,8] He also developed the idea of an historical psychological analysis to reconstruct the development of an illness. His nosology rested on the existence of two basis neuroses: hysteria and psychasthenia. Psychasthenia consisted of those neuroses that showed obsessions, phobias, and other neurotic manifestations and resulted from a generalized lowering of mental activity, while in hysteria there was a dissociation of a particular activity from the conscious personality.

Emil Kraepelin (1856–1926), best known for his delineation of the two major psychoses, also used the neuroses as a diagnostic group. In his first classification, in 1893, he included a category of "psychic weakness" with such disparate conditions as idiocy, obsessions and phobias, and homosexuality. Hysteria is described elsewhere along with hypnosis, stupor, epilepsy, and acute dementia as a "twilight state." Menninger attributes the appearance of the terms *psychoneuroses* and *character disorders* in the 7th edition of his textbook to Kraepelin's becoming the director of a large city (Munich) university clinic and his exposure to a wider range of clinical material.[9] Kraepelin divided the neuroses into two groups: (1) those of psychogenic origin, hysteria, fright neuroses (traumatic neuroses), and expectation neuroses (anxiety neurosis) and (2) those conditioned by a constitutional predisposition, which included neurasthenia, constitutional ill humor and excitement, compulsive states, impulsive states, and sexual abnormalities.[10] This changed again in his later work. Kraepelin, like Freud, constantly struggled with the concept of the neuroses and finally settled on a division that separated out those neuroses that seemed predominantly psychological from those that seem predominantly constitutional.

A full exposition of the contribution of Freud and his followers to the neuroses would require an outline of psychoanalytic theory in its entirety, since it is predominantly a theory of the neuroses. In his "Introductory Lectures," Freud writes[8]: "The theory of neurosis is psychoanalysis itself." His interest was in the psychological mechanisms that underlie mental diseases and is reflected in his nosology that separates the actual neuroses (anxiety neuroses and neurasthenia) from the psychoneuroses. The distinction rests on what Freud believed to be a difference in the pathophysiology of symptom formation between the two groups. The symptoms of the actual neuroses seemed to be the physiologic expression of either the frustration of sexual excitement as a result of abstinence (anxiety neurosis) or the incomplete discharge of it in masturbation or coitus interruptus (neurasthenia). The symptoms of the psychoneuroses, in contrast, were a symbolic expression of a psychological conflict. The cause of the actual neuroses was somatic, that of the psychoneuroses was psychic.[11]

The psychoneuroses were subdivided into transference neuroses and the narcissistic neuroses. In the transference neuroses (anxiety hysteria [phobic neuroses], conversion hysteria, and obsessional neurosis), the individual's libido or sexual interest is directed toward real or imaginary objects, forming a "transference." In the narcissistic neuroses (paranoia, hallucinatory confusions, and certain forms of melancholia) there is a withdrawal of libido from objects, real or imaginary, and a redirection of it to the self. The distinction was considered vital because only the transference neuroses

were believed to be amenable to psychoanalytic treatment.

Freud's original classification of the neuroses is no longer widely accepted. The concept of the actual neuroses was discarded in response to the findings of subsequent investigators that there were conflicts in these disorders that were no different from those found in the transference neuroses. Also Freud's distinction between the narcissistic and transference neuroses proved to be only partially valid. Psychotic individuals did establish transferences, albeit of a very different type than those found in the neuroses.

Epidemiology

Excellent surveys of the epidemiology of the neuroses are provided by Marks[12] and by Katschnig and Shepherd.[13] They agree that the pertinent studies are difficult to compare because of the different populations studied, the different methods of case identification, and finally, the different definitions of neuroses. The most widely cited investigation is that of Hagnell,[14] who personally interviewed the entire population of the small Swedish parish of Lundy and found a lifetime prevalence for neuroses of 13.1 per 100. He employed a broad definition of neurosis as a nonpsychotic mental disease in the absence of organic brain disease.

In general, the neuroses are the most common psychiatric disorders found in the community and in general medical practice. In institutional psychiatric practice, they are less frequent. Shepherd and colleagues reported that 63% of psychiatrically ill patients found in a general medical practice are neurotic. This corresponds to 40% for outpatients in a psychiatric clinic and 29% in mental hospitals.[13] The epidemiologic finding of a larger frequency of neurotic patients in nonpsychiatric populations has been described as an "iceberg effect," with psychiatrists seeing only a small percentage of those who are neurotic. The distribution of the different neuroses is highly dependent on the population, but anxiety and depression are the most frequent. Hysteria is usually next with obsessive-compulsive disorder being fairly rare.

Katsching and Shepherd,[13] in their summary of the epidemiologic literature, argue that no valid associations can be identified regarding neurosis and social class. Evidence suggests that the rates are higher for women in all age-groups up to 60 years. Young single women are reported to suffer a low rate of neurosis, while those who remain single all their lives have a high rate. This female preponderance is not true in certain categories such as obsessive-compulsive neurosis.

An intriguing finding is the periodic epidemics of neurosis, particularly hysteria, described since the Middle Ages. These have involved well-documented cases of towns and convents being "visited" by particular symptom complexes.[15] It is likely that Charcot's patients were probably strongly influenced by their physicians' theories and the epileptic patients with whom they were hospitalized.[7]

There is some clinical belief that the neurotic disorders relapse repeatedly and are chronic, but this has not been validated.[16] In Hagnell's study, 70% were better in 6 months and only 4% were still florid after 3 years.[14] In a study by Denker, quoted by Eysenck, 72% of neurotic patients spontaneously recovered in 2 years and over 90% after 5 years.[14,17] Rawnsley and Loudon reported that women who had exhibited hysterical seizures during an epidemic of hysteria on the island of Tristan da Cunha 20 years later suffered more frequently from psychogenic headaches when the island had to be evacuated because of volcanic eruption.[18]

Neurotic Process and Psychopathology

Freud initially attempted to develop a nosologic system that divided the nervous disorders into those without psychological conflict (actual neurosis) and those with conflict (the psychoneuroses). As was noted previously, this model was abandoned when later studies revealed conflicts associated with the symptoms of anxiety neurosis and neurasthenia.

The presence of neurotic process is characteristic of other psychological states as well. In the *Psychopathology of Everyday Life*, Freud examined in detail how the "symptoms" of normality such as momentary forgetting and slips of the tongue or pen reveal the operation of unconscious conflict and "symptom formation." Similar processes are found in the psychoses.[19] Burnham[20] has described a need/fear dilemma in schizophrenic patients in which the wish for intimacy conflicts with the profound fear of identity dissolution or loss of self-object separateness and results in such regressive psychotic symptoms as concrete thought or hallucinations.

Neurotic process is not specific to the neurotic disorders, although it is in the neuroses that it has been most widely studied. It can also be found to exert an influence on behavior in the psychopathology of everyday life, character disorders, organic disorders, and psychoses. In fact, it is a process that seems to be intrinsic to humans and to affect the entire range of their behavior. Kubie shows how neurotic process can result in remarkable achievements that contribute to personal and societal growth.[21] Some psychiatrists take the positions that neurotic process is more central or of greater etiologic significance in the neurotic disorders than it is in normal behavior or psychoses in which habit, conscious thought, and biological defect are the dominant determinants of behavior. Although this may be true, it is still inaccurate to describe a process as neurotic when it is at least an aspect of nonneurotic behaviors; therefore the term *psychodynamic process* is preferred.

Defense Mechanisms and Neuroses

An alternative approach to the study of different psychopathologic conditions uses defense mechanisms to distinguish them. Thus, in hysterical neurosis we find repression, conversion, and dissociation; in obsessive-compulsive neurosis, intellectualization, isolation of affect, and reaction formation; in depression, identification and retroflexion of anger; and in schizophrenia, denial, projective identification, splitting of objects, and self-object merger. Vaillant[21] has developed a useful hierarchy of defense mechanisms. Healthy or mature mechanisms of defense include humor, suppression, altruism, anticipation, and sublimations. Neurotic mechanisms of defense include displacement, dissociation, reaction formation, repression, and intellectualism. Immature and psychotic mechanisms include acting out, hypochondriasis, delusional projection, and denial. Vaillant is careful to emphasize that the context and events that call forth a particular defense must be evaluated before judging it as pathologic.[22] Denial of a fatal cancer in many circumstances would hardly be considered pathologic.

Personality Disorder and Neurosis

A basic discovery, first noted by Freud and then amplified by Reich, is the striking similarity between neurotic symptoms and character traits. These traits, although usually ego-syntonic and of no personal distress seem to be an expression of a defense caused by conflicts in seemingly the same manner that neurotic symptoms are. Thus, the symptom of dissociative-hysterical states in which an individual forgets his prior identity is remarkably similar to the character trait of superficiality in a hysterical man. Both patients "forget" the richness and complexity of their past experiences and fantasies so that every moment is lived emptily. In one patient the result is a "symptom neurosis," while in the other it is what is generally referred to as a "character neurosis." Similarly, the compulsive handwashing of the compulsive neurotic may represent conflict and choice of defense mechanisms similar to the overbearing neatness of the obsessive-compulsive character. What in the neurotic is an ego-alien symptom in the character disorder becomes a way of life, an ideal, or a preference. Its basically neurotic origins remain in the effect that the character trait has on others who more easily see its inflexible, driven, and self-defeating aspects.

An intermediate condition between the neurosis and character disorders is the perception as part of the self of a trait that is truly not ego-dystonic but that nevertheless provides distress to the individual. Excessive neatness, a tendency to eroticize all heterosexual relationships, a need always to tell the truth regardless of consequences, and perverse sexual preferences or object choices are all examples of such personality disturbances. Often in the treatment of personality disorders ego-syntonic character traits become neurotic symptoms of this kind. The examination of a patient's preference for the aisle seat in a plane and the regular pattern of relaxing with a novel and a drink during the flight lead to the recognition of a plane phobia, self-treated by avoiding the view from the window, by the distraction of the novel, and by the tranquilizing effect of the alcohol. Neurotic symptoms are frequently embedded in a personality structure in which the same defense is central to symptom and character trait. The analytic investigation of a plane phobia often reveals a host of "preferences" or "tastes" that are based on the same underlying defense mechanism of avoiding an activity or behavior that is conflictual.

Neurotic disorders are not always found in association with equivalent character disorder (*i.e.*, obsessive-compulsive neurosis in obsessive character or phobic neurosis in phobic character). The neurotic symptom does not necessarily predict the dominant character traits or character structure.

Conversion symptoms have been found not only in hysterical personalities but also in obsessive and antisocial personalities. These mixed clinical pictures, although not infrequent, will nonetheless alert the clinician to the possibility of a more severe underlying process. Hoch and Polatin described a syndrome of shifting neurotic symptoms in the presence of diffuse anxiety and a mixed homosexual/heterosexual sexual preference. This entity of pan-neurosis, pan-anxiety, and pan-sexuality, which they called "pseudoneurotic schizophrenia" and which would be described in the current nomenclature as a mixture of borderline and schizotypal personality disorders, draws attention to the significance of shifting neurotic symptoms in the diagnosis of severe character disorders.[23] Kernberg has maintained this clinical observation by including polysymptomatic neuroses as a criterion for the borderline personality.[24]

Etiology of the Neurosis

In the *DSM-III* glossary, *neurotic process* (psychodynamic process) is described as a "specific etiological process" with a characteristic sequence of behaviors that begins with an unconscious conflict and results in symptom formation. I have already objected to the implication in this definition that psychodynamic process is specific to the neurosis. It is also problematic to describe it as etiologic. The conflict may simply occur in association with the underlying disorder. For example, homosexual conflicts are often found in paranoid disorders and may explain some of the characteristic symptoms of these disorders, such as pathologic jealousy, erotomania, and delusions of homosexual attribution by others without explaining the etiology of the paranoid disorder in which they occur. Also, it is not clear why the conflict occurs in the first place and why it may result in a neurosis or character disturbance rather than a character trait within the normal range. Conflictual process and its relation to symptom formation may be analogous to the relationship of heart failure to dyspnea. Heart failure like psychodynamic process describes a sequence of events without really specifying what the cause of the heart failure might be. Beriberi, coronary occlusion, alcoholic myopathy, and rheumatic heart disease all result in heart failure and dyspnea through a similar pathophysiology, although the morbid pathology and etiology of the specific underlying conditions are quite different.

An alternate approach to the problem of etiology and the neuroses is to argue that the neuroses are not diseases or disorders but are closely related to normal behavior. Schneider, in his system of classification, includes the neuroses and personality disorders as "variants of normal behavior."[25] The traditional notion of a mental disease with abnormal pathologic findings exemplified by cerebral lues and presumed to be true on different level of brain organization in the major psychoses is not true for the neuroses. Jaspers writes of the neuroses: "The body only enters the picture as it does in relation to healthy psychological development."[26] A related viewpoint is found in Freud's view that neuroses are an inevitable and tragic dilemma of civilization; they are unsuccessful efforts to mediate successfully the conflicts between the demands of biological drives and the necessity of culture to tame these drives.[27] For Freud, the neuroses "shade off by easy transition into what is described as normal; and on the other hand, there is scarcely any state recognized as normal in which indication of neurotic traits could not be pointed out."[28] Neurotic disorders are disorders of degree rather than kind.

Yet another approach to the problem of etiology of the neuroses derives from the large number of theories that postulate that current neurotic symptoms can be traced to an earlier traumatic incident or series of traumata. Trauma occurs when the organism is overwhelmed and unable to master the event successfully. The result can be the repression of the memories of the event, the strangulation of affects stimulated by it, and/or the persistence of maladaptive learned behaviors attached to the event. An important variation on the traumatic model of neurotic etiology is to argue that instead of a single major trauma there can be a series of minor or even micro traumas. In this model the repeated withdrawals from an infant by a depressed mother could be as traumatic as the mother's death or abandonment of the child. The moment one proposes such a dynamic model (*i.e.*, that trauma produces neurotic symptoms), there is a tendency to track the psychopathology to its traumatic origins in order to release the individual from its toxic influence. Dynamic theories have emphasized a "return" to the traumatic event via suggestion, hypnosis, sodium amobarbital, psychoanalysis, primal scream therapy, and so on in order to accomplish this release. Behavior therapists have argued that this is not necessary if one attends to the current reinforcers of the symptom.

Whatever the treatment implications, the etiologic importance of the "trauma" remains to be clarified. Basically, there are the organic-biological and the environmental-psychogenic schools of thought regarding the way in which trauma produces a neurosis in some individuals. The organic-biological schools of thought usually pose the existence of an underlying defect that renders the individual vulnerable. Examples would include Charcot, who viewed the propensity to neurosis as related to hereditary degeneration of the brain, or Breuer, who maintained that the individual was susceptible to the trauma because of a "hypnoid state" induced by states of fatigue with protracted affects. More recent theories have proposed that hereditary regulatory defects in synaptic pathways could effect anxiety regulation.

The work of Kohut offers an example of the environmental-psychogenic school. He proposed that it is the tragic failure of parents to provide infants and children with empathic, phase-appropriate caring that results in subsequent neurotic difficulties. Freud, of course, emphasized the failure of the child to master the conflicts of the Oedipus complex but did not commit himself to an etiologic explanation of why this sometimes occurs. More recent theories integrate biological and psychosocial factors. Rodents and primates separated from their mothers at critical periods of infancy demonstrate "neurotic-like" behavior as adults and in addition suffered endocrine abnormalities somewhat similar to those found in depressed humans.[29]

The Death of the Neurosis: A Premature Obituary?

An important issue which the *DSM-III* implicitly addressed was the historically vexing problem of whether the neuroses as a diagnostic category were a valid medical classification. Largely, although not exclusively due to Freud's impact, the study of the neurotic disorders had become closely intertwined with the study of psychodynamic process and both had become an acceptable part of psychiatry. Since psychodynamic process or the psychological pathophysiology of symptoms did not require a knowledge of anatomy and its morbid variations, there appeared in psychiatry a dichotomy between those psychiatrists who allied themselves with the traditional basic sciences of medicine, pathologic anatomy, biochemistry, and physiology and those primarily psychoanalytically trained physicians who found helpful guidance from psychology, philosophy, and sociology.

In the United States, during the 1940s and 1950s, the predominant direction in psychiatry was that of psychoanalytic medicine. In the 1960s and 1970s, with the development of new and effective psychotropic medications, biological research, and competition for limited resources within the medical community, a retrenchment of psychiatry occurred, with a reemphasis of the speciality as a medical discipline. Alternative "roots" were sought and Kraepelin replaced Freud and Bleuler as a dominant influence.

It is not surprising that the troublesome category "neurosis" disappeared under these conditions. The study of neurosis had become the study of disorders of the mind increasingly infringed on by nonmedical specialists. For example, Marks argued that since the neuroses were learned behaviors, they fell within the domain of psychology rather than psychiatry, which had as its domain the disorders of the brain.[12]

Looked at in a broader perspective, the issue of what to do with the term neuroses and whether they appropriately belonged in a disease model was an issue of significance for all of psychiatry that the *DSM-III* resolved to everyone's dissatisfaction by distributing them in a classification that does not distinguish them as a unified category from the major psychoses and organic disorders.

In deciding to discard the concept of neurosis as a descriptive diagnostic category the writers of the *DSM-III* abandoned an historically valid category for new subgroupings defined by a particular symptom, anxiety, depression, personality, dissociation, and functional physical symptoms. The advantages in this splitting of the neuroses into smaller units is that it presumably has created groupings that are more homogeneous and easier to define reliably. This remains to be proven, however, and in the opinion of many may not represent a substantial enough gain in order to displace the use of the familiar and traditional category of neurosis.

A marked disadvantage is that it obscures possible relationships among the neurotic disorders. For example, conversion disorders and dissociative disorders are placed in separate and distinct categories instead of being closely related to each other as they were in the *DSM-II*, in which they were classed as subtypes of hysterical neuroses. The *DSM-II* classification has the merit of emphasizing the similarity of the two disorders—that they both "split off" a mental content from the rest of the personality, which is then transformed into a somatic or psychologic expression with symbolic meaning to the patient's mental life. Also conversion and dissociative symptoms are frequently found in the same patient, who is often but not always an individual with an hysterical personality. Conversion disorder, from this perspective, seems more closely related to dissociative disorder than to hypochondriacal neurosis, with which it is now associated under the general rubric of somatoform disorders.

Finally, use of neurosis to describe a diagnostic category that is thought to be heavily influenced by psychosocial factors has a long tradition. Psychoanalysis as a recent investigative technique in this tradition has demonstrated that neurotic symptoms can be viewed from the perspective of symbolic meaning that expresses unconscious conflict. This psychosocial viewpoint does not preclude the usefulness of other perspectives such as biological or genetic that might further elucidate the neurotic disorders. Freud himself looked forward to the day when the somatic contribution to the neuroses would be discovered. At the present moment, the historical, descriptive, and pathophysiologic validity of the neuroses argues for maintaining them as a category.

This has been done in the following chapters albeit in a somewhat loosely interpreted manner. The *DSM-III* categories of somatoform disorders and dissociative disorders have been retained. Obsessive-compulsive neurosis and phobic neurosis were given special chapters apart from the anxiety disorders. Depressive neurosis was also included as a neurotic disorder, which is distinguishable from an affective disorder. The impulse disorders were included as neuroses despite controversy regarding their appropriately being included in this section, since they were not included as neuroses in the *DSM-II*. Although some investigators have maintained that many of the gender identity and sexual preference disorders can be understood as neuroses here they have been placed in a separate section in keeping with most contemporary classification systems.[30]

REFERENCES

1. Frances A, Cooper AM: Descriptive and dynamic psychiatry: A perspective on DSM III. Am J Psychiatry 138:9, 1981
2. Diagnostic and Statistical Manual of Mental Disorders, 3rd ed. Washington, DC, American Psychiatric Association, 1981
3. Ackerknecht EH: Short History of Psychiatry, 2nd ed. New York, Hafner Publishing, 1968

4. Bowman KM, Rose M: A criticism of the terms "psychoses," "psychoneurosis," and "neurosis." Am J Psychiatry 108:161, 1951

5. Lopez Piner JM: Historical Origins of The Concept of Neurosis. Cambridge, MA, Harvard University Press, 1983

6. Janet P: The Relation of the Neuroses to the Psychosis. In A Psychiatric Milestone, Bloomingdale Hospital Centenary. New York, Society of The New York Hospital, 1921

7. Ellenberger HF: The Discovery of the Unconscious: The History and Evolution of Dynamic Psychiatry. New York, Basic Books, 1970

8. Freud S: (1916–1917) Introductory lectures on psychoanalysis. In Strachey J (ed): The Standard Edition of the Complete Works of Sigmund Freud, vol 16. London, Hogarth Press, 1963

9. Menninger K: The Vital Balance. New York, Viking Press, 1963

10. Kraepelin E: Clinical Psychiatry. Diefendorf AR (trans). New York, Macmillan, 1962

11. Freud S: (1894) The neuropsychoses of defense. In Strachey J (ed): The Standard Edition of the Complete Works of Sigmund Freud, vol 6. London, Hogarth Press, 1962

12. Marks I: Cure and Care of Neuroses: Theory and Practice of Behavioral Psychotherapy. New York, John Wiley & Sons, 1981

13. Katschnig H, Shepherd M: Neurosis: The epidemiological perspective. In Van Praag HM (ed): Research in Neurosis. New York, SP Medical and Scientific Books, 1978

14. Hagnell O: A Prospective Study of the Incidence of Mental Disorder. Sweden, Svenska Bokforlaget, 1966

15. Huxley A: The Devils of Loudun. New York, Harper & Row, 1970

16. Detre TP, Jarecki HG: Modern Psychiatric Treatment. Philadelphia, JB Lippincott, 1971

17. Eysenck HJ: The effects of psychotherapy. In Eysenck HJ (ed): Handbook of Abnormal Psychology. New York, Basic Books, 1961

18. Rawnsley K, Loudon JB: Epidemiology of mental disorder in a closed community. Br J Psychiatry 110:830, 1964

19. Arlow JA, Brenner C: The psychopathology of the psychoses: A proposed revision. Int J Psychoanal 50:5, 1969

20. Burnham DL, Gladstone AI, Gibson RW: Schizophrenia and the Need-Fear Dilemma. New York, International Universities Press, 1969

21. Kubie L: The distortion of the symbolic process in neurosis and psychosis. J Am Psychoanal Assoc 1:59, 1953

22. Vaillant GE: Theoretical hierarchy of adaptive ego mechanisms. Arch Gen Psychiatry 24:107, 1971

23. Hoch PH, Polatin P: Pseudoneurotic forms of schizophrenia. Psychiatr Q 23:248, 1949

24. Kernberg O: Borderline Conditions and Pathological Narcissism, p 9. New York, Jason Aronson, 1975

25. Schneider K: Clinical Psychopathology. Hamilton MW (trans). New York, Grune & Stratton, 1959

26. Jaspers K: General Psychopathology. Chicago, University of Chicago Press, 1963

27. Freud S: (1930) Civilization and Its Discontents. In Strachey J (ed): The Standard Edition of the Complete Works of Sigmund Freud, vol 21. London, Hogarth Press, 1961

28. Freud S: (1940) An Outline of Psychoanalysis. In Strachey J (ed): The Standard Edition of the Complete Works of Sigmund Freud, vol 23. London, Hogarth Press, 1964

29. Kumar R: Experimental Neurosis in Animals. In Van Praag HM (ed): Research in Neurosis. New York, SP Medical and Scientific Books, 1978

30. Stoller RJ: Psychoanalytic Diagnosis. In Rakoff VM, Stancer HC, Kedward HB (eds): Psychiatric Diagnosis. New York, Brunner/Mazel, 1977

26

Jack M. Gorman and Michael R. Liebowitz

Panic and Anxiety Disorders

All patients with psychiatric illness experience pathologic anxiety. Furthermore, anxiety reactions are ubiquitous phenomena of normal human life. These facts may explain the delay in recognizing anxiety disorders as distinct clinical entities instead of mere symptoms accompanying other conditions.

In the 1952 edition of the American Psychiatric Association's *Diagnostic and Statistical Manual of Mental Disorders* (*DSM-II*), an ill-defined condition called "anxiety neurosis" seemed to apply indiscriminately to any patient suffering from chronic tension, excessive worry, frequent headaches, or recurrent panic attacks. Several lines of evidence over the subsequent 30 years indicated that this was too broad a conception of anxiety disorder to be either clinically or experimentally useful.

Most important of these findings involved discoveries suggesting that spontaneous panic attacks may be qualitatively dissimilar rather then simply a more intense version of chronic, unremitting anxiety. Patients with panic attacks appeared sensitive to the effects of intravenously administered sodium lactate to the point that an actual panic attack could be precipitated during an infusion.[1] Strong familial links were found among patients with panic disorder.[2] Patients with panic disorder often developed agoraphobia, avoiding all situations in which they would not be able to get immediate help in case of a panic attack. Finally, the panic attacks seemed remarkably responsive to drugs previously believed to be exclusively useful for depression, such as tricyclic antidepressants[3] and monoamine oxidase inhibitors.[4]

Because of these findings, the third edition of the *DSM* splits the old diagnosis of anxiety neurosis into two distinct categories: panic disorder and generalized anxiety disorder. Only patients with re-current, out-of-the-blue panic attacks warrant the former diagnosis, while generalized anxiety disorder (GAD) is reserved for patients with more constant anxiety. This division, however, must still be regarded as provisional, since the clinical, biological, genetic, and treatment studies now considered necessary to validate a diagnostic entity have not been conducted in GAD patients. In particular, studies of lactate provocation, antidepressant therapy, family history, and course of illness should help clarify whether GAD is truly distinct from anxiety disorders involving panic attacks and also whether GAD is itself a homogeneous category.

Definition

The hallmark of panic disorder is the discrete, spontaneous panic attack. Essential to the definition of this syndrome is that the attacks are largely unprovoked by environmental stimuli. Later in the course of the illness patients may associate certain situations, like driving in a car over a bridge, with having a panic attack and attacks may be most likely to occur in such situations. However, careful history reveals that the condition usually begins with a flurry of unpredicted attacks occurring at random moments of everyday life.

Typically, during a panic attack, a patient will be engaged in a routine activity—perhaps reading a book, eating in a restaurant, driving a car, or attending a concert—when he will experience the sudden onset of overwhelming fear, terror, apprehension, and a sense of impending doom. Several of a group of associated symptoms, mostly physical, are also experienced: dyspnea, palpitations, chest pain or discomfort, choking or smothering sensations, dizziness, vertigo or unsteady feelings, feelings of unreality (derealization and/or depersonalization), paresthesias, hot and cold flashes, sweating, faintness, trembling and shaking, and a fear of dying, going crazy, or losing control of oneself.

It is clear that most of the physical sensations of a panic attack represent massive overstimulation of the autonomic nervous system. Some physical symptoms not listed in the *DSM-III* that occasionally occur include nausea, an urge to urinate or defecate, blurred vision, and extreme weakness.

Attacks usually last from 5 to 20 minutes, rarely as long as an hour. Patients who claim they have attacks that last a whole day may fall into one of two categories. Some patients continue to feel agitated and fatigued for several hours after the main portion of the attack has subsided. The other possibility is that the patient is suffering from some other form of pathologic anxiety.

Many people experience an occasional spontaneous panic attack and the diagnosis of panic disorder is only made when the attacks occur with some regularity and frequency. *DSM-III* criteria mandate at least three attacks in a 3-week period while the Research Diagnostic Criteria[5] call for six attacks in any 6-week period. It is not uncommon to find patients who have attacks daily. Some patients are awakened from sleep in the middle of an attack.

GAD is a residual category for anxiety disorders other than panic disorder. The essential feature of this syndrome is persistent anxiety lasting at least a month. The symptoms of this type of anxiety usually fall within four broad categories: (1) motor tension, (2) autonomic hyperactivity, (3) apprehensive expectation, and (4) vigilance and scanning. Patients should manifest symptoms from at least three of the four categories before making the diagnosis of GAD.

Motor tension involves feelings of shakiness, trembling, inability to relax, and being easily startled. Autonomic hyperactivity is characterized by sweating, heart pounding, dry mouth, lightheadedness, stomach upset, frequent urination, and diarrhea. Patients are constantly worried over trivial matters, fearful, and anticipating the worst. Difficulty concentrating, insomnia, irritability, and impatience are signs of vigilance and scanning.

Again it must be emphasized that the patient with GAD does not have discrete episodes of panic and terror; their illness is a more constant and insidious syndrome.

Epidemiology

Only one large epidemiologic survey has been reported that yields incidence and prevalence data for panic disorder and GAD separately. Earlier work in which distinctions among various forms of anxiety were not made yielded prevalence rates of 2.0 to 4.7/100 for anxiety disorder.

In Weissman's work, based on careful interviews of 511 persons living in New Haven, Connecticut, the following prevalence rates were obtained: any anxiety disorder, 4.3/100; GAD, 2.5/100; and panic disorders, 0.4/100.[6] The patients with current agoraphobia and panic attacks originally met criteria for pure panic disorder. Phobic disorders in general occurred in 1.4/100 persons surveyed.

It is generally believed that these disorders primarily afflict women. Once again, rigorous data are lacking. Taking studies on patients with neurocirculatory asthenia, anxiety neurosis, and panic disorder together, a female-to-male incidence ratio of 2 : 1 emerges. It is the experience of most clinicians that a majority of patients who present to psychiatric attention with panic disorder or GAD are female. However, recent work indicates that a greater proportion of men than women with these conditions abuse alcohol in attempts at self-medication. Such cases may register on community surveys as alcoholism, thus artificially lowering the incidence of primary anxiety disorder in males.

These illnesses are apparently uniformly distributed among all social classes. Weissman's data suggest a slightly lower rate of GAD in the upper social classes. Among Hispanic patients a condition commonly called the "ataque nerviosa" may be a form of panic disorder.

As is the case with all serious psychiatric illness, advanced and severe cases of both panic disorder and GAD are sufficiently debilitating to interfere markedly with the ability to earn a living. Hence, a form of "downward drift" may operate among these patients socioeconomically.

Clinical Description

PANIC DISORDER

In the typical beginning of a case of panic disorder, the subject is engaged in some ordinary aspect of life when suddenly his heart begins to pound, he cannot catch his breath, he feels dizzy, lightheaded, and faint and he is convinced he is about to die. This patient is usually a young adult, most likely in the third decade. However, we have seen cases that begin in the sixth decade.

Although the first attack generally strikes during some routine innocuous activity, there are several concomitant events that are often associated with the early presentation of panic disorder. Not uncommonly, the first panic attack occurs in the context of a life-threatening illness or accident or the loss of a close interpersonal relationship. Patients developing either hypothyroidism or hyperthyroidism may get the first flurry of attacks at this time. Attacks also begin in the immediate postpartum period. Finally, many patients have reported experiencing their first attacks while taking mind-altering drugs, especially marijuana, cocaine, and amphetamines.

Even when these concomitant conditions are resolved, attacks often continue unabated. Thus, long after the automobile accident, the correction of the thyroid condition, the postpartum period, or the complete cessation of drug abuse the patient continues to get panic attacks spontaneously. This situation gives the impression that some stressors may act as triggers to provoke the beginning of panic attacks in patients who are already predisposed.

The patient experiencing his first panic attack generally fears he is having a heart attack or stroke. Such patients often rush to the nearest emergency room where routine laboratory tests, electrocardiography, and physical examination are performed. All that is found is an occasional case of sinus tachycardia and the patient is reassured and sent home.

The patient may indeed feel reassured and at this point the diagnosis of panic disorder would of course be premature. However, perhaps a few days or even weeks later the patient again has the sudden onset of severe anxiety with all the associated physical symptoms. Again, he seeks emergency medical treatment. At this point, depending on the patient's finances and the attitude of his doctors, he may either be told the problem is "psychological," be given a prescription for a benzodiazepine tranquilizer, or be referred for extensive medical workup. The last generally involves sophisticated cardiac workups, including 24-hour Holter monitoring, stress tests, and echocardiograms. Neurologic consultation may be requested, and electroencephalography and computed tomography performed. Five-hour glucose tolerance tests are often obtained as well, and patients are sometimes told their problem stems from reactive hypoglycemia.

In general, after complete medical workup, no abnormalities except perhaps mitral valve prolapse are found and the patient is still ultimately told the cause of his problem is psychological. Characteristically, patients at this point begin shunning medical attention for their panic attacks. Out of desperation some begin abusing alcohol.

Some patients do not progress in their illness beyond the point of continuing to have spontaneous panic attacks. Most patients develop some degree of anticipatory anxiety consequent to the experience of repetitive panic attacks. The patient comes to dread experiencing an attack and starts worrying about them in the intervals between attacks. This can progress until the level of fearfulness and autonomic hyperactivity in the interval between panic attacks almost approximates the level during the actual attack itself. Such patients may be mistaken for GAD patients.

The most serious outcome of panic disorder is the development of phobic avoidance, which can progress to the full agoraphobic syndrome. Phobias probably develop in the panic disorder patient for two reasons: First, the patient comes to associate certain situations with the occurrence of a panic attack. Hence, for example, if a number of panic attacks occur while driving the car, a patient may give this etiologic significance and believe that actually being in the car causes the attack. Second, and probably more important, the patient comes to fear situations in which help is not immediately available in case an attack occurs. Being in crowds with strangers, far from the exit in a movie theater, or enclosed in a plane or in a car on the expressway becomes intolerable for such patients.

In the most extreme form, the patient becomes afraid to leave the house under any circumstances and may even be uncomfortable at home unless a trusted companion is present. Although cases of agoraphobia without a prior history of panic attacks have been described, it is our impression a careful history always reveals at least one uncomplicated panic attack preceding the development of the agoraphobia.

Attempts to correlate particular character types with panic disorder have not been systematically conducted. In our experience, patients with panic disorder, when seen shortly after the onset of the condition, do not manifest any particular form of character. Hysterical, compulsive, narcissistic, borderline, dependent, and avoidant character disorders seem randomly represented among patients with panic disorder, and some do not suffer any character pathology at all.

The course of the illness without treatment is

highly variable. At the present time there is no reliable way to know which patient will develop agoraphobia. The illness seems to have a waxing and waning course in which spontaneous recovery occurs, only to be followed months to years later by a new outburst. At the extreme, some patients become completely housebound for decades.

Treatment aimed at blocking the occurrence of the spontaneous attack, described in detail below, is appropriate at any point in the course of the illness. Results are often dramatic. Pharmacologic blockade of panic attacks early in the illness, before phobic avoidance has become an ingrained way of life, often leads to complete remission. Even years into the illness, effective disruption of the attacks with medication can lead to resolution of anticipatory anxiety and phobias without other treatment.

However, a substantial number of patients with significant phobic avoidance remain frightened of confronting feared situations even after the attacks have been blocked. Such patients require other forms of intervention, described elsewhere in this text.

One study has shown a higher incidence of premature death due to cardiovascular illness and suicide among patients with panic disorder compared with normals.[7] The group of patients studied had all been hospitalized at one point, raising the question that they may have been a more severely ill group of patients than is generally encountered in clinical practice.

However, the increased suicide rate may be related to the fact that patients with panic disorder are more prone to major depressive disorder at some point in their life than the normal population. In the New Haven study, 2.5% of patients with panic disorder had already had a depressive episode at some point in their lives.

Patients who meet criteria for panic disorder and are not currently depressed rarely voice suicidal ideas, and suicides are uncommon at this point in the illness.

The increased death rate from cardiovascular illness described in this one study is also not reflected in the usual status of patients undergoing treatment for panic disorder. Most such patients have normal medical workups. The one cardiovascular abnormality that has been found to occur at high rate in patients with panic disorder is mitral valve prolapse. This association, discussed in the section on diagnosis, could conceivably explain a higher incidence of cardiovascular-related death in patients with panic disorder; however, mitral valve prolapse itself is rarely a cause of premature death.

One other possible explanation for early cardiovascular death in patients with panic disorder may be the tendency of such patients to live relatively sedentary lives. Some patients with panic disorder report that vigorous physical exercise precipitates their panic attacks and they therefore avoid exertion of any kind.

GENERALIZED ANXIETY DISORDER

By contrast with panic disorder, our ability to sketch a complete clinical description of GAD is limited. Much of what follows is necessarily tentative, awaiting completion of several research studies.

No overwhelming, single event prompts the patient with GAD to seek help. Such patients seem only over time to develop the recognition that their experience of chronic tension, hyperactivity, worry, and anxiety is not normal. Often, they will state that there has never been a time in their lives as long as they can remember that they were not anxious.

In one study of a small number of patients, GAD appeared to be a more chronic condition than panic disorder,[8] with fewer periods of spontaneous remission.

It is also commonly observed that mild dysphoric symptoms are associated with GAD. Without manifesting the full range of vegetative signs, anhedonia, and unremitting dysphoria of major depressive disorder, the patient with GAD expresses a sense of frustration, disgust with life, demoralization, and hopelessness. Abuse of alcohol, barbiturates, and antianxiety medication is said to be common in this group.

Adequate data on the true age at onset of this condition, its natural history, and prognosis are not available at this time.

Etiology

The causes of pathologic anxiety have been considered from a wide variety of fronts, with some theories conflicting with others. We will divide this section into five main parts: psychoanalytic theories, learning and behavioral theories, the role of separation phenomena, biological theories, and genetic data.

PSYCHOANALYTIC THEORIES

Freud's earliest concept of anxiety formation, summarized in his 1915 book *Introductory Lectures on Psychoanalysis*,[9] categorized pathologic anxiety essentially as failed repression. Repression, Freud felt at the time, is the mechanism of psychic work that holds away from consciousness all unacceptable libidinal thoughts, impulses, memories, and desires. Whenever the psychic energy attached to these banished elements becomes too strong to be held back by repression, they break through into consciousness in distorted and disguised aspect. The conscious experience of this occurrence is anxiety.

It is fascinating to read the early phenomenologic descriptions of anxiety disorder that Freud used to formulate this etiologic theory. One of the cases presented in his *Studies On Hysteria*,[10] that of a young girl he meets while climbing in the mountains, sounds remarkably like a case of panic disorder. Freud believed this patient's panic attacks were caused by the incomplete repression of her sexual interest in her uncle. Rather than acknowledging this unacceptable impulse, the girl suffered a series of severe anxiety attacks.

Freud noted the sequence of panic disorder leading to agoraphobia, as this passage from an early work indicates[11]: "In the case of agoraphobia . . . we often find the recollection of an anxiety attack; and what the patient actually fears is the occurrence of such an attack under the special conditions in which he believes he cannot escape it." As Freud's thinking progressed and his own experience as a psychoanalyst presented more complex case material, the need for a less simplistic theory of anxiety production arose. In the landmark book *Inhibitions, Symptoms and Anxiety*, Freud presented in 1926 what remains the central tenet of modern psychoanalytic theory of anxiety.[12] Instead of being derived from dammed up, unconscious libidinal impulses, anxiety is now seen as a signal to the ego that it is in a dangerous situation. This so-called "signal anxiety" sets in motion a series of psychic events, including repression, that are aimed at both reducing the amount of anxiety and avoiding the dangerous situation. Neurotic symptoms are measures designed to ward off signal anxiety. In the revised theory, then, anxiety leads to repression, instead of the reverse.

Refinements in psychoanalytic theory have revised many notions of ego functioning and object relations. However, Freud's 1926 explanation of anxiety as the signal of danger and generator of defense and repression remains basically intact.

Although psychoanalytic theories are not universally accepted by psychiatrists today, it should be pointed out that Freud's theory of anxiety formation is not incompatible with biological theories of anxiety disorder. Freud maintained on numerous occasions that biological predispositions to psychiatric symptoms are undoubtedly operant in most conditions; therefore further knowledge about brain neurochemistry, he felt, would only help elucidate the mechanisms behind various pathologic symptoms. He also acknowledged a constitutional variation in the capacity to experience anxiety from individual to individual.

What psychoanalytic theory does not help us with is a better understanding of why anxiety symptoms are manifested in some patients by anxiety attacks, in others by more chronic forms of anxiety, and in still others by phobias, obsessions, or compulsions. Psychoanalytic theory also posits that unconscious psychological conflict is at the root of all cases of panic disorder, which has by no means been established.

LEARNING THEORIES

A similar problem arises when considering the behavioral theory approach to the etiology of panic disorder and GAD. Behavior or learning theorists hold that anxiety is conditioned by the fear of certain environmental stimuli. If every time a laboratory animal presses a bar it receives a noxious electric shock, the pressing of the lever becomes a conditioned stimulus that precedes the unconditioned stimulus—the shock. The conditioned stimulus releases a conditioned response in the animal, anxiety, which leads the animal to avoid contact with the lever, thereby avoiding the shock. Successful avoidance of the unconditioned stimulus, the shock, reinforces the avoidant behavior. This leads to a decrease in anxiety level.

By analogy with this animal model, we might say that anxiety attacks are conditioned responses to fearful situations. For example, an infant learns that if its mother is not present (the conditioned stimulus) it will suffer hunger (the unconditioned stimulus) and learns to become anxious automatically whenever the mother is absent (the conditioned response). The anxiety may persist even after the child is old enough to feed itself. Or, to give another example, a life-threatening situation in someone's life, for example, skidding in a car during a snowstorm, is paired with the experience of rapid heart beat (the conditioned stimulus) and tremendous anxiety. Long after the accident, rapid heart beat alone, whether during vigorous exercise or minor emotional upset, becomes capable by itself of provoking the conditioned response of an anxiety attack.

There are clearly multiple problems with such a theory. First, although we have pointed out some traumatic situations, such as thyroid disease, cocaine intoxication, or life-threatening event, that do seem paired with the onset of panic disorder, for many patients no such dramatic event can ever be located. For patients with GAD, attempting to find a precipitating event that makes sense as an unconditioned stimulus is even more difficult.

It is also the case that most conditioned responses ultimately extinguish in laboratory animals if they are not at least intermittently reinforced. Presumably, patients with panic disorder or GAD do not undergo repeat traumatic events and therefore should be able to ''unlearn'' their anxiety and panic attacks. This has no basis in clinical fact.

Hence, even though learning theories have a powerful basis in experimental animal research they do not seem to explain adequately the pathogenesis of human anxiety disorder. They do, however, explain the development and maintenance of agoraphobia once a sequence of panic attacks has begun.

SEPARATION ANXIETY

Klein has advanced an etiologic theory that panic disorder represents aberrant functioning of the biological substrate that underlies normal human separation anxiety.[13] Based on work by Bowlby, Klein advanced the notion that the attachment of an infant animal or human to its mother is not simply a learned response but is genetically programmed and biologically determined. It is of great importance to this theory that 20% to 50% of adults with panic disorder recall manifesting symptoms of pathologic separation anxiety, often taking the form of school phobia, when they were children. Furthermore, the initial panic attack in the history of a patient who goes on to develop panic disorder is sometimes preceded by the real or threatened loss of a significant relationship.

Infant animals demonstrate their anxiety when separated from the mother by a series of high-pitched cries called distress vocalizations.

Imipramine has been found effective in blocking distress vocalizations in dogs by Scott[14] and in monkeys by Suomi and co-workers.[15] Imipramine,

as will be discussed below, is a highly effective anti-panic drug in adult humans. Hypothesizing a link between adult panic attacks and childhood separation anxiety, Klein and Gittelman conducted a study of imipramine treatment for children with school phobia. In these children, fear of separating from their mothers is usually the basis behind refusing to go to school. The drug proved successful in getting the children to return to school.

Hence, there is good evidence that the same drug that diminishes protest anxiety in higher mammals also reduces separation anxiety in children and blocks panic attacks in adults. This is further confirmation of the link between separation anxiety and human panic attacks.

BIOLOGICAL THEORIES

There are a number of biological theories of both panic disorder and, to a lesser extent, GAD, that are prominent in the psychiatric literature. We will summarize the evidence for or against some of the most promising of these.

Many investigators have found anxiety reactions associated with increases in plasma catecholamine levels, especially epinephrine. Levels of the enzyme that catabolizes catecholamines, monoamine oxidase, have also been found to be elevated in patients with anxiety disorder.[16] These findings suggest that elevations in epinephrine play a role in anxiety disorder but do not resolve the question of whether the role is etiologic or simply a reaction to the anxiety state.

It is not clear whether administration of catecholamines can actually provoke anxiety reactions and whether, if they can, the reaction is specific only to patients with anxiety disorder. Researchers in the 1930s and 1940s did show that epinephrine infusion caused anxiety in human subjects, but methodologic and diagnostic issues limit the applicability of these studies to patients with GAD and panic disorder.

For many years the possibility that panic attacks are manifestations of massive discharge from the beta-adrenergic nervous system has been considered. During a panic attack the patient complains of palpitations, tremulousness, and excessive sweating, all symptoms that are characteristic of massive stimulation of beta-adrenergic receptors. Early support for this hypothesis came from the work of Frohlich and colleagues who studied a group of patients with a condition called the hyperdynamic beta-adrenergic circulatory state.[17] When given intravenous infusions of the beta-adrenergic agonist isoproterenol these patients, but not normal controls, experienced "hysterical outbursts" that sound remarkably similar to panic attacks. A number of other groups also showed that patients with spontaneous anxiety attacks, some even meeting criteria for the diagnosis of panic disorder, are more sensitive to the effects of isoproterenol than are normal controls.

The beta-adrenergic hypothesis receives further support from innumerable studies claiming that beta-blocking drugs, such as propranolol, have an ameliorative effect on panic attacks and anxiety. Most of the studies, however, are uncontrolled so that it is impossible to know what the placebo response rate might have been. Of even greater importance, most studies using beta-adrenergic blockers to treat anxiety have been done using poorly diagnosed patients, so that patients with social phobia, GAD, panic disorder, agoraphobia, depression, and adjustment disorder are grouped together. When the properly designed and controlled studies of beta-adrenergic blockers used in anxiety disorder are reviewed, only modest antianxiety effects can actually be demonstrated. No study has ever shown whether beta-adrenergic blockers are specifically effective in blocking spontaneous panic attacks.

A further blow to the beta-adrenergic theory comes from the finding that intravenously administered propranolol, in doses sufficient to achieve full peripheral beta-adrenergic blockade, is not able to block a sodium lactate–induced panic attack in patients with panic disorder.[18] As will be discussed below, lactate infusion is a standard method for provoking panic attacks in patients with panic disorder. From this experiment it was concluded that hyperactivity of beta-adrenergic receptors is not likely to be responsible for causing spontaneous panic attacks.

Another prominent hypothesis for the etiology of panic attacks involves the locus ceruleus. This tiny nucleus located in the pons contains more than 50% of all noradrenergic neurons in the entire central nervous system and sends afferent projections to a wide area of the brain, including the hippocampus, amygdala, limbic lobe, and cerebral cortex.

Support for this complex hypothesis comes from the fact that electrical stimulation of the animal locus ceruleus produces marked fear and anxiety response while ablation of the animal locus ceruleus renders an animal less susceptible to fear responses in the face of threatening stimuli.[19] Also, drugs known to be capable of increasing locus ceruleus discharge in animals are anxiogenic in humans, while many drugs that curtail locus ceruleus firing and decrease central noradrenergic turnover are antianxiety agents in humans. Yohimbine is an example of a drug that increases locus ceruleus discharge and has been shown to provoke anxiety in humans, while clonidine, propranolol, benzodiazepines, morphine, endorphin, and tricyclic antidepressants curtail locus ceruleus firing. In the latter group, there is obviously a range of drugs from those clearly effective in blocking human panic attacks, like the tricyclic antidepressants, to those of more dubious efficacy, like clonidine and propranolol, to those of no proven anti-panic effect, like benzodiazepines and morphine. The effect on locus ceruleus firing of the benzodiazepine analog drug alprazolam, which has definite anti-panic effects, is not yet known.

A controversy exists about the relevance of these animal models. Redmond and colleagues have produced abundant evidence that situations that provoke fear and anxiety in laboratory animals are associated with increases in locus ceruleus discharge and in central noradrenergic turnover.[19] This would, of course, support the idea that the locus ceruleus is a kind of generator for anxiety attacks. However, Mason and Fibiger state that there is no consistent pattern of increased locus ceruleus discharge associated with anxiety in animals.[20]

Despite these difficulties in proving the locus ceruleus hypothesis, it remains an intriguing theory that has helped guide research in the anxiety field. The fact that tricyclic antidepressants, which block panic attacks, do curtail locus ceruleus firing is a fairly powerful reason not to dismiss this hypothesis readily.

Indeed, the locus ceruleus theory may receive support from an unlikely source of research endeavor, the relationship of hyperventilation to anxiety attacks. Respiratory distress, manifested by rapid breathing, choking, and air hunger, are common symptoms of panic attacks. Hyperventilation leads to a reduced level of carbon dioxide in the blood and consequently alkalosis. This in turn produces symptoms of dizziness, nausea, lightheadedness, derealization, and paresthesias. The standard treatment for acute hyperventilation of psychogenic etiology, carbon dioxide rebreathing, quickly corrects alkalosis.

This situation has led some to believe that hyperventilation is actually a cause of panic attacks. According to this theory, the patient begins to hyperventilate, induces respiratory alkalosis, and consequently experiences the full range of panic symptoms. By teaching the patient better breathing habits, these authors contend, most spontaneous panic attacks can be aborted.

Others, however, believe the hyperventilation is simply a secondary consequence of whatever process begins a panic attack. According to this view, the same central nervous system event that drives the heart rate up, increases sweating, and induces trembling in the patient experiencing a panic attack also provokes tachypnea.

We have found that controlled hyperventilation and respiratory alkalosis do not routinely provoke panic attacks in most patients with panic disorder. Surprisingly, however, giving these patients a mixture of 5% carbon dioxide in room air to breathe causes panic almost as often as does a sodium lactate infusion.

This finding was perplexing until data from Svensson in Sweden became available, showing that carbon dioxide, when added to inspired air, causes a reliable dose-dependent increase in rat locus ceruleus firing.[21]

Of all the biological theories of panic disorder, those involving the sodium lactate provocation of panic attacks have captured the most attention. Cohen first noted that patients with neurocirculatory asthenia, a condition closely related to anxiety disorder, developed higher levels of blood lactate while exercising than do normal controls.[22] This finding stimulated Pitts and McClure to administer intravenous infusions of sodium lactate to patients with panic disorder, finding that most of the patients suffered an anxiety attack during the infusion.[1] The subjects all believed these attacks were quite typical of their naturally occurring attacks; normal controls did not experience panic attacks during the infusion. Having been replicated on numerous occasions under proper experimental conditions, the finding that 10 ml/kg of 0.5 molar sodium lactate will provoke a panic attack in most patients with panic disorder but not in normals is now a well-accepted clinical fact.

What attracts attention are the numerous theories that attempt to explain why lactate provokes panic in susceptible patients. Because lactate is metabolized to pyruvate in the liver, some of which enters the tricarboxylic acid cycle, lactate infusion ultimately results in a net increase in bicarbonate. Thus one theory of lactate panicogenesis is that the induction of a metabolic alkalosis causes the attack.

A second hypothesis involves the fact that lactate infusion results in a net reduction of serum ionized calcium, which could result in neuromuscular irritability. Indeed, during lactate infusions even normal volunteers routinely complain of perioral paresthesias, an early sign of tetany. Also, it was found that the addition of calcium carbonate to lactate reduced the severity of panic as compared with that induced by lactate alone. However, Pitts has reported giving panic disorder patients infusions of the powerful calcium chelator ethylenediaminetetraacetic acid almost to the point of producing frank tetany, but no panic attacks occurred.[23]

There is an active effort in a number of laboratories at the present time to identify the mechanisms by which sodium lactate causes panic attacks. Our findings suggest that the capability of lactate to induce panic attacks requires a combination of both clinical vulnerability, having a history of panic disorder, and increased psychophysiologic arousal at the time the infusion begins. Hence patients who go on to panic during the infusion have higher heart rates, diastolic blood pressure levels, and subjective anxiety scores prior to receiving lactate than do either patients who do not panic or normal controls.

As already discussed, sodium lactate–induced panic attacks were used as a model to test whether beta-adrenergic blockade is capable of blocking panic attacks. Many drugs thought capable of treating panic attacks, especially the monoamine oxidase inhibitors and tricyclic antidepressants, are also capable of blocking lactate-induced panic attacks. In addition to supporting the similarity of lactate-induced and naturally occurring panic attacks, this finding suggests that new drugs can be tested in the clinical laboratory by seeing if they are also able to block sodium lactate–induced panic. In addition, the notion that reactive hypoglycemia is a frequent cause of panic attacks was called into question by the finding that blood sugar always remained in normal range during lactate-induced panic attacks.

Most of the biological theories discussed to this point are best applied to panic disorder. At the present time it is not known whether beta-adrenergic hypersensitivity or increased locus ceruleus discharge could possibly be involved in the pathogenesis of GAD. Nor is it known if patients with GAD have an enhanced sensitivity to carbon dioxide or sodium lactate.

One area of inquiry that may relate specifically to the biological etiology of GAD is the study of the recently discovered brain benzodiazapine receptor. This receptor, which probably occurs in two types, is linked to a receptor for the inhibitory neurotransmitter gamma-aminobutyric acid (GABA). Binding of a benzodiazepine to the benzodiazepine receptor facilitates the action of GABA, effectively slowing neural transmission. The receptor is found in gray matter throughout the human brain.

Because benzodiazepines are effective antianxiety agents, the discovery of the benzodiazepine receptor poses two questions of etiologic significance: (1) do patients with conditions like GAD have receptors that are abnormal in number or sensitivity, and (2) is there an endogenously produced benzodiazepinelike substance that may be lacking in patients with GAD?

Research into these two questions is still in an early phase, but some interesting points can already be mentioned. Studies have shown that there are differences in the density of benzodiazepine receptors in rat brain mediated both by acute stress and genetically determined levels of anxiety.[24] These findings suggest that changes in anxiety state are reflected in changes in the number and sensitivity of the benzodiazepine receptor.

Innumerable candidates for the endogenous benzodiazepine receptor ligand have been proposed, including several purine compounds, thromboxane A_2, and nicotinamide. Evidence for any of these being the true ligand is limited.

One series of compounds, the beta-carbolines, specifically blocks the binding of benzodiazepines to the benzodiazepine receptor and when administered to laboratory animals produces an acute anxiety syndrome.[25] Caffeine may be a specific benzodiazepine receptor antagonist. Hence, the common wisdom that excessive coffee intake leads to jitteriness and irritability may have a basis in caffeine blockade of benzodiazepine receptors. This raises the possibility that some substance is produced by GAD patients that actually interferes with proper benzodiazepine receptor function and is the cause of their symptoms.

The final line of evidence for the biological etiology of anxiety is the presence of studies indicating its possible familial nature. Several family history studies of panic disorder have found a higher rate in relatives of probands with panic disorder than in relatives of normals. In the most recent of these studies, Crowe and colleagues found a morbidity risk for panic disorder of 24.7% among relatives of patients with panic disorder compared with only 2.3% among relatives of normal controls.[26]

This kind of study cannot, of course, rule out the possibility that environmental rather than genetic influences are operant. Only studies comparing rates of illness in monozygotic and dizygotic twins are acceptable for distinguishing these two components of familial transmission of a psychiatric illness.

Torgersen published a study in which he examined 32 monozygotic twins and 53 dizygotic twins in Norway. If a disease has a genetic basis, it should be found more often in both partners of a monozy-

gotic pair, who share identical genetic information, than in both partners of a dizygotic pair, who are similar only to the extent found in ordinary siblings. Indeed, the concordance rate for anxiety disorders with panic attacks was much higher in monozygotic twins in Torgersen's study than in the dizygotic twins. This is strong evidence in favor of a genetic component to panic disorder. Interestingly, in this study there was no such difference in concordance rate for GAD between monozygotic and dizygotic twins.[27]

Even twin studies are open to question because they assume that parents treat identical twins in the same way they treat fraternal twins. More definitive proof of a genetic component to a psychiatric illness can come from studies in which identical twins are adopted away from their biological parents and raised in separate homes. No such studies have been reported for anxiety disorder.

No family or twin studies specifically investigating patients with GAD have been reported.

Diagnosis and Differential Diagnosis

Before a diagnosis of anxiety disorder can be made in the patient whose presenting complaint is either panic attacks or chronic anxiety, one must first rule out medical conditions that occasionally manifest themselves with symptoms of anxious mood before any other physical stigmata appear.

Both *hyperthyroidism* and *hypothyroidism* can present with anxiety unaccompanied by other signs or symptoms. For this reason, it is imperative that all patients complaining of anxiety undergo routine thyroid function tests, including the evaluation of the level of thyroid stimulating hormone. It should be remembered, however, that thyroid disease can act as one of the predisposing triggers to panic disorder, so that even when the apparently primary thyroid disease is corrected panic attacks may continue until specifically treated.

Hyperparathyroidism occasionally presents as anxiety symptoms, warranting a serum calcium level before definitive diagnosis is made.

A variety of *cardiac conditions* can initially present as anxiety symptoms, although in most cases the patient complains prominently of chest pain, skipped beats, or palpitations. Ischemic heart disease and arrhythmias, especially paroxysmal atrial tachycardia, should be ruled out by electrocardiography.

Pheochromocytoma is a rare, usually benign tumor of the adrenal medulla that secretes catecholamines in episodic bursts. During an active phase, the patient characteristically experiences flushing, tremulousness, and anxiety. Blood pressure is usually elevated during the active phase of catecholamine secretion but not at other times. Therefore, merely finding a normal blood pressure does not rule out a pheochromocytoma. If this is suspected, the diagnosis is made by collection of urine for 24 hours for determination of catecholamine metabolite concentration.

Disease of the vestibular nerve can cause episodic bouts of vertigo, lightheadedness, nausea, and anxiety that mimic panic attacks. Rather than merely feeling dizzy, such patients often experience true vertigo in which the room seems to spin in one direction during each attack. Otolaryngology consultation is warranted when this is suspected.

Although many patients believe their anxiety disorder is caused by *reactive hypoglycemia,* there is no scientific proof at present that this is ever a cause of any psychiatric disturbance. Glucose tolerance tests are not helpful in establishing hypoglycemia as the cause of anxiety because up to 40% of the normal population will have a random low blood sugar during a routine glucose tolerance test. The only convincing way to establish hypoglycemia as a cause of symptoms is to document a low blood sugar level at the same time the patient is symptomatic.

The relationship of *mitral valve prolapse* to panic disorder has attracted a great deal of recent attention. This usually benign condition has been shown by a number of investigators to occur more frequently in patients with panic disorder than in normals. However, screening of patients known to have mitral valve prolapse reveals no greater frequency of panic disorder than is found in the overall population.

Although patients with mitral valve prolapse occasionally complain of palpitations, chest pain, lightheadedness, and fatigue, symptoms of a full-blown panic attack are rare. Several lines of evidence indicate that mitral valve prolapse cannot be cited as the cause of panic disorder: treatment for panic attacks works regardless of the presence of the prolapsed valve, and patients with both mitral valve prolapse and panic disorder are just as sensitive to sodium lactate as are those with panic disorder alone. Some have speculated that mitral valve prolapse and panic disorder may represent manifestations of the same underlying disorder of autonomic nervous system function. Others have suggested that panic disorder, by creating states of intermittent high circulating catecholamine levels and tachycardia, actually causes mitral valve prolapse.

In any event, it is clear that the presence of mitral valve prolapse in patients with panic disorder has little clinical or prognostic importance in the management of spontaneous panic attacks. What it may tell us about the underlying etiology of panic disorder is a question currently under vigorous investigation.

Although the medical conditions that mimic anxiety disorder are usually easily ruled out, psychiatric conditions that involve pathologic anxiety can make the differential diagnosis of panic disorder and GAD difficult. By far the most problematic is the differentiation of primary anxiety disorder from depression.

Patients suffering from depression often manifest signs of anxiety and agitation and may even have frank panic attacks. On the other hand, patients with both GAD and panic disorder, if untreated for significant amounts of time, routinely become demoralized as the impact of the illness progressively restricts the ability to enjoy a normal life. Further complicating the picture is the fact that some, but not all, studies have shown that patients with anxiety disorder have increased family history of affective disorder.

Although the differentiation of anxiety from depression can at times strain even the most experienced clinician, several points are helpful. Patients with GAD or panic disorder generally do not demonstrate the full range of vegetative symptoms that are seen in depression. Hence, anxious patients usually have trouble falling asleep, not early morning awakening, and do not lose their appetite or ability to concentrate. Diurnal mood fluctuation is uncommon in anxiety disorder. Perhaps of greatest importance is the fact that most anxious patients do not lose the capacity to enjoy things or be cheered up as endogenously depressed patients do.

The order of developing symptoms also differentiates depression from anxiety. In cases of panic disorder or GAD, anxiety symptoms usually precede any seriously altered mood. Patients can generally recall having anxiety attacks first, then becoming gradually more disgusted with life, and then feeling depressed. In depression, patients usually experience dysphoria first, with anxiety symptoms coming later.

Results of the dexamethasone suppression test, which may be useful in diagnosing some cases of depression, are generally normal in panic disorder. The test has not been systematically studied in patients with GAD. Patients with atypical depression, as those depressions accompanied by overeating, oversleeping, the feeling of leaden paralysis, and maintenance of reactive mood have traditionally been labeled, often give a history of panic attacks. These may range from an isolated attack to enough attacks to meet criteria for frank panic disorder. Regardless of the frequency, any association of panic attacks with atypical depression appears to predispose to an excellent therapeutic response to monoamine oxidase inhibitors but only modest responsivity to tricyclic antidepressants.[28]

A few other psychiatric conditions often need to be differentiated from panic disorder and GAD. Patients with somatization disorder complain of a variety of physical ailments and discomforts, none of which are substantiated by physical or laboratory findings. They can appear like GAD patients because of their constant worry but are distinguished from GAD by their almost exclusive preoccupation with physical complaints. Unlike panic disorder patients, their physical problems do not occur in episodic attacks but are virtually constant.

Patients with depersonalization disorder have episodes of derealization/depersonalization without the other symptoms of a panic attack.

Although patients with panic disorder often fear they will lose their minds or go crazy, psychotic illness is not an outcome of anxiety disorder. Reassuring the patient on this point is often the first step in a successful treatment.

There is no question that some patients with anxiety disorder abuse alcohol and illicit drugs in attempts at self-medication. In one study, after successful detoxification, a group of alcoholics with a prior history of panic disorder were treated with medication to block spontaneous panic attacks.[29] These patients did not resume alcohol consumption once their panic attacks were eliminated. Therefore, in evaluating any patient with substance abuse the possibility that their illness began with spontaneous panic attacks or chronic anxiety should be considered.

Treatment

The central feature in treatment of panic disorder is the pharmacologic blockade of the spontaneous panic attacks. Several classes of medication have been shown effective in accomplishing this goal. The most widely used and studied are the tricyclic antidepressants, especially imipramine, desipramine, and clomipramine. Other tricyclics, including nortriptyline and amitriptyline, have not

been systematically studied. Monoamine oxidase inhibitors are effective anti-panic drugs and are usually reserved for patients who do not respond to tricyclic antidepressants. The presence of depressed mood is not a requirement for any of these drugs to be effective in blocking panic attacks.

Although benzodiazepines *per se* have not been shown to be useful in blocking panic attacks, the new benzodiazepine derivative alprazolam appears to be an effective anti-panic drug. Long-term efficacy and possible dependency on alprazolam are still under investigation. This medication has fewer side-effects than tricyclic antidepressants and monoamine oxidase inhibitors and may eventually prove to be a popular drug for panic disorder.

Beta-adrenergic blocking drugs, like propranolol, are said by some to be useful in a variety of anxiety disorders, but there is no scientific proof that they are specifically effective in blocking spontaneous panic attacks. Our impression is that they work less well than tricyclic antidepressants, monoamine oxidase inhibitors, or alprazolam.

Clonidine, which quiets locus ceruleus discharge, would seem for theoretical reasons to be a good anti-panic drug. Although in a small series two thirds of patients responded,[30] for several the therapeutic effect was lost in a matter of weeks despite continuation of dose. This, plus a number of bothersome side-effects, makes clonidine a poor initial choice for panic disorder.

When initiating a drug regimen for a patient with panic disorder, it is crucial for the patient to understand that the drug will block the panic attacks but not necessarily decrease the amount of intervening anticipatory anxiety. Patients may need to take a benzodiazepine as well for a short time to reduce the level of anticipatory anxiety. Alprazolam is unique in this regard in that it does reduce anticipatory anxiety as well as block panic attacks.

Some patients with panic disorder display an initial hypersensitivity to tricyclic antidepressants and monoamine oxidase inhibitors in which they complain of jitteriness, agitation, a "speedy" feeling, and insomnia. This is transient, but it is recommended that patients with panic disorder be started on lower doses of tricyclic antidepressants or monoamine oxidase inhibitors than would be given to depressed patients.

One regimen is to start the patient at a dosage of 10 mg qhs of imipramine and increase the dose by 10 mg every other night until 50 mg is reached. The dosage can be given all at once. If 50 mg is inadequate for full panic blockade, the dosage is raised by 25-mg increments every 3 days or by 50 mg weekly to as high as 300 mg. In some cases, a dosage of imipramine over 300 mg is necessary. This requires monitoring of the electrocardiogram. Patients who experience excessive anticholinergic side-effects to imipramine can be given desipramine instead.

Doses of phenelzine up to 90 mg daily are often needed to block attacks completely. Alprazolam in doses as high as 10 mg daily may be required, although 3 mg to 5 mg given in two divided doses daily is generally sufficient.

Once full remission of panic attacks has been accomplished, it is recommended that the patient be kept on medication for a full 6 months to prevent early relapse. After this, it is reasonable to taper the patient from medication. Although for many, panic disorder tends to be a recurrent condition, a high proportion of patients will not relapse immediately after cessation of medication.

The pharmacologic treatment of GAD is less well established. Traditionally, chronically anxious patients have been placed on benzodiazepines. However, no study has yet shown benzodiazepines to be more effective than other drugs or treatment methods in patients specifically diagnosed with GAD.

Although generally safe, with side-effects limited mainly to sedation, there is growing concern that some patients may become tolerant or even addicted to benzodiazepines. Available data indicate that most patients are able to stop taking them without serious sequelae and that the problem of frank addiction is overestimated and probably limited to an addiction-prone population or to patients with panic disorder who often escalate benzodiazepine usage in unsuccessful attempts at self-medication. Withdrawal symptoms of insomnia, agitation, irritability, and sensory disturbances can occur and are considerably lessened by gradual tapering of the medication. The distinction between actual withdrawal and a simple recrudescence of the original anxiety symptom when the benzodiazepine is stopped remains controversial. A few preliminary studies have shown continued efficacy of these drugs at the same dose level up to 6 months after beginning treatment, but shorter treatments are clearly preferable.[31]

Preliminary studies have indicated that tricyclic antidepressants may also be effective in treating chronically anxious patients without the presence of depressive symptoms. However, even here the patients did not specifically have GAD. An experimental drug, buspirone, is a nonbenzodiazepine antianxiety agent that appears to have less sedative property than the benzodiazepines and less potential for abuse.

Behavioral treatments for both panic disorder and GAD have centered on the various relaxation approaches. It is not known whether these treatments are as effective as benzodiazepines; they have not been shown to block panic attacks, although research into the area of behavioral treatment of panic attacks is currently underway.

Relaxation training is sometimes done using electromyographic (EMG) feedback. In this method, the patient learns to reduce his own EMG output, usually by monitoring his frontalis muscle recording. Progressive muscle relaxation, another method, involves teaching the patient to tense and then relax each muscle group sequentially. This is sometimes done in conjunction with breathing exercises. The theory behind both EMG-feedback-assisted relaxation and progressive muscle relaxation is that anxious patients can learn to relax their muscles, which will lead to an overall reduction in somatic tension and, secondarily, in anxiety level.

Other behavioral treatments, such as cognitive restructuring and transcendental meditation, have been tried and found useful by some patients. No systematic studies have been done of these treatment methods.

Probably the most useful behavioral treatment at this time is called anxiety management training. In this method, relaxation training is specifically applied to both imagined and real-life anxiety-provoking situations.

Traditional psychodynamic psychotherapy may be necessary for some patients with anxiety disorder, including some with panic disorder who respond to medication. Significant unconscious conflict over separations during childhood sometimes appears to operate in patients with panic disorder, causing a renewal of symptoms in adult life each time a new separation is imagined or threatened. Even after medication has blocked the actual panic attacks, such patients remain wary of independence and assertiveness.

Psychotherapy may even be the treatment of choice for some cases of GAD in which unconscious conflict is believed by the clinician to be the cause of the patient's chronic anxiety. At present, no firm scientific data indicate which form of treatment, behavioral, psychodynamic, or pharmacologic, is truly best for GAD.

Pharmacotherapy is in no way incompatible with behavioral or psychodynamic treatment for patients with GAD and panic disorder. The notion that eliminating the symptoms of anxiety disorder with medication will disturb a successful psychotherapy has never been proven and is largely dogmatic. Successful psychotherapy often cannot take place until the more debilitating aspects of these syndromes have been eliminated pharmacologically.

REFERENCES

1. Pitts FN, McClure JN: Lactate metabolism in anxiety neuroses. N Engl J Med 277:1328–1336, 1967
2. Crowe RR, Pauls DL, Slymen DJ et al: A family study of anxiety neurosis. Arch Gen Psychiatry 37:77–79, 1980
3. Klein DF: Delineation of two drug-responsive anxiety syndromes. Psychopharmacologia 5:397–408, 1964
4. Tyrer P, Candy J, Kelly DA: A study of the clinical effects of phenelzine and placebo in the treatment of phobic anxiety. Psychopharmacologia 32:237–254, 1973
5. Spitzer RL, Endicott J, Robins E: Research Diagnostic Criteria: Rationale and reliability. Arch Gen Psychiatry 35:773–783, 1978
6. Weissman MM, Myers JK, Harding PS: Psychiatric disorders in a U.S. urban community. Am J Psychol 135:459–462, 1978
7. Coryell W, Noyes R, Clancy J: Excess mortality in panic disorders. Arch Gen Psychiatry 39:701–703, 1982
8. Raskin M, Peeke HVS, Dickman W et al: Panic and generalized anxiety disorders. Arch Gen Psychiatry 39:687–689, 1982
9. Freud S: Introductory Lectures on Psychoanalysis. In Strachey J (ed): The Standard Edition of the Complete Psychological Works of Sigmund Freud, vol 15. London, Hogarth Press, 1961
10. Breuer J, Freud S: Studies on Hysteria. In Strachey J (ed): The Standard Edition of the Complete Works of Sigmund Freud, vol 2. London, Hogarth Press, 1961
11. Freud S: Obsessions and Phobias. In Strachey J (ed): The Standard Edition of the Complete Works of Sigmund Freud, vol 3. London, Hogarth Press, 1961
12. Freud S: Inhibitions, Symptoms and Anxiety. In Strachey J (ed): The Standard Edition of the Complete Works of Sigmund Freud, vol 20. London, Hogarth Press, 1961
13. Klein DF: Anxiety reconceptualized. In Klein DF, Rabkin JG (eds): Anxiety: New Research and Changing Concepts. New York, Raven Press, 1981
14. Scott JP: Effects of psychotropic drugs on separation distress in dogs. Proceedings of the IX Congress Neuropsychopharmolology. Amsterdam, Excerpta Medica, 1974
15. Suomi SJ, Seaman SF, Lewis JK et al: Effects of imipramine treatment of separation-induced social disorders in rhesus monkeys. Arch Gen Psychiatry 35:321–325, 1978
16. Mathew RJ, Ho BT, Kralik P et al: Anxiety and platelet MAO levels after relaxation training. Am J Psychol 138:371–373, 1981
17. Frohlich ED, Tarazi RC, Duston HP: Hyperdynamic beta-adrenergic circulatory state. Arch Intern Med 123:1–7, 1969
18. Gormam JM, Levy GF, Liebowitz MR et al: Effect of acute beta-adrenergic blockade on lactate induced panic. Arch Gen Psychiatry 40:1079–1083, 1983
19. Redmond DE: New and old evidence for the involvement of a brain norepinephrine system in anxiety. In Fann WE, Karacan I, Pokorny AD et al (eds): Phenomenology and Treatment of Anxiety. New York, Spectrum Publications, 1979
20. Mason ST, Fibiger HC: Anxiety: The locus ceruleus disconnection. Life Sci 25:2141–2147, 1979
21. Elam M, Yoat TP, Svensson TH: Hypercapnia and hypoxia: Chemo-receptor-mediated control of locus ceruleus neurons and splanchnic, sympathetic nerves. Brain Res 222:373–381, 1981
22. Cohen ME, White PD: Life situations, emotions and neurocirculatory asthenia. Res Nerv Ment Dis Proc 29:832–869, 1950
23. Pitts FN, Allen RE: Biochemical induction of anxiety. In Fann WE, Karacan I, Pokorny AD et al (eds): Phenomenology and Treatment of Anxiety. New York, Spectrum Publications, 1979
24. Tallman FJ, Paul SM, Skolnick P et al: Receptors for the age of anxiety: Pharmacology of the benzodiazepines. Science 207:274–281, 1980
25. Skolnick P, Paul SM: Benzodiazepine receptors in the central nervous system. Int Rev Neurobiol 23:103–140, 1982
26. Crowe RR, Noyes R, Pauls DL et al: A family study of panic disorder. Arch Gen Psychiatry 40:1065–1069, 1983
27. Torgersen S: Genetic factors in anxiety disorders. Arch Gen Psychiatry 40:1085–1089, 1983
28. Quitkin F, Rabkin J: Hidden psychiatric diagnosis in the alcoholic. In Solomon J (ed): Alcoholism and Clinical Psychiatry. New York, Plenum Publishing, 1982
29. Liebowitz MR, Fyer AJ, McGrath P et al: Clonidine treatment of panic disorder. Psychopharm Bull 17:122–123, 1981
30. Rickels K: Benzodiazepines: Use and misuse. In Klein DF, Rabkin JG (eds): Anxiety: New Research and Changing Concepts. New York, Raven Press, 1981
31. Liebowitz MR, Quitkin FM, Stewart JW et al: Phenelzine versus imipramine in atypical depression: A preliminary report. Arch Gen Psychiatry (in press)

27

Abby J. Fyer and Donald F. Klein

Agoraphobia, Social Phobia, and Simple Phobia

Phobias first appeared as a separate clinical entity in the psychiatric literature at the latter part of the 19th century. Classification systems developed at that time focused on the nature of the phobic stimulus and were without etiologic reference or conceptual framework. Each newly discovered phobic stimulus was dignified by a Latin or Greek name.

Freud,[1] in 1894, separated phobias, or phobic neurosis, from the other psychoneuroses on the basis of clinical phenomenology and response to analysis. Although initially Freud did not consider phobias to have a psychogenic etiology, in his later and still widely accepted theory of anxiety published in 1926, phobias were defined as a psychological symptom occurring as part of the ego's defense against internally and externally produced anxieties.[2] This theory implicitly assumed that all phobic disorders were etiologically uniform.

A second development, which took place in the 1920s, was the demonstration by behavioral psychologists that avoidant behaviors could be conditioned in the laboratory in both animals and humans. From these findings the behaviorists hypothesized that phobic behavior was the result of inadvertent maladaptive learning. The efficacy of treatment procedures derived from this principle reinforced belief in this hypothesis.

Phobias first appeared as a separate category in the American Psychiatric Association classification in the 1952 *Diagnostic and Statistical Manual of Mental Disorders* (*DSM-I*) under the title of "Phobic Reaction." No subtypes of phobic disorder were listed either in this edition or in the second edition of the *DSM*, reflecting the assumption of qualitative unity implicit in both the psychoanalytic and behavioral

approaches. In the *DSM-II* the term *phobic reaction* was replaced by the original Freudian term *phobic neurosis*.

The classification of phobic disorders in the *DSM-III* departs widely from previous versions because it contains four distinct subtypes and a perspective that acknowledges the possibility of qualitative distinctions between these disorders.

The *DSM-III* subdivisions are based on empiric findings of the past 20 years. Marks,[3] drawing on his experience in clinical, descriptive, and behavioral treatment studies, delineated four subtypes of phobias of external objects and situations: (1) agoraphobia, (2) social phobia, (3) animal phobias, and (4) miscellaneous specific phobias. These subtypes were observed to differ not only in clinical phenomenology but in course, age of onset, and distribution in the population.

Klein,[4] on the basis of his pharmacologic dissection studies, suggested that patients whose phobias are secondary complications of recurrent spontaneous panic attacks be diagnostically separated from phobic patients who did not have spontaneous panic attacks. This distinction is now supported by several lines of evidence.

In this chapter we will focus on the avoidant behavior manifested in simple and social phobias and in agoraphobia. Following the current *DSM-III* guidelines, a discussion of agoraphobia with panic attacks is included in this chapter rather than the chapter on panic and anxiety disorders. This is somewhat arbitrary as current research indicates that this disorder has more in common with panic disorder than with the other phobic disorders. Studies on panic and anxiety disorders are reviewed elsewhere in this volume.

Definitions

A *phobia* is defined as a "persistent and irrational fear of a specific object, activity or situation that results in a compelling desire to avoid the dreaded object, activity or situation (phobic stimulus). The fear is recognized by the individual as excessive or unreasonable in proportion to the actual dangerousness of the object, activity or situation."[5] Irrational fears and avoidance behavior are seen in a number of psychiatric disorders. However, in the *DSM-III* the diagnosis of phobic disorder is made only when single or multiple phobias are the predominant aspect of the clinical picture, a source of significant distress to the individual, and not the result of another mental disorder.

Phobic disorder is divided into three subtypes: (1) agoraphobia, (2) social phobia, and (3) simple phobia. Agoraphobia is further subdivided into agoraphobia with panic attacks and agoraphobia without panic attacks, depending on whether there is a history of spontaneous panic attacks in association with the development of the avoidant behavior.

AGORAPHOBIA

The *DSM-III* criteria for agoraphobia are as follows:

---

1. The individual has marked fear of and thus avoids being alone or in public places from which escape might be difficult or help not available in case of sudden incapacitation (*e.g.*, crowds, tunnels, bridges, public transportation).
2. There is increasing constriction of normal activities until the fears or avoidance behavior dominate the individual's life.
3. Not due to a major depressive episode, obsessive compulsive disorder, paranoid personality disorder, or schizophrenia.

The vast majority of agoraphobics either currently experience or give a history of having had spontaneous panic attacks in association with the development of their avoidant behavior.

Klein[8] has hypothesized that spontaneous panic attacks rather than multiple phobias are the core symptom of agoraphobia with panic attacks and that patients who develop agoraphobia in association with spontaneous panics suffer from a tertiary complication of panic disorder. Interestingly this was one of Freud's early observations on agoraphobia but was not incorporated into his later theories.[1]

In the *DSM-III*, agoraphobic patients who have had panic attacks are given the diagnosis of agoraphobia with panic attacks. The small minority of patients who present with similar fears and phobias but do not report a history of panic attacks is given the diagnosis of agoraphobia without panic attacks.

Accumulated evidence from provocative, biological, family, and pharmacologic treatment studies supports the relationship of panic disorder and agoraphobia with panic attacks. In light of this, it has recently been recommended that in the revised *DSM-III* "Agoraphobia with Panic Attacks" be renamed "Panic Disorder complicated by Agoraphobia" and classified as an anxiety state. The simple term *agoraphobia* would be used for those agoraphobic patients with no panic history. This category would remain under "Phobic Disorders."

SOCIAL PHOBIA

The *DSM-III* criteria for social phobia include the following:

---

1. A persistent, irrational fear of, and compelling desire to avoid, a situation in which the individual is exposed to possible scrutiny by others and fears that he or she may act in a way that will be humiliating or embarrassing.
2. Significant distress because of the disturbance and recognition by the individual that his or her fear is excessive or unreasonable.
3. Not due to another mental disorder, such as major depression or avoidant personality disorder.

The definition given in the *DSM-III* states that "generally an individual has only one phobia" of this type. In contrast, other investigators have described patients with both single and multiple social phobias. To answer the question as to whether patients with one social phobia differ from those with multiple phobias requires further research. It is our opinion that patients whose central fear is of humiliation or embarrassment in front of others be considered as social phobics even if they have a number of phobic behaviors.

Patients who develop avoidance of social situations secondary to recurrent spontaneous panics are not included in this diagnosis.

SIMPLE PHOBIA

The *DSM-III* criteria for simple phobia are listed below:

> 1. A persistent, irrational fear of, and compelling desire to avoid, an object or a situation other than being alone, or in public places away from home (agoraphobia), or of humiliation or embarrassment in certain social situations (social phobia). Phobic objects are often animals, and phobic situations frequently involve heights or closed spaces.
> 2. Significant distress from the disturbance and recognition by the individual that his or her fear is excessive or unreasonable.
> 3. Not due to another mental disorder, such as schizophrenia or obsessive-compulsive disorder.

A simple phobia is defined as a circumscribed fear and desire to avoid an object, situation, or activity that is not included in the categories of agoraphobia or social phobia. Anxiety symptoms are limited to situations involving actual or possible confrontation with the phobic stimulus. There are no spontaneous panic attacks.

Two additional aspects of the *DSM-III* diagnostic criteria for phobic disorders have been the subject of some discussion in the literature.

Although clinically important, evidence of significant distress may not be a useful criterion for diagnosis in all contexts. For example, Carey and Gottesman[6] have noted that certain phobic traits that individuals do not consider either distressing or signs of illness appear to be intergenerationally transmitted. They have coined the term *phobic features* to describe these characteristics and recommend that data on these types of behaviors be routinely collected in family studies.

The use of hierarchical exclusion conventions in the *DSM-III* diagnostic criteria for phobic disorders has also been questioned. For example, in a family study of probands with affective disorder, Leckman and co-workers[7] found that a lifetime diagnosis of anxiety disorder in the proband predicted an increased risk of major depressive disorder (MDD) and anxiety disorder in the first-degree relatives of probands as compared with relatives of probands with MDD but no anxiety disorder diagnosis. This finding was irrespective of the time relationship between the anxiety and affective disorders. The authors argue that the *DSM-III* convention that certain anxiety disorders not be diagnosed if they occur during an episode of MDD may obscure heritable relationships between disorders. They suggest that this hierarchy be discarded and a convention of multiple diagnosis be used for concurrent anxiety and affective disorders.

Epidemiology

Relatively little is known about the epidemiology of phobic disorders. There are almost no data about the prevalence and incidence of phobic disorders as defined by *DSM-III* in the general population. Studies using these criteria are in process. Two general population studies using specific diagnostic criteria for phobic disorders are available.

Agras and co-workers[9] found the prevalence of phobias in a probability sample of the population of Greater Burlington, Vermont, to be 76.9/1000 population. The 325 persons in the study were surveyed by trained interviewers using a fear questionnaire. A psychiatrist then clinically interviewed all individuals identified by the screening procedure as phobic or possibly phobic. Diagnosis of phobia was made using *DSM-I* criteria. Of the total 76.9/1000 prevalence of phobias, 74.7/1000 were considered to have mildly disabling illness. The remainder, 2.2/1000, were so severely disabled as to lead to absence from work or inability to carry out housekeeping routines.

The most common types of phobias were those of illness or injury (42%), followed by storm (18%) and the animal phobias (14%). Agoraphobia was relatively uncommon in the general population, having a prevalence of only 6/1000 and accounting for only 8% of phobias.

This general population prevalence pattern of types of phobias differed markedly from prevalence patterns of types of phobia seen in a sample of treated patients drawn from a hospital in the same community at the time of the study. Agoraphobics made up 50% of the clinical population. Illness and injury phobias (34%) were the next most common. There were no storm phobias in the clinical sample, and only 4% had animal phobias.

Agras and co-workers[9] found that incidence (rate of new cases) of phobias was highest in early childhood, considerably lower but stable between ages 10 and 30, and declined steadily after age 30. In contrast the total point prevalence of phobias at any given age increased steadily until the sixth decade. These data suggest that many phobias have a chronic course. However, as the incidence data were retrospectively collected no definite conclusions can be drawn. Agras and co-workers did not comment on the sociodemographic characteristics of their sample of phobics.

More recently, Weissman and associates[10] reported a prevalence of phobic disorder of 1.4/100 in a probability sample of the population of New Haven, Connecticut. In this study, 511 persons were evaluated by trained interviewers using a structured interview schedule. Diagnoses were made by research psychiatrists using Research Diagnostic Criteria.[11]

Prevalence rates for specific types of phobic disorders are not reported. Prevalence of phobic disorder was 1.4/100 in persons aged 26 to 45 and 2.1/100 in those aged 45 to 65. No phobic disorder was found in the 111 subjects over 66 years of age. Prevalence rates for women were twice those for men (1.7/100 versus 0.9/100). However, as the authors point out, these data can only be viewed as suggestive since sample sizes are too small to allow interpretation of rates by sociodemographic characteristics.

The considerable difference in rates reported by these two studies is probably due to the variation in methodology and diagnostic criteria used. Further studies are needed before epidemiologic conclusions can be drawn.

Clinical Presentation

AGORAPHOBIA

The clinical picture in agoraphobia consists of multiple and varied fears and avoidance behaviors that center around three main themes: (1) fear of leaving home, (2) fear of being alone, and (3) fear of being away from home in a situation where one cannot suddenly leave or help is not easily available in case of incapacitation.

Typical fears are of using public transportation (buses, trains, subways, planes), crowds, theaters, elevators, restaurants, supermarkets, department stores, waiting in line, or traveling a distance from home. In severe cases patients may be completely housebound, fearful of leaving home without a companion or even of staying home alone.

Most cases of agoraphobia begin with a series of spontaneous panic attacks. If the attacks continue the patient usually develops a constant anticipatory anxiety characterized by continued apprehension about the possible occasion and consequences of the "next attack." Agoraphobic symptoms represent a tertiary phase in the illness in which the individual attempts to cope with his fears of sudden incapacitation by panic by avoiding situations where either panic attacks are thought to be more likely, help would not be readily available, or escape would be difficult.

Many patients will causally related their panic attacks to the particular situations in which the attacks occurred. They then avoid these situations in an attempt to prevent further panic attacks. For example, a man who has had several attacks while taking the train to work may attribute the attacks to the train and in order to avoid the train, start driving to work. If he still experiences panic attacks in the morning while driving to work rather than on the train he interprets this as a sign that the attacks have spread to driving situations rather than as an indication that they were not, in the first place, caused by the train.

Agoraphobics also fear situations in which they feel they cannot leave abruptly if an attack occurs. Examples of this are dental and hairdressing appointments, medical procedures, waiting in line, and certain social occasions. Situations that once entered cannot be easily retreated from (*e.g.*, tunnels and bridges) are also frequently avoided for this reason.

Some individuals continue to have spontaneous panic attacks throughout the course of the illness. In other cases, after the initial phase of the illness, attacks may occur rarely or only (but not always) when the patient ventures into a phobic situation.

One interesting aspect of agoraphobia is the effect of a trusted companion on phobic behavior. Many patients who are unable to leave the house alone can travel long distances and partake in most activities if accompanied by a spouse, family member, or close friend. It is unclear if panic attacks are actually decreased in frequency in this situation or whether the patient feels less helpless and isolated.

In addition to panic attacks, multiple phobias, and chronic anxiety, these patients frequently exhibit symptoms of demoralization and multiple somatic complaints.

The multiple somatic complaints described by agoraphobics are often a mixture of the fears of death or collapse during panic attacks and the multiple physical symptoms that occur as part of both panic and anticipatory anxiety. Thus a patient who has chest discomfort, dyspnea, palpitations, or fears of dying or having a heart attack during panic attacks may respond to every muscle ache in his left arm or momentary difficulty catching his breath as signs of an incipient heart attack. Often these individuals have an alarmist attitude about even the smallest and most routine physical complaints. For example, every headache is a brain tumor and normal fatigue becomes a muscle wasting disease.

In individuals whose activities are restricted by the illness demoralization is common. Patients will often state "I'm depressed," but closer inquiry usually reveals no vegetative signs of an affective syndrome and an intact ability to have pleasurable responses.

Another complication noted by Quitkin and colleagues[12] is drug and barbiturate abuse. Patients often use drugs and alcohol to help alleviate chronic anxiety. Since alcohol and barbiturates do not have a specific anti-panic effect, although they may mitigate chronic anxiety, a vicious cycle can develop in which the individual, in a misguided effort to get better relief from his panic symptoms, escalates his self-medication to the point where he becomes addicted.

There is very little systematic data on the natural history of agoraphobia.

The usual age of onset of agoraphobia is between 18 and 35 years. Mean age of onset in most clinical series is between 24 and 25 years. There are no studies of age of onset of agoraphobia in general population samples.

Although in the case of those patients who eventually seek treatment the overall course of the illness is thought to be chronic, the general impression of experienced clinicians is that the illness waxes and wanes and that most patients have at least brief periods of remission.

There are no follow-up studies of untreated agoraphobics. Follow-up studies of treated patients are discussed in the section on treatment.

SIMPLE PHOBIA

Simple phobias are circumscribed fears of specific objects, situations, or activities. This syndrome has three components: an anticipatory anxiety that is evoked by the possibility of confrontation with the phobic stimulus, the central fear, and the avoidance behavior by which the patient minimizes anxiety.

In simple phobia the fear is usually not of the object itself but of some dire outcome that the individual believes may result from contact with that object. For example, driving phobics are afraid of accidents; snake phobics, that they will be bitten; and claustrophobics, that they will suffocate or be trapped in an enclosed space.

Simple phobic fears have a preprogrammed, noncognitive quality and are not modified by input at a symbolic level. Although most simple phobics will readily acknowledge that they know "there is really nothing to be afraid of," reassuring them of this does not diminish their fear. For the simple phobic, just the knowledge that he may come in contact with the avoided object or situation seems to set off an automatic anxiety response of an intensity that would be expected if his worst fears about the possible consequences of such contact came true.

When surprised or forced into confrontation with the phobic stimulus the simple phobic experiences intense anxiety accompanied by symptoms of autonomic hyperactivity (*e.g.,* trembling, sweating, palpitations). This anxiety can be so intense that its quality resembles that of a panic attack. However, these patients, unlike agoraphobics, do not experience spontaneous panic attacks. Their anxiety is attached wholly to the phobic stimulus.

Simple phobics generally experience little anxiety from their disorder as long as they are able to avoid their phobic stimulus and feel sure that this safe situation will continue. Individuals whose phobias are of situations or objects that are less predictably avoided (*e.g.,* thunderstorms, pigeons, or medical procedures) will have more frequent episodes of anticipatory anxiety and may even be chronically anxious.

In his epidemiologic study of a Vermont town, Agras and co-workers[9] found that the most common phobias in the general populations were of medical procedures, storms, animals, death, crowds, and heights. Other common simple phobias are of driving, sharp objects (*e.g.,* knives, scissors, razors), and enclosed spaces (claustrophobia).

Simple phobias of animals usually begin in early childhood and follow a chronic course. In contrast, simple phobias of objects and situations other than animals have been found to have a varied age of onset. Marks[3] found the mean age of onset for animal phobics to be 4.4 years. Patients with other situational phobias (*e.g.,* claustrophobia, acrophobia, or fears of darkness or thunderstorms) had a mean age of onset of 22.7 ($\pm$16) years.

SOCIAL PHOBIA

In social phobia the individual's central fear is that he will act in such a way as to humiliate or embarrass himself in front of others. Social phobics fear and/or avoid a variety of situations in which they would be required to perform a task while in the presence of other people. Typical social phobias are of speaking, eating, or writing in public; using public lavatories; and attending parties or interviews. An individual may have one social phobia or many.

As in simple phobia the anxiety is stimulus bound. When forced or surprised into the phobic situation the individual experiences profound anxiety accompanied by a variety of physiologic anxiety symptoms (*e.g.,* palpitations, sweating, tremor, stuttering, faintness). Spontaneous panic attacks are not part of social phobia.

Individuals who have only one social phobia may be relatively asymptomatic unless confronted with the necessity of entering their phobic situation. When faced with this necessity they are often subject to intense anticipatory anxiety. For example a businessman with phobias of eating and speaking in public was insomniac, irritable, and suffered from constantly sweating palms for 1 week prior to a 2-day trip during which he would be required to eat all his meals in restaurants with co-workers.

A common fear of socially phobic individuals is that other people will detect and ridicule their anxiety in social situations. These patients are often caught in a vicious cycle in which their phobic anxiety leads to poor performance (*e.g.,* faltering voice during public speaking), which in turn reinforces their anxiety and avoidance of the situation.

Multiple phobias of this type can lead to social isolation. Such patients may be chronically demoralized. Alcohol and sedative drugs are often helpful in alleviating at least the anticipatory component of this anxiety disorder, and abuse of these substances may be seen in severe cases or in those cases where the phobia is particularly problematic to the patient's life-style. For example a young man with a fear of speaking in public who comes from a family where all the sons become lawyers may find himself dependent on alcohol after using it to make his way through law school.

Social phobias are thought to have their onset mainly in adolescence and early adulthood. Mean age of onset in two clinical series was 19 years. Onset of symptoms may be acute following a humiliating social experience but is more usually insidious over months or years and without a clearcut precipitant. Men and women are thought to be equally affected.

The course of the illness has not been well studied but appears to be chronic in cases entering treatment.

Differential Diagnosis

Before the diagnosis of phobic disorder can be made the presence of other disorders that may cause irrational fears and avoidance behaviors must be ruled out.

AGORAPHOBIA

Widespread fears and avoidance of being alone or leaving home can be seen in psychotic states and major depressive disorders.

Psychotic states (schizophrenia, paranoid psychosis, schizophreniform psychosis) can be differentiated from agoraphobia by the presence of their defining symptoms, such as delusions, hallucinations, and thought process disorder. Although agoraphobic patients are frequently afraid that they are going crazy, they do not exhibit psychotic symptomatology.

The distinction between depressive disorders and agoraphobia is more difficult. Both groups commonly experience spontaneous panic attacks. Patients with agoraphobia are frequently demoralized and will state that they feel depressed. Closer questioning, however, usually does not reveal either vegetative symptoms or a loss of pleasure or interest in activities. Early morning awakening and pervasive anhedonia, which are common symptoms in endogenous depression, are rare in agoraphobia. Agoraphobics will usually say they would love to leave home and engage in a variety of activities if only they could be sure of not panicking. In contrast, depressed individuals usually see no point in going out because nothing gives them any pleasure and they feel that people will be better off without them.

Atypical depressives (*i.e.,* depression characterized by hypersomnia, hyperphagia, extreme low energy, and depressed but reactive mood) frequently have panic attacks but rarely have agoraphobia as part of their life history or current symptomatology. These patients can also be distinguished from agoraphobics by the presence of reversed vegetative signs (overeating, leaden paralysis, oversleeping), which are uncommon in agoraphobia. This is an important distinction since there is evidence that patients with atypical depression and a history of panic attacks respond preferentially to monoamine oxidase (MAO) inhibitors.[13]

SOCIAL PHOBIA

Avoidance of social situations is seen as part of avoidant and paranoid personality disorders, agoraphobia, obsessive compulsive disorder, depressive disorders, schizophrenia, and paranoid disorders.

In paranoid personality disorder and paranoid psychoses, the individual avoids social situations because of a mistrust of others and a fear that something unpleasant will be done to him by "them." In contrast, social phobics do not generally mistrust or dislike other people. The social phobic's fear is that they themselves will act inappropriately and cause their own embarrassment or humiliation.

In avoidant personality disorder the central fear is also rejection, ridicule, or humiliation by others. However, individuals with avoidant personality disorder have a long-term widespread avoidance of all social relationships and interactions as well as pervasive low self-esteem.

In general social phobics, although dismayed by their limitations in certain areas, do not have a negative overall self-assessment. Their fears are more circumscribed, and most have some close interpersonal relationships. However, there may be an overlap between the current definition of avoidant personality and an individual with multiple severe social phobias.

Individuals with obsessive-compulsive disorder will sometimes avoid social situations that are involved in their obsessional thoughts or compulsive rituals. For example, patients with contamination fears may avoid eating with others.

Some agoraphobic patients will say that they are afraid they will embarrass themselves by losing control if they panic while in a social situation. Agoraphobics may also avoid social situations because they are afraid the situation will trigger a panic attack or that they will just be too nervous about the next attack to act in a socially appropriate fashion. These patients are distinguished from social phobics by the presence of spontaneous panics, the typical agoraphobic avoidance patterns, and the fact that their fear of humiliation is not general but limited to the circumstance of having a panic attack.

Patients with psychotic disorders leading to social avoidance are distinguished from social phobics by the presence of delusions and/or hallucinations that lead to their avoidance. Panic anxiety or fears of humiliation leading to social avoidance are not diagnosed as social phobia when occurring in the context of schizophrenia, schizophreniform or brief reactive psychoses, and major depressive disorder.

Social withdrawal, which is seen in depressive disorders, is usually associated with a lack of interest or pleasure in the company of others rather than a fear of scrutiny. In contrast, social phobics generally express the wish to be able to interact appropriately with others and anticipate pleasure in this eventuality.

SIMPLE PHOBIAS

Simple phobia is the residual diagnostic category for phobic disorders in the *DSM-III*. The diagnosis is given only when phobic avoidance is not attributable to any other disorder.

One group of patients who deserve special mention are the "mixed phobics" described by Klein.[8] These are individuals who have spontaneous panic attacks and phobic avoidance of a limited number of situations or activities that developed in association with the panic disorder.

In the *DSM-III* it is not clear whether these patients are to be given a diagnosis of panic disorder only or diagnoses of both panic disorder and simple phobia. It has been suggested that the revised *DSM-III* include under anxiety states an additional category (panic disorder with limited phobic avoidances) to describe these patients.

Etiology

The etiology of phobic disorders is unknown. Current approaches to understanding the origin of phobias can be grouped under four headings: (1) psychoanalytic theory, (2) learning (behavioral) theory, (3) genetic data, and (4) biological and ethological theories. A brief summary of the major aspects of each of these is given below.

LEARNING THEORIES

In learning theory phobic anxiety is thought to be a conditioned response acquired through association of the phobic object (the conditioned stimulus) with a noxious experience (the unconditioned stimulus). Initially, the noxious experience, for example, an electric shock, produces an unconditioned response of pain, discomfort, and fear. If the individual frequently receives an electric shock when in contact with the phobic object, then by contiguous conditioning the appearance of the phobic object alone may come to elicit an anxiety response (conditioned response). Avoidance of the phobic object prevents or reduces this conditioned anxiety and is therefore perpetuated through drive reduction.

This classical learning theory model of phobias received much reinforcement from the relative success of behavioral (deconditioning) techniques in the treatment of many phobic patients. However, more recently the model has been criticized on the grounds that it is not consistent with a number of empirically observed aspects of phobic behavior in humans. Among the major criticisms are the following:

1. Most cases of phobia do not appear to have begun with a traumatic incident in which the phobic object is associated with an unpleasant unconditioned stimulus.
2. Although the learning theory model suggests that any object or situation that is regularly associated with noxious stimuli has an equal likelihood of becoming a phobic object, empiric observation indicates that the range of phobic objects is relatively small and is neither random nor predominantly made up of those items that in a modern industrial society might be most likely to be frequently associated with noxious stimuli (*e.g.*, electric switches, stoves).
3. Learning theory does not account for the qualitative distinctions between panic and anticipatory anxiety delineated by pharmacologic and sodium lactate infusion studies.
4. Learning theory does not explain the efficacy of different types of behavior therapy. For example, the learning theory model predicts that ungraded exposure or flooding should produce no effect on phobic behavior unless the individual remains in the phobic situation until anxiety begins to wane (habituation). However several studies have found that exposure treatments in which the patient removes himself from the phobic situation when his anxiety level becomes uncomfortable may be as effective as those in which prolonged exposure is required.[14]
5. Laboratory-conditioned avoidance behavior on which the learning theory model is based is easily extinguished. In contrast, clinical phobias are highly resistant to extinction and are well known for their refractoriness to cognitive interventions (*i.e.*, rational explanations of the harmless nature of the phobic object do not cure phobias).

PSYCHOANALYTIC THEORY

The development of Freud's thinking on the causes of anxiety has been discussed elsewhere in this volume. In this chapter discussion of psychoanalytic theory will be limited specifically to those theories explaining the origin of phobic behavior.

During his early work Freud observed that in analysis of phobias "nothing is ever found but the emotional state of anxiety. . . . In the case of agoraphobia we often find the recollection of an anxiety attack; and what the patient actually fears is the occurrence of such an attack under the special conditions in which he believes he cannot escape it."[15] At this time Freud did not consider phobias to have a psychological origin. Rather he understood them to be, like anxiety neurosis, manifestations of a physiologically induced tension state.

However, with the 1909 publication of the case of Little Hans, Freud reversed these earlier opinions and adopted a psychological theory of phobic symptom formation.[16] This theory was restated in a more refined version in the 1926 paper *Inhibition, Symptoms and Anxiety*.[2]

Little Hans was a 5-year-old boy who developed a phobia of horses. Through an analysis of the boy's conversations with his parents over a period of months Freud concluded that the phobia was a symptom of an unresolved unconscious Oedipal conflict. Freud hypothesized that Little Hans sexually desired his mother but feared the retribution of his father (in the form of castration) were he to act on these sexual feelings. The unacceptable conflict between his love and reverence for his father, the desire for sexual gratification with the mother, and the guilty fear of the father's retribution was repressed into the unconscious. The fear of the father's retribution was displaced onto an external and avoidable object: horses. Avoidance of horses permitted both avoidance of the anxiety caused by the intrapsychic conflict and avoidance of the real external danger, the father's anger. Little Hans' separation anxiety was seen as a secondary epiphenomenon.

Generalizing from this case, Freud hypothesized that phobic symptoms occur as part of the resolution of a conflict between the impulses for libinal or aggressive gratification and the ego's recognition of potential external danger that could result from this gratification. Mobilized by way of signal anxiety and acting according to the pleasure principle, the ego uses repression and displacement to avoid the anxiety produced by both intrapsychic conflict and potential external danger. The libidinal and/or aggressive impulses are repressed, and the threat of external danger is displaced onto a less cathected external object that can be avoided. Together, repression of the conscious impulse and avoidance of the "phobic" object eliminate signal anxiety and fear of retribution.

Freud does not appear to have reconciled his early clinical observations with this later theory in which all phobias have a unitary etiology and distinctions between types of anxiety are quantitative rather than qualitative.

GENETIC DATA

Only a few studies have addressed the question of the role heredity plays in etiology of phobias. Early studies usually included mixed groups of patients, and their results are difficult to interpret in terms of current diagnostic categories.

Harris and associates[17] compared the prevalence of psychiatric disorder in the first-degree relatives of 20 patients with agoraphobia with panic attacks (AgP), 20 patients with panic disorder (PD), and 20 normal controls using the direct interview method. The risk for any anxiety disorder in the relatives of AgP (32%) and PD (33%) patients was equivalent and significantly greater than that for relatives of controls (15%). These data suggest a familial component in development of agoraphobia, but the numbers are too small for definite conclusions and as in all family studies environmental factors cannot be ruled out.

No family studies of social or simple phobias have been reported.

Comparisons of concordance of traits in monozygotic (MZ) and dizygotic (DZ) twins can be used to distinguish between environmental and familial contributions to etiology. Three twin studies have found a higher rate of concordance for anxiety disorders among MZ twins than among DZ twins.[6,18] In only one of these studies was the sample of phobic patients large enough to look specifically at intergenerational transmission of phobic symptoms. Carey and Gottesman[6] studied 21 twin pairs (8 MZ and 13 DZ) in which the index twin had a primary or secondary diagnosis of phobic neurosis. Concordance rates for phobic symptoms or features with or without treatment were 88% for MZ twins and 38% for DZ twins.

These findings are consistent with a hereditary contribution to the etiology of phobias but again the numbers of subjects are small and replication is needed using larger samples and current diagnostic criteria. In addition there are no studies of phobias in twins separated at birth (adoption studies). The latter would rule out possible contributions of differential family treatment of twins to occurrence of phobic disorder.

ETHOLOGIC AND BIOLOGICAL APPROACHES

Some interesting recent hypotheses about the origin of phobias have resulted from integration of ethological, biological, and learning theory approaches.

Klein,[8] paralleling Bowlby's work, hypothesized that recurrent spontaneous panic attacks occur when the threshold of an innate mechanism that controls the young child's response to separation from its caretakers is pathologically lowered. Klein has further suggested that transient episodes of situationally predisposed rudimentary panics (formes frustes of the full-blown spontaneous panic attack) may serve as the original unconditioned stimulus for the conditioned response of fear and avoidance that form the clinical picture in simple phobia.

The occurrence of situationally predisposed rudimentary panics would explain the specific situational avoidance and absence of a remembered initial trauma in the history of most simple phobics. A possible explanation for the persistent, nonextinguishable, and noncognitive aspects of phobic behavior and the relatively narrow range of common phobic objects can be drawn from Seligman's[19] recent critique of learning theory. Seligman suggested that these characteristics can be understood if one considers phobias to be an example of evolutionarily prepared learning. The concept of "preparedness" refers to the observation that certain responses to stimuli are more easily learned than others and that the ease of learning in any one instance varies from species to species. Preparedness is a measure of the ease with which a particular stimuli becomes paired with a particular response. In the case of phobias, preparedness is the ease with which certain stimuli that are paired with fear are subsequently reacted to as though intrinsically dangerous.

One might speculate that at least some simple phobias originate when situationally predisposed rudimentary panics occur transiently in association with objects or events for which there is a prepared association to fear.

Treatment

In the past 30 years a variety of psychotherapeutic, behavioral, and drug treatments for phobic disorders have been developed. The choice of treatment or combination of treatments for a particular patient may depend on several factors: the specific diagnosis, the degree of motivation of the patient, and the time and resources available to patient and therapist.

In this section the major current treatment techniques for each type of phobic disorder are described and the literature on their efficacy reviewed.

SIMPLE PHOBIAS

The treatment of choice for simple phobias is exposure. The problem is to persuade the patient that exposure is good for him. A wide variety of persuasive techniques are available. Several of the most commonly used and best studied are described here. However, any treatment the patient finds convincing will probably go well.[20]

Exposure treatments may be divided into two groups depending on whether exposure to the phobic object is *"in vivo"* or "imaginal." *In vivo* exposure involves the patient in "real life" contact with the phobic stimulus. Imaginal techniques confront the phobic stimulus through the therapist's descriptions and the patient's imagination.

The method of exposure in both the *in vivo* and imaginal techniques can be graded or ungraded. Graded exposure uses a hierarchy of anxiety-provoking events, varying from least to most stressful. The patient begins at the least stressful level and gradually progresses up the hierarchy. Ungraded exposure begins with the patients confronting the most stressful items in the hierarchy.

Most exposure techniques have been used in both individual and group settings. In a group setting both the example and the exhortations of other members are often particularly helpful in persuading the patient to re-enter the phobic situation.

Systematic Desensitization

Systematic desensitization is a graded imaginal exposure technique based on the classical learning theory of phobias. Described by Wolpe in 1958, it was the first widely used exposure technique.

At the start of treatment a hierarchy of anxiety-producing situations related to the phobic stimulus is developed by therapist and patient. Then the patient is trained in the technique of deep muscle relaxation. At the start of each session, the patient is put into a state of deep relaxation. While in this state he is asked by the therapist to visualize the first scene in the hierarchy. If the visualization provokes any anxiety the patient stops and immediately proceeds with the deep muscle relaxation. When he is relaxed the scene is revisualized. When a scene has been visualized twice without provoking anxiety the patient proceeds up the hierarchy to the next most anxiety-producing scene.

Imaginal Flooding

Imaginal flooding is an ungraded exposure technique that is thought to work by causing habituation of phobic anxiety through prolonged imaginal exposure to the phobic stimulus.

The patient visualizes scenes involving the phobic stimulus that are at the most stressful part of his hierarchy and are extremely anxiety provoking. The exposure is maintained until the anxiety begins to decrease.

After repeated sustained exposure the patient is usually able to visualize, without anxiety, any realistically non-anxiety-provoking situation involving the phobic stimulus.

Imaginal flooding is a highly stressful technique that requires a highly motivated and well-prepared patient to be effective.

Prolonged *in Vivo* Exposure

Prolonged *in vivo* exposure is an ungraded exposure technique that has also been called flooding *in vivo*. It operates on the same principle as imaginal flooding—that repeated, prolonged exposure to the phobic stimulus extinguishes phobic anxiety by habituation.

At the start of treatment the patient is asked to go as close to the phobic object or situation as possible and remain there until his anxiety begins to diminish. The therapist then asks him to move a little closer and stay at this new point until his anxiety diminishes. This procedure continues until the patient is able to enter the phobic situation without anxiety.

Prolonged *in vivo* exposure is an extremely stressful technique. Patients must be both highly motivated and well informed about the treatment in order for it to succeed.

Because of its stressfulness patients with medical conditions in which stress or extreme anxiety are contraindicated (*e.g.*, certain seizure disorders, cardiovascular and respiratory illnesses) are not suitable candidates for prolonged *in vivo* exposure treatment.

Participant Modeling and Reinforced Practice

Participant modeling and reinforced practice are graded *in vivo* exposure techniques in which various combinations of supportive psychotherapy, vicarious and *in vivo* exposure are used to gradually encourage the patient into increasing contact with the phobic situation or object. In these two techniques, in contrast to prolonged *in vivo* exposure, the patient's anxiety is maintained at an elevated but still comfortable level throughout treatment.

A preliminary step in both methods is the construction of a graded hierarchy of fear-relevant tasks of increasing difficulty.

In participant modeling the patient first observes the therapist in various degrees of contact with the phobic situation. Then with the encouragement of the therapist and/or other group members the patient himself gradually undertakes "participation" in the exposure.

The major components of the reinforced practice program are practice in the phobic situation, praise for improvement, precise feedback of amount of improvement, and expectancy of success. The patient, accompanied by the therapist, approaches the phobic situation by steps in the graded hierarchy. If undue anxiety is experienced, the exposure is terminated. After a rest the patient again attempts exposure. Each increased approach is acknowledged and praised. The underlying principle of this program is that by positive reinforcement of repeated and increasingly close successive approximations, the patient will be conditioned to appropriate approach behaviors.

Treatment Outcome

The empiric literature indicates that the majority of simple phobics show a significant improvement with exposure treatment. Unfortunately most studies have reported outcome in terms of mean change scores rather than global clinical condition. This reporting makes it difficult to tell how many patients were cured and how many were not responsive to the treatment.

Consistent outcome differences between the different types of imaginal exposure techniques have not been found. The various techniques that include "real life" exposure also do not appear to differ from each other in efficacy. There has been some controversy as to whether *in vivo* exposure techniques are more effective than those using imaginal exposure.

Marks[21] and Gelder[22] have both stated that the essential therapeutic requirement for phobic patients is uninterrupted exposure to the phobic object for an hour or more. However, Mathews and associates[23] found no long-term difference in improvement between imaginal and *in vivo* exposure as long as between-session real life exposure practice was explicitly encouraged.

Klein and colleagues[24] hypothesized that psychotherapeutic treatments of phobias operate in the following way:

through nonspecific expectancy effects that incite the specific remedial action, i.e., maintained exposure in vivo. One must grasp the nettle. The pa-

tient engages in formerly avoided, fearful experiences in real life, experiences success, and thereby extinguishes paralyzing anticipatory anxiety engendered by the fear of intense discomfort, failure, and punishment.

From this point of view, imaginal and *in vivo* exposure as well as supportive and psychodynamic psychotherapy are all different ways of persuading the patient to reenter the phobic situation. Further research is needed to determine if particular groups of patients are more or less responsive to any one technique.

AGORAPHOBIA

There is some disagreement as to the best method of treatment of agoraphobia with panic attacks. One widely employed strategy is the use of medication to block panic attacks followed by a psychotherapeutic intervention that encourages the patient to reenter phobic situations. A second strategy uses behavioral psychotherapy alone in treatment of these patients.

The treatment for agoraphobia without panic attacks is behavioral psychotherapy that includes or encourages exposure to phobic situations.

Combined Use of Anti-panic Medication and Psychotherapy

The combined use of anti-panic medication and psychotherapy is based on Klein's theory of the pathogenesis of agoraphobia with panic attacks. Anti-panic medication is given to block the occurrence of panic attacks. Once the attacks are blocked, patients are encouraged to reenter phobic situations and activities to demonstrate to themselves that they will no longer have attacks. Repeated experience of *not* having an attack leads to a gradual decrease in anticipatory anxiety and avoidance.

The tricyclic antidepressant imipramine (Tofranil) and the MAO inhibitor phenelzine (Nardil) have been shown to be effective blockers of spontaneous panic attacks. Although controlled studies have not yet been done, clinical experience indicates that other drugs in these two classes are also effective in blocking spontaneous panics. Alprazolam (Xanax), a recently marketed benzodiazepine derivative with a triazolo ring, has been used in the treatment of panic attacks and appears effective in many cases. It has been suggested that alprazolam, in contrast to tricyclic antidepressants, may also have an effect on anticipatory anxiety.

The use of these drugs in the treatment of patients with agoraphobia with panic attacks is identical to their use for the treatment of panic disorder.

The goal of the psychotherapeutic intervention in this treatment technique is to get the patient to reenter the phobic situation and demonstrate to himself that he will no longer have panic attacks and therefore may give up both his avoidance and his worry, or anticipatory anxiety, about having attacks.

At the start of treatment the therapist explains to the patient the three-stage development of the illness and the fact that the medication will block the spontaneous panics but will not alleviate anticipatory anxiety or the desire to avoid. Some patients, once the frequency of spontaneous panics has abated, will begin to try out previously avoided situations on their own. Others will need structured encouragement in some form of psychotherapy. Supportive as well as imaginal and *in vivo* behavioral psychotherapies have been used in conjunction with anti-panic medication in the treatment of agoraphobia with panic attacks. Supportive psychotherapy may be non-directive or may take the form of active encouragement and education. In the former the therapist treating the bus-avoidant agoraphobic might wait until the patient mentioned a possible bus ride and then in response to the patient's suggestion agree that it sounded like a good idea. In the latter, more active, method the therapist would bring up the possibility of the bus ride in a statement such as: ''It's been a couple of months since you had a panic attack. We both agree that the reason you began avoiding buses was your fear that you might have a panic while stuck in a bus. Your panics are now blocked by the medication so you don't have to be afraid of the bus rides any more. You could try one this week.'' If the patient is reluctant, more exhortation may be required.

Efficacy of Treatment

Six studies have compared the efficacy of imipramine combined with some form of psychotherapy to that of psychotherapy and placebo in the treatment of agoraphobia. In five of these studies imipramine-treated patients did significantly better. In the sixth study there was no difference in outcome.

In four of six studies, MAO inhibitors have been found to be superior to placebo in reduction of anxiety in phobic patients.[25] Sheehan and co-workers[26] found that phenelzine and imipramine were equally effective in treatment of patients with panic and multiple phobias.

Behavioral Treatments

Most behavioral programs for treatment of agoraphobia use a combination of education, supportive psychotherapy, and one or more of the exposure techniques described under the section for treatment of simple phobias.

Interpretation of results is often limited by the fact that outcome is reported in terms of mean change scores rather than number of patients who achieve different levels of functioning at the end of treatment. It is also unclear whether or not patients in behavioral programs continue to have panic attacks in spite of treatment but deal with them differently or actually have fewer attacks after successful treatment.

Significant improvement effects have been found for a number of behavioral techniques in treatment of agoraphobia. However, overall results are moderate and many patients retain a substantial degree of symptomatology. The crucial factor in patient improvement appears to be practice of prolonged *in vivo* exposure to the phobic situation. The context in which the prolonged exposure occurs, with or without the therapist, in combination with other forms of behavioral treatment, during or between sessions, does not appear to affect outcome.

Recent reviews of the literature have found that from 60% to 75% of patients improve in treatment programs that include *in vivo* exposure.[27] Improvement rates for programs without *in vivo* practice are slighly less 50% to 60%. However it is not clear if the apparent higher percentage of improved patients in programs using *in vivo* exposure techniques is due to the method itself or to the fact that *in vivo* treatment gets the patient into the situation more rapidly. In time-limited treatment trials the more rapid effect of *in vivo* treatment could be mistakenly interpreted as an absolute superiority of this treatment over others.

For example, Zitrin and co-workers[20] found no significant difference in outcome at 26 weeks between agoraphobic patients who had received behavior therapy and imipramine (BT + IMI) as compared to those who received supportive psychotherapy and imipramine (ST + IMI). The outcome for either of these treatments also did not differ significantly from that in a study in which agoraphobic patients received imipramine and group *in vivo* exposure. Patients given *in vivo* exposure showed a greater improvement at 13 weeks, but outcome at 26 weeks was the same for all groups.

Several studies indicate that imaginal desensitization in conjunction with explicit instruction to practice exposure between sessions is as effective as *in vivo* exposure. Mathews and co-workers[23] have developed a home-based programmed practice treatment procedure based on the hypothesis that practice in the real-life situation is the essential factor in the treatment of agoraphobia. In this program the therapist and client have only a few initial sessions of evaluation and education. The major responsibility for the management of the treatment is given to the client and partner. The therapist serves as a consultant and troubleshooter. Studies by Mathews and co-workers indicate that a home-based program with as few as eight therapist-patient contact sessions can be an effective treatment for some patients. However preliminary data from work by Mavissakalian and Michelson[28] suggests that combining self-exposure assignments with imipramine, therapist-accompanied *in vivo* flooding, or both, greatly increases the number of patients who make a functional recovery. Specifically, these authors found that exposure alone gave a recovery outcome of 33% while combination treatment lead to recovery of roughly three fourths of patients.

Most follow-up studies have found that the great majority of patients treated with behavioral methods maintain their treatment gains over time. Furthermore post-treatment gains are not reported. Exceptions are the self-exposure program of Mathews and co-workers[23] and Emmelkamp and Wessels[29] in which patients continued to improve over the follow-up period. These studies do not report the actual numbers or percentage of patients who clinically relapsed. In their study of imipramine and behavioral and supportive psychotherapy, Zitrin and associates[20] found a relapse rate of 15% two years after treatment. There are no systematic studies of relapse rates following other types of drug treatments. It is not known if patients treated behaviorally have a significantly different relapse rate than those treated with drugs.

Further systematic follow-up studies are needed before any definite conclusions can be drawn.

SOCIAL PHOBIA

Since social phobia is the most recently defined of the phobic disorders, specific treatments for it have been less well studied than those for agoraphobia and simple phobias. Behavioral, drug, and psychotherapeutic approaches have been used with varying degrees of success. However, although some patients can be helped to a certain extent, there is at present no uniformly and predictably effective treatment for this disorder.

Behavioral Treatments

Systematic desensitization and social skills training have been used in the treatment of social phobics. Systematic desensitization is described above (see Simple Phobia). Social skills training is an approach to interpersonal difficulties that employs a combination of supportive and exposure therapy, modeling, rehearsal, role playing, and assigned practice to help individuals learn appropriate behaviors and decrease anxiety in social situations. The treatment is usually done in a group setting. As in reinforced practice, specific feedback on behavior and positive reinforcement for change are used to gradually reshape behavior.

Results of studies of behavioral treatment of social phobias are difficult to evaluate due to heterogeneous phobic patient samples, lack of operational definitions of disorder and improvement ratings, and the presentation of outcome data in terms of mean change scores rather than level of achieved functioning. In addition much of the research in this area was done in nonpatient populations.

There are six studies in the literature that specifically address the question of the efficacy of behavioral treatments in socially anxious or phobic individuals. Five found slight-to-moderate improvement after treatment, and one found no treatment effect over that in the waiting list controls. Most patients showed some improvement either in number of social contacts or quality of social skills, but all remained significantly symptomatic. It is important to note that the subjects in these studies are described as having multiple social anxieties and phobias.

Drug Treatments

There are no systematic studies of pharmacologic treatment of social phobias in clinical populations.

Recent studies of beta-adrenergic blockers as a treatment for "stage fright" in normal individuals has led to an interest in their possible use in patients with social phobia.[30] Two studies looked at effects on performance anxiety in professional musicians and two at public speaking anxiety in normal volunteers. In all cases the beta-adrenergic blocker was given in one acute dose prior to the anxiety-provoking stimulus. In three of four studies, subjects had both decreased anxiety by self- and independent-evaluator assessment and improved performance by objective assessment on active medication as compared with placebo. In the fourth study there was no difference between objective assessment of performance when subjects were on placebo or active medication, but decreased self-report of anxiety was reported by individuals during the active medication trial.

No studies of beta-adrenergic blockers in treatment of social phobia have been reported. Beta-adrenergic blockers have not been approved by the Food and Drug Administration for use in the treatment of social phobia. However, we believe that in situations where a beta-adrenergic blocker is not medically contraindicated and behavioral treatments are either unfeasible, or have failed, a trial of a beta-adrenergic blocker may be merited for the patient with social phobia.

REFERENCES

1. Freud S: Obsessions and Phobias. In Strachey J (ed): The Standard Edition of the Complete Works of Sigmund Freud, vol 3. London, Hogarth Press, 1961

2. Freud S: Inhibitions, Symptoms and Anxiety. In Strachey J (ed): The Standard Edition of the Complete Works of Sigmund Freud, vol 20. London, Hogarth Press, 1961

3. Marks I: Fears and Phobias. New York, Academic Press, 1969

4. Klein DF: Delineation of two drug responsive anxiety syndromes. Psychopharmacologia 5:397–408, 1964

5. Diagnostic and Statistical Manual of Mental Disorders, 3rd ed, p 225. Washington, DC, American Psychiatric Association, 1980

6. Carey G, Gottesman I: Twin and family studies of anxiety, phobic and obsessive disorders. In Klein, DF, Rabkin JG (eds): Anxiety: New Research and Changing Concepts. New York, Raven Press, 1981

7. Leckman JF, Weissman MM, Merikangas RR et al: Panic disorder and major depression. Arch Gen Psychiatry 40:1055–1060, 1983

8. Klein DF: Anxiety reconceptualized. In Klein DF, Rabkin JG (eds): Anxiety: New Research and Changing Concepts. New York, Raven Press, 1981

9. Agras SW, Sylvester D, Oliveau D: The epidemiology of common fears and phobias. Compr Psychol 10:151–156, 1969

10. Weissman MM, Myers JK, Leckman JL et al: Anxiety disorders: Epidemiology and familial patterns. Paper presented at Research Conference on Anxiety Disorders, Panic Attacks and Phobias, sponsored by Sanley Cobbs Psychiatric Research Laboratories, Psychiatric Service, Massachusetts General Hospital and Department Of Psychiatry, Tufts-New England Medical Center. Sonesta Beach Hotel, Key Biscayne, Florida, December 9–11, 1982

11. Spitzer RL, Endicott J, Robins E: Research Diagnostic Criteria: Rationale and reliability. Arch Gen Psychiatry 35:773–783, 1978

12. Quitkin F, Rifkin A, Kaplan J et al: Phobic anxiety syndrome complicated by drug dependence and addiction. Arch Gen Psychiatry 27:159–162, 1972

13. Leibowitz MR, Quitkin F, Stewart JW et al: Phenelzine versus imipramine in atypical depression: A preliminary report. Arch Gen Psychiatry (in press)

14. Mavissakalian MM, Barlow DH: Phobia: An overview. In Mavissakalian MM, Barlow DH (eds): Phobias. New York, Guilford Press, 1981

15. Freud S: Obsessions and phobias. In Strachey J (ed): The Standard Edition of the Complete Works of Sigmund Freud, vol 3. London, Hogarth Press, 1961

16. Freud S: The analysis of a phobia in a five-year old boy. In Strachey J (ed): The Standard Edition of the Complete Works of Sigmund Freud, vol 10. London, Hogarth Press, 1961

17. Harris EL, Noyes R, Crowe RR et al: Family study of agoraphobia. Arch Gen Psychiatry 40:1061–1064, 1983

18. Torgersen S: Genetic factors in anxiety disorders. Arch Gen Psychiatry 40:1085–1089, 1983

19. Seligman ME: Phobias and preparedness. Behav Ther 2:307–320, 1971

20. Zitrin CM, Klein, DF, Woerner MG et al: Treatment of phobias: I. Arch Gen Psychiatry 40:125–138, 1983

21. Marks IM: Behavioral psychotherapy of adult neurosis. In Garfield S, Bergin A (eds): The Handbook of Psychotherapy and Behavior Change. New York, John Wiley & Sons, 1978

22. Gelder M: Behavior therapy for neurotic disorders. Behav Mod 3:469–495, 1979

23. Mathews AM, Gelder MG, Johnston DW: Agoraphobia: Nature and Treatment. New York, Guilford Press, 1981

24. Klein DF, Zitrin CM, Woerner MG et al: Treatment of phobias: II. Arch Gen Psychiatry 40:144, 1983

25. Zitrin CM: Combined pharmacological and psychological treatment of phobias. In Mavissakalian MM, Barlow DH (eds): Phobias. New York, Guilford Press, 1981

26. Sheehan DV, Ballenger J, Jacobsen G: Treatment of endogenous anxiety with phobic, hysterical and hypochondriacal symptoms. Arch Gen Psychiatry 37:51–59, 1980

27. Mavissakalian MM: Exposure treatment of agoraphobia. In Psychiatry Update, The American Psychiatric Association Annual Review, vol 3. Washington, DC, American Psychiatric Association (in press)

28. Mavissakalian MM, Michelson L: Agoraphobia: Behavioral and pharmacological treatments. Psychopharm Bull 18:91–103, 1982

29. Emmelkamp PMG, Kuipers ACM: Agoraphobia: A follow-up study four years after treatment. Br J Psychol 134:352–355, 1979

30. Cole JO, Altesman RI, Weingarten CH: Beta blocking drugs in psychiatry. In Cole J (ed): Psychopharmacology Update. Lexington, MA, Collamore Press, 1980

28

M. Katherine Shear and William A. Frosch

Obsessive-Compulsive Disorder

While bathing her new infant, a young woman was overcome by fear that the baby would slip from her fingers into the water and drown. She called for her mother to help. Hounded by dread that something terrible would happen, she thought that walking to and from the mailbox in exactly 89 steps each way would ward off danger. Her mother cared for the child, while the woman spent the next week in this activity, with each attempt wrecked by concern that she miscounted. She was aware of the irrationality of her behavior but felt compelled to continue.

The day of onset of this behavior had been difficult. She had fought with her husband, had fought with her mother, and had been overworked. Just preceding the sequence of fear, avoidance, and compelled ego-alien behavior, she had the thought, rapidly put out of awareness, "if I didn't have this goddam kid, I wouldn't have all this work."

Obsessive-compulsive disorder (OCD) is a debilitating and chronic psychiatric illness. Symptoms can be so bizarre and upsetting that they seem psychotic, and associated mood disturbances can be as painful as those in affective disorders.

Patients with this disorder experience prominent obsessions and/or compulsions that cause distress and disrupt daily life. Obsessions are unwanted, repetitive, irresistible thoughts or urges. In spite of their ego-alien, senseless, and repugnant qualities, attempts to banish them are to no avail. Compulsions are stereotyped repetitive behaviors designed to produce or prevent something magically connected to the behavior. There is a subjective sense of being compelled that is often associated with a stimultaneous desire to resist.

Patients with OCD experience intrusive thoughts that interfere with concentration or perform ritualized behaviors that invade long periods of the day and interfere significantly with daily life. Obsessive themes of dirt, disease, or contamination and thoughts of harming oneself or others are common. Much compulsive behavior can be categorized into checking or cleaning behaviors. The disorder has been thought to be rare, with a prevalence in the general population around 0.05% and an incidence in the range of 0.1% to 4.6% in psychiatric populations.[1] However, the incidence may be considerably higher. One explanation for underreporting may be the shame many patients experience in connection with the repugnant nature of the symptoms or with the upsetting inability to control or banish them.

History

Medieval descriptions of demonic possession include early records of obsessive-compulsive behavior. In the 15th century, the *Maleus Maleficarcum* (cited by Nemiah[2]) describes a young man who cannot restrain himself from protruding his tongue or shouting obscenities whenever he tried to pray. The first medical account of obsessive-compulsive illness is generally attributed to Esquirol[3] in 1838 and the first use of the term to Morel in 1866. Westphal[4] defined obsessions as ideas that come to mind in spite of and contrary to the will of the patient. Janet[5] made the first attempt to describe a clinical syndrome in his two-volume work *Les Obsessions et la Psychasthenia*. He believed obsessional symptoms resulted from a diminution of mental energy. He emphasized lack of perseverance, indecision, checking, hesitancy, and the tendency to introspection. Lewis[6] reviewed previous definitions of obsessive illness and stated that the cardinal feature of the disorder is the fruitless struggle to resist experiences viewed by the patient as alien.

Freud[7,8] noted an association of obsessive-compulsive symptoms with certain personality traits: obstinancy, parsimony, and orderliness. He theorized that these traits and symptoms share psychogenetic origins and psychodynamic meanings and that they represent developmental disturbances of the anal-sadistic phase. Regressive energies provide impetus for urges to violence or to dirty and mess. The emergency defense mechanisms of isolation, undoing, and reaction formation are activated to control these dangerous and unacceptable impulses and lead to symptom formation. Three further consequences of the regression to the anal-sadistic phase are ambivalence, magical thinking, and the activation of an archaic, harsh, and punitive conscience. Clinical descriptions by Freud and other psychoanalysts contain some of the most vivid delineations of the obsessive-compulsive syndrome, and psychoanalytic theories provide the best explanation for the association of obsessive-compulsive symptoms and compulsive personality. However, learning theory and psychobiology have added to understanding obsessional psychopathology, and a full understanding of the disorder will undoubtedly require synthesis of data from each discipline.

Current Definition

The *Diagnostic and Statistical Manual of Mental Disorders*, 3rd ed (*DSM-III*) categorizes OCD among the anxiety disorders because of the frequency of anxiety, the association of its symptoms with other anxiety disorders (especially phobias), and the use of these symptoms to control anxiety. However, recent findings suggest that compulsions do not necessarily decrease anxiety. Rachman and Hodgson[9] and others have suggested that OCD might be placed with affective disorders.

The *DSM-III* defines OCD as obsessions or compulsions that cause significant distress or interfere significantly with social and vocational function. A third criteria, that symptoms not be attributed to another psychiatric disorder, is now controversial.

The *DSM-III*, as did its predecessors (*DSM-I* and *II*), stresses the occurrence of persistent, repetitive, and unwanted ideas and thoughts, images, or actions recognized as senseless and resisted by the patient. Obsessive rituals are distinguished from other stereotyped behaviors by being "seemingly purposeful" and "designed to produce or prevent some future situation or event." Obsessive-compulsive symptoms are also distinguished from repetitively impelled activities such as eating, sexual behavior, gambling, or drinking that are experienced as pleasurable.

Other classification systems subdivide OCD patients according to content (types of obsessions) or form (presence of obsessions, compulsions, or both). There is evidence that behavioral treatment is more successful for compulsions than for obsessions[10] and that outcome is different for compulsive checkers and compulsive cleaners.[9] Thus, subtyping may prove clinically useful.

Epidemiology

Studies of the incidence of OCD suggest that it is one of the rarest of mental disorders. Woodruff and Pitts[11] reasoned from population and available incidence figures and concluded that a maximum of 5 of 10,000 persons in the United States have obsessional neurosis. This figure includes children, in whom the diagnosis is also made. Although the reported incidence of OCD in children is generally even lower than in adults, the latter often report having suffered from obsessional symptoms during their childhood.

Sex distribution shows a striking prevalence in men (73%) versus women (27%) in some studies and the opposite, men 26%, women 74%, in other studies. Black[1] tabulates 1336 patients in 11 studies and reports a ratio of men to women of 49:51. Some authors suggest that the sex distribution of obsessive illness is similar to that of the general psychiatric caseload in any given setting.

The issue of heredofamilial contribution to obsessional illness has not been settled. Black[1] summarizes reports of 20 pairs of monozygotic twins viewed as concordant for obsessional illness. Of these, he notes that only 3 pairs can be said to have had both zygosity and diagnosis reliably established. However, considering the rarity of the obsessional syndrome (.05%) and of monozygotic twins (1/132−200 adults) the chance probability of even one concordant twin pair is extremely low.[12] Twin studies of dizygotic pairs show a lower incidence of concordance. The study of Rapaport and co-workers[13] of nine young obsessional patients and their families revealed a variety of psychopathologic disorders in relatives with only one sibling diagnosed as having OCD. Woodruff and colleagues[14] conclude that obsessional illness and other psychiatric illness probably occur with increased incidence in the families of obsessional patients but that the extent of increased family risk is uncertain. Black[1] warns that current studies "do not provide sufficient evidence of a genetical contribution to obsessional neurosis."

Clinical experience generated the idea that patients with OCD tend to be of high intelligence, a finding supported by several studies comparing intelligence testing in obsessional patients versus other neurotics (hysterics or anxiety neurotics). It is possible that a higher capacity for abstract thought might predispose an individual to obsessional ruminations.

There is some evidence suggesting obsessional illness is more prevalent in higher socioeconomic classes, although this was not the case in a Chinese sample.[15] Such a finding might be consistent with reports of higher intelligence among obsessional persons. Patients with OCD also have an unusually high rate of celibacy, approximately 40%. Some studies of obsessional illness have found celibacy higher in male patients (50% to 70%) than female patients (35% to 40%).[1] Obsessional illness occurs in all Western cultures, and available rates for non-Western cultures are similar to those reported in US studies. Moreover, the form and content of obsessions and compulsions seems to be strikingly similar in England, Scotland, Germany, Canada, the United States, and India.[15]

Clinical Descriptions

OCD patients suffer from unwanted, intrusive, repetitive thoughts or behaviors or both. These symptoms have been categorized in many ways. For example, Woodruff and co-workers[14] delineate six types of obsessional thoughts (ideas, images, convictions, ruminations, impulses, and fears) and one category of obsessional behaviors (rituals or compulsions). Obsessional ideas are repetitive thoughts that interrupt the normal train of thought. Often these are words, phrases, or rhymes with violent, blasphemous, or nonsensical content. Obsessional images are repeated vivid visual imaginings that are often described as violent, sexual, or disgusting. Obsessional convictions are thoughts based on magical ideas that the person consciously

both believes and disbelieves: "If I don't finish breakfast in less than five minutes, my mother's aunt will have a heart attack." Obsessional ruminations involve prolonged inconclusive thinking about unanswerable questions. Such ruminations may refer to metaphysical questions or to endless doubting about ordinary matters. Obsessional impulses relate to insistent unwanted urges that often involve injury to self or others or embarrassing behavior.

Obsessional fears are similar to phobias but typically involve dirt, disease, contamination, or potential weapons and are present even in the absence of the phobic stimulus. Obsessional fears may also relate to fear of some embarrassing and out of control behavior. Akhtar[16] cites a teacher in the classroom who was plagued by the fear that he would refer to his unsatisfying sexual relationships.

Obsessional behaviors (also called compulsions) have been categorized in a variety of ways. Stern[17] lists different kinds of rituals, including repeating, checking, cleaning, avoiding, striving for completeness, and being meticulous. Patients with repeating compulsions must do everything by numbers. One woman felt that whenever she had a certain thought she must repeat what she was doing at the time five times. A compulsive checker must repeatedly check that everything is in order. A man could leave his home only after spending several hours checking that windows were closed, the furniture was placed properly, the electric appliances were turned off, and the refrigerator door was closed. Often, after he left, he would be compelled to return to recheck. Patients with cleaning compulsions are compelled to scrub themselves for long periods after touching anything remotely dirty. Compulsive avoidance is seen in people who must avoid objects or situations for magical reasons. A woman felt she must avoid anything remotely like chocolate, for example anything brown. Compulsive striving for completeness relates to overconcern for perfection in small tasks such as buttoning a button. The task may be repeated over and over to "get it right." Similarly, compulsive meticulousness is seen when there is an urge to have objects "just so." Such a person may spend hours arranging pencils in his desk or making sure that scissors, pencils, and letter openers are all pointed in the "proper direction." Marks[18] notes a category of compulsive hoarders who find it impossible to throw rubbish away, making it difficult to live in a home thus cluttered. He also notes the frequency of requests for reassurance among obsessional patients. Such patients may demand to be repeatedly told if they are contaminated, if they have harmed someone, or if they are ill. Marks regards such repeated requests as a form of compulsive ritual.

Stern[17] studied 45 obsessional patients over 16 years of age. He found compulsive cleaning (51%), avoiding (51%), repeating (40%), and checking (38%) were the most common problems. Completing rituals (1%), meticulousness (9%), and slowing (4%) were considerably less common. Most patients had three or more compulsions. This hierarchy of problems is similar in several other studies.[15]

In Stern's sample, 46% had slight or no resistance to their rituals, while only 30% exerted a great effort to resist. Sixty-five percent rated their rituals as absurd, and 35% did not. Roughly a third of the patients performed rituals exclusively or predominantly in one place (usually home). Seventy-one percent of the time, compulsive behavior was rated as causing moderate to heavy family distress. Among patients who resisted rituals, it was frequently the repeating component that was resisted.

The relationship of obsessions to delusions is complex. Insight into the senselessness of obsessional thoughts may wax and wane, and the distinction between obsession and delusion may be blurred. However, delusional thinking in obsessionals is circumscribed and of short duration. Only a small percentage of patients diagnosed as OCD are eventually rediagnosed as schizophrenic. Retrospective studies of schizophrenic patients reveal that only a small percentage have premorbid obsessional symptoms. Most of these patients continue to experience their obsessions after the onset of schizophrenia.

The relationship of OCD to depression is an interesting and provocative one. An increased incidence of depression is found in obsessional persons, obsessional traits are commonly found in the premorbid history of depressed patients, and depression is frequently accompanied by obsessive-compulsive symptoms. Biological measures support an association of OCD with depressive illness. There is also evidence for a relationship of obsessive-compulsive symptoms with anxiety disorders (especially phobias), compulsive personality disorder, and with Gilles de la Tourette syndrome. Insel[19] suggests that OCD represents a heterogeneous syndrome that is in need of further biological and psychological delineation.

OCD in children is a recognized but rare illness. Adams[20] outlines eight types of increasingly pathologic obsessional behavior:

1. Ritualized collective play
2. Phase appropriate rituals seen in the 2 and 3-year old and sporadically in older children
3. Ritualized solitary play in children over 3 years of age
4. Obsessive collecting with avidity that suggests a driven quality
5. Circumscribed interests (implosions) seen in children who "go nuts" over specialized and often slightly unusual interests
6. Obsessive character (seen in 10 of 49 children he describes)
7. Obsessional neurosis
8. Obsessive-compulsive symptoms secondary to psychosis or brain damage.

Rapaport and colleagues[13] studied nine children with OCD, hoping to find the illness in "pure form." Instead, they found that children resembled adults with obsessional disorder in several ways: biological similarity to affective illness (depressive symptoms, shortened rapid eye movement [REM] latency), mildly abnormal neuropsychological testing, a lack of strong genetic loading, and discontinuity from compulsive personality traits.

Course

OCD typically begins early in life. Several series find the mean age at onset in the late teens or early 20s. Black[1] reviewed these series and concluded that 31% of first episodes occur between the ages of 10 and 15, with nearly three fourths of patients developing symptoms by age 30 and fewer than 10% after age 35. In most studies, obsessional patients report rituals during childhood, but surveys show that most normals also report these childhood behaviors. Although many clinicians believe that OCD occurs almost exclusively in patients with an obsessive-compulsive character, studies of OCD patients fail to substantiate this impression. Of 47 OCD patients studied, Rosenberg[21] found 53% had obsessional personality styles, 17% were schizoid, 13% were immature, 4% were hysterical, 2% were cyclothymic, and 11% were not classifiable. Black,[1] summarizing seven studies done between 1953 and 1968, concluded that it is likely that not all OCD patients show preexisting obsessional personality traits. Blacker and Levitt[22] and Insel[19] argue that obsessional symptoms have different meanings and treatment implications depending on the patient's personality type.

No particular "stressor" events occur with greater frequency in OCD patients than in control groups. Most patients report insidious onset of symptoms, although some patients do describe a sudden onset of symptoms. Ingram (cited by Black[1]) studied natural history and outcome in 89 obsessional patients in Scotland and concluded that the illness course may be characterized as constant, with progressive worsening; constant and static; fluctuating but never completely symptom free; or phasic. Black also reviewed three studies that found 11% to 14% of 219 patients had phasic courses, 24% to 33% had fluctuating courses, and 54% to 61% had constant (either static or worsening) courses.

Often the disorder has a major impact on daily life, with virtually all waking hours spent avoiding, ruminating, or ritualizing. In other cases people with OCD "succeed in making a productive and satisfying life for themselves, in spite of their obsessional disorders."[9] Rachman and Hodgson provide a vivid description of the invasiveness of symptoms:

> A patient who had been "a competent, trained secretary" became house bound. She "feared" contamination by germs and as a result she engaged in prolonged intensive washing and cleaning rituals. Her young child was restrained in one room of the four bedroom house, as it was the only one she could keep satisfactorily free from germs. Three rooms were kept permanently locked . . . she used extraordinary amounts of disinfectants to clean her house, to wash herself and her child. As is common . . . she was particularly agitated by contact with doors and doorknobs, and therefore learned how to open a door with her feet in order to avoid contaminating her hands. The large and complicated series of rituals that had to be carried out in preparing food meant that the family was kept on a restricted diet. Meals were seldom complete and rarely ready on time. The patient's fear of contamination made her virtually housebound, and her child was not permitted to leave the house except on a very few essential occasions. On returning from work each day, her husband was obliged to go through a series of decontamination-cleaning rituals. Their sexual relationship, never satisfactory, had been abandoned because of her fears of contamination. Their social life was damaged beyond repair, and they had lost all but one of their friends; even the members of their families could neither visit them nor be visited by them.

Occasionally a patient manages to contain compulsive activities and "live a normal life." Another of Rachman and Hodgson's patients, a schoolteacher, did so. She suffered from fears of disaster such as fire or gas leak and each night performed elaborate checking rituals, but during the day she could successfully inhibit her impulses to check.

Goodwin and co-workers[23] outline predictors of favorable outcome in patients with OCD, which include mild or atypical symptoms, including predominance of phobic-ruminative ideas and the absence of compulsions; short duration of symptoms prior to treatment; and good premorbid personality. Ingram[1] suggests there may be a correlation between early age at onset and poor prognosis.

Depression and anxiety are common complications of OCD. Depressive episodes may be severe enough to warrant diagnosis of a major depressive disorder. It is interesting that suicide is rarely a complication of OCD, in spite of the frequent presence of depression and of the common self-mutilative content of obsessional thoughts. On the contrary, the presence of obsessional symptoms in a depressive episode is associated with a lower incidence of suicide attempts. Obsessional symptoms may appear, disappear, or remain constant during a depressive episode.[24]

Etiology

The etiology of OCD is poorly understood. Learning theory, psychodynamic, and biological thinkers have contributed hypotheses, some of which have been useful, discarded, or untested.

Although classical conditioning does not adequately explain the onset of most obsessional illness, anxiety reduction is thought to play an important role in the persistence of ritualistic behavior. In a series of interesting experiments, Rachman and colleagues attempted to test the anxiety reduction theory in patients. They provoked compulsive behavior and measured subjective physiologic and behavioral responses. They then intervened to delay or interrupt the performance of the ritual and measured the effects of the intervention. They found that anxiety and discomfort increase significantly following exposure to a contaminated object and decrease following completion of a washing ritual, interruption of the ritual once it had started did not further increase anxiety, and provoking an urge to check resulted in increase in anxiety and performance of a checking ritual usually led to decreased anxiety. In a minority of instances, checking was reported to lead to increased anxiety. Rachman and Hodgson[9] conclude that the anxiety reduction model is probably applicable to OCD in some circumstances, specifically those in which the compulsive urge is elicited by circumscribed anxiety/discomfort-provoking stimulation and in which the execution of the ritual is followed by a noticeable reduction in anxiety discomfort. Some rituals (especially checking behavior) are probably perpetuated in an attempt to avoid anxiety. Other rituals lead to increased anxiety. It is postulated that such rituals are maintained in order to prevent still further increases in anxiety or possibly to prevent some other even more painful affect, such as severe guilt or depression.

Animal experiments using avoidance learning may be relevant to the anxiety reduction theory. Conditioned avoidance responses occur when an animal is taught to engage in some behavior (active avoidance) or to refrain from some activity (passive avoidance) in order to avoid an unpleasant stimulus. Compulsive behaviors such as performance of cleaning rituals and systematic refusal to touch "contaminated" objects might be conceptualized respectively as active or passive avoidance. Animal experimenters working in the past 30 years have investigated many aspects of the avoidance learning paradigm. Some authors attempt to use this model to explain OCD symptoms. The interested reader is referred to the work of Teasdale[25] for a more comprehensive review. However, the prominent use of language and symbols in OCD symptoms suggests that animal models could never be more than partially explanatory.

Interest in the neurobiology of OCD has been stimulated, in part, by the observation of the relationship of OCD to depressive symptoms. Insel[26] found that in OCD patients 18 years or older, who were sick at least a year, 25 of 28 patients showed dexamethasone nonsuppression and 15 of 17 OCD patients showed decreased REM latency, including some patients without depressive symptoms. REM density (found to be increased in major depressive disorder) was not altered in OCD patients. They also found that OCD patients showed attenuated growth hormone response to clonidine, which was again similar to depressed patients, but not all the patients were depressed. This group's attempt to use biological markers of depression to predict clomipramine response in OCD patients has been unsuccessful so far. They conclude that some patients with biological features of depression fail to improve while other patients who show neither biological nor clinical features of depression may show substantial improvement.

Other researchers have focused on identifying brain pathology in OCD. Obsessive symptoms have been described in patients with epidemic encephalitis. Some studies of electroencephalograms in patients with OCD report abnormalities, while others do not confirm this finding. Some evidence suggests that individuals with obsessive styles may have left hemispheric predominance. A report of exacerbation of OCD by naloxone[27] suggests that the opiate receptor system may play a role in symptom formation. Stereotypic, compelled, perserverative behaviors are also seen in some amphetamine users.[28] On the other hand, short-term relief of obsessional symptoms using D-amphetamines has been reported.

Rachman and Hodgson[9] have summarized the physiology of obsessional symptoms. Findings include increased heart rate, increased heart rate variability, and increased skin conductance on presentation of real or imagined obsessional stimuli; prompt decrease in these measures on performance of rituals; and more modest and gradual decrease even if no ritual is performed. This is similar to findings reported in phobic patients.

The eerie image of the typical obsessional patient as a rational individual engaged in irresistible senseless behavior is one of the most compelling examples of the presence and power of unconscious mental processes. Psychoanalytic explanations of obsessional phenomena focus on the uniquely human aspects of the symptoms: the use of human symbolic capacities in the psychological transformation of biological urges into mental or motor behavior. Although behavioral theorists tend to group obsessional symptoms (Rachman's "checkers" and "cleaners"), psychoanalysts focus on the details of each individual situation to explain symptom formation. The obsessive or compulsive symptom is a derivative or partial manifestation of an unconscious wish or fear and of the defense against it. The symptom may serve to distract the patient from unacceptable ideas that would otherwise emerge.

The instinctual urges and prohibitions that underlie OCD symptoms are those prominent in the anal stage of development. In early psychoanalytic thinking, the central and pathognomonic feature of obsessive compulsive neurosis was regression from a genital level of sexual interest to an earlier, never fully relinquished, psychosexual stage. The resulting symptoms reflect the characteristic behaviors and concerns of a child at this developmental phase. For example, the defense mechanisms of isolation, undoing, and displacement are used and ambivalence, magical thinking, and a harsh, insistent, and punitive superego are apparent. Other phase-related functions also contribute to the character of the symptoms.

Isolation, undoing, and displacement help determine the character of obsessional symptoms. Isolation (splitting off of ideas from the feelings originally associated with them) removes the possibility of contact. When a neurotic isolates an impression or an activity by interpolating an interval, he is letting it be understood symbolically that he will not allow these thoughts to come into associative contact with other thoughts.

Undoing attempts to reverse a psychological event, such as a thought, gesture, or word, and involves magical thinking. Undoing can take different forms in obsessional symptoms. An act itself can be "undone" by its opposite. A gas jet may be turned on and then turned off; an imagined act may be "undone" by a behavioral opposite act. Undoing is evoked in obsessive patients and also frequently fails: "What has been warded off returns in the very measure of warding off."[29] Seemingly senseless compulsions can sometimes be explained in this way:[29]

> A patient with scruples in regard to the unnecessary expenditure of money bought a newspaper for a nickel; unconsciously to him this was equivalent to a visit to a prostitute. He regretted it and, wishing to undo the act, decided to return to the newsstand. He was uncertain what to do because he would have been ashamed to return the paper to the boy and to ask for the money. Then it occurred to him that the purchase of a second paper might ease his mind. But the stand was already closed. Thereupon he took another nickel out of his pocket and threw it away.

In displacement, a substitution is made for the object of an unacceptable affect. An obsessive patient preoccupied with "dirty thoughts" relating to sexual urges may feel compelled to wash his hands incessantly. Intrusive hostile thoughts toward strangers on the street may substitute for unconscious hostility toward a loved parent.

Feelings of ambivalence characterize relationships with love objects in obsessional patients. In normal development the aggressive urges are neutralized and loving feelings predominate. Strong aggressive impulses reemerge in the obsessional patient and may lead to the displaced ambivalence and paralyzing doubt that characterize some obsessional symptoms. The anal-stage child believes in the omnipotence of thought. In the obsessional person, magical thinking can lead to anxious concern that thoughts of harm to others may actually cause harm: a patient had the persistent thought that he might stab someone on a subway with a scissors and had to repeatedly reassure himself that he had not done so.

The realistic standards, ideals, and conscience of the normal adult are foreign to the obsessional patient. Under internal tyrannical rule the obsessional person may spend increasingly painful hours attempting to do penance through rituals for thoughts, feelings, or behavior that might seem harmless or inconsequential to an outside observer. Insel[19] suggests that the overworked superego of the OCD patient may become fragmented. He cites a patient who demanded orderliness and cleanliness of himself and others but whose clothes were in continual disarray and whose room was "a den of (contamination)." Other patients may appear clean on the surface but avoid bathing and wear dirty underwear.

More recently, some psychoanalysts have rephrased the conflict as one between obedience and defiance resulting in an "alternation between the emotions of fear and rage—fear that he will be caught at his naughtiness and punished for it, rage at relinquishing his desires and submitting to authority."[30] The obsessional patient thinks rather than feels and particularly avoids tenderness and love, which connote dependency and danger. In the absence of an unconscious magical omnipotent partner (originally the mother), the obsessional person is overwhelmed with feelings of helplessness, inadequacy, and dependence. In the obsessional patient, secret expectations of omnipotence and perfection join forces with a brutal retaliatory conscience to provoke painful feelings of anxiety and guilt, which are feebly defended against by defensive maneuvers. Failing defenses lead to repetitions of rituals and encroaching symptoms that may eventually engulf the patient's life.

Psychoanalytic theory has been criticized for generating untested and perhaps untestable hypotheses, but still, nevertheless, psychoanalytic ideas facilitate empathic understanding of the haunted, lonely, obsessional patient. Although the theory has considerable explanatory power and is internally consistent, psychoanalytic concepts may often be more useful in understanding the person who suffers from OCD than in treating the symptoms themselves.

Diagnosis

The diagnosis of OCD is usually clear-cut. Although diagnositic criteria have changed little in the past century, sometimes problems do occur in distinguishing OCD from major affective disorder or schizophrenia. Patients with OCD frequently have complicating depression that may be difficult to distinguish from a depressive episode with complicating obsessive-compulsive symptoms. When such a distinction cannot be clearly made, treatment of both disorders is indicated. Differentiation of OCD from schizophrenia can also be difficult. Obsessional patients can lose reality testing and become convinced of the necessity to perform a ritual, but delusional ideas do not involve other aspects of the patient's thinking. Moreover, OCD can be a chronic debilitating disease that resembles schizophrenia in its impact on social and occupational functioning. Intrusive thoughts or compulsive urges and *"made thoughts or actions"* typical of schizophrenia seem to be a continuum. Nevertheless most OCD patients can be clearly differentiated from schizophrenics if current (*DSM-III*) criteria for schizophrenia are carefully applied. In rare instances OCD may occur in a patient with diagnosed schizophrenia. Revised criteria for OCD might allow for diagnosis of both disorders. OCD must also be differentiated from Gilles de la Tourette movement disorder. Other organic disorders, such as amphetamine intoxication, may occasionally present as OCD symptoms. Rachman and Hodgson[9] suggest that the organically induced symptoms typically lack intellectual content and intentionality and have a mechanical quality. Similarly, addictive behaviors have a compelled quality but are pleasurable and often are not ego dystonic while they are being performed and not spontaneously resisted. OCD must be differentiated from compulsive personality, which consists of traits that are ego syntonic, is seldom associated with a sense of compulsion, and seldom provokes resistance.

Obsessional thoughts and compulsive behavior are sometimes seen in a mild form in adults with no psychiatric disorder. Meticulous tidiness is common, for instance, and may be adaptive. Group ritualistic behaviors occur in many religions. Obsessional intrusive thoughts occur after stressful events.

Obsessions and ritualistic behaviors are seen commonly in children. A small child may insist on a specific story at each bedtime or demand that his toast be cut in a particular way. Older children develop games with counting or checking themes. Obsessive-compulsive disturbances have been described in children[13,20]; however, their relationship to adult OCD is not known.

Assessment concerns of those working behaviorally with OCD patients focus on details of the obsessional experience. Beech and Vaughn[31] suggest considering ten areas relevant to treatment:

1. Number and nature of obsessions and rituals
2. Environmental eliciting stimuli
3. Emotional response to contact with eliciting stimuli

4. Avoidance of eliciting stimuli
5. Frequency and duration of rituals
6. Emotional response associated with rituals
7. The frequency of thoughts associated with fear
8. Mood state
9. Moderating environmental cues
10. Marital, family, social, and sexual problems

Assessment for psychodynamic psychotherapy includes a detailed standard psychiatric history. In addition, suitability for exploratory therapy must be considered, as outlined by Nemiah.[2]

Assessment of OCD patients for research purposes presents a particularly difficult problem. Self-rating scales may become part of a ritual or the focus of an obsession; observer rating can be complicated by the variable willingness of obsessional patients to reveal their symptoms. Nevertheless, rating scales are used. Two of the more popular ones are the Leyton Obsessional Inventory[31] and the Maudsley Obsessive Compulsive Inventory.[9] Other assessment methods include graded ratings of individual target symptoms are derivation of obsessional subscales from a general psychopathology scale.

Treatment

Psychotherapy, behavioral therapy, pharmacotherapy, and psychosurgery have all been used to treat OCD. This disorder has been notoriously difficult to treat. Careful treatment outcome studies have demonstrated the effectiveness of behavioral and psychopharmacologic methods. The outcome of psychodynamically based treatments has not been systematically studied. Psychosurgery has been used to treat severe intractable cases with apparently good success.

Psychotherapy, frequently used to treat obsessive-compulsive patients, is probably helpful. Classic psychoanalysis is done with some patients, and individual analysts have reported success.[2] The decision as to whether psychoanalysis will be helpful must be based on the consideration of both the prominence of situational precipitating events and of general personality characteristics, such as good capacity for interpersonal relationships and effective work, psychological mindedness and motivation for change. Salzman and Thaler[33] suggest that classic psychodynamic methods should be altered in treating obsessional patients. They advocate an emphasis on the present while analyzing the patient's defensive maneuvers. They warn that the obsessive's introspective stance and tendency to ramble can be strengthened inadvertently by overuse of free association and focus on the past. They believe the therapist must intervene actively when clouds of details mask the issue, and they further claim that the patient may need encouragement, pressure, guidance, or drugs in addition to insight therapy. Sifneos[34] described treatment of patients with mild obsessional neurosis using short-term, dynamically oriented treatment. In one case a 32-year-old man on his honeymoon developed symptoms of "a need to pick up papers or pieces of metal from the floor or from the street . . . to be sure he picked up everything and that everything was clean" and had a disturbing obsessional thought that he had killed his father. Brief treatment led to symptom remission. In other cases treatment was effective in relieving distress even when full symptom remission was not achieved. Patients selected for this form of treatment should be intelligent, reasonably well-related people who have an acute onset of symptoms with a clear precipitating event. They should have anxiety and strong motivation for treatment.

Behavioral treatments of OCD center on exposure of patients to ritual-eliciting stimuli and preventing the usual compulsive response.[9,18] Assessment focuses on details of thoughts, feelings, and behavior during symptomatic periods and on the details of the stimuli that evoke responses. Exposure techniques can be ordered on a continuum related to the degree of approximation of the actual ritual eliciting stimulus. On one end of the spectrum (systematic desensitization), initial exposure is brief and imaginal. Treatment progresses stepwise and slowly, with the patient experiencing minimum distress. On the other extreme (maximal flooding), the patient is exposed to actual ritual-evoking stimuli for a long period of time. Patients often experience severe discomfort during flooding, but the technique is rapidly effective in reducing symptoms. In actual treatments, exposure is usually done in the mid range of this continuum and techniques used vary according to patient needs. A variation in which the therapist "models" exposure (such as contamination) is sometimes used.

Steketee and colleagues[34] studied effects of exposure *in vivo*, systematic desensitization, and response prevention on treatment outcome. They found that exposure *in vivo* reduces anxiety/discomfort related to eliciting stimuli, response prevention reduces ritualizing behavior, and *imaginal* exposure solidifies treatment gains. It was also shown that attention focusing during exposure treatment sessions leads to better between-session habituation than distraction during exposure, that severely depressed patients and patients with poor reality testing failed to respond to behavioral treatment even when they cooperated with treatment protocols, and that long-term outcome was improved in patients with less pretreatment depression or anxiety, lower baseline physiologic reactivity, better habituation to eliciting stimuli within and between sessions, younger age at onset, and better posttreatment outcome.

Obsessional thinking is more difficult to treat using behavioral techniques. Thought stoppage, aversive conditioning, or exposure in fantasy have been used with some success, but studies to date have not shown predictably effective treatment.[18]

Jenicke[35] reviews reports of psychopharmacologic treatment of OCD patients using a variety of medications. Successful case reports include anxiolytic drugs, antipsychotics, lithium, tricyclic antidepressants, monoamine oxidase inhibitors, LSD, and tryptophan. Other drugs that have been tried, without success, include propranolol, clonidine, and antiseizure medication.

The use of antidepressants in OCD is a source of considerable recent interest. Clomipramine has been most studied using controlled double-blind methods, and significant effectiveness has been shown in comparison to placebo control groups.[36] Studies using amitriptyline, nortriptyline and clorgyline have shown some effectiveness but statistically nonsignificant difference from placebo. The relationship of effectiveness of antidepressant treatment to clinical depression is unclear. Some authors claim medication is effective only in the presence of depression. However, Insel and co-workers[36] find improvement of rituals and obsessions even in the absence of depression. This group also suggests that the maximum effect may occur later than 6 weeks. Monoamine oxidase inhibitors may also be effective in treating some OCD patients, especially those with associated panic attacks, phobias, or severe anxiety,[35] although selective monoamine oxidase inhibition using clorgyline produced little improvement in the study of Insel and co-workers.[36] Several studies showing improvement with the use of medication have reported relapse after the drug therapy was stopped.

Psychosurgery has been used with some success in OCD patients. Surgical results have not been examined in controlled clinical trials and have generally been reported for patients with severe intractible illness. Small lesions in the cingulum and/or lower medial quadrant of each frontal lobe are used. Psychosurgery may have a role as a treatment for patients with severe, distressing life-threatening illness who have failed adequate trials of behavior therapy, medication, and psychotherapy.

REFERENCES

1. Black A: The natural history of obsessional neurosis In Beech HR (ed): Obsessional States. London, Methuen Press, 1974
2. Nemiah JC: Obsessive compulsive disorder. In Kaplan H, Freedman AM, Sadock BJ (eds): Comprehensive Textbook of Psychiatry, vol 3, 3rd ed. Baltimore, Williams & Wilkins, 1980
3. Esquirol JED: Des Maladies Mentales, vol II. Paris, Ballière, 1838
4. Westphal C: Zwangsvortellungen. Arch Psychiatr Nervenkr 8:734–750, 1878
5. Janet P: Les Obsessions et la Psychasthenie. Paris, Ballière, 1903
6. Lewis AJ: Problems of obsessional illness. Proc R Soc Med 29:325–336, 1936
7. Freud S: The disposition to obsessional neurosis. In Strachey J (ed): The Standard Edition of the Complete Works of Sigmund Freud, vol 12. London, Hogarth Press, 1961
8. Freud S: Transformation of instincts as exemplified in and eroticism. In Strachey J (ed): The Standard Edition of the Complete Works of Sigmund Freud, vol 17. London, Hogarth Press, 1961
9. Rachman S, and Hodgson RJ: Obsessions and Compulsions. Englewood Cliffs, NJ, Prentice-Hall, 1980
10. Marks IM: Review of behavioral psychotherapy: I. Obsessive compulsive disorders. Am J Psychiatr 138:584–592, 1981
11. Woodruff R, Pitts FM: Monozygotic twins with obsessional neurosis. Am J Psychiatr 120:1075–1080, 1964
12. McGuffin P, Mawson D: Obsessive compulsive neurosis: Two identical twin pairs. Br J Psychiatr 137:285–287, 1980
13. Rapaport J, Elkins R, Langer DH et al: Childhood obsessive compulsive disorder. Am J Psychiatr 12:1545–1555, 1981
14. Woodruff RA, Goodwin DW, Guze SB: Psychiatric Diagnosis. New York, Oxford University Press, 1974
15. Emmelkamp PMG: Phobic and Obsessive Compulsive Disorders. New York, Plenum Press, 1982
16. Akhtar S, Wig NH, Verma VK et al: A phenomenologic analysis of symptoms in obsessive compulsive neurosis. Br J Psychiatry 127:342–348, 1975
17. Stern RS, Cobb JP: Phenomenology of obsessive compulsive neurosis. Br J Psychiatry 132:233–239, 1978
18. Marks IM: Cure and care of neuroses. New York, John Wiley & Sons, 1981
19. Insel TR: Obsessive compulsive disorder: Five clinical questions and a suggested approach. Compr Psychiatry 23:241–251, 1982
20. Adams P: Obsessive Children. New York, Penquin Books, 1973
21. Rosenberg CM: Personality and obsessional neurosis. Br J Psychiatry 113:471–477, 1967
22. Blacker KH, Levitt M: The differential diagnosis of obsessive compulsive symptoms. Compr Psychiatry 20:532–547, 1979
23. Goodwin DW, Guze SB, Robins E: Follow up studies in obsessional neurosis. Arch Gen Psychiatry 20:182–187, 1969
24. Gittelson WL: The effect of obsessions in depressive psychosis. Br J Psychiatr 112:253–259, 1966
25. Teasdale JD: Learning models of obsessional compulsive disorder. In Beech YR (ed): Obsessional States. London, Methuen Press, 1973
26. Insel TR, Mueller EA, Gillin CJ: Biological markers in obsessive compulsive and affective disorders. (in press)
27. Insel TR, Pickar D: Naloxone administration in obsessive compulsive disorder: Report of two cases. Am J Psychiatry 140:1219–1220, 1983
28. Ellinwood EH: Amphetamine psychosis: I. Description of the individuals and process. J Nerv Ment Dis 144:273–283, 1967
29. Fenichel O: The Psychoanalytic Theory of Neurosis. New York, WW Norton and Co, 1945
30. Mackinnon R, Michels RM: The Psychiatric Interview in Clinical Practice. Philadelphia, WB Saunders, 1971
31. Beech HR and Vaughan M: Behavioral Treatment of Obsessional States. New York, John Wiley & Sons, 1978
32. Cooper J: The Leyton Obsessional Inventory. Psychol Med 1:48–64, 1970
33. Salzman L, Thaler FH: Obsessive compulsive disorders: A review of the literature. Am J Psychiatry 138:286–296, 1981
34. Sifneos P: Psychoanalytically oriented short term dynamic or anxiety producing psychotherapy for mild obsessional neurosis. Psychiatr Q 40:271–282, 1966
35. Steketee G, Foa E, Grayson JB: Recent advances in the behavioral treatment of obsessive-compulsives. Arch Gen Psychiatry 39:1365–1371, 1982
36. Jenicke M: Obsessive compulsive disorder. Compr Psychiatry 24:99–115, 1983
37. Insel TR, Murphy DL, Cohen RM et al: Obsessive compulsive disorder. Arch Gen Psychiatry 40:605–612, 1983

Somatoform and Factitious Disorders

The somatoform and factitious disorders are a group of behavioral disturbances in which persons speak not with feelings or words but with their bodies. In chronic hypochondriasis the disturbance involves a persistent mode of experiencing oneself and one's life and of relating to others through body symptoms. In contrast, the conversion reactions are sporadic, unconsciously determined symptomatic expressions of such communications. Then there are the malingerers, who consciously use real or feigned body symptoms to achieve defined and conscious but unexpressed wishes. Finally, there is that fascinating but indeterminant group of factitious disorders in which individuals more or less consciously feign illness or actively create even dangerous pathophysiologic disturbances to achieve ends of which they are only dimly aware and usually which are related to the wish to obtain the gratifications implicit in the sick role.

How does it come about that some people use such aberrant means of relating to the world? There are a number of ways of approaching this problem. Katon and his associates[1] propose an interesting idea about communication as it pertains to bodily symptoms although they limit their discussion to hypochondriasis. They suggest that the existence of psychological man—individuals who examine their states of feelings, their inner motivations, and their fantasies and who relate to the world through an understanding of the impact that the outer world has on their inner world—is a historically recent phenomenon and limited to Western society. The authors cite extensive evidence to indicate that in most non-Western societies individuals communicate inner distress by means of

bodily symptoms. Racy's[2] study of manifestations of depression in traditional Arab groups is illuminating. These patients presented with the classic somatic complaints of depression such as gastrointestinal symptoms, loss of appetite, and loss of weight but rarely were aware of guilt or self depreciation. As they became more westernized they began to describe mood changes characteristic of depression and similar to those changes found in Western society. This finding seems to be generally true in the non-Western world and extends to certain unsophisticated, rural, lower-class subcultures in the United States itself. Katon and associates[1] point out that most non-Western cultures influence the expression of depression in three major ways: (1) in many cultures there are no words to describe the affective state of depression adequately; (2) many cultures have strong sanctions against expressing painful feeling states like depression and anxiety and encourage the expression of inner distress through the presentation of somatic symptoms; and (3) in many cultures the affective state of depression has evil connotations and negative values attached to them, such that individuals are actively discouraged from describing anything but the somatic manifestations of painful affective states. Hence, the psychological description of internal distress may be more a Western aberration than a universal phenomenon.

Nonetheless, in the Occident these somatic expressions are deviations from the norm and require special explanation. Under what conditions does somatization "become a metaphor for personal distress" in our culture? Katon and associates' description of the non-Western patient is similar to that subsumed by the concept of alexithymia.

Alexithymia literally means the inability to put feelings into words. This concept was elaborated by Sifneos and Nemiah after the French psychosomaticians Marty and M'Uzan who called the phenomenon pensíe opératoire. These patients appear to be unable to describe their inner feeling states and are likely to infer that they are angry, for example, by noting that they are acting in an angry fashion. Their inner lives are empty, devoid of imaginative fantasy, and they tend to see and describe the world in concrete terms. Although this concept has been applied by Nemiah to the so-called psychosomatic diseases, it is my impression that it is much more consistently found in the somatoform disorders, with the exception of conversion phenomenon. Although Sifneos and Nemiah understand the origin of this phenomenon as a neurophysiologic defect, the thesis of Katon and associates suggests that cultural factors may be of predominant importance.

Psychoanalytic conceptualizations of the development of affect may also contribute to the understanding of these aberrations. Basch[3] takes note of Darwin's work on the phylogenetic origins of affect and presents data to suggest that infants are born with the biological capacity to express seven different affective states. Although these are primitive expressions, they act as important signals to guide the mother in response to the child. In an average "expectable" and healthy dyad, the mother, by responding appropriately to the infant's expression of affect, helps it to distinguish and define these varying affective states. With development they become labeled, more nuanced, and associated through memory traces with particular experiences that color them. In this way the child begins to define what he is feeling and as his verbal capacity increases to be able to describe these states in verbal terms. When the mother is incapable of appropriately interpreting these signals, either because of some defect in the child or because of some psychopathology of her own, a nondifferentiated inner state evolves in the child with confusion of feeling. A number of authors have described pathosis that relates to this phenomenon. Bruch describes mothers who respond to every signal from the child by feeding him. Such children have difficulty in distinguishing hunger from other painful affects and may be a subset of obese patients. Other authors have seen this a causal factor in schizophrenia. Munichin's "psychosomatic families" seem unable to differentiate feelings and intrapersonal and interpersonal conflicts. Members of these families tend to communicate through somatic symptoms. The somatization disorders may reflect early developmental abnormalities of this sort.

Cultural and social factors also play a role in structuring the families' reaction toward the expression of painful feelings and inner distress. Zborowski[4] has demonstrated that different cultural groups have different attitudes toward painful symptoms. Anglo-Saxons require stoicism and nonexpression of feeling, whereas Jewish and Italian groups are highly emotive, encourage the expression of such feelings, and demand relief of symptoms and an understanding of the causes of these symptoms, respectively. Mechanic has pointed out that family attitudes differ in the degree of sanction offered for the expression of these feelings in boys and girls.

The concept of the "sick role"[5] and "illness behavior"[6] also has pertinence to the somatization reactions. Parsons has conceptualized the sick role as follows: (1) the sick person is required to recognize that he is ill and relinquish his adult responsibility; (2) he is obliged to place himself in the hands of a caretaker and to obtain care, by implication, a sanction of regressive dependency; and (3) he is required to take on his former responsibilities when he regains his health. Relinquishment of responsibility and the expectation of care seem to be central features of the behavior of many patients with somatoform disorders. As long as they are designated as sick, they have no obligation to fulfill the third requirement of the sick role, to resume adult responsibilities. Although it is a matter of considerable dispute as to whether the assumption of the sick role is a primary motivation (primary gain) or a secondary motivation (secondary gain or adventitious extra gratification), it is apparent that aspects of the sick role are of critical importance in understanding the patient who somatizes.

The majority of these patients are seen by internists and are often resistant to psychiatric referral. Because they do not have disease in the usual sense and because their communication is so indirect and often tainted with manipulation, they are a source of great frustration to the treating physician. Almost by definition these patients "do not wish to become well." And yet, in one form or another, they constitute a high percentage of the practices of nonpsychiatric physicians and, as such, constitute an important public health problem. In many situations, the patterns manifested by these patients are so fixed that they are unmodifiable and the physician must change his goals and expectations. They resist psychiatric referral and even when they accept it their psychological incapacity makes them reluctant patients who reveal little about their inner states. Psychodynamic theories about the origin of these disorders are therefore highly speculative and often based on the unusual case.

Although absolute distinctions between these groups of disorders is not always easy, they will be discussed below in the categories suggested by the *Diagnostic and Statistical Manual of Mental Disorders (DSM-III)*. It is to be noted, however, that, as is the case with all of human behavior, the categories are not absolute and human behavior is often so richly varied as to defy them.

Conversion Disorder

Psychoanalysis was born with the discovery of the conversion reaction, but as interest turned from symptom neuroses to character disorders, attention to conversion waned. In the context of this transition, it became less the province of the psychoanalyst than that of the psychiatrist working in the general hospital. This change coincides with an important change in its epidemiology, namely, the fact that these phenomena are now observed more frequently in less sophisticated persons of lower social class origin. However, along with "Psychogenic Pain Disorder," a subcategory of conversion reactions in which pain is the symptom, they are unique in the *DSM-III* nomenclature in that etiologic considerations are included as diagnostic criteria and are psychological in origin.

The concept of conversion has undergone considerable modification through the years. Originally the term *conversion* was used synonymously with hysteria. Although Charcot demonstrated that these symptoms could be induced by suggestion, he viewed "hysteria" as a hereditary degenerative disease. It was Freud's work with Breuer that led to a new etiologic concept of "hysteria" in which traumatic factors of psychological origin were the etiologic causes. This was later changed to emphasize the role of intrapsychic conflict. Freud coined the term *conversion*, a step that would permit the ultimate dissociation between the symptom conversion and hysterical personality disorder.

Historically, it is to be noted that there have been three main modifications and clarifications of the concept of conversion over the past 80 years: (1) its differentiation from the "classic psychosomatic disorders"; (2) the modification of the view of the nature of the etiologic intrapsychic conflict; and (3) a tendency by some to view the unconscious moti-

vation of the conversion symptom as an attempt to communicate or to effect a change in the environment rather than as the product of an intrapsychic conflict. These historical modifications will be discussed below since they have pertinence to the manner in which the concept is used currently.

The *DSM-III* diagnostic criteria of conversion disorder (or hysterical neurosis, conversion type) are as follows:

1. The predominant disturbance is a loss of or alteration in physical functioning suggesting a physical disorder.
2. Psychological factors are judged to be etiologically involved in the symptom, as evidenced by one of the following:
   a. There is a temporal relationship between an environmental stimulus that is apparently related to a psychological conflict or need and the initiation or exacerbation of the symptom.
   b. The symptom enables the individual to get support from the environment that otherwise might not be forthcoming.
3. It has been determined that the symptom is not under voluntary control.
4. The symptom cannot, after appropriate investigation, be explained by a known physical disorder or pathophysiologic mechanism.
5. The symptom is not limited to pain or to a disturbance in sexual functioning.
6. Not due to somatization disorder or schizophrenia.

The classic definition of conversion is that of a symptom that is psychological in origin, reflective of an unconscious conflict, having no definable or clearly observable anatomic basis or physiologic change in function. The symptom reflects the fantasy of an unconscious conflict or its resolution. The original implication of the word *conversion* was that the symptom binds the psychic energy generated by the impulse in intrapsychic conflict by converting it into a disturbance of body functioning.

During the 1940s and 1950s, when Alexander was formulating his theories of psychosomatic medicine, it became important to distinguish between conversion reactions and the so-called classic psychosomatic disorders. Conversion disorders appeared to manifest themselves predominantly through the voluntary (sensorimotor) nervous system. They led to no immediate structural (tissue) changes, and there were no evident pathophysiological processes. Alexander hypothesized that certain diseases such as peptic ulcer, hypertension, and ulcerative colitis were the product of intrapsychic conflicts, with each conflict having a specific etiologic relationship to a particular disease. Important to this conceptualization was the idea that specific conflicts activated functional disturbances in the autonomic nervous system that led to symptoms and ultimately to structural change. The symptoms did not symbolically represent intrapsychic conflict in these diseases. This conceptualization led to a categorical distinction between conversion symptoms and "psychosomatic disease," the former involving the voluntary nervous system, the latter, the autonomic nervous system. This dichotomy was maintained in spite of the fact that it had been long known that conversion symptoms such as vomiting are mediated by autonomic function. Engel[7] resolved this dilemma by suggesting that any sensation in the body that achieves psychic representation including those generated by the autonomic nervous system can become the locus of a conversion symptom if it becomes secondarily associated with intrapsychic conflict even though the sensation originally had another origin. With the reactivation of the conflict, the body sensation and its physiologic substrate also became activated and come to represent the conflict symbolically. Hence intrapsychic conflict can activate the autonomic nervous system and lead not only to symptom formation but also to structural change. In particular, diseases related to allergic and immune functions, especially vascular and skin disorders, may be seen as conversion disorders and may represent etiologic links between intrapsychic conflict and physical disease. This is an area for future research.

The *DSM-III* etiologic criteria are not limited to intrapsychic conflict and include other unconscious motivations for the development of conversions. The manual notes that the symptom may enable the individual to avoid some activity that is noxious or may enable the individual to obtain support from the environment that might otherwise not be forthcoming. In traditional psychoanalytic thinking, this involves the distinction between primary and secondary gain. Primary gain is the gain of the symptom and implies that the symptom symbolically represents a compromise solution to the conflict. Secondary gain implies all the other advantages that accrue to the situation of being ill, such as dependency care, special consideration from others, and avoidance of adult responsibility. It remains to be determined whether this distinc-

tion is absolute and whether the primary motivation for the development of a conversion symptom can include interpersonal etiologies exclusive of intrapsychic conflict. Hollender has reinterpreted Freud and Breuer's case of Anna O. to suggest that Anna O.'s motivation for falling ill and maintaining her illness had much to do with the attention that she received from Breuer and the relief it afforded this imaginative woman who was leading a constricted, isolated, and tedious life.

EPIDEMIOLOGY AND INCIDENCE

Since conversion reactions vary from fleeting and unrecognized reactions to chronic and severely disabling disorders, it is difficult to determine their incidence and distribution. Definitive diagnosis is difficult, and some studies have reported that as many as 50% of patients who presented with disturbances of the voluntary nervous system diagnosed as conversion ultimately were determined to have neurologic abnormalities. Moreover, many patients with neurologic disorders have conversion reactions as well.

An important theme that had dominated the literature has been the relationship between conversion disorder and hysterical personality style. In the 19th century, these patients were regularly called hysterics and were considered to be highly suggestible. In the past few decades it has become apparent that conversion reaction occurs in a wide variety of personality types and is not limited to histrionic personality disorder.[8] It also occurs in all of the major psychotic disorders and frequently accompanies physical illness, particularly neurologic disorders.

Conversion is not uniquely a disorder of women, as was previously thought, but is probably more common in women. It is important to distinguish conversion from Briquet's syndrome, which is diagnosed predominantly in woman. There is some disagreement in the literature as to whether the incidence of conversion has diminished over the past century. It seems apparent that the most flagrant conversion symptoms previously evident in the upper middle class society of Freudian Vienna are now rare, but they are frequently observed in less educated populations of rural areas and inner city emergency rooms. It is not clear whether Engel is correct in inferring that subtle conversion symptoms, difficult to diagnose, afflict the urban middle class population.

The overall incidence of conversion reaction is

difficult to determine because of the variety of its manifestations, the different settings in which it is observed, and the fact that many of these patients do not reach psychiatrists and are treated for physical symptomatology. Engel[9] estimates that there is a 20% to 25% life time incidence of conversion symptoms. Various studies have reported that anywhere from 5% to 16% of consultations done on consultation-liaison services involve the diagnosis and management of conversion reactions. In an early study, Ljungberg[10] reports a 0.5% incidence in the general population of Sweden. The confusion of hysteria and Briquet's syndrome with conversion disorder and the fact that many apparent conversion reactions are ultimately determined to be of organic origin make it difficult to interpret the early reports on incidence and prevalence.

This is compounded by uncertainty of diagnosis and the wide variety of symptoms being evaluated. Watson and Buranen[11] report that the most common manifestations of conversion are non-headache pain, dizziness, weakness, headache, and nausea. This contrasts to the dramatic symptoms such as blindness, mutism, tics, and so on reported in most textbooks.

CLINICAL DESCRIPTION

Attitude Toward Disability

Patients with conversion symptoms tend to describe these symptoms in unusually rich and dramatic ways. They often will elaborate endlessly on the symptom that becomes a primary focus in their lives. The language they use may be highly suggestive of the unconscious meanings that underlie the symptoms. For example, a patient preoccupied with painful sensations may describe the pain as stabbing, shearing, or annoying, if anger appears to be an important unconscious element.

In spite of the rather flamboyant and extremely elaborate descriptions of their symptoms, patients with conversion disorders often seem inappropriately unconcerned about the potential threat of these symptoms to their life and physical well-being. This has been described in the early French literature as *la belle indifférence*. This is a frequent, but not absolute characteristic of conversion reactions. This indifference often extends to the implications of the symptom as it relates to the disruptions that ensue in their life activities. In cases of persistent chronic conversion, the symptom and the ensuing disability become the central focus of their lives and their *raison d'être*.

Somatic Compliance

Conversion reactions tend to crystallize in areas of the body that have been previously afflicted by physical disease or have been the focus of special attention. It is as if these bodily parts lend themselves to utilization by the conversion symptom for the expression of an unconscious intrapsychic conflict.

Freud noted that the site of a conversion reaction may be established by contiguity as well as by symbolization. The former implies that a body part or sensation can come to represent the conflict if by chance it is the focus of attention at the time the conflict emerges.

Hysterical Identification

The conversion symptom frequently patterns itself after a symptom observed in some other person. The identification with this other person is facilitated by the recognition of a similar motivation inferred in the person who originally experienced the symptom. Freud,[12] in an amusing example, describes how a young girl in an all girls' school swooned upon receiving a love letter from her boyfriend. Within a day, an epidemic of swooning developed in the school, presumably based on the wish of the other girls to receive similar letters. Dramatic examples of the development of conversion symptoms occur not infrequently after the death of a person with whom the patient had a highly ambivalent relationship.

In eliciting a history in patients thought to have conversion reactions, it is important to determine whether other important people in their lives have had similar disturbances in bodily functioning. An examination of the nature of the previous relationship often reveals important data about the motivations for the development of the symptom.

The Phenomenology of Conversion

Detailed descriptions of the phenomenology of conversion reaction have been published by Walsh,[13] Woolsey,[14] and Weintraub.[15] Characteristic is the fact that they do not follow anatomic or functional patterns that would be anticipated by a knowledge of pathophysiology. These will be briefly summarized to offer the reader a sense of how such discriminations are made.

CONVULSIONS. Walshe[13] offers an excellent description of the conversion fit:

There is no ordered sequence of events, there is no true loss of consciousness, there are no changes in the reflexes, no incontinence or tongue biting, and the patient does not sustain injuries in his fall, nor fall in a dangerous place. The eyes are not passively closed as in true coma, but shut, and the attempt to open them with the finger is usually met with a tightening of the lids. The convulsion is not a matter of tonic and clonic stages but a wild struggling, which is aggravated by attempts at restraint . . . The hysterical fit may appear to last for hours, phases of apparent unconscious swooning intermitting with the phases of violent activity.

Individuals with conversion seizures not infrequently have true epilepsy (somatic compliance) and are often responsive to the environment during seizures.

SENSORY DISTURBANCES. Sensory disturbances are inconsistent with the anatomic patterns expected on a basis of our current understanding of nervous system function. The boundaries of the affected area are sharply defined, usually at gross anatomic areas such as foot, knee, or hand. Often all sensory modalities (touch, pain, temperature, and position sense) will be affected at the same level, whereas spinal cord lesions are likely to involve unique sensory modalities and, if multiple modalities are affected, to manifest disturbances at different levels. The patterns of sensory disturbance vary at different moments of testing. In conversion, loss of vibration sense maintains a strict midline separation in spite of the fact that vibrations are normally perceived on the ipsilateral side through bone conduction.

A hemisensory loss, including all modalities of hearing, vision and taste, may occur as a conversion reaction. The patient will be able to perform a finger-to-nose test accurately with his eyes closed in spite of an apparent disturbance in position sense. Sensory disturbances are often associated with disturbances in the motor system. Patients who have bilateral conversion blindness negotiate their environment reasonably well. They do not walk into obstacles and may be able to reach out accurately for objects. They are likely to have tracking responses to a rotating drum. Less complete visual impairment occurs in conversion with narrowing of the visual fields and tunnel vision. In unilateral blindness of a conversion origin the direct pupillary response in the affected eye is intact. Patients with conversion aphonia are likely to be able to whisper intelligibly.

MOTOR DISTURBANCES. Conversion reactions may manifest themselves as paraplegias, hemiple-

gias, or monoplegias. The affected limb tends to be flaccid but may be easily lifted by the examiner and will fall less heavily when dropped than with organic disturbances. Reflexes are generally intact and no Babinsky reflex is present. Inconsistencies in muscle strength are to be noted and on examination, when the patient is asked to lift the sound limb, the heel of the paralyzed limb can be felt to press down on the observer's hand. On examination the antagonistic muscles of the afflicted limb will contract when the limb is moved in the opposite direction. Weakness in conversion reactions more often appears in the proximal muscles than in the distal ones. Hence, in a hemiplegic conversion reaction, the patient will drag his leg behind him rather than swing it in a circumduction. Tremors in conversion reactions tend to be gross rather than fine and are likely to disappear at rest.

INVOLVEMENT OF THE AUTONOMIC NERVOUS SYSTEM. Engel[7] proposed that the autonomic nervous system may be the site of conversion symptoms. Recurrent vomiting that is not self induced may represent a conversion symptom and, according to Engel, certain skin lesions and allergic conditions may also involve conversion mechanisms.

What characterizes conversion reactions is their extraordinary variability. Fleeting conversion reactions have a higher incidence than is generally noted. Extensive and disabling conversion reactions are frequently observed on neurologic wards. Patients with the best prognosis have good object relations, minimal psychopathology and live in stable environments. Recent symptoms associated with definable emotional conflict and precipitating events suggest better outcome.

Slater[16] reports that 50% of patients are free of symptoms after 1 year but that 20% retain them for 15 years or more. Carter's[17] study indicates that 83% are well or improved at 4 to 6 years. It should be noted that severely disabling conversion symptoms that persist for a significant length of time have a poor prognosis and are likely to lead to permanent total disability.

ETIOLOGY

Although there is a general agreement about the psychological origin of conversion disorders, there are differences of opinion as to whether the conversion phenomenon reflects predominantly an intrapsychic conflict, an interpersonal communication, or behavior unconsciously motivated to obtain gratification from the environment. These views are complementary. The symptoms occur in a wide variety of people at different times of their lives, and there is no uniformity in developmental history or early family environment. There is some evidence to suggest that a certain percentage of patients with conversion seizures may have been the objects of childhood incest.

Psychodynamic Hypothesis

Freud's first traumatic theory of neuroses presumed that hysterics (at this point not differentiated from patients with conversion reactions) were the passive victims of childhood parental incest. The traumatic theory of neuroses rapidly gave way to the instinctual theory of motivation, and it was postulated that conflicted infantile wishes led to conversion. Freud's interest in symptom choice led him to the conclusion that hysterical patients were fixated at the phallic-genital level of development, that they used denial and repression, and that the threat of castration was the danger situation associated with the disorder. Gradually, it became apparent that symptom choice could not be so precisely defined. The personality structure of patients with conversion reactions was noted to be more primitive than originally assumed. The current view is that conflict may be related to unconscious sexual wishes, dependency wishes, and aggressive impulses. Often the symptom itself represents a punishment for a prohibited aggressive or sexual wish.

Interpersonal Communication and Psychosocial Adaptation

With increasing recognition of oral dependent characteristics of many patients who experience conversion reactions, there has been a renewed focus on the use of the conversion symptom to effect a dependency adaptation and to obtain attention. In the psychodynamic framework this behavior is considered the secondary gain of illness. Clearly immature, dependent individuals find in their symptom a powerful and coercive weapon to influence their environment. Helplessness can be used to control doctors and family.

Engel's[18] complementary categorization of the multiple motivations underlying a conversion reaction is most useful. The motivations are to permit the expression of an unconscious and forbidden wish; to achieve punishment for such a wish; to remove the person from a threatening life situation; and to offer a new mode of relating to others. The degree of inference required to assess the motivations of individual patients will vary depending

on the personality structure, intelligence, and psychological capacity of the patient.

DIAGNOSIS AND DIFFERENTIAL DIAGNOSIS

The history is of central importance in the diagnosis of conversion reactions. The patient, unaware of his unconscious conflicts or the special meanings of his symptom, must be questioned carefully about the context in which the symptom developed. Detailed inquiry about the events of the day and associated fleeting fantasies considered in the light of the patient's history will often suggest possible motivations for the development of the symptom. The patients's affect should be noted as the story emerges, and areas of potential conflict should be pursued. The history should include information about the patient's relationship with individuals who have similar symptoms (hysterical identification) and inquiries should be made about previous afflictions at the site of the conversion symptom (somatic compliance). Determination of what activities or responsibilities become impossible because of the symptom are often revealing. *La belle indifference* may be helpful but is not a dependable indicator of the presence of the conversion reaction.

Conversion reactions must be differentiated from organic disease. Careful physical examination is indicated. The details of differentiation between neurologic disease and conversion reactions have been described previously. Ancillary evaluative procedures, such as electroencephalograms for epilepsy or evoked potentials in the cases of conversion blindness, should be done. Sodium amobarbital (Amytal) interviews will often reveal new motivational material, particularly data about intrapsychic conflict, and symptoms may disappear with suggestion and encouragement.

TREATMENT

Many conversion reactions are fleeting and require no treatment. When a conversion symptom becomes consolidated, treatment should be active and rapid. Chronicity of symptoms often leads to intractable disability. Mature, psychologically minded individuals with significant conflict should be referred for intensive psychotherapy. In acute crisis, active engagement of the patient may be useful. A warm, affirmative, and reassuring attitude by the physician, with an explanation of the symptom, and strong suggestion that the symptom will resolve is often useful. Mild sedation may be helpful. Behavioral techniques and biofeedback may be useful and should be recommended in an affirmative and suggestive way so that the magical authority of the physician is brought into play. In the acute situations parenteral diazepam (Valium) may be useful in demonstrating to the patient that the symptom can be relieved.

Psychogenic Pain Disorder

The "Psychogenic Pain Disorder" has emerged as a new diagnostic heading in the *DSM-III*. It is the analog of the conversion disorder but limited to pain as a symptom. Although it has only recently achieved separate diagnostic respectability, it was described in a classic paper by Engel,[18] to which repeated reference will be made in this discussion. Theories of pain, acute pain, or chronic benign, or malignant pain of known source will not be included.

DEFINITION

The *DSM-III* criteria for psychogenic pain disorder are as follows:

---

1. Severe and prolonged pain is the predominant disturbance.
2. The pain presented as a symptom is inconsistent with the anatomic distribution of the nervous system; after extensive evaluation, no organic pathology or pathophysiologic mechanism can be found to account for the pain; or, when there is some related organic pathology, the complaint of pain is grossly in excess of what would be expected from the physical findings.
3. Psychological factors are judged to be etiologically involved in the pain, as evidenced by at least one of the following:
   a. A temporal relationship between an environmental stimulus that is apparently related to a psychological conflict or need and the initiation or exacerbation of the pain
   b. The pain's enabling the individual to avoid some activity that is noxious to him or her
   c. The pain's enabling the individual to get support from the environment that otherwise might not be forthcoming
4. Not due to another mental disorder

EPIDEMIOLOGY

Devine and Merskey[19] found pain a predominant symptom in 137 of 182 consecutive general medical patients. Seventy-five percent of those with pain had no discernable organic disease. There is a high incidence of alcoholism and depression in the families of these patients, a finding not surprising since psychological testing often reveals "masked depression."[20] The disorder may be more common in women. A large sample presenting to a neurosurgical division[21] were individuals of lower middle class families who had begun work at a very early age and had stoically continued to work until their illness became manifest.

CLINICAL DESCRIPTION

The clinical description will address itself to two main issues: (1) the way in which these patients describe their pain and (2) their overt personality characteristics.

Pain Description

Pain generated by organic disease usually has well-defined characteristics relating to site, quality, and variation in intensity of symptom. The diagnosis of coronary disease, cholecystitis, renal colic, and so on usually is facilitated by a characteristic description of the pain. In most cases of psychogenic pain disorder, the description of the pain does not conform to the pattern characteristic of a particular disease. In some cases, patients may imitate the patterns of others with known disease. Psychogenic pain patients tend to describe their pain as of the highest intensity, often only partially relieved by strong analgesics, with very little variation through the day and not subject to changes in position or other influences. The pain is overwhelming, unrelieved, and a source of constant preoccupation. They describe it as something that prevents them from sleeping rather than as something that awakens them. The anatomic area affected by the pain tends to be wide and often extremely variable. The rich description of the pain often reveals its unconscious meaning. It may be described as stabbing, jabbing, "like someone jumping up and down upon me," burning and twisting, or biting or tearing. These descriptions reflect underlying aggressive content. The described intensity of the pain seems inconsistent with the minimal distress that is apparent as the patient tells his story. With encouragement the patient is likely to amplify the description with more florid adjectives. There is often a history of extensive use of medications, including analgesics, muscle relaxants, and antianxiety agents, without success. The patients complain of sleeping poorly. Multiple previous surgical interventions have resulted in little or temporary relief, but the patient will often press for further surgical intervention.[21] Frequently they describe close friends or family members with similar pain disturbances.

Personality Characteristics

No single personality constellation can adequately encompass the entire group of pain-prone patients. However, the group studied by Blumer and Heilbron[21] showed a remarkable uniformity in their personality presentations. All of their patients idealized their relationships with others and appeared to present "supernormal pictures of mental health." They were stoic, action oriented, and over controlled—two thirds had never lost control of their tempers. They were hard workers who had worked since adolescence and made strong efforts to conceal interpersonal and intrapsychic conflict.

A substantial number of these patients have the characteristics of what has been described as alexithymia. They are devoid of fantasy, are unaware of their feelings, seem incapable of introspection, and describe their lives in concrete terms. History taking designed to elicit areas of conflict is frustrating, and the patient prefers to offer detailed descriptions of his pain. A variant of this is the histrionic personality who reveals considerable affect although he dissociates the pain from emotional events.

The outlook for this disorder is poor. If untreated, these patients persist with severe and often debilitating pain and are unable to work. They seek some immediate concrete treatment for their disorder, particularly repeated surgical interventions. The pressure on physicians to offer narcotics is great, and frequently they become addicted to narcotic analgesics.

ETIOLOGY

The psychogenic pain disorders are, by definition, of emotional origin, although the focus of the pain may have originated in a defined physical disease. The psychodynamic, psychosocial, and interpersonal considerations described for conversion disorder apply to this group as well. However, certain consistent developmental and psychodynamic constellations characterize the group.

Developmental considerations that pertain to the meaning of pain in childhood may be helpful in understanding the use of pain in these patients. Pain is an organizer of body image and is an impor-

tant factor in the development of self–object differentiation.[22] The experience of pain in the child becomes an indication of danger and the threat of bodily damage. As such it becomes a focus in the relationship with a comforting mother, and the association of pain with obtaining comfort from a maternal object may be established. Pain may be perceived as a punishment for the expression of forbidden sexual and aggressive wishes, and therefore may be a product of guilt over the expression of these wishes. In some types of masochism, for example, pain becomes the contingent requirement for the expression of forbidden sexual and aggressive impulses. The association is established thereby between pain, sexuality, aggression, and guilt—all of which are related to psychogenic pain disorders.

Engel[18] has spelled out some of the elements present in the developmental history of patients with this disorder:

> Suffice it to say that we often find that aggression, suffering and pain played an important role in the early family relationships. These may include: (1) parents, one or both of whom were physically or verbally abusive to each other and or to the child; (2) one brutal parent and one submissive parent, the former sometimes an alcoholic father; (3) a parent who punished frequently but then suffered remorse and overcompensated with a rare display of affection, so that the child became accustomed to the sequence; pain and suffering gained love; (4) a parent who was cold and distant, but who responded more when the child was ill or suffering pain, even to the point that the child invited injury to elicit response from the parent; (5) the child who had a parent or other close figure who suffered illness or pain for which he came to feel in some way responsible and guilty, most commonly because of aggressive impulses, acts or fantasies; (6) the child who was aggressive or hurting until some event suddenly forced an abandonment of such behavior, usually with much guilt; (7) the child who deflected the aggression of a parent away from the other parent or a sibling onto himself, usually an early manifestation of guilt.

The strong masochistic tendencies associated with guilt often lead to the development of symptoms when some burden in life is relieved. Pain as a reflection of an aberrant grief response suggests a highly ambivalent relationship with the lost object. The arousal of any forbidden aggressive impulse may proceed the onset of pain.

Pain as a signal of distress becomes a communication likely to evoke a nurturent response from the environment. A concerned and responsive family may share the patient's frustration and anger at the medical establishment that seems unable or unwilling to help. Alternately the patient's pain may reflect past and present deprivation and may evoke hostile responses from the family.

DIAGNOSIS AND DIFFERENTIAL DIAGNOSIS

As is the case of the conversion disorder, the diagnosis should be made if at all possible by eliciting details of the patient's past life and current onset situation that suggest the presence of conflict and its expression through pain.

Certain principles in approaching the patient are important. The psychiatrist should be introduced directly by the referring physician, and he should be presented as part of a team. The interview should begin by obtaining a careful, detailed history of the pain in all of its ramifications so that the patient understands that the psychiatrist believes the pain is genuine. He should convey the sense that he has no preconceived notion as to the origin of the pain. This should be followed by an exploration of the patient's history and current life situation.

An important problem in the differential diagnosis of patients with psychogenic pain disorder involves the determination of whether there is a defined, organic source of pain that is treatable. This may be especially complicated because the disorder may evolve after a physical illness. Frequent operations complicate the clinical picture. Abdominal surgery in particular may result in adhesions that lead to pain.

Patients with psychogenic pain disorder have in addition a wide spectrum of Axis I and Axis II diagnoses although their Axis II diagnosis includes mixed personality features with masochistic and immature traits predominating.

TREATMENT

With rare exception, insight-oriented therapy is of little value with such patients. Supportive therapy can be of value in those patients with less impairment in their object relations. The therapist must emphasize his acceptance of the "genuineness" of the pain and it may be useful to convey to the patient that any pain, even pain with a very precise peripheral origin, will vary significantly depending on the degree of attention to it and the special circumstances surrounding its exacerbation. I frequently comment to patients on Beecher's observation of how severely wounded soldiers in war time experienced little pain because of the relief generated by the awareness that the wound would remove them from the life-threatening battle situation. It should be emphasized to the patient that considerable time will be required before the pain can be diminished and that careful observation of the physical status of the patient will continue so as to be sure that no threatening pathology will be overlooked. Biofeedback may be a useful adjunct because it offers a changed focus of attention and some sense of control. Referral to a multidisciplinary pain center may be helpful. Pinsky[23] found that group therapy with other pain patients can lead to pain reduction as well as improvement in psychosocial functioning. Conjoint family therapy is indicated when the pain syndrome becomes an important systems problem in the family.

Hypochondriasis

Hypochondriasis has been observed since the beginning of civilization. Aristotle described it, Galen commented on it, and Burton wrote an extensive treatise about it in 1651. It was described in 1733 by Cheyne as "the English malady," and Boswell wrote at least four essays associating melancholy with hypochondriasis, a theme that has persisted to modern times. Molière immortalized the hypochondriac in *La Malade Imaginaire* and, ironically, died playing the role of the protagonist Aragon. Gillespie, in the late 1920s, offered a rich description of the syndrome and separated it from other psychiatric entities. Psychoanalysts have shown some interest in this disorder, although most of these patients are unanalyzable. Freud first viewed it as an actual neurosis associated with anxiety neurosis, neurasthenia, and melancholia. In the Schreber case he related it to paranoia and later, with the development of the concept of narcissism, interpreted hypochondriasis as a reflection of the decathexis of objects and the return of object libido onto the ego with cathexis of the body. These three themes, namely, the association with depression, with paranoia, and with disturbed object relations, remain important themes in the current conceptualization of hypochondriasis.

DEFINITION

The following are the *DSM-III* diagnostic criteria for hypochondriasis:

1. The predominant disturbance is an unrealistic interpretation of physical signs or sensations as abnormal, leading to preoccupation with the fear or belief of having a serious disease.
2. Thorough physical evaluation does not support the diagnosis of any physical disorder that can account for the physical signs or sensations or for the individual's unrealistic interpretation of them.
3. The unrealistic fear or belief of having a disease persists despite medical reassurance and causes impairment in social or occupational functioning.
4. The disorder is not due to any other mental disorder such as schizophrenia, affective disorder, or somatization disorder.

The diagnostic criteria as stated well encompass the special criteria for hypochondriasis. Important are the presence of bodily symptoms without organic cause, the intense preoccupation with such symptoms, and the general failure of the patient to respond to reassurance.

One must distinguish between first, hypochondriasis as a chronic adaptation to life closely allied with personality and, second, acute hypochondriacal reactions that occur in the context of acute stress, such as the death of a loved one or rejection. Another common group of situational hypochondriacal reactions is found among medical students and house staff. Although some argue that significant pathology characterizes this group, it is my impression that these reactions are generally amenable to reassurance or brief psychotherapy.

In addition to the group of chronic hypochondriacs, it is important to separate what Strain[24] calls the "pseudohypochondriasis of old age."

EPIDEMIOLOGY

As is the case with the other somatoform disorders, statistics on the incidence and distribution of hypochondriasis present many problems. Apart from differences of view with regard to diagnosis, sample selection has been a major problem. The majority of such patients are never seen by psychiatrists, and those who are, probably represent a special subset. Much more is known about the frequency of nonorganic somatic symptoms in various medical care facilities. It has been reported that in primary care facilities anywhere from 68% to 92% of people are without serious physical disease. The incidence of hypochondriasis in the general population has been estimated at from 4% to 14%. Although the figures are quite unreliable, it is clear that hypochondriasis is a major public health problem that places significant demands on health care facilities.

Age at onset is generally considered to be early, often in childhood and adolescence. The sex difference is equally unclear. Tradition has it that conversion reactions were the province of women and hypochondriasis the equivalent in men. Kenyon,[25] in an extensive review of the literature, indicates that the majority of writers consider hypochondriasis a male condition, although more recent writers have contested this. Obviously, much depends on how one views somatization disorder (Briquet's syndrome), which is considered to occur predominantly in women. Broad surveys have indicated that it is more common in lower social classes and certainly in the elderly, where it is commonly the presenting symptom of depression.

CLINICAL DESCRIPTION

The typical hypochondriac assaults the physician with a complex and detailed chronologic history of multiple symptoms that he is convinced have an organic basis. Often obsessional in style, the patient will consult his notes and may even present a written outline. The symptoms evoke considerable anxiety, and the patient is insistent on proper diagnosis and treatment because he is fearful that the "disease" is dangerous and potentially life threatening. His presentation of symptoms is pressured and he is often impatient as the physician attempts to interrupt or crystallize his own view of the difficulty. The focus is on symptomatology and its implications, and the patient is disinclined to offer any psychosocial data. Questions about his life situation are usually viewed as irrelevant distractions and unless tactfully presented confirm his view that the physician is unlikely to take his symptoms seriously. He is presenting himself to the physician for the cure of a physical malady.

As the history unfolds, it becomes apparent that the symptoms dominate the patient's life and are the center of an intense preoccupation. The patient expects that others will afford him the gratification of the sick role, namely a release from responsibility and an expectation of care, and he becomes angry when these demands are not met. The designation of narcissistic self-involvement is not ill placed.

Although studies have indicated that the areas of symptomatology pertain particularly to the gastrointestinal tract, the musculoskeletal system, and the central nervous system, the symptom complexes often change. The symptoms themselves do not have primary symbolic meaning.

ETIOLOGY

There are multiple models for the understanding of hypochondriasis, some of which have been elaborated by Barsky and Klerman.[26]

Hypochondriasis as a Result of a Perceptual or Cognitive Abnormality

Barsky and Klerman present the thesis that hypochondriasis may be a product of a perceptual or cognitive abnormality. This issue has been addressed in the introduction to this chapter in a discussion of the work of Katon and his collaborators,[1] who suggest that communication of distress through somatic symptoms is characteristic of non-Western cultures. In our culture hypochondriasis could be viewed as a developmental abnormality reflective of a psychopathologic interaction with the mother who does not help the developing child to define and label constitutionally given feeling states and thereby encourages the expression of psychological distress by somatic means. This conceptualization is closely related to the concept of alexithymia, which characterizes many hypochondriacs.

However, Barsky and Klerman define this category in a way that poses logical problems. They suggest that hypochondriacal patients may amplify normal body sensations or misinterpret bodily sensations of normal intensity. In view of the fact that bodily sensations are entirely subjective phenomena, it is unclear how one could experimentally determine whether either of these hypotheses are correct. Experiments that involve measurements of response to external stimuli cannot reproduce subjective states. Hypochondriacal patients are misinterpreting internal stimuli by definition. Although one can roughly measure intensity of subjective reports, it would appear impossible to measure intensity of internal stimuli objectively.

Social Learning Theories

Social learning theories are complementary to psychodynamic developmental theories of hypochondriasis. They focus heavily on the rewards that ensue from the "sick role" and the particular modes of child–caretaker interactions that occur early in

life. Clearly, parents who are excessively concerned about the dangers of injury and illness in childhood and are excessively responsive to minor illnesses and complaints are likely to engender similar anxieties in children, which may become translated into adult hypochondriacal behavior. Parents indifferent to the emotional needs of their children and inclined to respond predominantly when the child is physically ill inevitably teach the child that physical symptomatology will be a vehicle for care when emotional distress is ignored. Special life experiences also may play a role. The presence of a sick sibling or parent in the household and the special attention directed toward this person may leave the child feeling deprived and invested in obtaining similar ministrations. Zborowski's study of different cultural attitudes toward illness and pain has been discussed previously.

Disturbed Object Relations

Freud's view that hypochondriasis is a reflection of narcissism and disturbed object relations appears to have considerable merit. These patients are intensely preoccupied with themselves, relate to others through their symptoms, and have marked defects in empathetic capacity that lead to shallow interpersonal relationships. Their developmental histories reveal a general lack of awareness of their emotional needs by caretaking figures.

Aggression and Masochism

Brown and Vaillant[27] define hypochondriasis as "the transformation of reproaches toward others arising from bereavement, loneliness or unacceptable aggressive impulses first into self-reproach and then complaints to others of pain or somatic illness. In lieu of open complaining that others have ignored or hurt him, the hypochondriac settles on belaboring those present with his genuinely felt, but misplaced, bodily pains, or discomforts." The authors' contention that hypochondriacal complaints are reproaches against others is suggested by the intense hostility generated in others by the constant complaints. This constellation may be viewed as a manifestation of projective identification in which the patient first projects his own anger onto another person who introjects the angry part of the patient and who in turn becomes angry and treats the patient in an angry way. In response to the anger and ensuing deprivation the patient gratifies masochistic needs related to guilt about his own anger. Myers[28] has described masochism and the presence of beating fantasies in hypochondriacal patients.

Pathology Rooted in Conflict versus Self-Pathology

Anna Freud[29] described bodily preoccupation in motherless, institutionalized children. She stated "the child actually deprived of the mother's care adopts the mother's role in health matters, thus playing 'mother and child' with his own body." "What child analytic studies seems to make clear is that in the staging of the mother-child relationship, they themselves identify with the lost mother, while the body represents the child (more exactly, the infant in the mother's care)." It appears that these patients care for their bodies as they hoped that their mothers would have cared for them both emotionally and physically. Kohut[30] proposed that hypochondriacal anxiety reflects a regressive reactivation of anxiety about disintegration, a dread of the loss of the self that cannot be verbalized, a "fragmentation of and the estrangement of the body and mind in space, the breakup of the sense of continuity and time." Richards[31] argues that this conceptualization is unnecessary and describes the analysis of a patient whose hypochondriasis was understood in traditional conflictual terms.

Unfortunately, these contrasting psychoanalytic views of hypochondriasis cannot be easily generalized or verified because the vast population of patients are unsuited for exploratory psychotherapy or psychoanalysis. Those patients actually analyzed are probably an unrepresentative subset of hypochondriacal patients. The vast majority of these patients have a poverty of affective experience, an emptiness in their inner lives, and a shallowness in their relations with others, both past and present.

Depression

There appears to be good evidence that the symptoms of some hypochondriacal patients reflect the vegetative signs of a depression without obvious mood change. Pilowsky[32] distinguish primary and secondary hypochondriasis, the former a pure state of hypochondriasis, the latter a reflection of an underlying, "masked depression." Two of the largest studies differentiating primary and secondary hypochondriasis[32,33] appear to demonstrate that there is a subgroup of hypochondriacs who have significant degrees of depression and anxiety and are effectively treated by antidepressants.

DIAGNOSIS AND DIFFERENTIAL DIAGNOSIS

Hypochondriasis is relatively easy to diagnose. The physician must be aware of the possibility of concurrent organic disease that is readily overlooked. Depression should be considered in patients with psychomotor and vegetative signs.

The *DSM-III* diagnosis excludes the diagnosis of hypochondriasis in the presence of a definite diagnosis of affective disorder or schizophrenia. This blurs the concept of secondary hypochondriasis as a manifestation of depression. A rigidly held belief of a bizarre nature about the interior workings of the body or of bodily disintegration suggests somatic delusions and a psychotic process. If pain is the predominant symptom, psychogenic pain disorder should be considered. Conversion reactions tend to be focal and relatively constant and may be accompanied by *la belle indifference*.

The pseudohypochondriasis of the aged must be differentiated from hypochondriasis *per se*. Aging is often accompanied by an increased preoccupation with the body, particularly in the context of a constricted social world accompanied by personal loss. Such patients seek help and reassurance from physicians but unlike the true hypochondriac they are appreciative and responsive to reassurance that no serious illness exists. Depression frequently presents as hypochondriacal symptoms in the aged, and the physician should be alert to this diagnosis.

Bishop[34] outlines three categories of monosystematic hypochondriasis: (1) delusions of parasitosis (the belief that one is infested with vermin); (2) dysmorphal phobia (the belief that one is physically misshapen and unattractive); and (3) reference syndrome (the belief that one emits an offensive body odor). Although these conditions are well defined, they are rare, specific, and not truly encompassed by the general term *hypochondriasis*.

TREATMENT

With the rare exception of those patients who have some degree of psychological mindedness, any insight-oriented approach is unlikely to be accepted by the patient and, if accepted, to succeed. The hypochondriacal patient is best treated by a patient and caring internist who is aware of the limitations of what he can do and intent on management of the disorder rather than cure. Such a treatment must be of long duration. The physician offers an object relationship, limited but durable over time in which the currency is a discussion of the patient's symptoms. This gratifies the isolated patient's need for a relationship on terms that he can accept. Gentle inquiries about the patient's psychosocial situation may be helpful in an exploratory way and occasionally after long periods of time cautious interpretations and connections of conflicts to symptoms may be made. The physician must commiserate with the patient's misery and convey his admiration for the patient's forebearance and capacity to tolerate suffering.

When available, an "integration clinic"[35] where the psychiatrist works in a medical setting, acting as both a consultant and a therapist, can be useful. Antidepressants are indicated if there is evidence of an underlying affective disorder. Other medications should be avoided if at all possible. There have been some reports of success with group therapy for some hypochondriacal patients. These groups provide a structure for social interaction and encourage relatedness.

Briquet's Syndrome

The designation somatization disorder as a separate diagnostic entity occurs for the first time in the *DSM-III*. However, the description of the disorder has a long history enmeshed in all of the other syndromes included under the designation of somatoform disorders. It began to emerge as a designated syndrome in 1951 with the work of Purtell and his associates[36] and was given credibility as a separate diagnostic category in 1962 by Purley and Guze.[37] The latter group has continued to elaborate its descriptive diagnostic criteria and has shown its epidemiologic relationship to alcoholism and sociopathy.

Of special interest is Briquet's monograph on the subject.[38] Briquet formulated a psychogenic hypothesis of the disorder in susceptible personalities and emphasized that the physical symptoms had no organic basis. His hypothesis was that this was a traumatic neurosis with repeated subsequent trauma involving cognitive and affective elements. This hypothesis had some similarity to Breuer and Freud's concept of retention hysteria. The personality characteristics of these women, for in Briquet's large sample there was a ratio of women to men of 20:1, resembles the histrionic personality described in the *DSM-III*. Briquet described cases of hysteria in men, disputed Sydenham's hypothesis that hysteria was limited to women and hypochondriasis to men and eliminated female genital difficulties as the etiology. His view was concordant with an earlier view of Whytt, described in 1764, that ideas or emotions could create bodily changes. It is not without irony that Briquet's name should be attached to a purely phenomenologic entity when his original treatise involved the subtle and nuanced development of a biopsychosocial model

for this disorder. Also noteworthy is the fact that many of Briquet's patients had symptoms that would be more readily classified today as conversion disorders. Breuer and Freud's[39] early case of Anna O. descriptively could be called Briquet's syndrome.

DEFINITION

The *DSM-III* diagnostic criteria for somatization disorder are as follows:

> 1. A history of physical symptoms of several years' duration beginning before the age of 30
> 2. Complaints of at least 14 symptoms for women and 12 for men, from the 37 symptoms listed below. To count a symptom as present the individual must report that the symptom caused him or her to take medicine (other than aspirin), alter his or her life pattern, or see a physician. The symptoms, in the judgment of the clinician, are not adequately explained by physical disorder or physical injury and are not side-effects of medication, drugs or alcohol. The clinician need not be convinced that the symptom was actually present (*e.g.*, that the individual actually vomited throughout her entire pregnancy); report of the symptom by the individual is sufficient.
>   *Sickly:* believes that he or she has been sickly for a good part of his or her life.
>   *Conversion or pseudoneurological symptoms:* difficulty swallowing, loss of voice, deafness, double vision, blurred vision, blindness, fainting or loss of consciousness, memory loss, seizures or convulsions, trouble walking, paralysis or muscle weakness, urinary retention or difficulty urinating.
>   *Gastrointestinal symptoms:* abdominal pain, nausea, vomiting spells (other than during pregnancy), bloating (gassy), intolerance (*e.g.*, gets sick) of a variety of foods, diarrhea.
>   *Female reproductive symptoms:* judged by the individual as occurring more frequently or severely than in most women: painful menstruation, menstrual irregularity, excessive bleeding, severe vomiting throughout pregnancy or causing hospitalization during pregnancy.
>   *Psychosexual symptoms:* for the major part of the individual's life after opportunities for sexual activity, sexual indifference, lack of pleasure during intercourse, pain during intercourse.
>   *Pain:* Pain in back, joints, extremities, genital areas (other than during intercourse); pain on urination; other pain (other than headaches).
>   *Cardiopulmonary symptoms:* Shortness of breath, palpitations, chest pain, dizziness.

Guze's diagnostic classification[37] is somewhat more elaborate. It offers ten symptom groups and requires that a patient have a minimum of 25 symptoms in at least nine of the ten groups. Guze also requires that the symptomatology begin before the age of 35. There is controversy about whether this syndrome should be separated from the broad category of hypochondriasis. This will be discussed in greater detail in the section on clinical description.

EPIDEMIOLOGY

Ford[40] offers an excellent summary of the epidemiologic data on Briquet's syndrome. He reports that Farley and Woodruff estimated the prevalence to be 1% to 2% of the female population based on examination of hospitalized postpartum women. This extremely high prevalence may be a reflection of the nature of the sample. It is highly questionable whether such a high prevalence would be noted in a large urban hospital. Briquet's syndrome is more common in rural populations of lower socioeconomic status and lower educational achievement. Purley and Guze[37] indicate that there is considerable stability in the diagnosis so that at follow up, 6 to 8 years later, 90% of patients diagnosed as having Briquet's syndrome still fell in this diagnostic category and no other diagnosis was evident. This may simply reflect the persistence of chronic hypochondriacal reactions in a deprived social group.

Of interest are Guze's epidemiologic studies that suggest that male relatives of patients with Briquet's syndrome have an extremely high incidence of alcoholism and sociopathy (33%). Female relatives have a considerably higher incidence of Briquet's syndrome. Studies of convicted male criminals indicate that many of their female relatives have somatization disorders, and imprisoned women have a high incidence of Briquet's syndrome. Interesting is the observation that those convicted females who have Briquet's syndrome appear to be devoid of guilt and tend to deny their criminal behavior, unlike the imprisoned women without Briquet's syndrome.

CLINICAL DESCRIPTION

Briquet's syndrome occurs predominantly in women, and symptoms appear well before 35 years of age. These patients present the usual litany of physical complaints involving multiple systems and for the most part have histrionic personalities with exhibitionism, dramatization, and emotional color. The stories they tell are often vague and contradictory. They have had frequent hospitalizations and unsatisfactory treatment, and there is a high incidence of what Menninger first called "the polysurgery patient," implying multiple surgical operations often without defined cause and frequently including hysterectomy.

These women often come from highly disorganized families in which one or both parents are alcoholic and/or sociopathic. They frequently have been the object of abuse, have had poor school and social adjustments in childhood and adolescence, and have had difficulty with menarche. Their current lives are joyless and focused on their physical symptomatology, and they reveal little interest in sex. They have long histories of involvement with doctors from whom they have received many medications, including habituating drugs that often lead to iatrogenic complications.

Ford distinguishes Briquet's syndrome from hypochondriasis in three ways:

1. Sex ratio. Briquet's syndrome is almost predominantly found in women whereas hypochondriasis occurs equally in men and women.
2. Cognitive style. Patients diagnosed as having Briquet's syndrome are typically histrionic in style, whereas hypochondriacs tend to be more obsessional.
3. Multiplicity of symptoms. Briquet's syndrome is characterized by multiple symptoms whereas hypochondriasis may involve more limited symptomatic expression.

In my view these are not definitive differentiations. What is called somatization disorder may be a more severe form of hypochondriasis found in hysteroid women who have been brought up and live in a chaotic social world.

ETIOLOGY

Since Briquet's syndrome is currently a descriptive diagnosis, little can be said about etiology. Its frequent occurrence in severely disrupted families involving alcoholism, sociopathy, and physical abuse would suggest that these factors play an important part in the use of bodily symptoms to express distress. In many respects the considerations detailed under hypochondriacal reactions may be pertinent to this disorder. The strong familial association with alcoholism and sociopathy suggests genetic factors.

TREATMENT

The prognosis for significant improvement in this disorder is poor. Some suggest that the physician should pay little attention to the patient's somatic complaints for fear of increasing attention to them. I believe that the patient is more likely to be engaged if the physician is willing to use the currency of the patient's own communications. Only later, after a relationship is established, can the more conflictual aspects of the patient's life be explored. Attention should be paid to possible organic illness masked by the syndrome and medications, and surgery should be avoided in the absence of definite indications. Morrison reports some success with behavior modification. Group therapy may be of some value in this condition if the patient is amenable to such a referral.[41]

Factitious Illness

Factitious illness has fascinated, frustrated, and irritated internists and psychiatrists. Although relatively rare, it poses difficult diagnostic and ethical problems and not infrequently places the patient at serious risk. The understanding of these disorders is limited because of the confabulatory behavior of the patients: they are inclined to lie and to discontinue treatment when confronted with the factitious nature of their disease. The spectrum of syndromes that will be discussed here has been called pathologic malingering, peregrinating problem patients, hospital hoboes, Munchausen syndrome, and polysurgical patients. "Factitious Illness" should be separated from "Munchausen Syndrome" in classification.

DEFINITION

It is to be noted that factitious illness is represented in the *DSM-III* as a separate group of disorders from the group of somatoform disorders. The diagnostic criteria listed by the *DSM-III* are as follows:

1. Plausible presentation of physical symptoms that are apparently under the individual's voluntary control to such a degree that there are multiple hospitalizations.
2. The individual's goal is apparently to assume the "patient" role and is not otherwise understandable in light of the individual's environmental circumstances (as is the case in malingering).

It has been pointed out previously that all of the somatoform disorders tend to merge with one another and rarely exist in pure culture. Hence, it is not unusual to find some degree of hypochondriasis or conversion reactions in this group of patients. Factitious illness is to be distinguished from malingering, in which case the patient simulates illness with conscious intent to obtain a precise and definable material goal such as lodging or freedom from prosecution by the law. Although it is difficult to delineate the precise motivations of the patients with factitious illness, the wish to attain the "sick role" seems central.

Within the spectrum of the factitious disorders, recent evidence suggests that there are two subtypes not yet differentiated in the *DSM-III*. Patients who fall into the first group, factitious illness proper, maintain more stable social and professional lives and develop personal attachments to individual physicians who for long periods of time do not suspect the factitious nature of their illness. This group appears to consist predominantly of young women, who are often unmarried and who work in the medical profession. A high percentage are nurses. In contrast, the classic patient with Munchausen syndrome is an impostor, lies and confabulates more frequently, has marked sociopathic tendencies often with a history of incarceration, and has an array of factitious illnesses that extend to every body system. This syndrome, less common than the first, appears to predominate in men. Although the two groups may be on a spectrum, the distinction is important because there is evidence that the prognosis is different in the two groups.

EPIDEMIOLOGY

Both factitious illness and Munchausen syndrome are relatively rare disorders. In a 16-year study of 343 patients who were participating in a prospective study of prolonged fever of unknown origin, 9% were determined to have factitious fevers usually of greater than 1 year's duration. Twenty-five of the patients were women and only seven were males, with an average age of 23 years.[42] Reich[43] found a greater preponderance of women (39 of 41 patients). Twenty-eight of these 39 patients worked in medically related jobs. The predominant medical presentations of these factitious disorders were sepsis, nonhealing wounds, fever, and electrolyte disorders. Ford[40] found that the most common categories were factitious blood disease, factitious endocrine disease, and factitious gastrointestinal diseases.

The classic Munchausen syndrome is probably much less common than factitious illness. It appears to be predominantly a disorder of men, but epidemiologic data are extremely limited.

CLINICAL DESCRIPTION

The clinical description of these syndromes is confounded by the fact that the distinction between factitious illness proper and Munchausen's disease is relatively recent.[44,45]

Chronic Factitious Illness

The discovery of chronic factitious illness often comes as a surprise to the treating physician who has known the patient over a considerable period of time. The patient is most frequently a young adult woman when the disorder first begins (although cases in childhood have been reported often with the complicity of the parent), working in some medical discipline such as nursing, who appears before the discovery of the illness to be knowledgeable and cooperative and struggling to overcome the illness. The inexplicable persistence of symptoms and its recurrence when the patient is discharged from the hospital appears as a source of constant puzzlement to the physician until he begins to suspect that the symptoms of the illness are either feigned or self-induced.

The phenomenology of factitious diseases is so diverse that it cannot be described in detail in this chapter (see Shafer and Shafer[45] for such a discussion). In order to convey a sense of the behavior of such patients, variants of factitious fevers and self-induced infections will be described. Patients elevate thermometer measurement by shaking the thermometer until the mercury rises, touching its bulb to a hot object, rubbing against gums, or the anal sphincter. Hot tap water may be used. The patient may induce fever by self-injection of pyrogenic substances such as vaccines, toxoids, and pyrogenic materials. Aduan and associates[41] indicate that the following signs are useful in the diagnosis of factitious fever:

1. Fever without evidence of active disease at physical examination or with screening diagnostic tests
2. Absence of tachycardia with abrupt temperature spikes
3. Discrepancy between the patient's physical examination findings and apparent very high temperature, particularly in the absence of skin warmth
4. Apparent rapid defervescence unaccompanied by diaphoresis

5. Marked hyperpyrexia greater than 41°C
6. Lack of diunal variation in temperature or other unusual temperature pattern
7. Marked discrepancy between oral and rectal temperatures taken simultaneously
8. No fever with nurse or physician attending
9. Other associated factitious disease

Self-induced infections may be produced by self-inoculation with bacteria, both in the skin subcutaneously or through body orifices such as the urethra. Infectious skin lesions may be constantly reinoculated to interfere with the healing process by persistent intentional manipulation. Chronic wounds are a major source of difficulty, and in Reich's[43] study "willful interference with wound healing was suspected when 1) wounds that appear to be healing normally broke down for no apparent reason, 2) wounds that had not been healing improved under casts or protective dressings, 3) wounds remained open chronically in the absence of vascular impairment or infection, and 4) when the physical nature of the wounds themselves suggested that the lesions were factitious."

Other reported factitious illnesses include factitious kidney stones and hematuria, factitious urinary disease, factitious dermatitis, factitious nausea, vomiting and diarrhea, factitious anemia, factitious bleeding disorders (often induced by the use of anticoagulants), factitious water intoxication, factitious seizures (which must be differentiated from conversion seizures), and factitious endocrine disorders, including disorders evoked by self-medication with thyroid preparations, insulin, adrenalin, and so on.

Munchausen Syndrome

Typically the Munchausen patient is a man who has a history of a wide variety of medical illnesses involving all systems who has undergone many surgical procedures. The Munchausen patient is very knowledgeable about medical matters, is familiar with medical terminology, and describes the symptomatology of various illnesses so precisely that medical and surgical interventions often seem to be required as emergency procedures. These patients often are impostors; they lie repeatedly both about their illness and their previous roles in life. Pseudologia fantastica is characteristic. They have long medical charts and when adequate history is obtained are often revealed to have multiple hospital admissions (often in the hundreds) in hospitals all over the country. They are wanderers, ever seeking medical attention. For the most part confrontation of these patients with the feigned or self-induced nature of their illnesses leads to rage, rapid flight, and a continuation of the behavior at other hospitals. The prognosis for such patients is very poor.

Unusual was a 37-year-old man presenting himself for psychiatric hospitalization indicating that he needed treatment for Munchausen syndrome. He was an isolated and pathetic man with a history of severe early deprivation. The patient indicated that he wished to maintain an honest relationship with one medical center where he could be treated for real medical disease if he became ill. He readily admitted that he felt compelled to present himself at other centers with false or self-induced symptoms for reasons that he could not understand. This man had had a thoracotomy, bilateral femoral vein ligations for "pulmonary emboli," as well as a laparotomy. He could express only the vague sense that he felt safe and cared for when he was in the hospital.

There has been considerable attention in the literature to this personality diagnosis in these syndromes. Nadelson[44] emphasizes the borderline features of these patients although he does not distinguish between chronic factitious illness and Munchausen's disease. Reich,[43] who was describing factitious illness as distinct from Munchausen syndrome, found that although most of the 33 patients who were studied showed evidence of having personality disorders, none fell readily into the classifications in the *DSM-III*. His group did not

> demonstrate the intense anger, impulsivity, identity disturbances or instability of interpersonal relationships associated with a borderline personality. They tended to be immature, sometimes hysteroid and remarkably inhibited in their personal relationships, especially in the area of sexuality. Of particular interest was . . . his observation . . . that there were marked hypochondriacal concerns often traceable to childhood and that they were motivated by deeply ingrained hypochondriacal beliefs and fears as well as by wishes for the attention and gratification associated with medical care.

A subgroup of patients who create conditions for surgical intervention apparently are motivated at least in part by the conviction that surgery will reveal a defined physical disease.

The Munchausen subgroup of patients clearly have strong sociopathic tendencies and often have criminal records reflective of major antisocial behavior.

ETIOLOGY

Certain broad developmental and psychodynamic patterns emerge as one examines the literature on patients with chronic factitious illness and Munchausen syndrome. The difficulties in establishing a therapeutic alliance with such patients makes it difficult to determine what underlying fantasies accompany this unusual behavior. Reports on etiology are contaminated by the failure to distinguish between chronic factitious illness and Munchausen syndrome.

Chronic Factitious Illness

Early maternal deprivation with failure to receive proper care and nurturance associated with abusive parental behavior and a frequent history of abandonment or loss in childhood is common in the histories of these patients. An early pattern of relatedness through physical abuse by the parent may lead to masochistic tendencies in which the induction of pain may be equated with caring. Often there is a history of childhood illness and hospitalization. This may have been the only setting in which the child received appropriate care and may become a prototype for adult behavior in which gratification of dependency needs occurs through self-induced or feigned illness and the treatment thereby obtained. Menninger[46] views the self-mutilating behavior of these patients as equivalent to an act of suicide, since the self-destructive behavior of many of these patients may lead to death. The element of guilt may play an important role in this regard.

The most meaningful general statement that can be made about the motivation of these patients has to do with their unconscious need to assume the sick role with its attendant relief from responsibility and entitlement to care. In deprived individuals with poor interpersonal relationships, physical illness becomes a powerful instrument to obtain dependency gratification and nurturance that is otherwise unavailable.

An interesting variant on chronic factitious illness is what Meadow[47] calls "Munchausen syndrome by proxy." In this situation mothers induce illness in their children. In the context of the child's hospitalization the mothers obtain a great deal of attention from the hospital staff by their constant presence and active participation in the treatment.

Munchausen Syndrome

The early history of patients with Munchausen syndrome is similar to what has been described above for chronic factitious illness. The typical adult Munchausen patient is frequently an impostor and manifests sociopathic and often criminal behavior. Spiro[48] summarizes the dynamics of the impostor that apply to the typical Munchausen patient. He emphasizes the marked discrepancy between the patient's self-representation and his ideal self-representation. The grandiose roles that the patient assumes conceal markedly damaged self-esteem. Often there is a marked discrepancy between the patient's scholastic achievement and the grandiose presentation of himself. The impostorship also has a hostile component in which the patient obtains satisfaction in deceiving the physician and therefore being superior and more powerful. Childhood hospitalizations may be experienced by the patient as traumatic, and the subsequent recreation of this event may be in the service of the attempt to master an earlier trauma.

DIAGNOSIS AND DIFFERENTIAL DIAGNOSIS

When the physician is first confronted with manifest symptoms or signs, he does not naturally consider the possibility of feigned or self-induced illness. Only with the persistence of bizarre and inconsistent signs and symptoms will he begin to consider factitious illness as a possible diagnosis. Once considered, the procedure for accurate diagnosis will depend on the nature of the factitious illness. Careful observation then becomes central to diagnosis. In situations where self-medication is the primary source of the difficulty, it has been recommended by Reich that the patient's room be searched when the patient is not present. Although this clearly poses important ethical issues, Reich argues persuasively that the serious nature of the illness, the need for a definite diagnosis, and the fact that a direct confrontation implemented in a supportive way may lead to the disappearance of the behavior justifies this approach.

Patients with Munchausen syndrome may be suspected of having this disorder by the complicated medical history they present, elaborated in a knowledgeable way but characterized by inconsistencies. Their behavior in the hospital is often erratic, and they may shift from agreeable compliance to angry outbursts that alienate staff. Grandiose past histories that are inconsistent with the patient's ward status are also suggestive.

As with all of these disorders, the physician must distinguish factitious illness from physical disease. Hypochondriacal patients may at times be difficult to distinguish from patients with factitious illness.

The former are more consistent in their behavior and develop institutional transferences that make them frequent visitors at multiple clinics in the same hospital.

Patients with conversion disorders, unlike those with factitious illness, present symptom complexes that are inconsistent with known diagnostic entities. Patients with body delusions may be very insistent on surgical intervention, but their delusional belief is associated with great anxiety and careful examination usually reveals a psychotic state.

Treatment

After establishing the fact that the illness is factitious, supportive confrontation of the patient by both internist and psychiatrist is indicated, emphasizing to the patient that his need to engage in such behavior must reflect extreme distress and is an indication for treatment. Reich comments on the fact that although patients rarely accept the recommendation for psychotherapy, in a surprisingly large number of cases the behavior disappears without recurrence. This finding is rarely reported in the literature.

The confrontation with a patient with Munchausen syndrome frequently results in an angry outburst and the patient's decision to sign out of the hospital against advice. A few case reports suggest that prolonged psychiatric hospitalization and a confrontational psychotherapy may be of some usually limited value although the cost–benefit ratio would appear to be very high, and it is questionable whether the investment in such a treatment is indicated even if possible.

REFERENCES

1. Katon W: Depression and somatization: A review: I and II. Am J Med 72:127–135, 241–247, 1982
2. Racy J: Psychiatry in the Arab East. Psychiatr Scand Suppl 21:1–171, 1970
3. Basch MF: The concept of affect: A reexamination. J Am Psychoanal Assoc 24:759–777, 1976
4. Zborowski M: Differences and similarities. In Monat A, Lazarus RS (eds): Stress and Coping, pp 95–107. New York, Columbia University Press, 1977
5. Parson T: The Social System. Glencoe, IL, Free Press, 1951
6. Mechanic D: The concept of illness behavior. J Chronic Dis 15:189–194, 1962
7. Engel GL: A reconsideration of the role of conversion in somatic disease. Compr Psychiatry 9:316–329, 1968
8. Chodoff, Lyons: Hysteria. Am J Psychiatry 114:739, 1958
9. Engel GL: Conversion symptoms. In MacBride CM (ed):

Signs and Symptoms, pp 650–688. Philadelphia, JB Lippincott, 1970

10. Ljungberg L: Hysteria: A clinical, prognostic and genetic study. Acta Psychiatr Neurol Scand 32. Suppl 112:1–162, 1957

11. Watson CG, Buranen C: The frequency of conversion reaction symptoms. J Abnorm Psychol 88:209–211, 1979

12. Freud S: Group Psychology and the Analysis of the Ego, 18:67–143. London, Hogarth Press, 1955

13. Walsh FMR: Diseases of the Nervous System. Baltimore, Williams & Williams, 1952

14. Woolsey RM: Hysteria: 1875–1975. Dis Nerv Syst 37:379–386, 1976

15. Weintraub MI: Hysteria: A clinical guide to diagnosis. Clin Symp 29(6):2–3, 1977

16. Slater E: Hysteria. J Ment Sci 107:359, 1961

17. Carter AB: The prognosis of certain hysterical symptoms. Br Med J 1:1076–1079, 1949

18. Engel GL: Psychogenic pain and the pain prone patient. Am J Med 36:899–918, 1959

19. Devine R, Merskey H: The description of pain in psychiatric and general medical patients. J Psychosom Res 9:311–316, 1965

20. Lesse S: Hypochondriasis and other psychosomatic disorders masking depression. Am J Psychother 21:607–620, 1967

21. Blumer D, Heilbron N: The pain prone disorder: A clinical and psychological profile. Psychosomatics 22:395–402, 1981

22. Frances A, Gale L: Proprioceptive body image in self-object differentiation. Psychoanal Q 44:107–125, 1975

23. Pinsky J: Chronic and intractable benign pain: A syndrome and its treatment with intensive short term group psychotherapy. J Human Stress 4:17–21, 1978

24. Strain JJ, Grossman S: Psychological Care of the Medically Ill. New York, Appleton-Century-Crofts, 1975

25. Kenyon FE: Hypochondriacal states. Br J Psychiatry 129:1–14, 1976

26. Barsky A, Klerman GL: Overview of hypochondriasis: Bodily complaint and somatic styles. Am J Psychiatry 140:273–283, 1983

27. Brown HN, Vaillant GE: Hypochondriasis. Arch Intern Med 141:723–726, 1981

28. Myers WA, Broden AG: Hypochondrial symptoms as derivatives of unconscious fantasies of being beaten or tortured. J Am Psychoanal Assn 29:535–558, 1981

29. Freud A: The role of bodily illness in the mental life of children. Psychoanal Study Child 7:78–80, 1952

30. Kohut H: The Restoration of the Self. New York, International Universities Press, 1977

31. Richards A: Self theory and conflict theory. Psychoanal Study Child 319, 337, 1981

32. Pilowsky I: Primary and secondary hypochondriasis. Acta Psychiatr Scand 46:273–285, 1970

33. Kenyon FE: Hypochondriasis. Br J Psychiatry 110:478–488, 1964

34. Bishop ER: Monosystematic hypochondriasis. Psychosomatics 21:731–747, 1980

35. Lipsett DR: Medical and psychological characteristics of "crocks." Psychiatr Med 1:15–25, 1970

36. Purtell JJ, Robino E, Cohen ME: Observations on clinical aspects of hysteria. JAMA 146:902–909, 1951

37. Purley MG, Guze SB: Hysteria: The stability and usefulness of clinical criteria. N Engl J Med 266:421–426, 1972

38. Mai FM, Merskey H: Briquet's concept of hysteria. Can J Psychiatry 26:57–62, 1981

39. Breuer J, Freud S: Studies on hysteria. In Strachey J (ed): The Standard Edition of the Complete Works of Sigmund Freud, vol 2. London, Hogarth Press, 1955

40. Ford CV: The Somatizing Disorders. New York, Elsevier, 1983

41. Valko RJ: Group therapy for patients with hysteria. Dis Nerv Syst 484–487, 1976

42. Aduan RP, Fauci AS, Pale DC: Factitious fever and self-induced infection. Ann Intern Med 90:230–242, 1979

43. Reich P: Factitious disorders in a teaching hospital. Ann Intern Med 99:240–247, 1983

44. Nadelson T: The Munchausen spectrum. Gen Hosp Psychiatry 1:11–17, 1979

45. Shafer N, Shafer R: Factitious diseases including Munchausen's syndrome. NY State J Med 80:594–604, 1980

46. Menninger KA: Polysurgery and polysurgical addiction. Psychoanal Q 3:173, 1934

47. Meadow R: Munchausen by proxy: The hinterland of child abuse. Lancet 2:343, 1977

48. Spiro H: Chronic factitious illness. Arch Gen Psychiatry 18:569, 1968

SUGGESTED READING

BARSKY A, KLERMAN GL: Overview of hypochondriasis: Bodily complaint and somatic styles. Am J Psychiatry 140:273–283, 1983

ENGEL GL: Conversion symptoms. In MacBride CM (ed): Signs and Symptoms, pp 650–688. Philadelphia, JB Lippincott, 1970

ENGEL GL: Psychogenic pain and the pain prone patient. Am J Med 36:899–918, 1959

FORD CV: The Somatosizing Disorders. New York, Elsevier, 1983

KENYON FE: Hypochondriacal states. Br J Psychiatry 129:1–14, 1976

REICH P: Factitious disorders in a teaching hospital. Ann Intern Med 99:240–247, 1983

Margaret M. Gilmore and Charles Kaufman

Dissociative Disorders

For centuries, philosophers, physicians, and the lay public have observed and struggled to label and understand the phenomena of dissociation, and have even employed them therapeutically (*e.g.*, as in "sleep therapy" or the Greek Aesculysian medical cult).[1] The earliest medical report of a case of multiple personality dates at least to Paracelsus in the 17th century, who observed a woman whose secondary personality stole her money.[2] Carlson attributes the first reports in American medicine of both psychogenic amnesia and multiple personality to Benjamin Rush in the early 19th century.[3] The case of Reverend William Tenent as recorded by Rush is illustrative of early observations.

CASE STUDY

William Tenent fell ill while studying for the Presbyterian ministry. Despite medical care, he became emaciated, finally collapsed, and was considered dead. However, when the attending physician felt warmth in the patient's body, he cancelled the funeral. After 3 days, the apparent corpse "opened its eyes, gave a dreadful groan, and sunk again into apparent death."[3] After the third such awakening, William remained conscious. He made a gradual recovery over the next year, but was amnestic for his life prior to his deathlike state. His brother began to teach him to read and write. One day during a Latin lesson, William felt shock in his head. He suddenly remembered he had read the book before. Subsequently, he regained his complete memory. He also recalled that during the 3 days of his deathlike state, which had felt to him like 5 or 10 minutes, he had believed he was "transported by a superior being to a place of ineffable glory."[3] For the next 45 years, William's physical health was good. He married, had three sons, and functioned as a successful pastor.

Despite such early reports, the major surge of medical interest in dissociative disorders occurred in the late 19th century when physicians began more systematic studies of hysteria and hypnosis.[4] The recognition that patients under the influence of posthypnotic suggestion could perform complicated tasks without any conscious memory of why they were doing so led to concepts of an unconsciousness which contained thoughts and feelings capable of influencing a person without his knowledge. Thereafter, observations and concepts on hysteria, hypnosis, and dissociation became entangled. In their book *Studies on Hysteria*, Freud and Breuer claim that ideas that are kept out of conscious awareness are the cause of somatic symptoms seen in hysteria.[5] Freud used the term *repression* to label the phenomenon of ideas kept out of conscious. However, the model proposed was essentially one of dissociation.

The initiation of the term *dissociation* is usually attributed to Janet who hypothesized a model of *idea complexes existing outside of consciousness* as the cause of symptoms seen in hysteria and multiple personality.[4] Prince developed a similar theory of co-consciousness in which different conscious states exist in a person without his awareness as his attention is not focused on them. Prince used the state of co-consciousness as an explanation for phenomena seen in both multiple personality disorders and symptoms of hysteria. Thus, most of the investigators on hysteria and multiple personality attributed the symptoms to the existence of ideas outside of consciousness. There was major disagreement only on the mechanism of dissociation. Freud preferred a purely psychological explanation of dissociation. He saw it as the result of ideas having been actively banned from consciousness by the patient in order to ward off painful affects. Breuer was inclined to a model of *hypnoid states* in which ideas that were registered in an altered state of consciousness become unavailable to the person in his normal conscious state. Janet thought dissociation was the result of neurophysiologic weakness in the patient.

There are two important observations to be made from this historical review. First, the different investigators used both the term and the concept of dissociation with different meaning. For Janet, *dissociation* was a term used to describe the phenomenon of the split in consciousness. In Freud's writings, the concept of *dissociation* referred to both the observation of the phenomenon of split in consciousness and the description of a defense mechanism. Finally, some recent psychiatrists, as exemplified in *Diagnostic and Statistical Manual of Mental Disorders, 3rd Ed. (DSM-III)*, have used the term as a diagnostic label specifying a set of disease entities.[7] The second important observation is that the investigators derived their observations and theories from work with patients suffering from widely different symptoms. Freud and Breuer were studying patients who they diagnosed as suffering from hysteria, which to them meant somatic symptoms without clear organic cause. Janet, Prince, and later others, such as Fisher, were studying patients with fugue states, somnambulism, amnesias, and multiple personalities.[4,6,8] However, since in each case dissociation was the postulated underlying mechanism, the authors tended to lump observations on the phenomena of amnesia, multiple personalities, somnambulism, fugue, and hysteria together.

The influence of these varying definitions and concepts of dissociation on diagnosis is reflected in the different versions of the *Diagnostic and Statistical Manual*, written by the American Psychiatric Association (APA).

DSM-I separated amnesia and its related memory disorders from somatic conversion symptoms by creating a new diagnostic category—dissociative reactions.[9] This category included amnesia, stupor, fugue, somnambulism, dream states, and depersonalization. *DSM-I* assigned somatic symptoms to the conversion reaction category. *DSM-II* reunited the memory disorders with the hysterical conversion symptoms by creating the diagnosis of hysterical neurosis, which was split into two categories—hysterical neurosis (conversion type) and hysterical neurosis (dissociative type). *DSM-III* separated the disorders once again by eliminating the hysterical neurosis category.[7] Conversion symptoms were placed under somatoform disorders.

Dissociative disorder was established as a separate diagnostic category, including psychogenic amnesia, psychogenic fugue, multiple personality, depersonalization disorder, and atypical dissociative disorder.

The diagnostic arrangement of *DSM-III* deviates from previous approaches in several ways. First, depersonalization is raised to the category of a disorder and not treated as a symptom occurring in other disorders. Second, somnambulism is excluded from the category of dissociative disorder and is established as a separate entity, sleep walking disorders, under the disorders of infancy and childhood. Third, psychogenic amnesia and psychogenic fugue are treated as separate disorders rather than as symptoms that occur on a continuum of altered levels of overlapping and merging consciousness in a single individual suffering from dissociative disorder. These changes are all consistent with the *DSM-III's* overall approach to diagnosis as based on similarities in clinical signs and symptoms or known organic etiology rather than on postulated underlying psychological mechanisms. However, it is important to note the above diagnostic changes in order to interpret data properly on the incidence, prevalence, signs, symptoms, genetics, prognosis, and treatment of the disorders. The reader must first understand that in the past one psychiatrist's fugue was another's psychogenic amnesia. Therefore, papers purporting to describe characteristics of psychogenic fugue have often included cases which under *DSM-III* would be diagnosed as psychogenic amnesia. Rosenbaum suggests a second way in which the changing fashions of diagnosis may have influenced data on these disorders.[11] He attributes the decline in case reports of multiple personalities since 1910 to the rise in the popularity of the diagnosis of schizophrenia as introduced by Bleuler at that time. Bliss also claims that a careful review of published clinical reports indicates that cases of multiple personality have been misdiagnosed as schizophrenia.[2]

With full understanding of the complicated history of the diagnosis of these disorders, the author will now approach further discussion of dissociative disorders using definitions found in *DSM-III*.

Psychogenic Amnesia

DEFINITION

DSM-III defines *psychogenic amnesia* as a sudden inability to recall important personal information, an inability not due to an organic mental disorder."[7] Four specific subtypes are delineated. *Localized amnesia* is a "failure to recall all events during a circumscribed period of time," usually a few hours following a traumatic event.[7] *Selective amnesia* is a "failure to recall some, but not all, of the events occurring during a circumscribed period of time."[7] *Generalized amnesia* is a "failure of recall which encompasses the individual's entire life."[7] *Continuous amnesia* is a "failure to recall events subsequent to a specific time up to and including the present."[7] Episodes of amnesia in which the person pursues organized travel to a new locale or assumes a new identity are called psychogenic fugues and are specifically excluded from the category of psychogenic amnesia.

Although the general definition of psychogenic amnesia as given by *DSM-III* is in agreement with the literature,[8,12,13,14] the breakdown into separate and specific subcategories and the exclusion of episodes of organized travel during the amnesia are not. *DSM-III* considers as separate disorders what many authors describe as stages of memory disturbance in single patients.[12,14,15] For example, Fisher and Joseph describe cases of psychogenic loss of personal identity as occurring in stages.[12] In stage one, the subject suddenly enters an altered state of consciousness in which he is either stuporous or delusionally preoccupied with a single idea or affect, and in which he is unaware of memory loss. During this stage, the subject can perform complicated acts and travel long distances without assuming a new identity. After minutes to weeks, the subject enters the second stage, where he simultaneously becomes aware of loss of personal identity and becomes amnesic for the events of stage one. According to *DSM-III*, this amnesia for the events of stage one would be classified as psychogenic amnesia, localized. During stage two, the subject is capable of ordered cognition and of remembering events of stage two, but remains amnesic for personal identity. According to *DSM-III*, this amnesia for personal identity would be classified as psychogenic amnesia, generalized. Thus, according to *DSM-III*, the single subject would be suffering from two disorders—psychogenic amnesia, localized, and psychogenic amnesia, generalized. Furthermore, the episode of stage one in which the patient pursues organized travel over long distances without the assumption of a new identity cannot be classified under *DSM-III* other than as an atypical dissociative disorder. The organized travel disqualifies the diagnosis of psychogenic amnesia and the lack of assumption of a new identity eliminates the diagnosis of psychogenic fugue. A second problem with *DSM-III's* classification is that case reports indicate that many patients evolve from psychogenic amnesia, generalized, to psychogenic amnesia, localized (loss of memory for events of stage one), in which the localized amnesia remains permanent.[12] The irretrievability of the localized amnesia disqualifies the patient from a diagnosis of psychogenic amnesia, localized, because *DSM-III* distinguishes psychogenic amnesia from organic memory disturbance by the criterion of complete memory recovery in psychogenic amnesia.

These diagnostic difficulties are important for three reasons. First, *DSM-III's* diagnostic system is unrealistic in that it ignores the fact that the majority of reported cases of psychogenic amnesia show such overlaps of memory disturbance. Second, the diagnostic difficulties contribute to confusion in epidemiologic and descriptive data. Thus, studies purporting to report data on fugue often combine data from cases of psychogenic amnesia with cases of psychogenic fugue. Finally, these diagnostic distinctions reflect differences in conceptualization of the disorders. Psychoanalytic authors see these dissociative phenomena as symptoms on a continuum of severity of memory disturbance.[12,13,15] For them, the amnesias—selective, localized, and generalized—as well as fugues and some multiple personalities are different manifestations of either the severity of the trauma or the severity of disturbance of ego functioning and do not represent diagnostic entities with their own specific epidemiology, genetics, prognoses, and treatments. *DSM-III* approaches these phenomena as separate diagnostic disorders with the expectation of finding differences in epidemiology, genetics, prognoses, and treatments.

CASE STUDY—PSYCHOGENIC AMNESIA, GENERALIZED

Ms. A., a 30-year-old mother of four, was brought to the emergency room by her husband. Her chief complaint was, "I don't know who I am." Although Ms. A. was alert, oriented, and could remember the events of the previous 36 hours, she had no recall for earlier events. She did not know her name nor recognize her family. Her thoughts were goal-directed. She showed no hallucinations or delusions. She was mildly depressed. Neurologic examination was completely normal.

Mr. A. provided the following history. Two nights earlier, Ms. A. became furious with him when he returned home drunk. She awoke the next morning depressed, with a headache, and took 45 mg of diazepam. When Mr. A. later returned home from work, he found his wife sitting in a chair, staring into space. His questioning her revealed the memory disturbance.

During the 6 days of amnesia following her presentation to the emergency room, Ms. A. functioned successfully as a housewife, doing laundry, making meals, and caring for her children. When her memory for personal identity spontaneously returned, she gave the following history. Six months earlier, while depressed over her marriage, she had attempted suicide. On recovering, she resolved that since suicide meant abandoning her children, she would not try again. She considered divorce as a solution to her marital problems, but was afraid of being on her own. Just prior to the onset of her amnesia, she had once again felt overwhelmed with anger and helplessness.

During the 4 months following this initial amnesic episode, Ms. A. experienced four more amnestic episodes. Each episode was preceded by increased depression and irritability, and was initiated either on awakening from sleep or after prolonged sleeplessness. Three episodes seemed to occur in response to threatened abandonment. Two episodes were associated with prodromal headache.

Formal psychological testing was conducted on Ms. A., both in her normal state (following recovery from her first episode of amnesia), and in her state of amnesia (during the second episode of amnesia). Baseline testing revealed Ms. A. to be a woman of average IQ who was suffering from considerable feelings of helplessness and hopelessness. Retesting during amnesia showed a similar IQ, with a marked reduction in feelings of anger and helplessness. Her cognitive testing revealed a diminished ability to retrieve personal information, but no decrease in memory for general information. Although Ms. A's capacity for integrative thinking declined in the amnestic state, there was no psychotic ideation observed in either test situation.

This case demonstrates several typical features of psychogenic amnesia. First is onset of the episode in a setting of intense internal psychological turmoil combined with what the patient sees as an impossible but inescapable environmental situation. Second is the prodromal headache. Third is onset in a setting where the patient's level of consciousness may already be altered—either on awakening from sleep, after prolonged sleep deprivation, or in a setting of tranquilizing medication. Fourth is the patient's unawareness of the memory loss until confronted by an outsider. Fifth is the memory disturbance occurring in stages with stage one characterized by memory loss without awareness of it and the second stage characterized by an awareness of loss of memory. Sixth is the fact that during stage two, the patient is often capable of conducting his or her business as usual, despite profound memory loss for past life and personal identity. Seventh is the typical transition from one stage to another. The subject may return from stage two to premorbid functioning either suddenly and completely,[13] or gradually.[15] The subject may recall both past life and stage two events simultaneously

(as did Ms. A.), or retrieve past life and personal identity while becoming amnestic for events of stage two.[16] The amnesia for stage two may then resolve spontaneously or be terminated with hypnosis or barbiturates. According to Fisher and Joseph, the amnesia for stage one often persists and becomes permanent.[12] Eighth, the recurrence of episodes of amnesia when the subject is in similar emotional turmoil is frequent. Finally, the episodes of amnesia are usually short-lived (hours to days).

A report of two more cases of psychogenic amnesia, one case of localized variety and a second of the continuous type, may help to clarify the diagnoses. Fisher reports the case of a 21-year-old soldier who "blacked out" at the instant when he was aiming his gun at an enemy plane that was diving directly at him.[8] The soldier "came to" 32 days later in a hospital hundreds of miles away with no memory of the events subsequent to the instant when the plane was diving at him. The patient reported that he had joined the army to avenge the deaths of his parents who were killed in a bombing raid. He had resolved to kill as many enemy soldiers as possible. Under hypnosis, the patient recalled the events at the onset of his amnesia. At the moment when he saw the enemy plane diving towards him, he thought, "I can't take it. I have to get out of here. I'm yellow; I'm a coward."[8] He escaped, stole money, and took flight to the rear of the battleline. After wandering the country for days, he was rescued by soldiers who brought him to the hospital. On followup, this patient suffered from three subsequent amnestic episodes, all of which were precipitated by strong reminders of enemy attack.

Fisher also reports a case of psychogenic amnesia, continuous.[8] The patient was an 18-year-old merchant seaman who was admitted to the hospital with loss of memory for all events in the previous 2 years up to and including the present. He reported the date to be 2 years prior and thought he was located in a different city. The patient accurately recalled his name and past life history up to 2 years previous. Under hypnosis, the patient revealed that he had become amnestic for the last 2 years when he became frightened about his new naval assignment and "blacked out" only to awaken on shore after his ship left port.

As these cases demonstrate, the literature supports *DSM-III's* claim that the onset of such episodes is usually abrupt and precipitated by intense affective states.[8,12,14] Also, most case reports indicate some clouding of consciousness at the onset of the amnesia. Patient complaints of having felt dizzy, having a headache, or experiencing unusual sleepiness are the most frequent manifestations of such altered states of consciousness. Patient reports of experiencing hallucinations or preoccupation with single delusional thoughts during this period are frequent, but not mentioned in *DSM-III*. Reports of hallucinations and delusional preoccupations are particularly frequent in war neuroses.[8] According to Fisher, the difference between these hallucinations and delusions and those seen in schizophrenia is their complete disappearance when memory is restored.[8]

EPIDEMIOLOGY

There are few specific data available on the incidence of psychogenic amnesia in the civilian population. In military population studies as cited by Fisher,[8] Torrie found that 8% of all battle neuroses included amnesia, and Henderson and Moore reported a prevalence of 5% amnesia in combat soldiers. While *DSM-III* claims that the disorder is most often observed in young females,[7] Kanzer reported that more men than women developed the symptom.[17] Both Parfitt and Kanzer noted the average age of onset to be between 20 and 40 years of age.[14,17] In two cases, the first episode occurred after age 40, and in three cases the first episode occurred in individuals under 20 years of age. In a report on 30 cases of hysterical amnesia in Royal Air Force (RAF) men, Parfitt[14] claimed that the disorder most frequently occurred in overly dependent, immature personalities. Twenty subjects were given the diagnosis of hysterical personality disorder; six were diagnosed as antisocial personality disorders; and four were diagnosed as schizoid. Parfitt found no organic etiology in any of the patients, but did find signs of increased anxiety such as dilated pupils, increased perspiration, increased reflexes, and tremors.[14] Parfitt points to the fact that many patients who suffered amnesia during wartime duty reported earlier episodes of amnesia during civilian life for which they had never sought medical attention as evidence of underreporting in civilian populations.[14] Bliss and Rosenblum claim that clinicians' misdiagnosing those cases which experience hallucinations and delusions as schizophrenia are another source of civilian underreporting.[2,11]

ETIOLOGY

There have been three major models proposed for understanding psychogenic amnesia—the purely psychological model, the physiologic model, and a psychosocial model. Freud proposed the original psychological model in which amnesia was seen as the result of repression of unacceptable thoughts and wishes which, if they were conscious to the patient, would cause painful feelings.[5] Fisher and Josephs, Luparello, and Rapaport later updated the psychological model to consider the amnesia as a result of patient's use of regression to an altered state of consciousness as a compromise formation to solve a painful internal psychic conflict.[12,15,16] In this model the patient in fugue could both *express prohibited feelings and impulses* (thus they are *not* repressed) and simultaneously deny authorship of them. For example, the soldier in Fisher's example of psychogenic amnesia, localized, could act on his fear by running away from the front lines while at the same time defend himself against self-accusation of cowardliness by denying authorship of the running away.[8]

The model of amnesia as the result of the patient's unwitting use of autohypnosis is a variant of the psychological regression model. Here the patient enters the altered state of consciousness by suggesting it to himself and the amnesia is the result of posthypnotic state.

Mayer-Gross, Janet, and Breuer proposed a physiologic model of amnesia.[3–5] They see the patient as having an inborn neurologic susceptibility to entering altered states of consciousness in response to intense stimuli. The patient is then unable to recall in his normal state experiences and feelings that were registered during the altered or hypnoid state.

Kirshner first articulated the social role model of amnesia.[4] He claimed that psychogenic amnesia is a well-defined social role which the patient uses to protect himself from social criticism.[4] Citing the wide variety of precipitants and psychosexual conflicts reported in cases of psychogenic amnesia, he felt that it is unlikely that psychogenic amnesia is the result of specific psychosexual conflicts. The explanation of amnesia as malingering is a variant of the psychosocial model. Here the subject is seen as adopting the sick role to escape social responsibilities or legal punishment. For example, the sailor who does not wish to honor his contract to go to sea complains of amnesia when found to be AWOL.

DIAGNOSIS AND DIFFERENTIAL DIAGNOSIS

The difficulty in making the diagnosis of psychogenic amnesia is to differentiate it from amnesia secondary to an organic mental disorder. Psychogenic amnesia is usually typified by abrupt onset in the context of severe psychosocial stress. There is usually a clear-cut boundary to the beginning and end of the lost memory. The decreased cognitive functioning is restricted to the memory loss, and the patient is capable of new learning as well as of conducting complicated mental tasks during the interview. Although it is often claimed that full recovery of memory is typical of psychogenic amnesia,[7] many case reports indicate a permanent memory loss for events of stage one of the fugue.[12]

A complete history and physical examination, including EEG, are necessary to differentiate psychogenic amnesia from organic mental disorders. Even then it may be difficult to sort out a psychogenic component of the memory loss from an organic basis; patients with known head trauma may later totally regain what was thought to be memories lost as a result of organic inability to register events at the time of the trauma.[14] Substanced-induced intoxication is differentiated by the history of substance ingestion or laboratory evidence of intoxication, as well as inability to attain full memory recovery. However, as mentioned above, full memory recovery is not achieved in many cases of psychogenic amnesia. In alcohol amnestic disorder, immediate recall is preserved while intermediate memory is lost. This pattern of short-term memory disturbance is not reported in psychogenic amnesia. Epilepsy can be differentiated by abnormal EEGs, as well as by the character of the episodes. Epileptic episodes are usually briefer and involve simpler motor behaviors occurring in subjects with clouded consciousness. Malingering is a common differential diagnostic consideration as the memory disturbance is often of immediate psychosocial benefit to the patient.

TREATMENT AND PREVENTION

While early treatments were oriented toward recovery of the lost memory through hypnosis or amytal interviews, later approaches have stressed the need to treat the whole patient in his psychosocial predicament.[8,14] These later approaches recommend temporary removal of the patient from the stressful environment, accompanied by psychotherapy. The psychotherapy is oriented not only to uncovering the lost memory, but also to exploring the psychological conflicts that engendered the memory loss in order to help the patient accept the feelings that he found intolerable. For example, the soldier who tried to counteract his fear of the enemy by taking flight into a fugue had to be helped to consciously accept his fear of the enemy.

As to the effectiveness of such treatment, Parfitt found that while the majority of cases were able to return to active duty, more than 20% of the men remained chronically incapacitated.[14] Recurrences of amnestic episodes are frequent in both military and civilian case reports with and without treatment.

Psychogenic Fugue

DEFINITION

DSM-III considers the essential features of *psychogenic fugue* to be sudden unexpected travel away from home or customary work locale with assumption of a new identity and an inability to recall one's previous identity.[7] In the author's opinion, the requirement that the patient assume a new identity makes this a rather restrictive definition. As mentioned above under psychogenic amnesia, many case reports describe the patient's sudden organized travel away from work or home but where the patient is initially unaware of loss of personal identity and never assumes a new identity.

EPIDEMIOLOGY

There are no reliable data available on the incidence, prevalence, sex ratio, or genetics of this disorder. Most case reports are from military literature, in which predisposing factors include immature, dependent personalities under severe psychosocial stress.[8,14] The baseline rates of prevalence of psychogenic amnesia in military personnel reported previously under psychogenic amnesia include cases that would be diagnosed as psychogenic fugue by *DSM-III*.

CLINICAL DESCRIPTION

The case of the Reverend Ansel Bourne as cited by Nemiah is an excellent example of Psychogenic Fugue as defined by *DSM-III*.

CASE STUDY
The Reverend Bourne disappeared from his home in Rhode Island in 1887. Two months later, a Mr. Brown awoke from sleep in Pennsylvania to find himself confused as to where he was and what he was

doing, as nothing around him appeared familiar. He had no memory for Mr. Brown. He insisted his name was Rev. Bourne and that he lived in Rhode Island. As the story unfolded, it appeared that the Reverend Bourne had withdrawn money from the bank in Rhode Island, traveled to Pennsylvania, and set up a small dry goods store there under the name of Mr. Brown. There he had lived quietly with few social contacts.

This case shows several typical features. The fugue had an abrupt onset and termination. The recovery on awakening from sleep is typical in that often both onset and recovery are reported to occur at times when the patient is in an altered state of consciousness. Also, the Reverend's recovery of his past identity as Reverend Bourne was accompanied by an amnesia for the events that occurred during the fugue (Reverend Bourne did not know Mr. Brown nor recognized his store or acquaintances). In the case of Reverend Bourne, there were no reported recurrences of fugue, which is in accord with *DSM-III's* claim that recurrences are rare.[7] However, Reverend Bourne was reported to have experienced earlier trance states without assumption of a new identity or travel. The cases of fugue reported in soldiers during wartime indicate a higher rate of recurrence.[8,14] Also, the pattern of recovery of original identity without treatment is typical.

ETIOLOGY

The models proposed for understanding psychogenic fugue are the same as those cited above for psychogenic amnesia and are not be repeated here. Suffice it to say that the question of malingering to avoid social responsibilities or condemnation is more prominent in discussions of psychogenic fugue, as it is typical that during the fugue, the patient travels away from either a dangerous or stressful situation.

DIAGNOSIS AND DIFFERENTIAL DIAGNOSIS

The differential diagnosis of psychogenic fugue includes organic mental syndromes, psychogenic amnesia, and multiple personality. Although dramatic personality changes with loss of memory can occur in organic mental syndromes, neither the symptom of assuming a new identity nor that of complex organized travel are frequently reported.

Also, memory loss in organic brain syndromes is usually, but not always, accompanied by clouding of consciousness, is more severe for recent than remote memory, and is accompanied by decreased attention span. Although the patient with psychogenic fugue may experience a period of clouding of consciousness at the onset of the fugue, during fugue his recent memory, attention span, and level of consciousness are normal. Because the differential diagnosis includes organic mental syndrome, a complete physical examination, an EEG, and blood toxicologies are indicated. It should be noted that the relationship between temporal lobe epilepsy and dissociative phenomena is complex. In a report of 40 patients followed in a neurology clinic for temporal lobe epilepsy, Shenk and Bear found that 33% of patients exhibited some dissociative phenomena, several showing aspects of multiple personality with altered identities.[19] However, these authors point out that the dissociative phenomena occur interictally and thus are not direct manifestations of the seizure activity. Rather, they propose that the dissociative phenomena seen in temporal lobe epilepsy are the result of psychological defenses against intense affects produced interictally by the limbic epileptic focus.[19] The differential diagnosis of psychogenic fugue from multiple personality disorder can usually be based on the fact that the secondary personality in multiple personality is aware of the primary personality, whereas in psychogenic fugue the new identity is amnestic for the primary personality.

TREATMENT AND PREVENTION

Because the patient is unaware of the amnesia during the fugue, he usually seeks treatment only after the episode has ended. The problem is then one of recovering memory for events during fugue. Hypnosis, amytal interview, and psychotherapy have all been successful techniques to recover these memories. However, psychiatrists have recently cautioned against the use of hypnosis or amytal interviews. They fear that such techniques might foster further episodes of fugue because the patient may perceive the therapist as sanctioning dissociative states. The usual recommendation is for psychotherapy to explore the psychosocial stresses that led to the fugue. The goal of the therapy is to help the patient tolerate the painful affects being warded off.

Multiple Personality

DEFINITION

According to *DSM-III,* the essential features of *multiple personality disorder* are the existence within the individual of two or more distinct personalities, each of which is dominant at a particular point in time; two, the personality that is dominant at any particular time determines the individual's behavior; and three, each individual personality is complex and integrated with its own unique behavior patterns and social relationships. This definition is in agreement with the literature.[20,21,22]

EPIDEMIOLOGY

Multiple personality is a rare disorder with a total of about 200 cases reported in the literature.[2,20] There are more case reports in females than in males, although many detailed reports of multiple personality in males exist. As mentioned above, some researchers believe that multiple personality is often misdiagnosed as schizophrenia,[2,11] and thus that underreporting accounts for some of the apparent rarity of the disorder.

CLINICAL DESCRIPTION

The chief complaint of a patient suffering from multiple personality usually focuses on "losing periods of time," or being accused of misdeeds that he does not recall committing. Although varying degrees of amnesia between the personalities are reported,[20] typically the primary personality is amnestic for the secondary personalities, while the secondary personalities remain aware of both the primary personality and the other secondary personalities.[23] Switches from one personality to another are abrupt and dramatic and are usually described as precipitated by intense affect. The history reveals onset of separate personalities in childhood, although the diagnosis is rarely made before adolescence.[2] The disorder is usually chronic and the prognosis is guarded. The patient may do better with psychotherapy focused on attempts to make the patient aware of his tendency to use dissociation to deal with frightening impulses and affects. The case of "Jonah," as reported by Ludwig and co-workers, exemplifies the typical features of this disorder.[23]

CASE STUDY

Jonah, a 27-year-old, Black, married man was admitted to the hospital with the chief complaint of severe headaches accompanied by amnestic periods. Jonah's wife described that during these periods, he became violent and referred to himself by another name, Usoffa Abdulla, Son of Omega.

Through questioning, the psychiatrist found Jonah to have three secondary personalities—Sammy, King Young, and Usoffa Abdulla. Jonah, the primary personality, was unaware of the secondary personalities. The psychiatrist described Jonah as shy, polite, and highly conventional. Sammy described himself as purely intellectual, rational, and legalistic. He stated that his duty was to help Jonah with legal problems. Sammy stated that he first appeared when Jonah was 6 years old and had witnessed his mother stab his father. After that episode, Sammy always appeared when Jonah's parents fought, so that Jonah no longer witnessed the battles. King Young described himself as a pleasure seeker and ladies' man, and that his duty was to secure sexual gratification for Jonah. King Young claimed to have first appeared when Jonah was 6 or 7 years old and struggling with a confused sexual identity. The psychiatrist described King Young as a very charming, glib talker. The third personality, Usoffa Abdulla, was described as a cold, belligerent person who claimed to have emerged to protect Jonah when he was beaten by a neighborhood gang at 8 years of age. At the moment when Jonah was most frightened, Usoffa appeared, fought viciously, and freed Jonah.

The results of a battery of psychological and neurophysiologic tests on Jonah and his secondary personalities were consistent with both the observations of the psychiatrist and the claims of the personalities. The Minnesota Multiphasic Personality Inventory (MMPI) and adjective checklist portrayed strong affective differences between the personalities. Usoffa was angry and violent; King Young, sexual and charming; and Sammy, rational and conventional. The differences in affective responsiveness were also confirmed by differences in galvanic skin response measurements to word lists. The authors found a blurring of personalities with information exchange in affectively neutral areas. For example, the personalities obtained similar IQ scores and showed improved learning on tasks across personalities. One interesting finding was the difference on neurologic examination. Usoffa showed considerable areas of hypalgesia which were consistent with his claim "not to feel pain." The authors considered the hypalgesia a conversion symptom. EEG results, while normal for each personality, showed significant differences among the personalities.

The case of Jonah demonstrates several features

of multiple personality. The onset of the secondary personalities dating from childhood, the amnesia of the primary personality for the secondary personalities, the automatic switchover from one personality to the other under conditions of affective stress, and the chief complaint of headaches and memory loss are all typical. The finding that the primary personality is restricted in affective and behavioral scope, whereas the secondary personalities are uninhibited in aggressive or sexual behavior, is also characteristic. The history of severe trauma in childhood is frequent. Finally, the recurrence of the secondary personalities when Jonah was under stress even after treatment is not unexpected. Multiple personality disorder is usually chronic.

ETIOLOGY

The major theories on the etiology of multiple personality disorder are psychological. The first theory proposed by Prince was that multiple personality was the result of blocked emotion that came about when a severe emotional shock was dealt with by amnesia.[24] The repressed emotion led to the secondary personalities. Later, Taylor and Martin theorized that the secondary personalities represented the breakthrough of drives which the primary personality could no longer repress.[20] Subsequent authors elaborated on this model by stressing the primary personality's inability to cope with psychological stress other than by dissociation.[25] Autohypnosis is another psychological model that has been proposed to explain multiple personality disorder.[2,20] In this model, the subject, at an early age, unwittingly induces a trance in himself in order to deal with stress. The trance states result in the secondary personalities, as well as account for the amnesias of the primary personality. Many authors consider that severe psychosocial stress in childhood leads to early splits in the personality either through dissociation or autohypnosis, and thus to a vulnerability in the patient to use dissociation to deal with later life crises.

DIAGNOSIS AND DIFFERENTIAL DIAGNOSIS

The differential diagnosis of multiple personality disorder includes Psychogenic Amnesia, Psychogenic Fugue, Schizophrenic Disorders, and Malingering. Although there is a second organized personality in psychogenic fugue, this second personality is amnestic for the primary personality and appears only in one episode rather than in frequent shifts of identity in a chronic course. While the person with psychogenic amnesia may be less inhibited during the episode, the differential diagnosis can be made in the fact that a secondary organized personality does not emerge. The differential diagnosis of multiple personality from malingering is more difficult. It is particularly difficult when the patient has committed illegal acts and claims amnesia for the events. In cases of multiple personality, the secondary personality should be able to recall the events and accompanying affect. As mentioned above, the differentiation of multiple personality disorder from schizophrenia has been the subject of recent attention.[2,11] Because the patient with Multiple Personality Disorder may overhear conversations between different personalities, as well as develop paranoid ideas about being influenced by other personalities, these symptoms may be confused with the hallucinations and delusions of schizophrenic disorders. The lack of a formal thought disorder plus the history of amnesia usually serve to differentiate the disorders. However, the psychiatrist must inquire after the amnesia as it is often not spontaneously reported. A full physical examination, including neurologic examination and EEG, are indicated. The EEG is important to uncover undiagnosed temporal lobe epilepsy, as dissociative symptoms are found in a high percentage of these patients.[19] The neurologic examination is important to determine presence or absence of conversion symptoms.

TREATMENT AND PREVENTION

The treatment most often recommended is psychotherapy. The goal of the therapy is twofold. First, the therapist tries to make the patient aware of his tendency to use dissociation and amnesia to deal with painful conflicts. Then he tries to help the patient understand and accept his individual conflicts so they can be integrated into the primary personality. The limited success of this therapy has been attributed to the patient's reverting to dissociation when under stress. Some therapists use hypnosis to uncover the secondary personalities and then suggest to the secondary personalities that they will be remembered by the primary personality. This is done to confront the primary personality with the warded off experiences. However, others caution against the use of hypnosis for two reasons. First, they claim that the therapist, by using hypnosis, is fostering the patient's tendency to dissociate.[25] Second, they point out that the anxiety induced by forcing the primary personality to face warded-off conflicts may increase the patient's use of dissociation to cope with anxiety. Most therapists agree that ego-supportive techniques should be used to help the patient lower his anxiety and thus prevent the need for dissociation.

Depersonalization Disorder

DEFINITION

DSM-III defines *depersonalization disorder* as the occurrence of "one or more episodes of depersonalization that cause social or occupational impairment," and in which the depersonalization is not considered a symptom of another disorder. Depersonalization itself is defined as an alteration in the patient's perception of the self so that one's sense of one's own reality is temporarily lost. According to *DSM-III*, manifestations of depersonalization may include self-perceptions such as "one's extremities have changed in size," seeing one's self as if from a distance or as "mechanical," or a feeling that one is not in complete control of one's actions.[7] *DSM-III* also considered derealization, an alteration in the perception of the reality of objects or people in the external world so that they seem strange or unfamiliar, as a common symptom associated with depersonalization.[7] The only major difference between the *DSM-III* definition and those in the literature is that *DSM-III* considers depersonalization as a disorder, whereas most of the literature considers depersonalization as a symptom occurring in many different disorders.[26] In the author's opinion, the data from case reports and studies on depersonalization, as reported below, support the concept of depersonalization as a symptom seen in many disorders and give little support for *DSM-III's* treating depersonalization as a disorder in its own right.

EPIDEMIOLOGY

Depersonalization was originally considered an early symptom of psychosis. However, in 1936 Mayer-Gross reported that he observed depersonalization not only in patients suffering from early schizophrenia but also in patients with obsessional and hysterical neuroses and in normals under extreme fatigue.[26] More recently, Brauer, Harrow, and Tucker reported two studies on the prevalence of depersonalization in hospitalized psychiatric patients.[27,28] They found that while 80% of 128 consecutive admissions reported depersonalization as one of their symptoms, in only 12% was it severe or long-lasting. In no case was depersonalization the chief complaint.[27] Other findings were that depersonalization was more frequent in both younger patients and patients suffering from schizophrenia.[27] They did not find a sex differential that is consistent with recent studies of depersonalization in normals,[29] but in contradiction with early claims that depersonalization is more prevalent among women.[30] Tucker and Harrow characterized the patient who experiences depersonalization as "a person with chronic anxiety, persistent depressive affect, and some degree of psychopathological thinking."[28] The association between depersonalization and disordered thinking was based on the results of Rorschach tests. They found no correlation between the presence of hallucinations and delusions and depersonalization.

The literature includes two studies on the incidence and characteristics of depersonalization in college populations.[29,30] Both studies found that one third to one half of students reported having experienced depersonalization. These findings may overestimate the incidence of depersonalization in college students because the methodology was a self-report questionnaire that could have led to students' mislabeling hypnogogic or other phenomena as depersonalization. But, these results should introduce a note of caution in the discussion of depersonalization as a disorder or as an early symptom of psychosis.

ETIOLOGY

Freud explained depersonalization as the result of a defense against feelings of guilt in which the patient attempted to deny the experiencing self and thus deny authorship of the feelings. He did not see the presence of depersonalization as indicative of a severe disturbance in ego functioning. However, many of his followers did see depersonalization as the result of primitive defenses and a fragile sense of self and thus associated depersonalization with psychosis. As mentioned above, Mayer-Gross and later others saw depersonalization as a nonspecific symptom of stress.

DIAGNOSIS AND DIFFERENTIAL DIAGNOSIS

The major differential diagnostic problem is to distinguish depersonalization as a symptom secondary to impending psychosis, fatigue, stress, organic mental disorder, or physical disorder from depersonalization as a disorder itself. Thus, a complete history, physical examination, and EEG are indicated. Again, the EEG is important to rule out temporal lobe seizure disorder as depersonalization is frequently found in this disorder.

TREATMENT AND PREVENTION

Data about the appropriate treatment for depersonalization disorder are few. Brauer reported that patients complained that phenothiazines worsened depersonalization and that minor tranquilizers had no effect.[27] Lehman followed the analytic tradition and recommended psychodynamic psychotherapy to uncover the underlying conflicts and help the patient deal with the painful affects.[32] He also reported that while electroconvulsive therapy (ECT) successfuly relieved the depression in patients with depression and depersonalization, ECT had no effect on the depersonalization itself.[32]

Summary

As the foregoing discussion demonstrates, case reports and theorizing on dissociative disorders have made a colorful and confusing chapter in the history of psychiatry. There has been little consensus on the definition of the syndromes and almost no systematic studies have been conducted on the phenomena. Perhaps now with the more specific diagnoses established by *DSM-III* and new epidemiologic approaches that stress gathering cases from wide geographic distributions, more will be learned about these fascinating and rare disorders. However, researchers using *DSM-III* as a diagnostic basis must remain alert to possible confusions of data caused by difficulty diagnosing patients with psychogenic amnesia who travel long distances. Otherwise, there is a possibility that many of the cases will be lost in the category of atypical dissociative disorder.

REFERENCES

1. Alexander FG, Selesnick ST: The History of Psychiatry, p 50. New York, The New American Library, 1966
2. Bliss EL: Multiple personalities: A report of 14 cases with implications for schizophrenia and hysteria. Arch Gen Psychiatry 37:1388, 1980
3. Carlson ET: The history of multiple personality in the United States: I, the Beginnings. Am J Psychiatry 138:666, 1981
4. Kirschner LA: Dissociative reactions: An historical review and clinical study. Acta Psychiatr Scand 49:698, 1973
5. Freud S, Breuer J: Studies on hysteria. In Strachey J (ed): The Pre-Standard Edition of the Complete Psychological Works of Sigmund Freud. London, Hogarth Press, 1955
6. Prince M: Dissociation of a Personality. New York, Longmans, Green and Company, 1906
7. American Psychiatric Association: Diagnostic and Statistical Manual-III, 1982
8. Fisher C: Amnesia states in war neuroses: The psychogenesis of fugues. Psychoanal Q 14:437, 1945
9. American Psychiatric Association: Diagnostic and Statistical Manual-I, 1952
10. American Psychiatric Association: Diagnostic and Statistical Manual-II, 1968
11. Rosenbaum M: The role of the term schizophrenia in the decline of the diagnosis of multiple personality. Arch Gen Psychiatry 37:1383, 1980
12. Fisher C, Josephs E: Fugue with loss of personal identity. Psychoanal Q 18:480, 1949
13. Abeles M, Schilder P: Psychogenic Loss of Personal Identity. Archives of Neurology and Psychiatry 34:587, 1935
14. Parfitt DN, Gall CM: Psychogenic amnesia: The refusal to remember. Journal of Mental Science 90:511, 1944
15. Luparello TJ: Features of fugue: A unified hypothesis of regression. J Am Psychoanal Assoc 18:379, 1970
16. Rapaport D, Gill MM: Amnesia and its bearing on the theory of memory. In Gill MM (ed): The Collected Papers of David Rapaport, pp 113–120. New York, Basic Books Inc, 1967
17. Kanzer M: Amnesia: A statistical study. Am J Psychiatry 96:711, 1939
18. Nemiah J: Hysterical neuroses: Dissociative type. In Friedman A, Kaplan H, Sadock B (eds): Comprehensive Textbook of Psychiatry, 2nd ed, pp 1220–1231. Baltimore, Williams and Wilkins, 1975
19. Schenk L, Bear D: Multiple personality and related dissociative phenomena in patients with temporal lobe epilepsy. Am J Psychiatry 138:1311, 1981
20. Taylor WS, Martin MF: Multiple personality. Journal of Abnormal and Social Psychology 39:281, 1944
21. Thigpen CH, Cleckley H: A Case of Multiple Personality. Journal of Abnormal and Social Psychology 49:135, 1954
22. Douglas-Smith R, Buffington PW, McCard RH: Multiple Personality: Theory, Diagnosis and Treatment. New York, Irvington Publishers, 1982
23. Ludwig AM, Brandsma JM, Wilbur CB: The objective study of multiple personality. Arch Gen Psychiatry 26:298, 1972
24. Winer D: Anger and dissociation: A case study of multiple personality. J Abnorm Psychol 87:368, 1978

25. Sutcliffe JP, Jones J: Multiple personality and hypnosis. Int J Clin Exp Hypn 10:231, 1962

26. Mayer-Gross W: On depersonalization. Br Med J Psychol 15:103, 1935

27. Brauer R, Harrow M, Tucker GJ: Depersonalization phenomena in psychiatric patients. Br J Psychiatry 117:509, 1970

28. Tucker GH, Harrow M, Quinlan D: Depersonalization, dysphoria and thought disturbance. Am J Psychiatry 130:702, 1973

29. Dixon JC: Depersonalization phenomena in a sample population of college students. Br J Psychiatry 109:371, 1963

30. Roberts WW: Normal and Abnormal Depersonalization. Journal of Mental Science 110:236, 1960

31. Freud S: A disturbance of memory on the acropolis. In Strackey J (ed): The Complete Psychological Works of Sigmund Freud, pp 239–248. London, Hogarth Press, 1964

32. Lehman LS: Depersonalization. Am J Psychiatry 131:1221, 1974

Depressive Neurosis

The diagnosis of depressive neurosis is complicated by the multiple and imprecise meanings attached to it. These include nonpsychotic, nonendogenous or reactive, characterologic, and responsive to psychotherapy. The list could be extended, but essentially the critical question regarding the diagnosis is its relation to the affective disorders on the one hand and the neurotic-characterologic disorders on the other.

If one views depressive neurosis as differing in degree but not in kind from the affective disorders, it will be no surprise that many patients with the initial diagnosis of neurotic depression, especially if seen in inpatient settings or special mood disorder clinics, will develop more florid and severe affective disorders of either the bipolar or unipolar type. Within this perspective, the depressive neurosis is regarded as a heterogeneous collection of mild affective disorders that include neurotic-characterologic depressions, depressions secondary to other psychiatric or medical disorders, as well as primary affective disorders, either unipolar or bipolar.[1,2]

If, however, one views the depressive neurosis as qualitatively distinct from the primary affective disorders and places it in the neurotic-characterologic category, then the specific diagnosis implies different treatment directions. It is not an uncommon error to mistake a cyclothymic or dysthymic disorder (the character or temperament equivalents of bipolar and unipolar disorders) for a depressive neurosis, with the unfortunate result that much time and effort is spent in a wasteful psychotherapy. The reverse situation may occur, with a depressive neurotic receiving a long course of exclusively biological treatments when what is required is a psychological intervention directed at a neurotic behavior.

Historical Overview

The diagnosis of depressive neurosis has been described in various forms, at least since Kraepelin.[3] He recognized a "psychogenic depression" that remained reactive to news, good or bad, and was unlike the autonomous depressions and character temperaments of manic-depressive insanity. Freud, his contemporary, did not include depressive neurosis in his original classification of the neuroses, but it was soon included by most psychoanalysts who distinguished it from the biological depressions on the basis of the lesser degree of regression and withdrawal from reality. Subsequent analytic investigators clarified the psychodynamics of neurotic depression, examined its relation to character structure, and more recently have focused on its narcissistic aspects.[4-6]

Kendell describes in illuminating detail the debate in English psychiatry during the first half of the 20th century between the Kraepelinian binary conception of two depressions, biological and psychogenic, and the unitary approach that viewed the apparent differences between the two as simply one of severity.[7] This clinical debate continued on a mathematic level without any real alterations in its nature as populations of patients with depressive states were factored into homogeneous subgroups. A large number of such investigations identified a bipolar endogenous-neurotic factor and another factor that related to severity. Andresean summarized 12 validation studies between 1965 and 1976, suggesting that endogenous depressions, unlike neurotic depressions, showed a good treatment response to antidepressants and electroconvulsive therapy (ECT), had a better progress and outcome, and differed on neurochemical and neuroendocrine measurements.[8]

American nosologists of depression, heavily influenced by Adolf Meyer and Sigmund Freud, included the diagnosis of neurotic depression in both the first and second editions of the *Diagnostic and Statistical Manual of Mental Disorders (DSM)* as a nonpsychotic and reactive depression that was grouped together with the other neuroses, all of which were defined as reactions to warding off anxiety associated with unconscious conflict. In the past 2 decades a paradigmatic shift in American psychiatry toward biological and phenomenologic research has been accompanied by increasing dissatisfaction with depressive neuroses as a nosologic category because of "ideological assumptions" and "clinical confusion."[9] The diagnosis of neurotic depression was initially discarded from the nomenclature by the *DSM-III* task force. After considerable controversy, they resurrected an obsolete term, *dysthymic disorder,* to describe a characterologic depression. A latter compromise added the modifier "(or depressive neurosis)" but was believed by many to be a meaningless addition.[10] At present the diagnosis of neurotic depression in the *DSM-III* can be made by major depression without melancholia, dysthymic disorder, or adjustment reaction with depression.

Epidemiology

Given the uncertain boundaries of the depressive neuroses, any epidemiologic data must be cautiously interpreted. Many recent studies have attempted to avoid nosologic confusion by distinguishing depressive symptoms, unipolar depression, and bipolar depression. Depressive symptoms are found to be remarkably common. Self-report inventories of depressive symptoms such as the Zung have found that 12% of a "normal" population obtains scores that are greater than or equal to the threshold level for depressive disorder.[11] Weissman and Myers in a recent community study found that 12% of men and 20% of women report depressive symptoms at any given time.[12] One cannot make any inference from this data regarding the incidence of depressive disorder. Risk factors for depressive symptoms include female gender, early adulthood for women and later in life for men, a low socioeconomic status, and divorce or separation. Weissman and Myers found a prevalence of 2.5% for minor depressions. This

might be regarded as a tentative but best available estimate for depressive neurosis. Marks[13] has summarized a number of studies that indicate that depressive neurosis is a frequent finding in primary care populations. He cites Cooper and Clyph's finding that 96% of all psychiatric morbidity in eight general medical practices in London took the form of anxiety–depression.

Definitions and General Considerations

DEPRESSIVE AFFECT AND MOOD

Depressive affect is commonly defined as the emotion that accompanies an uncomplicated grief reaction to a bereavement. Jacobson[14] has argued for the distinction between depressed affect and the affect of grief by noting the relief that depressed individuals feel when they are able to experience grief. Others have emphasized helplessness or a loss of self-esteem as the central feeling of depressive affect.[6,15,16]

Another group of investigators assume a more generalist view and regard depressive affect as embracing a wide range of dysphoric, painful, or unpleasant feelings.[17] Sadness, dejection, self-reproach, helplessness, despair, feeling rejected, pessimism, and boredom may all be included. This is the approach taken by most depression inventories. They include a general question regarding the presence or absence of depressive or "blue" feelings and then contain a list of other dysphoric affects.

Anxiety is a dysphoric affect that is usually distinguished from depression. Anxiety is accompanied by somatic evidence of arousal such as palpitations, dyspnea, and muscular tension as well as an apprehensiveness or fear of an imminent danger. Depressive affect in contrast is accompanied by somatic evidence of inhibition such as fatigue and loss of appetite and libido as well as a feeling of helplessness in the face of a loss or narcissistic injury. Anxiety and depression often occur together and patients frequently confuse them.

When an affect becomes pervasive and influences all aspects of behavior for a period of time it becomes a mood. Depressed moods are not uncommon, are easily identified, and need not be pathologic. The grief that follows a bereavement or the acute disappointment in failing to attain a wished for goal are examples of nonpathologic depressed moods. The moods are understandable and have an interpersonal communicativeness and responsiveness that is part of our ordinary relations with others.

Demoralization is a mood that has considerable currency in the current psychiatric literature.[18] It refers to a belief in one's ineffectiveness engendered by severe life defeat that can derive from intolerable situational factors as well as medical or psychiatric illnesses. It is descriptively similar to despair. There is of course no contradiction in maintaining that one can feel helpless and depressed about one's mental state, whether it be anxiety, obsessions, or depression. Kierkegaard[19] stated it simply, "the degree of consciousness potentiates despair."

Both anxious and depressive affects and moods are easily recognized, ubiquitous, and of probable adaptive value, with anxiety serving as a signal of imminent psychological danger and depression as a signal of psychological loss or defeat. Freud[20] viewed the depressed response to loss as an adaptive means of overcoming the loss by identification and growth. Bowlby[21] has suggested that it is a conservation mechanism that maximizes survival until attachment to another is reestablished. Brenner[22] regards the affects of anxiety and depression as the two basic danger affects, which together with pleasure guide all human behavior.

A critical question is whether the depressed affect or mood found in pathologically melancholic conditions is qualitatively similar or different from that found in normal depressive conditions. The controversy relates to the diagnoses of neurotic depression. Those who subscribe to the narrow definition of depressive neurosis believe that the affective experience that occurs in it is qualitatively similar to normal depressive moods and different from those found in the affective disorders. They then direct their attention to the learned or acquired behaviors believed to occur in the neurotic-characterologic disorders. Those who believe that the difference is simply quantitative are usually those who embrace a continuum or unitary theory of clinical depression in which depressive neurosis is viewed as a "mild" form. The distinctions in quality and quantity that are central to the controversy over the definition of depressive neurosis are to be found in the classic distinctions between endogenous/reactive and psychotic/neurotic.

ENDOGENOUS VERSUS REACTIVE DEPRESSION

Endogenous ("arising from within") is classically used to describe the severe "constitutional-like" retarded or agitated depressions seen frequently in manic-depressive or unipolar disorders. It is contrasted to exogenous or reactive depressions that can arise from toxins, infections, or psychological causes, although current usage confines the meaning to psychological. Endogenous and reactive depressions are believed to differ with regard to precipitants, reactivity, somatic symptoms, quality of mood, and severity.

Kraepelin recognized that endogenous depressions may also be precipitated by stressful events, but in his view these events were sparks that ignited a fundamentally morbid process.[3] Later clinicians neglected this observation and believed that endogenous depressions were without precipitants until Garmany[23] established that stressful events preceded both reactive and endogenous depressions. Somatic symptoms commonly reported in endogenous depression and believed not to occur in reactive depressions include insomnia, especially in the early morning, weight loss, decreased appetite and libido, fatigue, diurnal variation, and altered psychomotor behavior. These somatic symptoms were regularly reported to occur in association with the "endogenous factor" in most analytic studies of depressions. Nelson and Charney,[24] in their review of this topic, conclude that most of these symptoms with the exception of altered psychomotor activity may be nonspecific responses to stress and not specific to endogenous depressions. Roth[25] states that it is not unusual to find somatic symptoms in neurotic depression.

Reactivity was the pathognomonic symptom that Kraepelin[3] believed distinguished psychogenic depressions from endogenous-constitutional depressions. The depressed mood in the endogenous depression lost its responsiveness to environmental events while in psychogenic depression it remained. Gillespie[26] prefers the terms *reactive* and *autonomous* as modifiers because the neurotic group has as its central feature a "responsiveness to influence, both external and internal" while the autonomous endogenous group shares no such reactivity beyond, at most, an initial precipitation. Klein[27] has emphasized the anhedonia of the autonomous group as a distinguishing feature.

The severity of the depression is traditionally referred to as the psychotic-neurotic distinction where *neurotic* simply means the absence of florid symptoms such as hallucinations, delusions, or loss of reality testing. This distinction historically relates to the practical issue of certification and asylum treatment. Endogenous depressions tend to be more severe but not always. Many patients with a strong history of bipolar disease present with mild recurrent depressions or a persistent characterologic dysthmia.

In summary, endogenous depressions may have a precipitant, are autonomous and anhedenic, present with characteristic somatic symptoms, and may vary in severity. Reactive-neurotic depressions have a precipitant, are reactive, may have some somatic symptoms, and remain circumscribed in severity.

Eysenck[28] argues it is an error to regard the dichotomy between endogenous and neurotic depression as being between separate categorical diagnostic classes. He believes that each category measures dimensions present in all depressions and that each should be rated individually from mild to severe. This view is in accord with the finding of the large numbers of mixed endogenous-neurotic patients described in most factor analytic studies, an average of 33% in one overview.[29] Klein, in a widely cited paper,[27] has argued for a combined dimensional and categorical system. He views the endogenomorphic category as a dimensional factor since it predicts ECT and tricyclic response and finds that some neurotic depressions may have an endogenomorphic dimension. Akiskal[30] has defined subcategories of depressive neurosis (broadly defined) on the basis of tricyclic response, but it appears that his responders are primarily mild forms of endogenous depressions.

Response to biological treatments is one validating factor in an endogenous depression/neurotic depression distinction. Another is the responsiveness of neurotic depression to psychological interventions. The reader is referred to the chapter on neurosis (*please consult index*) in which responsiveness to psychosocial treatments is recorded as a distinguishing feature of the neuroses since, at least, Pinel's description of them as "moral" disorders. This is, of course, a major issue since one purpose of diagnosis is treatment.

CHARACTER STRUCTURE AND DIAGNOSIS

The relationship of character to the depressive neurosis begins with Kraepelin's observations of a depressive temperament "characterized by a permanent emotional stress in all experiences of life."

This disorder begins in late adolescence, and although it might progress "imperceptibly" to real attacks of melancholia, it need not.[3] Nevertheless, because of the genetic association of these patients with manic-depressive disease, Kraepelin viewed their character disorder as a "rudiment of the fully developed disease." He also described "cyclothymic" and "irritable" variations. This equivalence of character with an attenuated version of the manic-depressive disorder is believed by many to be what is meant by depressive neurosis and is reflected in the *DSM-III* diagnosis of dysthymic disorder "(depressive neurosis)." The term *dysthymic character* will be reserved to refer to this predominantly constitutional depressive character in contrast to depressive neurosis.

Another view points to the possibility that character modifies or affects the expression of the depression. This is called the pathoplasty view of depression and character by Hirschfeld and Cross.[31] Thus, the work oriented, obsessive patient emphasizes his inability to work effectively or efficiently while the dependent hysterical patient complains of feelings of insecurity and humiliation.

Additionally the character structure of the patient may predispose to depression. The psychoanalytic literature maintains that the depression-prone character is distinguished by difficulty in expressing anger without guilt, a tendency to be self-punitive or intolerant of personal failings, a narcissistic need for unqualified positive regard from valued others in order to feel good, and inflated aspirations and self-images.[32] These traits are not mutually exclusive, and some theorists have maintained that one or the other is primary. Traditional psychoanalytic theory emphasized a punitive superego or conscience with difficulties in accepting hostile impulses, as well as a tendency for severe self-reproach. More recent literature has emphasized the narcissistic grandiosity and vulnerability of the pre-depressive. His inflated self-image and aspirations are easily punctured or frustrated. Basch[6] maintains that depressive neurosis is a form of narcissistic personality reacting to a narcissistic injury. Roth[25] believes that if the depressed mood in the neurotic depressive cannot be traced to personality features or difficulties, the diagnosis is suspect. Hirschfeld and Cross[31] summarize a number of psychometric studies that suggest that nonmelancholic depressives may be predisposed to depressive episodes by a high degree of neuroticism.

For completeness, two other possible relationships between depression and character are that they are unrelated or that a depression may deleteriously affect the personality either as a result of chronicity or severity. Some have called this a demoralization syndrome. Kraines[33] has described a syndrome of postdepressive personality in patients with major affective disorders that might fit this category. A more likely possibility is that these patients develop a chronic mild residual depression.[30]

In summary, depression and personality can interact in several ways. In considering the diagnosis of depressive neurosis one must exclude the dysthymic character and chronic-residual affective states and be able to relate the depression to a personality predisposition to respond to stress with depression. Different personalities may express or modify the depression differently, but this is not as crucial to diagnosis as the personality predisposition.

NEUROTIC DEPRESSION

Neurotic depression is defined as a depressed mood that is inappropriate in duration and magnitude but that remains circumscribed and is reactive to both environmental and psychological events. The depression is qualitatively more related to normal depressive moods than to endogenous depression. It occurs in individuals with the character traits of difficulty in dealing with anger, tendency to self-reproach, excessively high expectations, and a dependence on the unqualified positive regard of others for the maintenance of self-esteem.

Clinical Description

The patient usually presents with a depressed mood and complains of depression, sadness, lowering of mood, emptiness or loss of spontaneity. Helplessness, loss of confidence and initiative, loneliness, self-disparagement, and regretful preoccupations are other common complaints. The precise description of the depression will be influenced by the patient's personality, gender, history, developmental phase, and cultural background. Men may be less likely to complain of depression than women because of the greater difficulty they have, probably because of cultural influences, in acknowledging the passive helplessness that is so integral to any experience of depression. They usually complain of secondary depressive phenomena, such as problems with work or difficulties with aggressive strivings. From a developmental perspective young adult patients are more

likely to emphasize existential aspects of depression, such as loss of meaning, while older patients more frequently complain of failure or disappointments in self, family, or career or focus entirely on somatic concerns.

The patient's depression may be accompanied by other affects, such as anxiety or anger. Anxiety is the most common accompaniment of depression so that most depressives present with what seem to be an anxious depression. Guilt in the forms of self-reproach, self-criticism, and self-devaluation is another common accompaniment of depression. In the past, guilt has been thought to correlate with the severity of the depression and to be more characteristic of psychotic or endogenous depression. Recent studies, however, suggest that this is not so.[34]

Apathy with some loss of interest in work, recreation, and social activity occur. These symptoms may be quite mild. Normal activities are continued, but with a mechanical and automatic aspect; they become more difficult and require greater energy than usual. At work, papers are shuffled and decisions requiring initiative and originality are not made because of the loss of confidence. This may not be apparent to colleagues because of pseudo-activity, which often gives the impression of busyness. The spouse may observe that the patient seems more subdued, less spontaneous, slightly withdrawn or more "mopy."

The patient's thoughts are characterized by worry, difficulty in concentration, and efforts at superficial and passive distraction, such as reading mysteries or watching television without really absorbing their content. The patient may wish passively for death or actively think of suicide, but these are usually accepted as passing thoughts or, in more insightful patients, as a means of providing temporary relief or to obtain revenge against specific targets. They are not, in most cases, seriously entertained.

One or two somatic symptoms such as insomnia, diurnal variation, appetite changes, decreased libido, and fatigue may be present. A common sleep disturbance in neurotic depression is hypersomnia with the patient escaping into sleep with frequent naps. This is particularly true when he is not able to occupy himself with work or some other activity, such as on weekends or vacations. Finally, somatic complaints are frequent and include bowel disturbances, headaches, neuromuscular aches and pain, and fears of serious diseases such as cancer or heart disease. The older the patient, or the more his self-esteem depends on physical attractiveness or health, the more likely are somatic or vegetative complaints to dominate the picture.

Depression in the neurotic remains contained, and its fluctuations can often be traced to changes in narcissistic support, reparative successes, distraction, or mastery as a result of increased psychological maturity. Insight is variably present. The patient is aware of his depression and usually has a sense of it being related to a specific situation, although this is not always the case.

With those who are initially unaware of a precipitant, obtaining a detailed anamnesis of the patient's depression against the background of his personal and work history will usually reveal a precipitant that will be recognized with insight and some abreaction by the patient. Often this may turn out to be an apparently trivial incident that will only be revealed in its full meaning by an understanding of the patient's personal history and intrapsychic dynamics. The full exposition of the precipitants may be quite complex and elusive as in the following case: A married woman became guiltily depressed after an affair. During treatment it became clear that the affair was an effort to ward off a depression that had begun several days prior to the affair as the result of an imagined rejection by a younger brother toward whom she still unconsciously turned, as she had as a child, for support and love. In the absence of a precipitating event, despite inquiry, the diagnosis of neurotic depression is suspect. The converse is not true. The presence of a precipitating event does not rule out an endogenous depression.

Course of Neurotic Illness

Neurotic depressions, like all depressions, are time limited, although they tend to recur. Because of characterologic predisposition, the neurotic depressive often responds with depression to the inevitable small frustrations and disappointments of work and family. These can last for hours or days. Many neurotic depressives show a lifetime pattern of fleeing depression through characteristic defenses and coping devices. Examples of these patterns include compulsive work, parenting, or play; substance abuse; defensive denial or inhibition of fantasy; and withdrawal from situations that might prove disappointing. However, when life events inevitably overwhelm the patient's usual coping mechanisms the underlying depressive tendency becomes

fully evident. Careful history should reveal the antecedent depressive tendencies.

Differential Diagnosis

In this chapter the position has been taken that the mild depressions may result from different etiologies and that it is possible to clinically distinguish neurotic depressive illness within this heterogeneous group. This conceptualization is at variance with the widely held belief that there are a large number of mild depressions that cannot be clinically differentiated and that one should precede on the assumption that one is dealing with a mild endogenous depression and prescribe pharmacologic treatment. Only after all such treatments have failed, and there is evidence that the patient is responding to psychotherapeutic intervention, is one on more firm ground in diagnosing neurotic depression. This method of diagnosis by exclusion, given the present state of knowledge, is not without merit. In the absence of any biochemical, physiologic, or pathognomonic symptoms, one is always on uncertain ground in defining a disease. Until we have a valid diagnostic test to distinguish via laboratory results the particular subgroups of depression, it is wise to proceed cautiously. With this cautionary note in mind, it is possible to consider the following differential diagnoses in the diagnosis of neurotic depression.

UNIPOLAR OR BIPOLAR DEPRESSION. A differential problem occurs in attenuated or mild forms of these syndromes. Often the patient's subjective experience of his depressions is that they are mysterious in origin, that they somehow "befall" him rather than occur in reaction to a disappointing event. The depression often feels qualitatively different from their normal depression because of greater fatigue or retardation and a sense of their apparent autonomy and absence of reactivity. A family history of bipolar disease, or a history of either spontaneous or tricyclic antidepressant–induced episodes of hypomania, will suggest a bipolar disorder.

MAJOR DEPRESSIONS WITH RESIDUAL CHRONICITY. This is a late-onset depression that is the sequela to one or more episodes of major (unipolar) depression in which the premorbid personality was not notably depressed. The major depressive episode usually results in hospitalization and ECT or tricyclic medication with an incomplete remission.

Endogenous symptoms of insomnia, fatigue, and psychomotor retardation persist, often with attitudes of helplessness, dependence, resignation, and pessimism. A strong family history of depression, an unhappy environmental situation, and secondary drug dependence are often present. Inadequate treatment and/or the presence of realistic stress adds a demoralization or reactive-neurotic component that may foster the persistence of the illness. Akiskal[30] has observed a decreased rapid eye movement (REM) latency in these patients similar to patients with major depressions. This, together with their genetic loading, suggests that the residual symptoms of these patients represent a true affective illness.

CHRONIC SECONDARY DEPRESSIONS. These patients suffer from a concurrent chronic medical or psychiatric disease. These may include alcoholism, opiate addiction, neurologic disease, schizophrenia, and obsessive-compulsive, panic, and phobic disorders. Patients usually experience these depressions as an aspect or reaction to their basic illness so that changes in the latter are accompanied by parallel mood changes.

"HYSTEROID DYSPHORIA" AND THE ATYPICAL DEPRESSIONS. Klein[35] has designated as hysteroid dysphoria a group of predominately female depressives whose mood is shallow and labile and who are overly sensitive to rejection from others. This "rejection sensitivity" results in frequent, painful, crashlike depressions that last for hours but may persist for days and that are usually nonautonomous in that depression can be terminated by attention and applause. The response is often associated with overeating, a craving for sweets, oversleeping, and a sense of extreme fatigue, leaden paralysis, or fatigue. Klein initially regarded hysteroid dysphoria as a borderline personality syndrome and more recently as an atypical depression. It seems more likely to be depressive neurosis in a severely hysterical or borderline personality.

The atypical neurotic depressions manifest prominent anxiety, hysterical features such as emotional overreactivity and lability, and somatic complaints that include fatigue, hypersomnia, and hyperphagia. The entire group is reported to be responsive to monoamine oxidase inhibitors. Their relationship to the depressive neuroses is unclear. Often the onset of a neurotic depression will be accompanied by anxiety, phobias, and obsessive-compulsive symptoms that disappear when the depression lifts. Equally true is the secondary development of depressions in patients with anxiety states and phobic or obsessive-compulsive neurosis that does not affect these symptoms or may intensify them until the depression remits.

BORDERLINE, NARCISSISTIC, MASOCHISTIC, SCHIZOID, AND SCHIZOTYPAL PERSONALITY DISORDERS. These personality disorders often present as depression. In many instances it is believed that these patients are also neurotic depressives who manifest problems described from different characterologic vantage points, such as from self-esteem regulation disturbance in the narcissistic personality disorder, or the intensely unstable object relations in the borderline personality disorder. Generally, the "pure" depressive neurotic will be less interpersonally exploitative or ruthless and more capable of caring and concern than patients with these other diagnoses. Other distinguishing features may include evidence of transient psychotic episodes in the borderline personality disorder and the haughty arrogance of the narcissistic personality disorder. The person with a narcissistic personality disorder often presents with a late midlife neurotic depression when he begins to appreciate the unattainability of some of his grandiose self-expectations. These patients are not infrequently misdiagnosed as unipolar depressions. The masochistic personality disorder is often diagnosed by an emphasis on the centrality of ego-syntonic self-destructive behavior that is not usually accompanied by a depressed affect. Both the masochistic personality disorders and neurotic depressive may turn a victory into defeat, but the depressive is likely to do this intrapsychically by experiencing depression rather than triumph; the masochist is more likely to provoke an external disaster that undermines the success. Schizotypal and schizoid personalities can often present with depression, but the bizarre delusional-like picture of the former and the social isolation of the latter are distinguishing features.

DYSTHYMIC CHARACTER. This diagnosis, introduced in the *DSM-III* as the equivalent of depressive neurosis, is defined there as a persistent depressive syndrome of subclinical severity ("neurotic") of at least 2 years' duration. It is probably best to use this diagnosis to refer to a personality disorder that is a rudimentary form of either bipolar or unipolar depression. These patients present with a long history of persistent depressions that imperceptibly move in and out of major depressive episodes of full syndromal severity. Often the distinction between such depressions is one of feeling "really awful" rather than my "usual terrible self." The cyclothymic personality in a depressed phase can be easily differentiated by the history of mild hypomanic episodes.

CHARACTER SPECTRUM DISORDER.   Akiskal[30] has described a group of patients who have a chronic low-grade depression all of their lives that he labels character spectrum disorder. "Their life is one of instability, impulsivity, and subtle interpersonal manipulativeness, with chronic dysphoria and low self opinion weaved into the character structure." Unstable character traits may include dependent, histrionic, antisocial, and schizoid features. The childhood history is often one of parental loss, alcoholism, and broken homes. Akiskal found none of the biological markers of affective disorders in these patients, such as decreased REM latency or genetic loading for depression in family members, and views these patients as the outcome of their exposure to parental alcoholism, sociopathy, and somatization disorders. This disorder seems to be closely related to the borderline personality syndrome with depressive and hysterical features.

Etiology

BIOLOGICAL STUDIES

Studies of endocrine function, REM latency, peripheral receptor assays, and response to antidepressant medications all offer exciting possibilities for the more precise definitions of disease subgroups and etiology. These and other biological studies of depression in humans have not focused on outpatient populations of neurotic depressives. When they have, it has usually been within the wide definition of the diagnosis so that the findings are difficult to interpret. Mother–infant separation studies in primates and rodents have provided animal models for the role of early maternal deprivation in the development of a vulnerability to dysphoria throughout life.[36]

PSYCHODYNAMICS

The psychodynamic contribution to the etiology of depressive neuroses has been in two major areas: The psychological pathophysiology of depressive symptoms and the developmental contribution to the adult vulnerability to depressive neuroses. Each will be discussed in turn.

Grief and Depression

Freud's major contribution to the understanding of depressive illness was an analysis of the distinctions between grief and depression. Grief occurs over time and in uncomplicated cases moves through a sequence of shock and disbelief, characteristic symptoms of depression and, finally, recovery. This process of grief or mourning involves the gradual relinquishment of the intense attachment to the lost object and the reappearance of an interest in and capacity for new relationships. Depression is characterized by a miscarriage in this process; the melancholic remains helplessly resigned to his loss and is unable to move on to a new attachment successfully. He also, unlike the grief-stricken individual, experiences an intense diminution of self-regard; the loss is felt as part of the self. "In mourning, it is the world which has become poor and in melancholia it is the ego itself; the patient represents his ego to us as worthless."[37]

Freud found that the shameless and insistent self-reproaches of the depressive do not really refer to the patient but are complaints and accusations directed at the lost object; it is as if the object has taken up residence within the ego of the melancholic. Freud illuminated this process by noting that it occurred when the attachment to the lost object was unconsciously ambivalent and narcissistic. The anger, usually not acknowledged, toward the ambivalently perceived object elicits a guilty response. The resulting conflict between rage and guilt is unconsciously resolved by internalizing the now angrily devalued object. He is "placed in the ego" where he can be freely attacked under the disguise of self-reproaches. A secondary identification with the lost object also occurs in depression, which was described by Rado.[38] In this identification the relationship with the positive gratifying aspects of the object is separated from the frustrating aspects of the same object by placing him in a different internalized location—the conscience or superego—where his criticisms are directed toward the self. The depressed individual through painful expiation and suffering can now regain the love and praise of this internalized, idealized, good object. The pathophysiology of neurotic depression is a miscarried grief in which the patient as a result of identifications with the ambivalent significant other participates in a secret drama of hostile attack and painful expiation.

Clinically, one may observe these phenomenon in patients. They often recognize in their self-reproaches, in their tone or contents, both an anger toward a significant person in their life or the angry criticism of a significant person toward them. In comparison, the bereaved individual also shows identifications with the deceased, but they are with more positive aspects of the lost object. An example is a woman who pursues a career in which her dying husband had encouraged her in and has the persistent feeling that he would admire or like what she was doing. In the analytic psychotherapy of the neurotic depressive, grief is a significant sign of the resolution of the depression that occurs as the patient experiences more positive feelings and identifications toward previously devalued and frustrating objects in his life.

This defense mechanism, "identification with the lost object," was later amplified by Freud[20] as a crucial process that accompanies the growth of the ego. Every step forward in growth and individuation is accompanied by the loss and increasing internalization of important aspects of ongoing relationships. The child, at each stage of development, assumes for himself functions that previously were performed by parents. In normal identification with the lost object, such as in uncomplicated grief or growth, the ego identified with positive adaptive aspects of the lost object. The losses, disappointments, and unhappiness of life are overcome by the growth of the ego.

Depression and Self-Esteem

As has been discussed, depression is often related to thoughts of real and/or fantasized object loss and grief. In other cases, however, there may be experiences of injury to one's sense of personal worth that lead to feelings of inferiority, inadequacy, sadness, and unworthiness. Bibring[15] argues that the loss of self-esteem or narcissistic vulnerability is by itself not depression. Only when there is a superimposed feeling of helplessness to live up to highly charged aspirations can one speak of depression. These aspirations will vary from individual to individual, and Bibring provides a classification developed along psychosexual developmental phases. The aspirations may be oral dependent—the wish to be loved, to receive narcissistic supplies, or to be cared for; it may be anal aggressive—the wish to be good, loving, clean; or the wish may be phallic narcissistic—the wish to be admired or to be strong and triumphant. Depressions will result in the individual with oral-dependent aspirations if there is a perception, real or imagined, of not being loved or independent; in the individual with anal-aggressive aspirations if there is a perception of lack of control over hostility, defiance, or dirtiness; and finally, in the phallic-narcissistic individual, over defeat, ridicule, and retaliation.

Depression and Object Relations

Bibring's theory of depression makes little mention of the role of aggression and object relations. There are, it is true, depressions in which aggression does not seem to play a significant part, but this may only be true of the manifest content of these depressions. Often there is an unacknowledged hostile fantasy that is expressed in indirectly manipulative or coercive behavior of the depressive toward his objects. The sulking or hurt expression that the neurotic husband casts toward his concerned wife carries with it an angry accusation as does his responding with a despairing "no" to her questions of whether there is anything that she can do to help. This anger usually becomes more explicit as the patient recovers from the depression, or when the patient can justify its presence as a secondary response to the annoyance and frustration that his depressed behavior evokes in family and friends.

More recently Kohut[39,40] and others of the school of self-psychology have emphasized the narcissistic attachments of individuals prone to depression. They emphasize the dynamic role of the valued object, the self-object in their terminology, in maintaining the depressive individual's self-esteem. Such an individual may react with depression when the self-object fails to supply necessary supplies for self-esteem maintenance. This can occur if the self-object fails to provide a "mirroring" or external confirmation of the depressive's grandiose but fragile self-image or fails to live up to an expected idealized state. The resulting "ego depletion" or depression is a manifestation of a problem in the self's regulation of self-esteem.

Related Psychological Theories

A current psychological theory of depression that has received much attention is "learned helplessness."[40] This is an operational construct used to describe a behavior pattern in animals repeatedly subjected to inescapable painful electric shocks. If they are then subjected to a new task, they cower passively and do not initiate new learning responses. This "learned helplessness" lasts for 72 hours at which time most of the experimental dogs recover.

Seligman and his associates[41] have argued that learned helplessness provides an animal model for depression. The symptoms are similar and include passivity, a negative cognitive set to learning responses that might produce relief, an apparent lack of aggression, weight loss, appetite loss, improvement over time, and finally, improvement by ECT.

The depressive patient believes or has learned that he cannot control elements of his life that provide relief or bring gratification. He feels helpless. This cognitive model is strikingly similar to Bibring's proposal that depression is a basic ego response to an awareness of its helplessness.

Another cognitive theory of depression is provided by Beck[42] and emphasizes specific distortions or "schema" in the thinking of a depressed individual that influence the way in which reality is processed. These include a negative view of world, a negative concept of self, and a negative appraisal of the future. This cognitive triad is considered to be the primary disturbance in depression. It is a filter through which life's events are perceived, experienced, and organized. Other symptoms such as fatigue or withdrawal are the results of an expectation of a negative outcome. Persistent sadness is the result of a chain reaction in which the sadness is intensified by the misinterpretation, "I will always be sad." Vegetative signs are thought to be physiologic concomitants of the psychological disturbance.

Early Developmental Contributions to Depressive Neuroses

A fundamental theme in the psychodynamic and most other psychological theories of depression is the vital importance of early childhood experiences to the development of adult depressive pathology. Numerous studies of children and adults have attempted either to document the existence of antecedent childhood depressive disorders or to describe failures in the organization and mastery of normal depressive affects in the course of development. Closely related to both investigative trends has been the etiologic role of loss and inadequate parenting through parental death, separation, deprivation, and overstimulation. It is a complex and uncertain field of study that nonetheless is rich in observation and theory although weak in conclusions.

A number of analytic investigators have suggested, on the basis of analytic work with adult depressive neurotics, that there is an infantile or childhood depression that creates a latent tendency for future adult depressions. Jacobson,[43] elaborating on an earlier hypothesis of Abraham, proposed that the adult depressive experiences an intense disillusionment as a child. Characteristically this is preceded by a sequence of spoiling, deficient mothering, precocious onset in the relationship to the father, and finally a strong oedipal disappointment in both parents that produces a resentful narcissistic retreat. This primal depression, at a time when the boundaries between object and self images are not firmly established, results in fragile object relations based on oral-dependent needs with overexpectations in both loved objects and the self that are easily frustrated in later life.

These hypothetical constructions of childhood depressions have been supplemented by direct observations of children. Spitz[44] described the syndrome of hospitalism in some infants deprived of maternal interaction, which was characterized by sadness, weepiness, withdrawal from the environment, developmental retardation, loss of appetite, insomnia, and death. He notes that expressions in these infants as difficult to describe, but in an adult, they would be called depressed. Poznanski[45] has summarized her work and others documenting the existence of later childhood and adolescent depressions. It is not clear from her work whether these develop into adult depressions.

Other theorists have argued that depression is a basic affect that all children must master. Developmental failures in this task would create a tendency in the adult toward neurotic depression. Zetzel[46] has argued that psychological maturity can be measured by the capacity to tolerate depressive affects in response to life's misfortunes without being overwhelmed and immobilized by the development of a depressive disorder or reacting with blame, denial, anger, or some other behavior intended to decrease the significance of the events.

A highly influential theory of the relationship between normal childhood depressive experiences and adult depression is the proposal by Melanie Klein of a universal depressive position in all infants. According to Klein, all children pass through a depressive phase evident in stranger anxiety between 6 and 12 months of age characterized by their growing awareness of their mother as a person who leads a life of her own and has relationships with other people. This is accompanied by fears that the infant's greed, envy, and jealousy have destroyed, or will destroy, this loved mother on whom he is so utterly dependent. During the depressive phase, the infant begins to experience an appropriate guilt at these destructive impulses, and if the mother is able to provide a suitably supportive environment the child will gradually become confident of his capacity to love and master his rage and guilt. This depressive position is not an actual prototype for adult depression but is more accurately conceived of as a normal childhood developmental achievement that provides the foundation for the mastery and tolerance of adult depressive affects. Klein[47] proposed that those infants with a constitutional excess of sadistic envy would find it more difficult to accomplish this and be vulnerable to symptomatic depressions.

Mahler and her collaborators[48] have described changes in affect associated with the development of the infant's establishment of "separateness" from the mother. Mahler describes the predominant mood of the child during the practicing period of separation-individuation as the child moves to and away from the mother as one of elation, grandeur, triumph, and conquest. The toddler is "intoxicated" with his mastery of locomotion. However, inevitable experiences of relative helplessness puncture his inflated sense of omnipotence and he attains a more realistic appraisal of his smallness in relation to the outside world at 15 to 18 months. In this new phase of "rapprochment," there is a mood of relative soberness or even temporary depression. The interaction of the child with the mother during this period is crucial in influencing the child's management of his injured self-esteem and basic depressive mood. Often a mood of low-keyedness can be assuaged by the mother's attentive "refueling" of the child at critical moments. If the child fails to work through the loss of his infantile omnipotence, Mahler speculates that he will be prone to respond to later disappointments with clinical depression, denial, or paranoid attributions of blame.

An important contribution to the theory of the relationship of childhood experiences to adult psychopathology has been made by Bowlby in his studies of childrens' and lower animals' reactions to separations.[49] Initially, the child or animal responds with weeping and aggressive actions that seem to be an automatic response aimed at the reclaiming of the mother. If successful, the result is a reunion and the cessation of what Bowlby calls the phase of protest and pining. If the mother does not appear, the protest diminishes and is replaced by despair and disorganization. The child becomes withdrawn and inactive, makes few demands on his environment, and appears to be depressed. Adaptationally, the child is conserving his energy. If the mother returns at this point the child responds with a renewal of the anger at her and an increase in clinging behaviors. If she does not return, there is a stage of detachment, during which there is a seeming reengagement and interest in the environment, but the persistence of a remoteness and apathy in regard to the mother.

Bowlby believes that repeated separation and rejections in childhood, parental death being an extreme form, provide the necessary condition for an adult pathologic reaction to loss. The child, as a result of such losses, has an unresolved protest and yearning for his mother that develops into a tendency toward object possessiveness and angry demands that the object not abandon him. These persist in latent form, and when losses occur as an adult a healthy grief response is aborted.

The hypotheses that variables in the child/parent relationship place a child at future risk for depression and other psychiatric illnesses has resulted in a large number of studies. Currently, there are at least 35 studies on the subject of affective disorder and specific losses in childhood due to death and separations. Only weak associations have been demonstrated, and a number of excellent current reviews have interpreted them differently. Akiskal and McKinney[50] maintain that any causal link remains unproved, but Lloyd[51] writes that although the results are conflicting, there are more positive than negative reports.

Efforts to study the qualitative aspects of the parent–child interaction in any systematic way are even more difficult. The predominant clinical consensus is that failures in this area, however conceptualized, lead to impaired object relations as an adult, fragile self-esteem, and an inability to bear depression without becoming symptomatic. Studies by Parker[52] on the perceived parental characteristics in adult depressives have established that depressive neurotics, unlike bipolar patients and matched controls, perceive themselves as having been exposed either to an insufficiency of parental care or to parental overprotection. Parker maintains that the representation of the parents as "affectionless and controlling" is not only specific to the depressive neuroses but is also a valid representation since many of the patients' parents rate themselves similarly.

In summary, there is a general clinical consensus, with some research support, that an impaired child–parent relationship contributes to an adult tendency to depression. We conceptualize that a basic depressive affect develops out of a biological substrate and gains increasing psychological representation as the capacity for symbolization, memory, and fantasy develops. Childhood trauma of the kinds described above by Spitz, Klein, Mahler, Jacobson, and Parker modify this process and create an adult vulnerability to depression. In examining the patient with depression, both current and past developmental experiences will be found to be relevant.

Treatment

Treatment choice in neurotic depression is usually determined more by training and bias than patient variables. For example, the cognitive therapist is more likely to recommend the treatment modality in which he is skilled than to cross ideological boundaries and recommend a pharmacologic or psychoanalytic treatment. The problem is more complex for the eclectic psychiatrist who is skilled in a number of treatments. He can select from a wide range of treatments for neurotic depression that include psychoanalysis, psychoanalytic psychotherapy, brief therapies, system treatments (couple or family), and pharmacologic treatments.

In general, the treatment of choice for a neurotic-characterologic disorder is a long-term psychoanalytic treatment. The tactics of treatment include the clarification of the symptoms, interpretation of unconscious conflicts, and working through. This is most effectively accomplished through analysis of transference, which refers to the patient's tendency to "attach" to the psychiatrist and the treatment, the core conflicts, and fantasies that underlie the neurosis. Current conflicts and relationships will prove to be heavily, but not exclusively, influenced by antecedent childhood experiences. The models for depression provided by Spitz, Klein, Mahler, Bowlby, and Jacobson provide useful schemas for the patient and therapist to frame the effect of childhood influences. Development, however, does not stop with childhood but extends throughout the life cycle. Adult depressions often occur during phase-specific crises such as becoming a parent, divorce, career failure, and retirement. The triangulation of current life situation, childhood experiences, and transference reactions provide the material for the mutative change in the patient during psychoanalytic psychotherapy.

Psychoanalytic psychotherapy requires not only a major commitment in time and money on the part of the patient but also the presence of specific psychological capacities such as trust, introspection, and tolerance for frustration and regression. Most crucial is the capacity of the patient to form a collaborative relationship with the psychiatrist while simultaneously being able to direct toward the same analyst a regressive transference reaction that reveals the full intensity of depressive affects and fantasies related to the core neurosis. Not everyone possesses this capacity and for those patients who do not, a more supportive and less regressive treatment is indicated.

Patients who are unsuitable for an analytic treatment because of circumstances or nonanalyzability may be suitable for a brief psychosocial treatment. More positive indications for a brief treatment include depressions that are strongly situational, such as might occur during a transitional life event such as childbirth, divorce, or bereavement. There are numerous brief treatments from which to choose.

Kovacs[53] provides an excellent overview of the theoretic perspectives, tactics, goals, and outcome studies of several brief therapies. She includes cognitive therapy, interpersonal therapy, behavior therapy, and psychoanalytic psychotherapy. Although there are no specific indications for any of these treatments, aspects of the patient will often suggest a specific technique. The developmental history, the character style, the environmental circumstances, or the symptom profile may suggest a "fit" between the patient and the theory and methods of the different treatments. Those who experience the depression as predominantly conflictual might benefit from a brief psychoanalytic therapy that elucidates and clarifies the conflict; those for whom the depression seems to focus on a dominant ambivalent relationship might better be directed to an interpersonal therapy; and those for whom depression is characterized by the assignment of a negative or gloomy value to events, a cognitive therapy. The skilled psychotherapist during the actual treatment will blend a number of techniques and approaches from different schools of brief therapy in order to arrive at an optimal therapeutic prescription.

Marital or family treatment is useful in elucidating important systems issues. Often it is useful to involve a spouse or parents initially in the treatment in order to allay fears of being scapegoated in the treatment or of jealousy of the patient's relation to the psychiatrist.

In general, the more medication-responsive mild depressions such as dysthymic character will have been separated out in the establishment of the diagnosis of neurotic depressive. Nevertheless, in certain doubtful diagnostic situations or when circumstances will not allow even a brief therapy, a trial of tricyclic antidepressants or monoamine oxidase inhibitors, either singly or in conjunction with psychotherapy, may be useful. In general, benzodiazepines are not indicated, although they may improve the patient's overall mood by decreasing anxiety without affecting the depression. Occasionally, methylphenidate or dextroamphetamine will prove useful.

REFERENCES

1. Winokur G, Pitts FN: Affective Disorder: I. Is reactive depression an entity? J Nerv Ment Dis 138:541, 1964

2. Akiskal HS, Bitar AH, Puzantian VR et al: The nosological status of neurotic depression: A prospective 3–4 year follow up examination in light of the primary-secondary and the unipolar-bipolar dichotomies. Arch Gen Psychiatry 35:756, 1978

3. Kraepelin E: Manic-Depressive Insanity and Paranoia. Edinburgh, E & S Livingstone, 1921

4. Fenichel O: The Psychoanalytic Theory of Neurosis. New York, WW Norton & Co, 1945

5. Nacht S, Racomer PC: Symposium on depressive illness II, depressive states. Int J Psychoanal 41:481, 1960

6. Basch M: Toward a theory that encompasses depression: A revision of existing causal hypotheses in psychoanalysis. In Anthony E, Benedict T (eds): Depression and Human Existence. Boston, Little, Brown & Co, 1975

7. Kendell RE: The Classification of Depressive Illnesses. London, Oxford University Press, 1968

8. Andreason NC: Concepts, diagnosis and classification. In Paykel ES (ed): Handbook of Affective Disorders. New York, Guilford Press, 1982

9. Klerman GL, Endicott J, Spitzer R et al: Neurotic depressions: A systematic analysis of multiple criteria and meanings. Am J Psychiatry 136:57, 1979

10. Bayer R, Spitzer R: Neurosis, psychodynamics and DSM-III: A history of the controversy, unpublished manuscript

11. Zung WWK: From art to science: The diagnosis and treatment of depression. Arch Gen Psychiatry 29:328–337, 1973

12. Weissman MM, Myers JK: Affective disorders in a US urban community. Arch Gen Psychiatry 35:1804, 1978

13. Marks I: Cure and Care of Neuroses. New York, John Wiley & Sons, 1981

14. Jacobson E: Depression. New York, International Universities Press, 1974

15. Bibring E: The mechanism of depression. In Greenacre P (ed): Affective Disorders. New York, International Universities Press, 1953

16. Sandler J, Joffee WG: Notes on childhood depression. Int J Psychoanal 46:68, 1965

17. Hamilton M: Symptoms and assessment of depression. In Paykel ES (ed): Handbook of Affective Disorders, p 3. New York, Guilford Press, 1982

18. Klein DF, Gittleman R, Quitkin F et al: Diagnosis and Drug Treatment of Psychiatric Disorders, p 258. Baltimore, Williams & Wilkins, 1980

19. Kierkegaard S: The Sickness Unto Death. London, Oxford University Press, 1941

20. Freud S: The Ego and the id. In Strachey J (ed): The Standard Edition of the Complete Works of Sigmund Freud, vol 19. London, Hogarth Press, 1963

21. Bowlby J: The making and breaking of affectional bonds. Br J Psychiatry 130:201, 1977

22. Brenner C: On the nature and development of affects: A unified theory. Psychoanal Q 43:532, 1974

23. Garmany G: Depressive states: Their aetiology and treatment. Br Med J 2:341, 1958

24. Nelson JC, Charney DS: The symptoms of major depressive illness. Am J Psychiatry 138:1, 1981

25. Roth M, Mountjoy CQ: The distinction between anxiety states and depressive disorders. In Paykel ES (ed): Handbook of Affective Disorders. New York, Guilford Press, 1982

26. Gillespie RD: The clinical differentiation of types of depression. Guy's Hosp Rep 79:306, 1929

27. Klein DF: Endogenomorphic depression: A conceptual and terminological revision. Arch Gen Psychiatry 31:447, 1974

28. Eysenck HJ: The classification of depressive illness. Br J Psychiatry 117:241, 1970

29. Levitt EE, Lubin B, Brooks JM: Depression: Concepts, Controversies, and Some New Facts, 2nd ed. London, Lawrence Erlbaum Associates, 1983

30. Akiskal HS: Dysthymic disorder: Psychopathology of proposed chronic depressive subtypes. Am J Psychiatry 140:11, 1983

31. Hirshfeld RMA, Cross CK: Personality, life events and social factors in depression. In Grinspoon L (ed): Psychiatric Update II. Washington, DC, American Psychiatric Press, 1983

32. Kulper PC: The Neuroses: A Psychoanalytic Survey. New York, International Universities Press, 1982

33. Kraines SH: Therapy of the chronic depressions. Dis Nerv Syst 28:577, 1967

34. Posen M, Clark DC, Harrow M et al: Guilt and conscience in major depressive disorder. Am J Psychiatry 140:839, 1983

35. Liebowitz MR, Klein DF: Hysteroid Dysphoria. Psychiatr Clin North Am 2:555, 1979

36. McKinney WT, Moran CT: Animal models. In Paykel ES (ed): Handbook of Affective Disorders. New York, Guilford Press, 1982

37. Freud S: Mourning and melancholia. In Strachey J (ed): The Standard Edition, vol 14. London, Hogarth Press, 1963

38. Rado S: The problem of melancholia. Int J Psychoanal 9:420, 1951

39. Kohut H: The Analysis of the Self. New York, International Universities Press, 1971

40. Kohut H: The Restoration of the Self. New York, International Universities Press, 1977

41. Seligman MEP: Helplessness: On Depression, Development and Death. San Francisco, WH Freeman, 1975

42. Beck AT: Depression: Clinical, Experimental and Theoretical Aspects, New York, Harper & Row, 1967

43. Jacobson E: The effect of disappointment on ego and superego formation in normal and depressive development. Psychoanal Rec 33:129, 1946

44. Spitz R: Anaclitic depression: An inquiry into the genesis of psychiatric conditions in early childhood II. Psychoanal Study Child 2:313, 1946

45. Poznanski EO: Depression in children and adolescents. In Val ER, Gaviria FM, Flasherty JA (eds): Affective Disorders: Psychopathology and Treatment. Chicago, Year Book Medical Publishers, 1982

46. Zetzell ER: On the incapacity to bear depression. In Schur

M (ed): Drives Affects, Behavior, vol 2. New York, International Universities Press, 1965

47. Klein M: A contribution to the psychogenesis of manic depressive states. Int J Psychoanal 16:145, 1935

48. Mahler M, Pine F, Bergman A: The Psychological Birth of the Human Infant. New York, Basic Books, 1975

49. Bowlby J: Attachment and Loss, vol 1. New York, Basic Books, 1969

50. Akiskal HS, McKinney WT Jr: Overview of recent research in depression: Integration of ten conceptual models into a comprehensive clinical frame. Arch Gen Psychiatry 32:285, 1975

51. Lloyd C: Life events and depressive disorder reviewed. Arch Gen Psychiatry 37:529, 1980

52. Parker G: Parental 'affectionless control' as an antecedent to adult depression. Arch Gen Psychiatry 40:956, 1983

53. Kovacs M: Psychotherapies for depression. In Grinspoon L (ed): Psychiatry Update II: Washington, DC, American Psychiatric Press, 1983

Stress-Response Syndromes: Post-Traumatic and Adjustment Disorders

Every individual in the course of a lifetime will experience stressful life events. The imposed stress may lead to emotional extremes. These subjective experiences will include very sad and fearful moods, as most of us learn to expect, as well as very apathetic, angry, guilty, chaotic, or ashamed ones, which are often more surprising. Such post-event responses are not necessarily pathologic. The clinician evaluating a person with a stress-response syndrome must appraise the degree of external stress imposed and the degree of distress experienced. He must evaluate how these interact with the person's preexisting personality characteristics, as well as how his response relates to typical responses in a representative population. For these tasks, it is essential that the clinician understand the processes underlying normal as well as abnormal psychologic responses. Therefore, general signs and symptoms of psychologic responses to traumatic life events will be discussed before the combination of these elements in the formal diagnostic nomenclature is considered.

Historical Background

For centuries physicians recognized emotional traumas as a possible cause of both psychological and physiologic syndromes. If a person has a heart attack, for example, there is a tendency to explain this physical episode as a part of an ongoing personal story involving such life events as recent losses, excessive work demands, or marital disrup-

tion. Awareness of this penchant for attributing physical illness to psychological causes has led to a debate among clinicians over the validity of hypotheses that relate disorders of any kind to antecedent stressful life events. In addition, the possibility of secondary financial or psychological gain to the patient from having a recognized disorder or disability related to stressful life events has added the issues of either malingering or unconsciously seeking gains to this debate.

In the late 19th century, the prevailing European view held that someone who developed symptoms after a stressful life event was predisposed to them by hereditary weakness of the nervous system.[1] Breuer and Freud[2] rejected this theory, proposing instead a theory that considered unconscious psychological processes. For decades, Freud[3] continued to focus on traumatization as one contributor to the formation of neurotic symptoms.

Studies in the 20th century[1] indicated that although malingering sometimes occurred, it was not a major factor in post-traumatic neuroses. As yet, hereditary predisposition has not been clearly demonstrated. Preexisting personality features have been found to be involved in individual responses to serious life events.[4] In addition, studies of large populations exposed to disaster or combat indicated that as the severity of the life event increased, so did the proportion of the exposed population manifesting disorders.[5] In some cases, personality factors predisposed the individual to greater resilience; in others, they predisposed the person to greater vulnerability. It became clear that some mental disorders followed traumatic life events and that psychological factors had an important place in the biopsychosocial explanatory matrix.[4,6–10]

Normal and Abnormal Psychological Responses to Stressful Life Events

Stress-response syndromes are composites of signs and symptoms occurring in relation to serious life events or threatening life circumstances. Some signs and symptoms tend to occur together, in coherent, empirically demonstrated clusters[9,11] and present themselves in two predominant states of mind, which may succeed each other: (1) the "intrusive" state (which features unbidden ideas, sudden rushes of feeling, and even compulsive actions) and (2) the "denial" state (characterized by ignoring implications of threats or losses, forgetting important problems, emotional numbing, withdrawal of interest in life, and behavioral constriction).

PHASES OF RESPONSE TO SERIOUS LIFE EVENTS

The immediate response to a serious life event when there is a sudden onset of recognition is often alarm, accompanied by strong emotion, most often fear. This initial appraisal leads to a short period of emotional outcry.[8] During the outcry phase, the person quickly processes the crude implications of

FIG. 1. Stress response and pathologic intensification.

Normal	Pathologic
→ Outcry	→ Panic, paralysis, exhaustion
→ Denial	→ Maladaptive avoidances: social withdrawal, suicide, drug or alcohol excesses, counterphobic impulsivity
→ Intrusion	→ Flooded, pressured, confused, distraught, or impulsive states, physiological disruptions
→ Working through—Blocked	→ Anxiety and depressive states, hibernative frozen states, psychosomatic changes
→ Completion—Not reached	→ Inability to work, create, or love

the event, has an alarm reaction that interrupts ordinary activities, and expresses warning signals. The person may call out a warning such as "Watch out!", scream for rescue—"God!" "Mama!"—or sob or grimace in anguish. In a precursor of what will occur more prominently in the later denial phase, he may exclaim passionately "Oh, no!" "It can't be true!" Outcry may also consist of only a stunned stare and the feeling of inability to comprehend the trauma.

An outcry phase is not invariably present. Some people continue to demonstrate effective, well-modulated behavior, with emotional expressivity, when confronted by severely stressful events. This does not mean there will not be an inward or outward "crying out" of emotional responses once immediate coping efforts are no longer required. Later, when such persons are alone and begin to relax and lower defensive barriers, phases of denial and intrusion may ensue (Fig. 1).

PERCEPTION AND ATTENTION DURING STRESS-RESPONSE SYNDROMES

Symptoms that may emerge during denial and intrusive phases of stress-response syndromes are listed in Table 1. In terms of perception and attention, the daze and selective inattention characterizing denial states are in stark contrast to the excessive alertness and startle reactions of intrusive states. Denial experiences may include such patterns as staring blankly into space, even avoiding the faces of others who can provide emotional support. Narrowing of focus and failure to react appropriately to new stimuli may also occur, with a sometimes stubborn adherence to tasks and stimuli considered important before the new and drastic changes in the life situation occurred. There may also be an accompanying inner sense of clouding of perception, with a feeling that the world has become grayer than before. This clouding of consciousness may include a diminished awareness of bodily sensations, even a feeling of being "dead in life."[12]

In contrast, intrusive phases are characterized by hypervigilance (excessive alertness for threatening stimuli), often evidenced by the subject's constantly scanning the environment for threatening cues.[7] This hypervigilance can prompt startle reactions to relatively innocuous stimuli, especially if loud noises or shocking visual stimuli were part of the traumatic event. These startle reactions may range from clenching a single muscle group to the

TABLE 1. Common Symptoms and Signs During Denial and Intrusive States

	Denial States	Intrusive States
Perception and attention	Daze Selective inattention Inability to appreciate significance of stimuli Sleep disturbances (*e.g.,* too little or too much)	Hypervigilance, startle reactions Sleep and dream disturbances
Consciousness of ideas and feelings related to the event	Amnesia (complete or partial) Nonexperience of themes implied as consequences of the event	Intrusive-repetitive thoughts, emotions, and behaviors (illusions, pseudohallucinations, nightmares, unbidden images, and ruminations) Feeling pressured, confused, or disorganized when thinking about event-related themes
Conceptual attributes	Disavowal of meanings of current stimuli in some way associated to event Loss of a realistic sense of appropriate connection with the ongoing world Constriction of range of thought Inflexibility of purpose Major use of fantasies to counteract real conditions	Overgeneralization of stimuli so that they seem as if related to event Preoccupation with event-related themes with inability to concentrate on other topics
Emotional attributes	Numbness	Emotional "attacks" or "pangs" of affect related to event
Somatic attributes	Tension-inhibition responses of the autonomic nervous system, with felt sensations such as bowel symptoms, fatigue, headache, muscle pain	Sensations or symptoms of flight or fight readiness) or of exhaustion from chronic arousal), including tremor, diarrhea, sweating (adrenergic, noradrenergic, or histaminic arousals) with felt sensations such as pounding heart, nausea, lump in throat, weak legs
Action patterns	Frantic overactivity Withdrawal Failure to decide how to respond to consequences of event	Compulsive repetitions of actions associated with the event or of search for lost persons or situations

sudden assumption of a globally protective position. The readiness to interpret a new stimulus as a repetition of traumatic events may in turn lead to illusions.

During the intrusive state, mental images in any sensory modality (visual, auditory, olfactory) may form as if they were real perceptions. In a hallucinatory experience, the person has sensations he interprets as real that have no external basis. In a pseudo-hallucination, the person appraises the vivid subjective images as not true signals of external reality but nonetheless responds emotionally as if they were real. These unbidden images, whether of hallucinatory, pseudo-hallucinatory, illusory, or mnemonic quality, include "sensing" the presences of others who may have died during the traumatic event.[13] These images may be the source of paranormal phenomena, such as seeing or hearing ghosts of the deceased.

Such unbidden images tend to occur most frequently when the person is relaxed, when he lies down to sleep, for example, or closes his eyes to rest. Vivid sensory images occurring during periods of rest or relaxation constitute a "hypnogogic" phenomenon. A similar occurrence when awaking is called a "hypnopompic" phenomenon. These frightening experiences may lead to anticipatory anxiety about their recurrence. They may also lead to secondary anxiety if the subject interprets the phenomenon as a sign of losing control or "going crazy." Patients can immediately be reassured that hypnogogic phenomena, and other unbidden perceptual experiences, are not serious portents of psychosis but are common in those who have experienced a traumatic event. Such reassurance is especially useful if denial states have created a latency period. In such instances, intrusive experiences come as a major surprise to a person who believes he has "mastered" the stressful life event.

A clinical example of a stress-response syndrome is presented below:

> A middle-aged man was involved in a head-on automobile collision that resulted in severe injuries to a passenger in his car and to the driver of the other car. The patient escaped with only bruises and cuts. In the period after the accident he felt he had recovered his equilibrium. It was important to him that he drive to carry out his work, and he did so without phobic anxiety.
>
> While driving several weeks after the accident, he had a severe startle reaction when a truck entered his peripheral vision as it passed him on the right. He swerved into the oncoming lane, which fortunately was unoccupied. He experienced intense panic and pulled off the road. Later that night, as he tried to go to sleep, he had intrusive, intense visual images of the oncoming car involved in the original accident. He became phobic about driving, and his work was impaired as a consequence.

EFFECTS OF STRESSFUL EVENTS ON THINKING AND FEELING

Persons often have a symptom of unproductive rumination about themes related to the serious life event during the intrusive phase. Themes related to the traumatic circumstances may overflow to incorporate ensuing and preexisting topics. The result is an apparent contamination of other themes by reactions to the trauma, a process called "overgeneralization." In normal reactions there is then a diminution of such wide-ranging associational linkages, a process called "extinction." Overgeneralization is the antithesis of symptomatic disavowal of the meanings of the event or constriction of associational width, often prominent during denial phases. Sometimes a contrived continuation of "life as usual" contains an altered subjective

quality; the person feels like an automaton, carrying out habitual patterns in an unspontaneous, devitalized manner.

This brings us to consider two important phenomena (1) the sense of numbness that may be present during the denial phase and (2) its opposite, pangs of strong emotion that may characterize an intrusive phase. Numbness is not simply an absence of emotions; it is a sense of being "benumbed." The individual may actually feel surrounded by a layer of insulation. Emotional blunting may alter patterns of interaction with support systems, affecting family life, friendship, and work relations. Members of the support network may be offended by this alteration in the nature of their relationship and withdraw, reducing the person's support just when he most needs it.

The opposite experience, that of emotional pangs, eventually becomes familiar to the person under stress. Such emotion occurs in an intense wave that seems almost unbearable at its peak. The subject comes to know these peaks will be followed by a reduction in intensity that makes it possible to "live through it."

Intrusive states sometimes contain reenactments of traumatic life events and fantasied responses. These compulsive repetitions may be only minor fragments of a larger complex—a complete reliving of the event. Increased activity may also occur during denial states, but the activity takes a different form. It may include excessive engagement in sports, in work, or in sexual activities in an attempt to jam thinking and feeling channels to such a degree that ideas and emotions related to the stressful event are stifled.

THE SEVERITY OF LIFE EVENTS AS POTENTIAL STRESSORS

Individuals vary in how stressful they find various life events. Assessing populations in general, however, one can determine which life events are relatively more stressful by subjective rating. This has been done through a life-events questionnaire, as reviewed by several authors.[14–17]

According to such field studies of basically normal populations, one of the most stressful life events is the death of one's child, with the death of a loved one such as a spouse also severely stressful. Other highly stressful life events have to do with a threat to one's own life, especially a threat seen as induced by the hostility and unjust behavior of others (*e.g.*, torture). Natural disasters such as earthquakes and floods are also highly stress inducing. Seemingly commonplace events such as automobile accidents can be devastating to the person who experiences them. Events such as rape, burglary, and insults to personal integrity all may assault the fundamental feeling of self-esteem and security of a person and lead not only to psychological stress-response periods but also to post-traumatic stress disorder or adjustment disorder.

NORMAL AND PATHOLOGIC GRIEF

In clinical practice the experiences most frequently observed as leading to stress disorders are injury, assault, or loss of a loved one. The discussion thus far has focused on personal traumatic assaults and injuries. Bereavement reactions follow many of the same forms and have a prototypical course of resolution that will be considered here before turning to issues of diagnosis, biopsychosocial processes influencing symptom formation, and treatment.

Freud[3] differentiated normal from pathologic grief. He characterized normal grief as feelings of painful dejection, with loss of interest in life functions and inhibition of activities. Pathologic grief reactions were marked by additional features such as panic, hostility toward the self, regression to narcissistic forms of self-preoccupation, and other

signs of deflated self-esteem. These additional features were explained by a theory of pathologic mourning, which postulated a preexisting ambivalent relationship with the deceased. After the death, this complex of ideas and feeling led to self-hatred, to attributes of the lost object being internalized, and to aggressive drives directed toward the self.

Subsequent field studies of bereavement and continued clinical investigations indicate that hostility toward the self is not an uncommon grief reaction in persons who do not otherwise warrant diagnosis as mentally disordered.[18,19] Self-blame, hatred, and disgust may normally occur. States of mind characterized by inertia, hypochondriasis, numbness, irritability, feelings of worthlessness, and apathy are also noted in normal grief reactions. These feelings are transient, however; the subject develops a sense of progressive mastery, which reduces secondary anxiety about being overwhelmed. When such subjective experiences persist, the reaction may be regarded as pathological. (My colleagues and I have studied this topic in detail.[20])

Bowlby[21] describes how the attachment bond functions as an expectation of continued self-involvement and how a traumatic separation requires a revision in mental schematization. There is set in motion a sequence of recognition and change after a loss, as modeled in Figure 2. This sequence

FIG. 2. Stages of mourning.

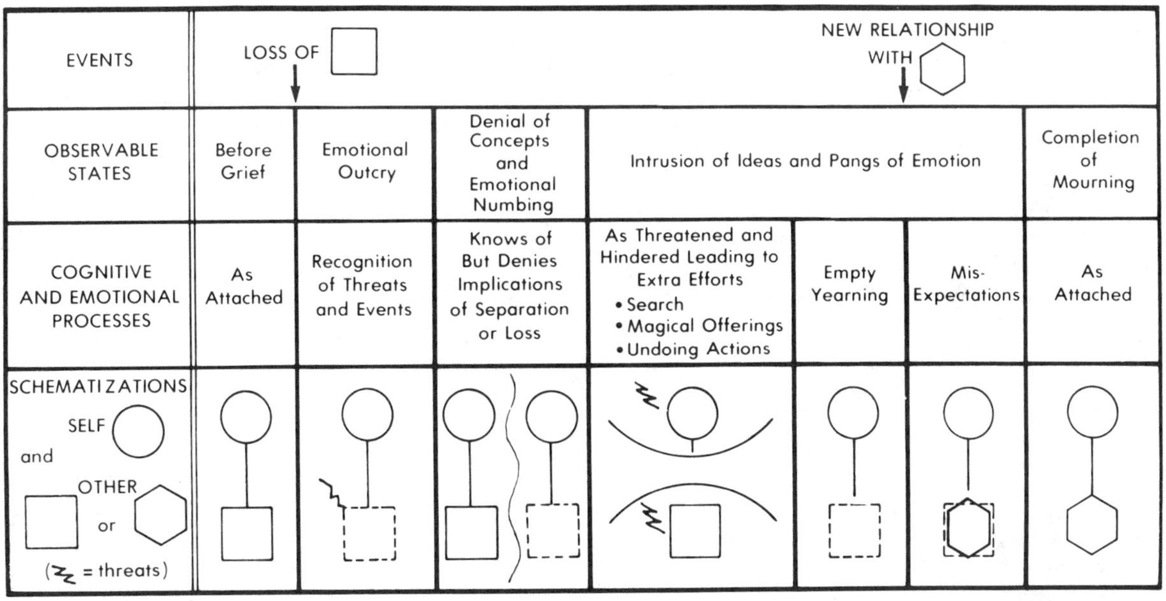

EVENTS	LOSS OF ☐			NEW RELATIONSHIP WITH ⬡			
OBSERVABLE STATES	Before Grief	Emotional Outcry	Denial of Concepts and Emotional Numbing	Intrusion of Ideas and Pangs of Emotion			Completion of Mourning
COGNITIVE AND EMOTIONAL PROCESSES	As Attached	Recognition of Threats and Events	Knows of But Denies Implications of Separation or Loss	As Threatened and Hindered Leading to Extra Efforts • Search • Magical Offerings • Undoing Actions	Empty Yearning	Mis-Expectations	As Attached
SCHEMATIZATIONS SELF ◯ and OTHER ☐ or ⬡ (⚡ = threats)							

is temporal and homologous to the phases of response already discussed. The figure models changes in schematic representations of self and other, where "other" can be a lost person, a body part, a work function, or an important aspect of the environment. Note that during the denial phase the person dissociates; that is, he knows of the loss yet maintains a schemata as if what has been lost continues to exist. In the next phase, threats are overgeneralized so that they assault the self. Later, as alternatives for what was lost are found, mistakes are made in which the old form is expected. Completion is reached when a new pattern of attachment is channeled into an enduring schemata.

THE STRESS OF RECOVERY FROM CHRONIC ILLNESS OR HANDICAPS

Sometimes the nature of loss is mysterious to others who know the subject, and sometimes the subject himself reacts to a loss without conscious recognition that he has sustained one. This state of affairs may occur when the "loss" is of something unpleasant, like an affliction. A person blind for decades has an operation and regains sight; an epileptic is relieved of seizures; a person with longstanding angina pectoris has surgery that relieves his pain; a person with trigeminal neuralgia (tic doloreux) has an injection that arrests the condition. In each instance conditions as they were mentally mapped are changed. This may also occur when a person taking care of a brain-damaged, unresponsive invalid is "freed" by the latter's death or a prisoner is released to return to his family. Even though good things, longed for things, are now possible, schematic revision, as modeled in Figure 2, is necessary. A mourning reaction for the "old, bad, but familiar" may occur. In pathologic form this odd form of grief may lead to a stress-response syndrome that is especially difficult to recognize as such. (Reports of such phenomena may be found in the works of Penman[22] and Sacks[23].)

The Formal Diagnoses

The diagnoses made most frequently in dealing with stressful life experiences are post-traumatic stress disorder, adjustment disorder, and brief reactive psychosis.

POST-TRAUMATIC STRESS DISORDER

A post-traumatic stress disorder characteristically includes reexperiences of the traumatic event, often as intrusive ideas accompanied by unbidden feelings. This reexperiencing may be associated with the other main set of symptoms seen in denial states. Denial, as explained earlier, is evidenced by numbness, unresponsiveness to, or reduced involvement with the external world. The stressor event producing the syndrome is usually one that would evoke significant symptoms in most people and that lies outside the range of such common experiences as simple bereavement, chronic illness, business loss, or marital conflicts.

As mentioned in the section on events, sudden helplessness and shocking perceptions are most prominent features of events that induce traumatic stress disorders. Rape, mugging, assault, military combat, torture, natural disasters, traumatically frightening or painful medical experiences, deaths of loved ones, and accidents such as airplane and car crashes can all evoke the reactions that characterize post-traumatic stress disorders.

Some stresses frequently produce the disorder in most persons who are exposed to them. For example, torture is likely to produce post-traumatic stress disorders in a larger proportion of victims than milder stress events. Only a few people who experience a car accident will have an ensuing post-traumatic stress disorder, although a period of stress and strain may ensue for most people, perhaps.

Intrusive experiences and psychic numbing (emotional anesthesia) are the two major symptoms that lead to the diagnosis of post-traumatic stress disorder. Unbidden images, dreams, and nightmares are frequent in post-traumatic stress disorders. In rare instances there may be dissociative states that last for hours or days. During these dissociative states there may be compulsive reliving of the event. Symptoms of depression, anxiety, guilt, shame, and rage are also common. (The word "symptoms" is used here to mean recurrent or prolonged episodes of very intense affect, experienced as beyond personal levels of self-regulation or endurance.) Increased irritability, common in persons under stress, may involve explosive, hostile behavior triggered by minor stimuli. In addition, the disorder may include components of sympathetic nervous system hyperarousal, such as difficulty relaxing or falling asleep, with persisting tachycardia, sweating, and pupillary dilation.

A latency period of months or even years may

intervene between the occurrence of the stressful event and the period of maximum symptomatic response, although this is less common than a direct response. When the symptoms begin within 6 months of the traumatic event and have not endured more than 6 months before the time of evaluation, the official diagnostic term is "acute post-traumatic stress disorder" according to the *Diagnostic and Statistical Manual of Mental Disorders (DSM-III)*. In such cases the prognosis for remission is good.

If more than 6 months have elapsed since the traumatic event and the first emergence of symptoms, the reaction is considered "delayed." If at least 6 months or more of symptoms have occurred before the evaluation diagnosis, the term *chronic subtype* is used. These forms of post-traumatic stress disorder (delayed, chronic, or both) are usually more difficult to treat.

In making both differential and comprehensive diagnoses, it is important to consider the possibility of concussion in acute physical traumas or malnutrition in prolonged stress responses. Very mild concussions may leave no immediate apparent neurologic signs but have residual long-term effects on mood and concentration.[1] Malnutrition during extended stressful periods may also lead to organic brain syndromes.

Persons with post-traumatic stress disorders commonly cope in ways that may lead to other disorders, such as excessive use of tobacco, alcohol, narcotics, sedatives, or food. If they present a mixed syndrome combining organic and psychological factors, one should make a diagnosis of each disorder concomitant with the diagnosis of post-traumatic stress disorder.

If the life event is not sufficiently severe to meet the criteria of the official nomenclature, the diagnosis of adjustment disorder may be made.

ADJUSTMENT DISORDERS

Adjustment disorders are defined by *DSM-III* as maladaptive reactions to identifiable psychosocial pressures. For this to be the correct diagnosis, signs and symptoms should emerge within 3 months of the onset of the change in life circumstances. The signs and symptoms, which are not as specifically defined as those of the post-traumatic stress disorders, include a wide variety of disturbances in interpersonal and work functions, as well as maladaptive extremes of anxiety, depression, rage, shame, and guilt. According to *DSM-III*, these signs and symptoms meet the criteria for another Axis I

mental disorder, such as anxiety disorder or depressive disorder, the diagnosis of adjustment disorder is not made.

The identifiable psychosocial pressures that may precipitate adjustment disorders include such changed life circumstances as divorce, difficulties with childrearing, illness or disability, financial difficulties, a new form of work, graduation, moving, retirement, and cultural upheaval.

DSM-III lists subcategories for adjustment disorders, organized by the patient's predominant complaint about his subjective experience. Among the subtypes are depressed or anxious mood, other out-of-control emotional states, disturbance of social conduct, work or academic inhibition, and withdrawal from others. This is a very open diagnostic entity, with subtypes classified by surface phenomena. In individual cases it is important to reach a specific formulation.

Neither post-traumatic stress disorder nor adjustment disorder should be regarded as "minor" mental disorders. In either instance, suicidal ideation may be high and severe disfunction found in such areas as work, social life, and parenting. Both disorders may cause high levels of personal distress. The prognosis for full recovery, however, is usually excellent.

BRIEF REACTIVE PSYCHOSES

Another diagnosis related to traumatic events is that of brief reactive psychoses. These conditions have a sudden onset immediately following exposure to stressful events. They may last for a few hours or as much as 2 weeks. The clinical picture includes emotional turmoil and the presence of at least one gross psychotic symptom, such as expressed delusions, which is what primarily differentiates this reactive psychosis condition from a post-traumatic stress disorder and adjustment disorder.

To be diagnosed as having a brief reactive psychosis, the patient should have experienced a recent traumatic life event that lies outside the range of usual human experiences. Epidemiologic studies suggest that brief reactive psychoses are less common than post-traumatic stress disorders. Studies are limited, however, by the fact that they are almost invariably retrospective. The absence of prospective studies means a lack of psychiatric assessments for diagnostic categories or dispositional characteristics existing prior to the occurrence of serious life events.[24]

UNCOMPLICATED BEREAVEMENT

Many persons react to bereavement in a resilient manner. In others, bereavement leads to a period of turbulent distress lasting 1, 2, or more years. At some time during the year following a death, a person may episodically experience signs and symptoms that would constitute a major depressive disorder were they not transient and clearly connected to grief. These reactions may constitute a disorder, in that professional treatment may be indicated, but they are not considered, in *DSM-III,* a mental disorder. There may be medical disorders as a component of such reactions. Clinicians should take a careful history for increased alcohol consumption, being alert for cirrhosis of the liver, organic brain syndrome, and accident proneness. Inquiry should also be made about suicidal impulses, increased cigarette smoking and its cardiorespiratory consequences, use of sedatives or tranquilizers with their potential for habituation, organic brain syndromes, paradoxic wakefulness, and other side-effects.

Some circumstances are likely to increase the severity or duration of grief reactions. These include preexisting high dependency on the deceased, preexisting frustration or anxiety in relating to the deceased, unexpected or torturous deaths, a sense of alienation from or antagonism to others, a history of multiple unintegrated earlier losses or simultaneous losses, and real or fantasied responsibility for the suffering or death itself. When several of these factors are present, a complicated bereavement reaction may result that warrants diagnosis as one of the anxiety or depressive disorders (including post-traumatic stress disorder), an adjustment disorder, reactive psychosis, or a flare up of a preexisting personality disorder.

Epidemiology

About 60% of persons diagnosed as having a mental disorder have experienced a severe life event in the weeks preceding the onset of that disorder, as compared with about 20% in comparison groups not diagnosed as having a mental disorder.[25] Paykel[26] summarizes such studies as indicating that in the months following a traumatic life event there is a six times greater risk of suicide, a two times greater risk for the onset of depressive disorders, and a somewhat slighter increase in the risk of developing a schizophrenic syndrome.

Stressful experiences lead, in the main, to the post-traumatic and adjustment disorders just described and to concomitant physiologic disturbances. They also contribute to other anxiety disorders. Preexisting episodes of separation trauma have been suggested as predisposition to panic disorders.[27] Serious or threatening life events have also been implicated in the onset of phobic disorders. For example, Weekes[28] reports that the majority of 528 agoraphobic men and women self-reported either sudden or prolonged stress created by difficult life situations as antecedents to the development of their anxious states of mind. Only 5% could offer no cause. Of course, these are impressionistic retrospective data. A more specific listing of ten types of stressful factors was reported by Sim and Houghton,[29] who found that the most common precipitants of phobic disorder in their sample of 191 patients with agoraphobia and other phobias were bereavement and "sudden shock." As pointed out by Rabkin,[24] the absence of control groups and a lack of precision in defining the terms for both stressors and diagnosis render such findings questionable. She described a more careful study by Buglass and colleagues,[30] in which 30 agoraphobic housewives were compared with 30 controls enrolled in a general medical clinic. Twenty-three percent of the patient sample could describe precipitating events.

These data on anxiety, depressive, and schizophrenic disorders do not indicate whether incipient mental disorder on the part of the patient may have contributed to the life events in question. It is probably best to view causation as interactional, with environmental, biological, and psychological causes and predispositions all involved. After all, many serious losses, injuries, and disasters do not lead to psychiatric disorders.[31] Most studies show marked individual differences, and it is not always the person who seemed most disturbed before an event who develops a disorder after. Nonetheless, it does seem to hold true that the more previous trauma experienced by the person, the more likely he is to develop symptoms after a stressful life event. Experimentally, persons with more previous trauma found vicarious stress more disturbing.

When stressors become extreme, as in extended combat or concentration camp situations, the rate of morbidity increases.[5,32–34] Chapman,[35] for example, reports that a post-disaster psychiatric syndrome may be found in from 0 to 30% of victims.

Physical sequelae may also be noteworthy. Faich and Rose[36] found that in the 5 days following a severe blizzard in Rhode Island, the rate of hospital admissions for myocardial infarction increased, along with mortality for ischemic heart disease and all other causes. Bennett[37] found many health differences between 316 respondents who had experienced the direct effects of a 1968 flood in Bristol, England, and 454 controls who had not for the year afterward. The differences included an increased likelihood of dying within 12 months, increased surgical rates for males, and overall poor health among flood respondents. Long-term physical health effects were noted 30 years after concentration camp imprisonment in World War II by Eitinger.[32] Such studies have been reviewed by Gunderson and Rahe[17] and Dohrenwerd and Dohrenwerd.[15]

An up-to-date and fairly comprehensive set of studies evaluated victims of the 1972 Buffalo Creek flood in West Virginia, which wreaked sudden, unexpected devastation, with considerable loss of life. Symptoms of intrusive recollection, reactive anxiety, depression, and social dysfunction comparable to levels of distress found in patients in mental health clinics with anxiety and depressive disorders were noted in survivors up to 2 years after the flood.[38–41] Workers exposed to dead and dismembered bodies after a disaster may themselves suffer post-traumatic stress disorders.[18] In children, there may be a long latency period with manifestation of traumatic reactions in altered social function.[42,43]

Perhaps the most studied personal disaster is the death of a loved one.[18,19] Reports of increased morbidity of surviving spouses have been questioned, but the death of a loved one clearly may lead to suicidal ideation and to increased use of potential toxins such as cigarettes, alcohol, and mood-altering drugs. A comparison of reactions to parental death in a group of volunteers and persons who sought brief therapy for symptomatic grief reactions after a parent's death was reported by Horowitz and colleagues,[44] and a summary of the levels of distress in both groups is shown in Table 2. High levels of distress were noted by some people in each group, but a significantly higher proportion of the patient group had such elevations in signs or symptoms. In spousal and parental deaths, there appears to be a greater tendency to pathologic grief reactions if the preexisting relationship was troubled by guilt and anger as well as strong attachment. Deaths that are unexpected, complicated, and experienced as in some way "unfair" are also harder to assimilate in mourning. Cascading consequences may include economic difficulties, social disengagement, and disruption of place of residence. Feelings of hopelessness and helplessness will increase the likelihood of depressive reactions. In general, human contact provides major sustenance in grief, and lack of such contact may make

TABLE 2. Percentages of Persons Who Sustained Parental Death at Three Levels of Distress

Primary Distress Variables	Patients Seeking Psychotherapy (N = 31)			Volunteer Field Subjects (N = 36)			χ^2	$P<:$
	LOW	MEDIUM	HIGH	LOW	MEDIUM	HIGH		
Self-rating:								
Intrusion (IES)	3	36	61	28	39	33	8.98	.011
Avoidance (IES)	10	32	58	61	17	22	19.02	.001
Depression (SCL-90)	7	32	61	46	31	23	15.23	.001
Anxiety (SCL-90)	23	26	51	65	6	29	13.32	.001
Total symptoms (SCL-90)	23	23	54	66	17	17	13.68	.001
Clinician rating:								
Intrusion (SRRS)	17	40	43	67	19	14	16.91	.001
Total neurotic signs and symptoms (BPRS)	3	52	45	42	47	11	17.56	.001

(IES, the Impact of Event Scale; SCL-90, the Symptom Checklist-90; SRRS, the Stress Response Rating Scale; and BPRS, the Brief Psychiatric Rating Scale) (Horowitz M, Krupnik J, Kaltreider N et al: Initial psychological response to parental death. Arch Gen Psychiatry 38:316–323, 1981. Copyright © 1981, American Medical Association) mourning difficult and lead to increased likelihood of psychological morbidity.[45]

Many reports indicate that childhood traumas may increase the rate of adult disturbances (*e.g.,* in the form of disposition to anxious states of mind) in part because of maladaptive characterologic formations. In terms of direct response, emotional disturbances tend to follow such stressful events in a child's life as surgery, the birth of a sibling, and parental divorce. These are generally short duration disturbances, and the majority of them will not be reflected in any later vulnerability to mental disorder.[46]

Divorce is a common but major stressful life event for children as well as for parents. Everyday events at the moment when one parent left the family remain etched in the child's memory in the same way that many persons recall exactly what they were doing when they heard that John Kennedy or Martin Luther King had been killed. Disturbed parental moods (rage, grief, or shame) have great impact on children. About 15% of families seeking divorce do not experience grave emotional upheavals following the separation, but the rest have very major disturbances in mood and behavior patterns.[47]

Epidemiologic studies have shown that traumas are followed not just by post-traumatic stress disorder, adjustment disorder, or brief reactive psychosis, but by multiform increases in morbidity in some of the exposed population.[48] These findings have been reviewed by a report from a committee of the National Institute of Medicine,[49] and an instructive example has been provided by Blank[50] for a group of war veterans. In his clinical experience with over 1000 Vietnam veterans, Blank[50] reported a wide variety of presenting phenomena. The first were psychological symptoms, including classic traumatic neurosis symptoms, depression, psychosomatic syndromes, violent paranoid states, addictive disorders, exacerbated character disorders, suicides and homicides, and psychotic syndromes. The second type of disorder was evidenced by a general alteration in life course, including underachievement, wandering life-style, and crime. The third type was characterized primarily by inability to relate to significant companions: difficulties in achieving intimacy with a wife or lover, special interferences relating to children, marked changes in relatedness to the country and its institutions, and general feelings of alienation. The fourth type involved men who had profoundly shattered images of themselves and of all humanity. These subjects seemed to have lost their basic faith in the capacity of humanity for goodness.[51]

Sex differences have been noted in response to stress, but these may be due to social gender stereotypes on what responses are appropriate to communicate. On life-events questionnaires, women rate similar events as more distressing than do men.[16] When it comes to children, however, a variety of studies find boys more vulnerable to stressful events.[52] The reasons for this are not known, but it is possible that because of cultural and sexual stereotypes, parents may be less supportive to boys manifesting emotional distress. It may also be that certain stress events pose a greater stress for boys or that they have less coping capacity than girls at a given age.[46,52]

High morale and imbeddedness in a valuable social context seem to increase resiliency in response to stressful life events, for both children and adults.[31,53] Therapeutic efforts, especially while the person is still exposed to stressor life events, may therefore be directed to restoring these psychological features as quickly as possible.

Clinical Description

The most frequent presenting symptom in posttraumatic stress disorders and in the more severe adjustment disorders is intrusiveness of and preoccupation with a complex of ideas and feelings (themes) related to the stressful event. These themes vary with the nature of the precipitating event and the preexisting history and development of the individual. Nonetheless, in clinical practice certain themes occur repeatedly in patients with stress disorders. These common presenting concerns are discussed briefly below.

FEAR OF REPETITION

An unpleasant event, associated with painful results, carries with it the threat of repetition. The person who has had one heart attack must come to grips with the idea that he may have another, potentially fatal, one. Since this is a realistic possibility, it is important to progress beyond denial, morbid preoccupation, or unrealistic and dreadful fantasies to a point where realistic consideration is possible.

SHAME OVER HELPLESSNESS

Most persons carry with them through much of their lives an unconscious sense of personal invulnerability. We believe that transience, illness, and death happen to all others, but not to ourselves. The experience of a stressful life event compels reconsideration of this belief in invulnerability, and that reconsideration often involves a period of feeling acutely vulnerable. In some persons this reaction is exaggerated, and, coupled with an attitude that vulnerability is bad, may lead to a sense of shame over their helplessness to prevent the serious life event or the loss of certain functions. In some cases there is a component in the precipitating life event that supports the sense of personal failure, as when the person has caused an automobile accident. Even when the person did not have any control over the events, he may ruminate, seeking to explain why he led himself into such a circumstance, why, for example, he took the particular plane that crashed.

RAGE AT "THE SOURCE" AND ENSUING GUILT

Any severe life event causes major frustration, because it involves a change in circumstances from what one thought them to be. One common reaction to this frustration is rage at any "source" that can be identified as involved in causing the event. The person may blame any companion available for an injury that occurred entirely without the companion's involvement. Displacement may extend to an accusation against God for allowing a tragically unnecessary bereavement. The expression of such rage reactions, in thought or in action, may then lead paradoxically to a guilt response. Anger at the perceived source of a serious life event usually has an irrational component and is often accompanied by destructive fantasies. Thoughts of enacting any of these fantasies lead to guilt or shame at expression of such hostility. Sometimes a person is frightened that he will lose control over his destructive fantasies. Someone who has been assaulted by a member of a specific cultural or racial group, for example, may be frightened that he will act out revenge fantasies on innocent members of the same group.

SURVIVOR GUILT

In events where others have been injured or killed, one often responds with immediate relief that one has been spared. The wish to be a survivor conflicts with a moral injunction that one should share the fate of others. At the level of magical thinking, relief at survival is not recognized as being a natural reaction, nor is the timing of the wish correctly considered. That is, the person may conclude that the wish to be spared occurred before the event, and thus he is to blame for others being killed or injured in order that he might be spared.

FEAR OF IDENTIFICATION OR MERGER WITH VICTIMS

A complementary theme to survivor guilt is the fear of sharing the fate of any victim they encounter. At a primitive level of thinking, people do not conceive of themselves as being separate; they do not conceive of life as having probabilities and improbabilities. If an event has hurt another, they fear they will discover they, too, have been hurt by it. This irrational but not unusual response occurs even when the victim is unknown. For example, a person who witnesses a suicide may become frightened that he himself is suicidal or will become so, perhaps by activation of some otherwise latent source of personal despair.

Some of these clinical issues will be reviewed in the following report of a complex case involving a delayed reaction to a traumatic event:

A middle-aged man presented for psychiatric evaluation on referral by an endocrinologist. He had been unable to work because of psychomotor retardation and constant feelings of fatigue. He had been tested for hypothyroidism and treated with thyroxin without effect. He had also been treated with antidepressants, which gave him side-effects but no improvement. The consulting endocrinologist had noted that the patient first experienced the syndrome suggestive of hypothyroidism 2 years earlier, when he had been mugged, and he referred the patient for psychiatric evaluation.

In psychiatric interviews, the patient indicated that he had felt fine, functioning well in both interpersonal and work situations, until the time of the mugging, and that his syndrome indeed dated from that experience. He nonetheless disavowed any continued psychological responsivity to the assault. He agreed, however, to accept exploratory psychotherapy.

In the psychotherapy, no medications were used. A trial intervention focused on all possible associations to memories of the assault. In his response, the patient reported a dream in which he was mugging another person, an obvious reversal of roles. He found no change in terms of his subjective experience while awake; however, he began to undertake interpersonal engagements and some work. He gradually became more in contact with a fear that he would lose control of a fantasy in which he assaulted members of the same cultural group as the men who had mugged him.

As this theme emerged, there occurred a period of increased turbulence in the patient's marriage, and he became irritable and short-tempered. This turbulence subsided, and he was gradually able to restore himself to work and social functioning.

OTHER CLINICAL FEATURES

In considering stress disorders, other clinical features that are of some importance in individual case formulation include the subsequent effect of shocking perceptions, the influence of preexisting neurotic conflicts or functional deficits, and the special phenomenon in which the person destroys social supports that might otherwise help him.

Shocking Perceptions

The subjective experience of memories of traumatic perceptions is that they are etched in memory with extraordinary intensity and permanence.[33] At the time of shocking perceptions, the overwhelming implication of what is seen cannot be fully assimilated; the person's information-processing systems are overloaded. This alters the state of consciousness and also affects thinking and memory encoding.[4] With the concomitant loss of a sense of volitional direction, the person may respond passively to instructions from others. He becomes "impressionable," which is one reason Breuer and Freud[2] called such states "hypnoid states." Recalling the traumatic memory may lead to a transition into that kind of mental state and, conversely, entry into that state of mind for some other reason may release the traumatic memory. The intensity of the representation and the sense of volitional passivity give the recollection a quality of reliving the experience.

At one time it was believed that these exceptionally vivid memories could be reduced in intensity by promoting vivid reliving experiences (abreaction). Such a technique was called "cathartic" (*i.e.*, it would expel the unwanted complex).[33] Unfortunately, it has not proved clinically possible to erase traumatic memories. The sense of passivity, however, can be changed. The memory can also be recalled in more composed states of mind, and the individual can learn to suppress deliberately a memory once it has been reviewed. This new learning renders the special vividness of the recollection less threatening.

The Influence of Preexisting Neurotic Conflicts or Functional Deficits

In some instances, pre-trauma neuroses may make a person unusually resilient. For example, the person used to anxious or sad states of mind will not be as surprised or secondarily frightened by them as a person who has no experience of distress. In the main, however, preexisting neurotic conflicts offer no advantages and may be impediments to processing stressful life events. Among the neurotic impediments to an adaptive response to stressful life events are the following:

Irrational but enduring attitudes that "bad thoughts cause real harm," "wishing makes it so," or "one must always be loved or protected by another in order to survive."

Active but incompatible sets of wishes whose content is associatively similar to the traumatic events.

Habitual use of pathologic defenses to prevent strong emotional responses by distorting memory and decision-making.

Excessive preoccupation with fantasy-based reparations of deficits, using fantasies related associatively to what was threatened or lost in the stressful life event.

Social support can protect the individual from some primary stressor effects, help him cope and thus avoid secondary stressors and strains, and provide restorative human contact. In most cases, people cope by activating and using a social network. In some cases avoidance, alienation, or outright destruction of relationships that might otherwise provide support occurs. When this happens, appropriate intervention can turn the situation around, and a falling social network can be regained.

Etiology

BIOLOGICAL RESPONSE SYSTEMS

A wide variety of studies have been made of biological responses to stress. Seyle[54] described a general physiological stress-response syndrome that begins with an increase in the release of corticosteroids, catecholamines, and growth and other hormones. The corticosteroids seem to have their main increase during the anticipation phase, with adrenergic responses occurring with each newly occurring external stimulus. There is, however, a high degree of individual variability, and other systems may be aroused in some individuals. Individuals also differ greatly in their physiologic capacity to maintain an alarm system at a high metabolic level for a sustained period.

Corticosteroids enable the body to increase responses, but they also interfere with the action of insulin, cause a loss of calcium from bones, suppress growth, and contribute to stomach ulcers and hypertension. Extended high output of corticosteroids may suppress immunologic mechanisms, such as the production of lymphoid tissue and gamma-globulin.[55] It is important that the organism learn to adapt to the life circumstances that have led to this alarm response before corticosteroid production "gives out" or causes morbidity. Adaptation involves developing a psychological structure that contains the new model of the world posed by the stressful changes, as well as new attributes for responding to the altered situation. How this occurs is discussed in the next section.

The catecholamines regulate blood pressure, heart rate, fat breakdown, and sugar metabolism. Because of their diffuse distribution throughout nerve cells, they act as both hormones and neurotransmitters in the brain and throughout the body. Neurons high in catecholamine content are found in networks that connect the limbic, cortical, cerebellar, and hypothalamic structures. Disturbances in these regions sometimes lead to increased disturbances in arousal level, regulation of emotional response as in rage attacks, reward- or gratification-seeking behavior, and motor functions.

Epinephrine is the principal catecholamine synthesized in the adrenal medulla. Activation of epinephrine production is a function of the sympathetic nervous system extending down the spinal cord from the brain. So far as we know now, dopamine and norepinephrine are the catecholamines most prominent in physiologic reaction to stress. As neurotransmitters they seem to be highly concentrated in the locus ceruleus and other neural clusters. Repeated alarms, traumas, or chronic stress may alter synaptic transmission of these alerting and arousing systems, leading to repeated "false alarms" (anxiety) or depressions of function.[56]

There is genetic control of dopamine receptors and the number of neurons in dopaminergic regions of the brain. This could lead to typologic differences and vulnerability to acute and chronic external stressors and possibly to different kinds of responses to antianxiety agents or other drugs. More research on these potential mechanisms of stress-induced morbidity may be expected during the next decade.[57]

Subjective estimates of the individual's capacity to maintain control or to cope with stressor events may affect the type of physiologic arousal that occurs. If a person feels threatened but capable, there tends to be activation of the sympathetic fight–flight mechanisms with catecholamine arousal, possibly testosterone elevation, and increased activity in the area of the amygdala. This leads to defensive behavior patterns, such as increased mobility and assertiveness.[58]

If the individual experiences the stressor events as overwhelming, with the self no longer competent to master them, there may be a conservation-withdrawal or hiding type of response, with restricted mobility and behavior that indicates a readiness to be subordinate. This may be associated with increased activity in the area of the hippocampus septum, with an increase in adrenocorticotropic hormone and corticosterone and a decrease in testosterone. The difference between a fight–flight state and a behaviorally frozen or subordinate state probably depends on event structure, on social circumstances, and on individual characteristics.

PSYCHOLOGICAL RESPONSE SYSTEMS

The earlier psychoanalytic theory of the effects of psychic trauma was summarized by Rangell.[59] According to that theory, a traumatic occurrence involved a high incursion of stimuli into the psychic apparatus. This breach of a hypothetic "stimulus barrier" set off an unconscious train of intrapsychic events called the traumatic process (so named because the overload of stimuli was seen as beyond the capacity of ego functions for mastery at that particular time). The result was an inferred traumatic state of mind, one in which the self is conceptualized as helpless. As a result of insufficient resources on the part of the ego, there was a lack of control over the entry of perceptual stimuli, which results in vulnerability to further excessive excitation.

We now discuss responses to traumatic events in terms of the amount of new information that is incongruent with preexisting inner schematizations or mental models, as illustrated earlier in Figure 2.[4,60,61]

Serious life events are by definition those that will eventually change cognitive maps, which are our inner schematic models of how the self articulates with the world. The processing of information that leads to such integrated change is slow. Time to review the implications of news inherent in stressful life events is essential. The mind continues to process the new information until reality and inner models are brought into accord. The tendency to persist in information processing until new external conditions match with inner mental models can be called a completion tendency.

THE COMPLETION TENDENCY AND ACTIVE MEMORY STORAGE

Until a traumatic event, represented as memories, can be integrated with mental schematizations, the memories are stored in an especially active form of coding. These memory contents tend toward repeated mental representation. Each repeated representation once again sets in motion information processing of the kind that may eventually revise schematizations. As new schematic meaning structures are established, the news about revised circumstances becomes a part of long-term memory and the codifications in active memory decay.

Codification in active memory tends to decay anyway, as is shown by experiments on short-term memory. Following a traumatic event, however, the news is so important that the active memory of the stressors involved does not, like ordinary short-term memory, undergo automatic erasure or replacement by other sets of information. Indeed, as discussed in the section on shocking perceptions, this decay to an ordinary form of memory may not occur at all.

The first processing of the news of the stressful life event entails a rapid appraisal of how best to cope with it.[8] A low level of inhibitory regulation leads to excitation of emotional systems and to the behaviors associated with emotional outcry. The amount of information requiring changes in schemata is usually so great that complete processing and integration are impossible in a short time. The emotional implications are too overwhelming. Inhibiting regulatory efforts are initiated so that the stressful information can be gradually assimilated, dose by dose. High excessively inhibitory controls may interrupt the assimilation and accommodation process. A high level of control in relation to the tendency of active memory toward repeated representation leads to the denial and numbing phases of stress-response syndromes. Failures of control lead either to a continuation of outcry, as in prolonged, panic-stricken states, or to the intrusive states. Optimally adaptive controls reduce ideational and emotional processing to tolerable levels. Periods of intrusion and denial allow a person to make new decisions gradually and record new intentions and beliefs as plans and schematizations and thereby come to the working through and completion phases.

Biological as well as psychological factors are involved in these sequences. One theory, as yet inadequately tested experimentally or empirically, is that the processing of psychological meanings of traumatic perceptions activates certain neural or neurohormonal networks in unusual ways. For example, continued strain of processing might lead to exhaustion in certain neurotransmitter systems, disposing the person to depressive states. Conversely, excessive arousal of certain neurotransmitter systems, such as the noradrenergic systems, could lead to perpetuation of anxious states of mind. Once certain biological systems are hyperaroused or depleted, other metabolic functions aimed at reestablishing equilibrium may be set in motion. During some states along this course toward equilibrium, it may be difficult for a person to process psychological meanings in a way that leads toward completion. For example, a person may become so depleted that until information-processing capacity is restored, only supportive treatment is indicated.

SOCIAL RESPONSE SYSTEMS

The social conditions in a community may either foster resiliency among community members or increase the likelihood of stress-response syndromes. Good leadership, high group affiliation, and strong, unambivalent ideologies seem to increase endurance.[31,53] Cultures providing support only after a threshold of illness is crossed will increase the likelihood that such illness will occur.

The most important social ingredients are shared values and value hierarchies. If a society promulgates the belief that fate distributes disasters according to a virtue calculus, then disaster victims are seen as receiving a deserved punishment. This dehumanization of victims increases their trauma and, if not offset by reactive group solidarity, probably increases the rate of stress disorders. At this writing, such an analysis applies to victims of acquired immune deficiency syndrome (AIDS).

Something of this sort occurred after the war in Vietnam. Returning American servicemen were sometimes socially ignored or treated as if they were responsible for unjustified combat.[51] The diagnosis of post-traumatic stress disorder in these men was at first underrepresented[62] and then became a major political issue.[63]

Treatment

Early intervention has distinct advantages. Immediate distress is reduced, chronic or delayed responses may be prevented, and pathologic responses may still be tentative, making for a briefer intervention.[6,64] In crisis work of this type, human relationship support is a powerful method of reducing distress and should be used as the first form of intervention. When insomnia produces fatigue and lowering coping capacity, sedation with one of the antianxiety agents may be used on a night-by-night basis. Smaller doses of the same agent may be prescribed, again on a dose-by-dose basis, during the day. The patient and persons close to the patient should be cautioned against the use of multiple mood control agents, especially against combining alcohol with prescribed medications. Antidepressive agents should not be prescribed to relieve immediate sadness and despondency responses to loss.

In the acute phase of responding to a traumatic event the patient may be advised to avoid driving, operating machinery, or engaging in tasks where alertness is essential for safety, as accidents are more likely to result when persons already under stress suffer lapses of attention, concentration, and sequential planning or have startle reactions that disrupt motor control. Intervention beyond transient support may be indicated where there is evidence of failure to progress well through adaptive phases of a stress response. Brief dynamic psychotherapy is one way to examine and change such blocks in recovery. Self-help groups may also be effective resources.[65]

Detailed expositions of treatment techniques for stress disorders are available elsewhere.[4,60,61] In this literature, a brief psychotherapy for recent stressful events has been advocated, both as an immediate treatment procedure and as a way of preventing chronic disorders. Several principles may be summarized here.

When a person seeks help, the therapist establishes a working alliance that allows him to assist the patient in working through his reactions. In addition, he may seek to modify preexisting conflicts, developmental difficulties, and defensive styles that rendered the person unusually vulnerable to traumatization by this particular experience.

Therapy begins with the establishment of a safe and communicative relationship. This, together with specific interventions, alters the status of the patient's controls. The patient can then proceed to reappraise the stressful life event, and the meanings associated with it, and make the necessary revisions of his inner models of himself and the world. As this reappraisal and revision takes place, the person is able to make new decisions and to engage in adaptive actions. He can practice desired behavioral patterns until they gradually become automatic. As the person achieves new levels of awareness, this process is repeated and deepened. That is, as the patient trusts the therapist more, he is able to modify controls further and assimilate more warded off thoughts about the current stress. Finally, he will need to work through reactions to the approaching loss of the therapist and the therapy.

Introduction of a plan for the termination of therapy (several sessions before the final one) leads to a reexperience of loss, often with a return of symptoms. This time, however, the loss can be faced gradually, actively rather than passively, and in the context of a communicative and helping relationship. Specific interpretations of the link between the termination experience and the stress event should be made, and the final hours of therapy center on this theme.

REFERENCES

1. Trimble MR: Post-traumatic neurosis. New York, John Wiley & Sons, 1981
2. Breuer J, Freud S: Studies in hysteria. In Strachey J (ed): The Standard Edition of the Works of Sigmund Freud, vol 2. London, Hogarth Press, 1975
3. Freud S: Mourning and melancholia. In Strachey J (ed): The Standard Edition of the Complete Works of Sigmund Freud, vol 4. London, Hogarth Press, 1957
4. Horowitz M: Stress-Response Syndromes. New York, Aronson, 1976
5. Grinker R, Spiegel J: Men under Stress. Philadelphia, Blakiston, 1945
6. Lindeman E: Symptomatology and management of acute grief. Am J Psychiatry 101:141–148, 1944
7. Janis I: Psychological Stress. New York, John Wiley & Sons, 1958
8. Lazarus R: Psychological Stress and the Coping Process. New York, McGraw-Hill, 1966
9. Horowitz M, Wilner N, Kaltreider N et al: Signs and symptoms of post-traumatic stress disorders. Arch Gen Psychiatry 37:35–92, 1980
10. Goldberger L, Bresnitz S: Handbook of Stress. New York, Free Press, 1982
11. Zilberg, Weiss, Horowitz M: Impact of event scale: A cross validation study and some empirical evidence. J Consult Clin Psychol 50:407–414, 1982
12. Lifton R: Death in Life. New York, Basic Books, 1967
13. Horowitz M: Image Formation and Psychotherapy. New York, Aronson, 1983
14. Holmes T, Rahe R: The social readjustment rating scale. J Psychosom Res 11:213–218, 1967

15. Dohrenwend B, Dohrenwend B (eds): Stressful Life Events. New York, John Wiley & Sons, 1974

16. Horowitz M, Schaefer C, Hiroto I et al: Life event questionnaires for measuring presumptive stress. Psychosom Med 39:413–431, 1977

17. Gunderson E, Rahe R: Life Stress and Illness. Springfield, IL, Charles C Thomas, 1974

18. Raphael B: The Anatomy of Bereavement. New York, Basic Books, 1983

19. Parkes C: Bereavement: Studies of Grief in Adult Life. London, Tavistock, 1972

20. Horowitz M, Wilner N, Marmar C et al: Pathological grief and the activation of latent self-concepts. Am J Psychiatry 137:1157–1162, 1980

21. Bowlby J: Loss: Sadness and depression. In Attachment and Loss, vol 3. London, Hogarth Press, 1980

22. Penman J: Pain as an old friend. Lancet 1:633–636, 1954

23. Sacks O: Awakenings. New York, Vintage, 1976

24. Rabkin J: Stress and psychiatric disorders. In Goldberger L, Bresnitz S (eds): Handbook of Stress: Theoretical and Clinical Aspects, pp 564–584. New York, Free Press, 1982

25. Brown G, Harris T: Social Origins of Depression: The Study of Psychiatric Disorder in Women. London, Tavistock Publications, 1978

26. Paykel E: Contribution of life events to causation of psychiatric illness. Psychol Med 8:245–254, 1978

27. Klein D: Anxiety reconceptualized. In Klein D, Rabkin J (eds): Anxiety: New Research Changing Concepts. New York, Raven Press, 1981

28. Weekes C: Simple, effective treatment of agoraphobia. Am J Psychother 32:357–369, 1978

29. Sim M, Houghton H: Phobic anxiety and its treatment. J Nerv Ment Dis 143:484–491, 1966

30. Buglass D, Clarke J, Kreetman N: A study of agoraphobic housewives. Psychosom Med 7:73–86, 1977

31. Hamburg D, Adams J: A perspective on coping behavior, seeking, and utilizing information in major transitions. Arch Gen Psychiatry 17:277–284, 1967

32. Eitinger L: Organic and psychosomatic aftereffects of concentration camp imprisonment. International Psychiatry Clinics 8(1):205–215, 1971

33. Furst S (ed): Psychic Trauma. New York, Basic Books, 1967

34. Krystal H: Massive Psychic Trauma. New York, International Universities Press, 1968

35. Chapman D: A brief introduction to contemporary disaster research. In Baker G, Chapman D (eds): Man and Society in Disaster. New York, Basic Books, 1962

36. Faich G, Rose R: Blizzard morbidity and mortality. Am J Public Health 69:1050–1052, 1979

37. Bennet BG: Bristol Floods, 1968. Br Med J 3:454–458, 1970

38. Titchener J, Kapp F: Family and character change at Buffalo Creek. Am J Psychiatry 133:295–299, 1976

39. Lifton R, Olson E: The human meaning of total disaster: The Buffalo Creek Experience. Psychiatry 39:1–18, 1976

40. Erikson K: Everything in its Path: Destruction of Communality in the Buffalo Creek Flood. New York, Simon & Schuster, 1976

41. Gleser G, Green B, Winget C: Quantifying interview data on disaster survivors. J Nerv Ment Dis 166:209–216, 1978

42. Newman C: Children of disaster: Clinical observations at Buffalo Creek. Am J Psychiatry 133:306–312, 1976

43. Terr L: Psychic trauma in children: Observations following the Chowchilla school-bus kidnapping. Am J Psychiatry 138:14–19, 1981

44. Horowitz M, Krupnik J, Kaltreider N et al: Initial psychological response to parental death. Arch Gen Psychiatry 38:316–323, 1981

45. Clayton P: The effects of living alone on bereavement symptoms. Am J Psychiatry 132:133–137, 1975

46. Garmezy N, Rutter M: Stress, Coping, and Development in Children. New York, McGraw-Hill, 1983

47. Wallerstein J, Kelly J: Surviving the Breakup: How Children and Parents Cope with Divorce. New York, Basic Books, 1980

48. Melick M, Logue J, Frederick C: Stress and disaster. In Goldberger L, Bresnitz S (eds): Handbook of Stress, pp 613–630. New York, Free Press, 1982

49. Elliot G, Eisdorfer C: Stress and Human Health, New York, Springer, 1982

50. Blank A: Stress of war: The example of Vietnam. In Goldberger L, Bresnitz S (eds): Handbook of Stress. New York, Free Press, 1982

51. Lifton R: Home from the War. New York, Simon & Schuster, 1973

52. Rutter M: Stress, coping, and development: Some issues and some questions. In Garmezy N, Rutter M: Stress, Coping, and Development in Children. New York, McGraw-Hill, 1983

53. Pearlin L, Schooler C: The structure of coping. J Health Social Behav 19:2–21, 1978

54. Seyle H: A syndrome produced by diverse noxious agents. Nature 138:32, 1936

55. Levine S: A psychobiological approach to the ontogeny of coping. In Garmezy N, Rutter M: Stress, Coping, and Development in Children, pp 107–132. New York, McGraw-Hill, 1983

56. Kandell E: From metapsychology to molecular biology: Explorations into the nature of anxiety. Am J Psychiatry 140:1277–1293, 1983

57. Ciaranello R: Neurochemical aspects of stress. In Garmezy N, Rutter M (eds): Stress, Coping and Development in Children, pp 85–106. New York, McGraw-Hill, 1983

58. Henry J: Present concepts of stress theory. In Usdin E, Kvetnansky R, Kopin I (eds): Catecholamines and Stress: Recent Advances. New York, Elsevier Press, 1980

59. Rangell L: The metapsychology of psychic trauma. In Furst S (ed): Psychic Trauma. New York, Basic Books, 1967

60. Horowitz M: States of Mind. New York, Plenum, 1979

61. Horowitz M, Marmar C, Krupnik J et al: Personality Style and Brief Psychotherapy. New York, Basic Books, 1984

62. Horowitz M, Solomon G: A prediction of stress response syndromes in Vietnam veterans. J of Social Issues 31(4):67–80, 1975

63. Figley C (ed): Stress Disorders among Vietnam Veterans. New York, Brunner/Mazel, 1978

64. Caplan E: Principles of Preventive Psychiatry. New York, Basic Books, 1964

65. Lieberman M, Borman L: Self-help Groups for Coping with Crises. San Francisco, Jossey-Bass, 1979

This chapter was written while I was a Fellow at the Center for Advanced Study in the Behavioral Sciences. I am grateful for financial support provided by the John D. and Catherine T. MacArthur Foundation.

Richard J. Frances and Michael H. Allen

The Interaction of Substance-use Disorders with Nonpsychotic Psychiatric Disorders

In psychiatry as in the rest of medicine, it is frequently the case that patients are affected by more than one illness at a time. The interactions between substance-use disorders and other psychiatric illnesses have diagnostic, treatment, and etiologic implications. There is a high prevalence of substance-use disorders; recent estimates reveal an 18% lifetime risk or a 6.3% risk in any 6-month period, and approximately two thirds of these persons will have an additional psychiatric disorder.[1-3] In order to illustrate the kinds of problems that occur, this chapter includes studies of interactions of substance-use disorders with affective disorder, anxiety disorders, organic disorders, and personality disorders and reviews the research literature on these interactions. There are a myriad of other disorders that interact with substance-use disorders (*e.g.*, schizophrenia, somatization disorder, anorexia nervosa, sexual orientation disorders, and familial tremor) that are not covered in this chapter. Substance-use disorders can mask, mimic, or result from a wide range of psychiatric and medical disorders. Psychiatrists have a central role in integrating a sophisticated understanding of substance-use disorders in relation to other psychiatric illnesses and to the full range of biopsychosocial factors.

The physiological, hereditary, psychological, familial, cultural, and social contributions to the etiology and manifestations of alcoholism should be taken into account in the treatment planning of each patient. The high prevalence of psychiatric symptoms in patients with addictive disorders and the difficulty of any form of treatment without abstinence point to the need for careful psychiatric assessment and treatment in all patients with substance-use disorders. A thorough substance-use history is crucial for all psychiatric patients.

Five years of experience with the *DSM-III* multiaxial diagnostic system has provided a data base with a focus on more careful assessment of patients who present with psychiatric disorders in association with their substance abuse. Longitudinal studies, adoption studies, epidemiologic studies, and family studies have not yet settled old questions as to cause and effect relationships between manifest psychopathology and addictive behavior. Although the trait of addiction may be primary to psychiatric illness or may exacerbate it, addictions may also develop as a way of coping with other vulnerabilities.

Our current treatment planning is based on an eclectic pragmatism that hopefully will become more exact when there is a greater understanding of pathophysiologic mechanisms, and when outcome studies demonstrate the right combination of treatment for the right patient. The research reviewed in this chapter sheds some light on, but does not yet resolve, the following questions: (1) Are substance-use disorders discretely inherited or do they interact with a broad-based genetic vulnerability to psychiatric illness? (2) To what degree do people "self-medicate," mask, or alter the expression of underlying psychiatric illness with a substance-use disorder? (3) What is the contribution of substance-use disorder to the exacerbation or causation of other psychiatric symptomatology? (4) What is the relationship of familial substance-use disorders to other psychiatric illness? (5) What is the mechanism or mode of inheritance that leads to vulnerability to substance-use disorders alone or in combination with other disorders?

Clinical Issues

The interactions between psychopathology and the addictions are often difficult to differentiate clinically because the picture is often clouded by overlapping signs and symptoms that can result from intoxication, withdrawal, mixed drug interactions, adverse drug responses, medical complications, and the organic and psychosocial effects of substance use on affective state, anxiety, or personality. All the above may interact with additional Axis I, II, and III disorders. The patient with substance-use disorders often demonstrates denial, dissimulation, and memory problems related to organicity, making it difficult to obtain a clear history. As a result of being socially isolated, the patient may have no family or friends who can be interviewed, and in the midst of intoxication or overdose, the patient may be unable to answer coherently. Frequently the patient with a substance-use disorder is coerced into seeking help by family, employer, the court, or family physician and is ambivalent about cooperating. The patient may have no trust in authority figures, lack insight of high dependency needs, and may have had bad experiences with physicians who did not understand substance-use problems.

An empathic, informed, nonjudgmental approach is needed to reassure the patient that with recognition of the problem and help, there is reason to be hopeful. Because the patient may not tell the symptoms, the clinician must be alert to observable signs, laboratory evidence, and a mental status characterized by high denial, projection, and rationalization.

Only a small fraction of the 18% of the population who will develop substance-abuse problems in their lifetime is ever diagnosed and treated by a health professional, and only a small fraction of that group ever sees a psychiatrist. Relatively few substance-use disorder treatment settings provide careful ongoing psychiatric evaluations with a team approach, and in many treatment programs, there is inadequate tailoring of treatment to the specific needs of patients.

The treatment of patients with substance-use disorders and other psychiatric disorders is made very difficult by the lack of integrated psychiatric and substance-abuse approaches in many facilities. Many psychiatric inpatient units, psychiatric halfway houses, outpatient clinics, and other support systems in the community are often unable or unwilling to treat psychiatric patients with a substance-use disorder. Patients with substance-use disorders and additional psychiatric problems are unlikely to receive adequate help in free-standing alcohol and drug rehabilitation facilities that are generally not equipped to deal with psychopathology. In these facilities, there is often minimal contact with a psychiatric consultant and relatively greater input by alcoholism counselors, who rarely have had psychiatric training.

If the need for medication is not well accepted and explained, the emphasis on abstinence can work antithetically to compliance with prescribed psychotropic medication. Many halfway houses for alcoholics will not accept patients on any medication. Frequently, when not tailored to the individual, confrontational methods found in therapeutic communities and self-help groups can be detrimental to the psychologically ill. Facilities that combine psychiatric treatment with rehabilitation for substance-use disorders are expensive and have yet to demonstrate that tailoring treatment to the patient is cost effective; however, they represent a healthy eclecticism and provide state-of-the-art treatment in the field. There have been well-controlled studies of poorly designed treatment programs that have found little connection between type of treatment and positive outcome. Poorly designed controlled studies in fine treatment programs have found positive results. Recently a well-controlled study by Woody found that treating additional psychiatric diagnosis along with substance-use disorders improves the outcome of these patients with a poor prognosis.[4] So far, the outcome literature reflects that factors such as stable family, stable job, less sociopathy, less psychopathology, and no family history of alcoholism weigh more heavily in positive prognosis than the type of treatment.[5] Studies investigating various treatment alternatives, either alone or in combinations, that are well controlled, well designed, and implemented by good clinicians are expensive and difficult to carry out, but are sorely needed.

Clinical Examples

A CASE OF DEPRESSION, ALCOHOLISM, AND DEPENDENT PERSONALITY

Mrs. P. is a 33-year-old married, upper-middle-class housewife with two children who drinks a fifth of vodka per day, is abusive to her husband, children, and family dog, and comes to treatment saying, "I am a failure as a mother." Although she occasionally drank abusively in college, her heavy drinking began 8 years ago soon after the birth of her first child.

Although a sought-after beauty, she always had a low opinion of herself and 10 years ago settled on her husband because he was a good provider and could be depended upon. Soon after the birth of her first child, she began to feel increasingly bored, empty, resentful of caring for the child, yet ashamed of herself for not being a better wife and mother.

She had difficulty falling asleep, gained weight, and lost interest in sex. Although she was thought of as competent, running a meticulous household, she was always unsure of herself, and as her drinking increased she let her housekeeper assume the responsibility for making important decisions. She became quarrelsome with her husband and alternately wished and feared that she would succeed in driving him away. At first, she drank to get to sleep and to socialize with a fast crowd of friends with whom she was afraid to compete. Although most of the time she could say no to no one for fear of rejection, she was often irresponsible and occasionally exploded with rage.

On several occasions she nearly kicked her dog to death. She alternated between trying constantly to entertain her children and screaming outbursts when they were irritating. Her drinking gradually increased during the day as she anticipated her husband's arrival home. She had periods of loss of memory for recent events, tremulousness, high blood pressure, vomiting, and diarrhea. Six months before presenting for treatment, the school notified her that her 8-year-old daughter appeared withdrawn, unable to make friends, inattentive at school, and fearful of talking with her teachers about her mother's abusiveness and drinking. After a meeting with her husband and the school counselor, Mrs. P. reluctantly agreed to go into a proprietary alcohol rehabilitation program that lasted 21 days. She seemed to make progress through alcohol counseling and Alcoholics Anonymous (AA) and admitted her drinking problems; however, she remained hopeless about her marriage, had difficulty taking care of her children, and continued to have trouble falling asleep. One month after leaving the hospital and still depressed, she stopped attending AA meetings and resumed her drinking. Her husband, having been sensitized to the problem through Alanon, began demanding that she again seek help or face losing the children and himself.

Mrs. P. is the only child of her mother's second marriage and has two older half-sisters. Her parents were divorced and abused alcohol; her maternal grandfather committed suicide, and her maternal aunt was hospitalized for depression. For the first 12 years of Mrs. P.'s life, her mother, who could be warm and entertaining at times, left most of the care of the patient to a loving housekeeper who was fired shortly after the divorce. Her mother was often intoxicated and extremely inconsistent in setting limits. Often bribed with presents and material things and told that she could get anything she wanted with her good looks, Mrs. P. was also told repeatedly that she was spoiled and ungrateful. Mrs. P. had her first episode of feeling hopeless, worthless, and despondent at age 12. It lasted 2 months, and there was a similar episode when she went away to college.

The patient is a strikingly beautiful woman, even with no makeup, and she has a distant fitful gaze. She constantly apologizes for needing help, blaming herself for drinking and being a terrible mother. She knows that she cannot stop drinking at home; however, she is furious at her husband's threat and afraid to return to the hospital. She denies suicidal intent but says she doesn't know what she would do if her husband took away the children. On physical examination, she is tremulous, has tachycardia, diaphoresis, elevated blood pressure, and an enlarged liver. Blood alcohol level is 110 mg/dl, and urine screen is negative for other drugs. Levels of serum glutamic-oxaloacetic transaminase (SGOT), serum glutamic-pyruvic transaminase (SGPT), and lactic dehydrogenase (LDH) are elevated. Her score on the Hamilton is 28, and her Minnesota Multiphasic Personality Inventory (MMPI) showed elevations in scales 2478 (D, Pd, Pt, and Sc). The *DSM-III* diagnosis is as follows: Axis I, 1) Alcohol dependence, continuous, 2) Alcohol withdrawal, 3) Major depression, recurrent; Axis II, Dependent personality disorder, narcissistic traits (provisional); Axis III, 1) Fatty hepatosis, 2) Hypertension; Axis IV (psychosocial stressors), alcohol's effect on marriage and relationship with children, severity: 5 (severe); Axis V, (highest level of functioning past year), 4 (fair).

TREATMENT PLANNING

The complex interaction between alcoholism and depression and characterologic problems makes a psychiatric evaluation necessary. Abstinence is required during treatment for both diagnostic and therapeutic reasons.[6]

Making the diagnosis of alcoholism early is especially hard because patients deny problems until their life situations have deteriorated. What the patient does not say is as important as what she does say. Initially the clinician must combine history gathering and evaluation of mental status with a confrontation of the denial of alcoholism and of other psychiatric illness by both the patient and her family in order to help them acknowledge and accept the problem.

Especially since Mrs. P. is being pressed by her family to see a therapist rather than seeking help on her own, it is essential that the therapist establish rapport with her. Motivation for treatment is initially low in many alcoholic patients, but it can be increased through a combination of confrontation, support, and education. When depression is also present, the therapist must explain the helplessness, hopelessness, poor self-esteem, and self-punitiveness to the patient as part of the reason for reluctance to accept help.

Mrs. P. is denying her intense dependency needs and the necessity to continue in treatment after she has stopped drinking. Her first treatment failed partly because her depression was not addressed. Confronting the patient with the severity of her problems with alcoholism and depression may create a beneficial crisis as she is forced to acknowledge the full impact that drinking has had on major areas of functioning. It is in this crisis context that the physician and patient begin to work out a treatment contract. The use of medical evidence, such as blood tests and liver scans, psychological tests, and the support of other physicians known by the patient may be very helpful. Outcome studies indicate that factors such as having a family and a stable job and the absence of sociopathy are better prognostic indicators than whether or not someone sought treatment or was pushed into it by an employer, family, or physicians.

The first phase of treatment for Mrs. P. is detoxification. In general, it is preferable to try outpatient rather than inpatient detoxification first. Patients who are reliable, have good family and social support systems, and are highly motivated for treatment are candidates for outpatient alcohol detoxification. The patient is started on Chlordiazepoxide hydrochloride (Librium), 25 mg to 50 mg four times per day, and multivitamins and makes daily outpatient visits; Librium is gradually decreased over the 3- to 5-day detoxification period.

Under certain conditions, inpatient detoxification is warranted: if there is severe concurrent medical and/or psychiatric illness; if outpatient detoxification cannot be done safely because of severe withdrawal symptoms or lack of a stable family system; or if the patient is unable to stop using substances outside the hospital or has failed to respond to less intensive forms of treatment, such as nonmedical alcoholism treatment. Patients admitted to a hospital usually require a slightly longer period of detoxification. They generally are started on chlordiazepoxide hydrochloride (Librium), 50 mg to 100 mg four times per day, multivitamins, folic acid, 1 mg, and thiamine, 100 mg four times per day, and are detoxified over a 5- to 7-day period. Those with a history of withdrawal seizures are given magnesium sulfate 50%, 2 ml IM three times per day for a total of eight to nine doses.

Mrs. P. had not done well in a previous detoxification program, is struggling with her husband, and is suffering from a major depression, all of which indicate a need for inpatient hospitalization for both detoxification and rehabilitation. In a hospital-based facility with psychiatric staff, it will be possible to develop a tailored treatment plan that addresses issues not effectively dealt with in her previous treatment.

Involvement of the family is mandatory if the treatment is to have a chance of success. Alcoholics present behavioral problems that directly affect the family, and the family may reinforce the patient's drinking. Awareness of the family's dynamics may aid in the patient's treatment and prevent relapses, and including the family in treatment increases the chances of engaging the patient.

Mrs. P.'s children are also in need of evaluation; they are at higher than usual risk for behavior problems, fetal alcohol syndrome, attention deficit disorders (ADDs), substance abuse, and child abuse. Her daughter has had to take care of her younger sister as well as her mother, whom she has experienced as inconsistent and irascible, while her father has offered her no protection.

Hospital rehabilitation allows an extended period of sobriety, thus breaking the cycle of addiction and encouraging the assumption of increasing responsibility for one's behavior. A hospital program offers a full schedule of activities including group therapy, lectures on alcoholism, study groups, and AA meetings, in addition to individual psychotherapy, family therapy, and occupational and alcoholism counseling. Mrs. P.'s family will be involved in a weekly family group and a children's group and will be encouraged to attend Alanon meetings. Mrs. P. will continue in treatment after discharge, through individual and group therapy and AA. Prevocational counseling, leading her to find a job, might help her self-esteem, channel her aggression, and allow her to feel more comfortable about less involvement with her children.

AA has been highly successful in helping patients like Mrs. P. accept their illness and in providing them with a network of social support, an auxiliary superego support, and an alternative means of meeting dependency needs. At AA the patient discovers that being an alcoholic does not mean being an immoral outcast, but that alcoholism is an illness that afflicts many fine people from all walks of life. She may also come to terms with her feelings about her parents' drinking problems. Although AA as an organization recommends following a physician's recommendations, some AA members may counsel against use of any drugs including antidepressants or disulfiram (Antabuse), and the patient may need to be prepared for this. AA may also serve as a healthier prosthesis than substance abuse for her dependent personality and provide a support system that never goes on vacation.

Disulfiram can be an important adjunct to treating alcoholism. The patient need make the decision about drinking only once a day, when she takes the medication. Thus, it gives her time to cope with the impulse to drink when it becomes very strong, eliminates the temptation of the high of drinking, and thereby reduces the craving for alcohol. Severe liver disease, heart disease, high suicide potential, and psychosis are all contraindications to disulfiram. In Mrs. P.'s case, it is necessary to wait 3 weeks for her liver enzymes to start returning to normal and to make a careful assessment of her suicide potential; if appropriate, she would then receive disulfiram, 125 mg/day. The usual dose is 250 mg/day, but for elderly patients or those with relative contraindications to disulfiram, half the usual dose is recommended.

Alcoholism can be the result of depression or can lead to a depression, which may remit at various intervals after abstinence. In Mrs. P.'s case, there had been recurrent depressive episodes prior to drinking and depression that had persisted 6 weeks after sobriety on a previous occasion. Mrs. P. requires a traditional diagnostic evaluation of mental status, course of symptomatology, a 2-week drug-free period, and medication trials with antidepressants when indicated. It is likely that she will need a tricyclic antidepressant, which may, through helping her depression, improve her ability to benefit from both AA and psychotherapy. Psychological screening tests for organicity, depression, and personality disorders are useful. Periodic checks with a breathalyzer will be made in the hospital. The dexamethasone suppression test is not likely to be useful for at least a month after admission because of the high incidence of false positives in patients with alcoholism. Close attention to her sobriety will be an important part of treatment both during and after hospitalization.

Mrs. P.'s individual therapy is likely to focus on her tendency toward repetition of self-defeating dependent relationships with men and women. She feels involved and somehow responsible for her parents' drinking and inconsistency. She fears that if she were to lose her beauty, she would have nothing left, yet she knows she does not take care of herself. Helping her to see how her own childhood is being repeated in her relationship with her daughter can be a beginning of change. It will be difficult for her to develop trust or closeness with a therapist. She should be encouraged to make new friends, both in AA and in her contacts with other mothers. She may need to distance herself from her drinking friends.

Much of the treatment program for Mrs. P. will be geared toward helping her achieve the experience of accepting herself as an alcoholic. She has used alcohol to ward off shame and guilt and, in giving up alcohol, will need to accept her own dependency needs, to admit to an illness, and to take better care of herself. This change in identity will come about through a combination of psychotherapy, education, social pressure, identification with her therapist, and counselors as role models. AA facilitates this process by providing normative social pressure, gratification of dependency needs, and a route for identification with an ego ideal of sobriety and self-honesty.

A CASE OF ATTENTION DEFICIT DISORDER, ALCOHOLISM AND ANTISOCIAL PERSONALITY

Mr. A., a 35-year-old divorced man, was readmitted to an inpatient alcohol treatment service with symptoms of anxiety and desperation following a blackout. He reported consuming 2 to 3 pints of rum daily during 7 years prior to admission and had been addicted to heroin prior to that time. He said that heroin and alcohol "helped to calm my nerves." During the 18 months before the readmission, he had had four admissions for detoxification and episodes of blackouts, delirium tremens, and withdrawal seizures.

Mr. A. was the product of a normal pregnancy and delivery but began to have problems with hyperactivity, impaired concentration, and learning difficulty early in school. He dropped out after the eighth grade and thereafter dealt drugs, worked as a bartender, and received public assistance. His marriage was short lived, and he had few relationships apart from his family.

On first admission to an alcohol rehabilitation service, Mr. A. had repeated outbursts of unprovoked temper, although at times he could be charming. He was anxious, fidgety, restless, and could not sustain concentration. He would walk out of lectures, groups, AA, and psychotherapy sessions. His disruptive behavior coupled with his pessimism about benefiting from the program resulted in the decision to discharge him after 2 weeks on oral disulfiram, 250 mg/day. He resumed drinking several weeks after leaving the hospital.

At the time of his readmission, Mr. A. had a normal neurologic examination, normal electroencephalogram (EEG), and normal physical examination. He continued to demonstrate impulsive behavior, emotional lability, and problems with concentration, and he frequently requested tranquilizers. He exhibited all the same behavior of his previous hospitalization. At that time, the following *DSM-III* diagnoses were made: Axis I, 1) Alcohol dependence, continuous, 2) ADD, residual type; Axis II, Antisocial personality disorder; Axis III, No diagnosis; Axis IV (psycho social stressors), unemployed, severity: 4 (moderate); Axis V (highest level of functioning past year), 5 (poor).

TREATMENT PLANNING

As in the case of Mrs. P., a careful psychiatric evaluation in an inpatient setting was helpful in making a diagnosis and designing a treatment tailored to this patient. A therapeutic trial of pemoline was begun. Although pemoline has fewer euphoriant properties than other stimulants, some potential for abuse remains, especially in persons who are already known to abuse alcohol and drugs. Mr. A.'s initial dose was 37.5 mg orally every morning. Within 10 days, this dose had been advanced to 37.5 mg twice per day. He became less restless and distractible and had fewer emotional outbursts. After 3 weeks he could watch an entire movie on television and could tolerate regular therapy sessions; he felt calmer and was better able to cope with stress. This observation was confirmed by members of his family. Neuropsychological testing done before and after he started taking pemoline revealed a marked change. During the first test he could not sit still or attend to the task at hand, becoming frustrated and exploding into a tirade. His visual and verbal memory was defective. The WAIS showed that Mr. A.'s potential cognitive functioning was in the average range. There were marked deficits in attentional skills and language comprehension. It was hard to distinguish the relative contributions of minimal brain dysfunction, poor school history, and chronic alcohol abuse to his cognitive functioning.

On the second test, Mr. A.'s tolerance of frustration had increased; his concentration had improved and his restlessness had lessened. His attentional skills were noted to be "dramatically improved." Continued use of pemoline was recommended. Mr. A. remained in the hospital for the entire 6-week program. He and the treatment team agreed that he had benefited from therapy groups, lectures, and AA meetings.

He was discharged and placed on a maintenance dose of oral pemoline 37.5 mg twice per day and oral disulfiram 250 mg hs. In a 13-month follow-up, he was taking his medication regularly and abstaining from alcohol. In a 15-month follow-up, he stopped attending AA meetings and had another slip.

This patient, with a combination of disorders, had had a poor history of treatment compliance, a poor work and social history, and severe behavior problems, all of which contributed to a poor prognosis. With the diagnosis of ADD and appropriate treatment, marked reduction in his behavioral symptoms was observed. His 15-month period of drug-free living represented the longest period of abstinence experienced by the patient since his early teens. Although he continued to have an antisocial personality, he was better able to control his behavior. Pemoline may have helped to improve his self-control by decreasing his impulsivity, emotional lability, and anxiety, which allowed him to benefit more from the rehabilitation program. He now had an explanation for his behavior problem that was medical rather than moral, and this increased his self-esteem. An improved understanding of the problem and a means of approaching it also helped reduce countertransference problems and improve cooperation on the part of the treatment staff. It is possible that Mr. A. had used heroin and alcohol as self-medication for the ADD and that earlier appropriate medication might have eliminated the need for these other substances.

Research Review

The prevalence of interaction between substance-use disorders, the issue of which is primary, the evidence for the role of heredity, the search for markers, and the contribution of psychosocial factors are all being actively studied. Methodologic problems in comparing these studies include lack of clarity in defining terms; use of different instruments and criteria for making diagnosis; difficulty of controlling other intervening variables such as socioeconomic status, sex, race, marital status, sources of sample from an inpatient, outpatient, or nonpatient pool; and difficulty obtaining accurate sequential histories from reliable sources. For example, the definitions of substance use versus abuse or dependency associated with sadness versus atypical depression or major affective illness must be clear in order to compare data.

Penick and others have pointed to the high prevalence of severe psychiatric symptoms in patients with addictive disorder and underline the value of careful psychiatric assessment in all patients with substance-use disorders.[3] In a large (N = 568) multicenter study of male alcoholics, Penick found that 68.5% of family-history–positive and 51.8% of family-history–negative alcoholics met diagnostic criteria for another psychiatric syndrome in addition to alcoholism. The mean number of positive syndromes including alcoholism was significantly higher for the familial alcoholics than for the nonfamilial alcoholics. The rather high incidence of carefully diagnosed psychopathology in family-history–positive alcoholics is as follows: depressive,

48.3%; manic, 24%; antisocial, 23.2%; panic attacks, 13.8%; drug abuse, 14.8%; obsessive compulsive, 14.3%; phobic, 11.1%; schizophrenic, 4.6%.

The work of McCord and McCord,[7] Vaillant,[8] and Pettinati, Sugerman, and Maurer[9] indicates that the majority of accompanying psychopathology is secondary to the substance-use disorder. Substance-use disorders can also be secondary to or symptomatic of other psychiatric disorders. The self-medication concept has emphasized the specific kinds of drug effects that particular patients may seek. Opiates may be used to defend against aggression, cocaine to lift mood, and hallucinogens to experience merging. The person may be seeking a chemical solution to a particular brain transmitter or receptor problem or deficit. Khantzian has hypothesized that patients whose childhoods were often dysphoric and out of control derive a considerable amount of masochistic reinforcement from their repeated attempts to gain mastery by titrating withdrawal symptomatology and dysphoria.[10] As addicts, they can control their pain as well as pleasure in divided doses. Khantzian has also suggested that cocaine may be used as self-medication for ADD.

Mental illness is often exacerbated by chronic drug use. In 1972, alcoholic men constituted 37.5% of all male inpatient admissions to psychiatric hospitals.[11] In a study of 250 young adult chronic patients, 55% were known to have used or abused other drugs alone or in combination.[12] Salzman has described a group of borderline patients who use large amounts of various drugs and often come to treatment after taking an overdose.[13] There is an increased risk of suicide in this population, who may not show signs of depression. Saxon found that 19% of drug abusers made suicide attempts.[14]

Recent research has almost confirmed a biological vulnerability to alcoholism based on heredity. Although adoption studies suggest inheritance of alcoholism apart from other psychiatric disorders, family-history studies indicate the possible association of alcoholism with mood disorder, hyperactivity in childhood, sociopathy, and phobic disorders. Currently the nature and mechanism of what is inherited is not known. The search for genetic markers may also have a bearing on alcohol's relationship to other psychiatric disorders. For example, platelet monoamine oxidase (MAO), the level of which is low in alcoholics and their first-degree relatives, is also low in patients with schizophrenia and bipolar affective disorders and, therefore, could be a marker of broad-based biological vulnerability.[15] Neuropsychological markers such as nondominant hemisphere–related test abnormalities or evoked potential P300 abnormalities found in alcoholics and their adolescent sons may or may not be specific for alcoholism.[16]

It is also possible that assortative mating could explain familial presence of other psychiatric disorders, since depressed and antisocial patients may frequently marry alcoholics. In addition to hereditary factors, psychological, social, and cultural factors also play a role. In Kaij's study, 53% of identical twins are concordant for alcoholism; however, the other 47% are not, indicating that if heredity plays a role, environment also contributes to phenotype.[17]

INTERACTIONS WITH AFFECTIVE DISORDERS

Alcoholism and substance-use disorders have long been thought to be related etiologically to disturbances of affect. Kraepelin describes alcoholism having its onset in a state of depression from which drinking serves as an escape.[18] In 1932, Rado described self-esteem problems of addicts as "tense depression," which could be relieved by use of substances.[19] Other writers who have continued along this line, such as Weider, Kaplan, Milkman, Frosch, and Khantzian, have written about depressive equivalents and self-medication for a variety of states, including mania, depression, tension, and aggression.[10] Schuckit and Vaillant have emphasized the preponderance of affective symptomatology that is secondary to substance use.[8] It is difficult to sort out the complex relationship between the two disorders and to specify whether one or the other is primary; the determination is usually based on a history of symptoms of one occurring before the other as well as positive family history.

The incidences of reported affective disorders vary depending on the criteria and instruments used for diagnosis. Keeler, Taylor, and Miller found varying percentages of depression among recently detoxified alcoholics depending on the instrument used: clinical interviews, 8.6%; the Hamilton Depression Rating Scale, 28%; the Zung Self-Rating Depression Scale, 66%; and the MMPI, 43%.[20] Rounsaville, in a study of narcotics addicts, found that 42% met criteria for major depressive disorder using the Schedule for Affective Disorders and Schizophrenia (SADS) interview as opposed to 9% using *DSM-III* criteria.[21] In a large sample of young males, Schuckit found that 60% of those who were depressed had had a substance-use–related problem prior to the depression. He also reports that of those who seek inpatient treatment, only 5% of male and 10% to 15% of female alcoholics have primary affective disorders, although a majority have quickly resolving secondary depressive symptomatology.[22]

Woodruff and co-workers found that alcoholics with secondary depression displayed more similarities to other alcoholics than to depressed patients and more frequently demonstrated delinquency, antisocial behavior, and criminal behavior than those who experienced depression alone.[23] In a court-referred group of narcotics addicts, Croughan and co-workers found no primary depression but up to 50% secondary depression in this group of largely sociopathic substance abusers.[24] The kinds of problems that force persons into inpatient treatment are more likely to be associated with sociopathy than with depression. It may very well be that those with primary depression are overrepresented in outpatients. The greater prevalence of depression in women compared with men parallels that of the general population.

It may be difficult to obtain an accurate history of onset. Clear-cut episodes of depression with intervals of normal mood prior to the onset of alcoholism would indicate that the recurrent depression is the primary disorder. Most studies have found an increase in alcohol consumption during manic episodes. Cassidy and associates found that approximately one third of patients drank more when ill and one third drank less when ill.[25] Mayfield found that of bipolar patients who were excessive drinkers, alcohol consumption increased in three times as many with elation as with depression and decreased in one quarter of the patients with depression.[26] Elation was never associated with decreased consumption. The increase in drinking during elation may be related to restlessness and impulsivity, while the decrease in drinking with depression may be a concomitant of constriction of interest and activity. Reich and colleagues similarly found that a high percentage of hospitalized bipolar patients abused alcohol and increased their consumption of alcohol before admission, primarily when elated.[27] Of those bipolar patients who were not hospitalized, none had used alcohol excessively. It was felt that alcohol might be symptomatic of more severe mania or that inordinate drinking might increase the morbidity and likelihood of hospitalization in bipolar patients.

Winokur's study of 100 manic episodes also revealed that alcohol abuse was a factor in admission for 32% of the males and 8% of the females.[28] Morrison found that among patients with bipolar disorder, those with alcoholism more frequently demonstrated orientation impairment and made more suicide attempts.[29] The combination of alcoholism and bipolar disorder increases the chance of attempted suicide. In summary, patients with bipolar illness exhibit more dramatic increases in alcohol consumption with elevated rather than depressed mood and in association with symptoms of hyperactivity and insomnia, which are being self-medicated with alcohol. Despite the increased consumption, there has been no clear-cut evidence of increased risk of addiction in bipolar patients.

One of the theories of the etiology of addiction relates to the psychopharmacology of the relationship between affect and addiction. The hypothesis is that alcoholics or other substance abusers have lowered levels of neurotransmitters and are trying to increase these levels by drinking. At first such an increase does occur, but then there is further depletion, which may lead to even more drinking. Goodwin has called this the reserpine hypothesis for addiction and has suggested the possibility that low serotonin levels might be involved.[30]

In experimental intoxication studies, it has been found that initially alcohol improves a number of mood variables, particularly in clinically depressed patients; however, this is only in the early phase of intoxication and only at low doses. With continued drinking, the effect is lost and chronic intoxication regularly leads to deterioration of affective state and the development of a depressive syndrome, often with suicidal ideation. Although patients may recall these experiences as being pleasant, when they can see themselves on videotape, they are able themselves to recognize how depressed they were. This kind of mood disturbance generally disappears with abstinence. Alcoholics tend to retain their expectations of a pleasant intoxicated state rather than remember what actually occurs.[23] Mayfield points out that although drinking improves mood, it does not encourage normal people to drink to excess; that it makes depression worse does not encourage alcoholics to stop. Alcoholics anticipate affective improvement; however, as they become more depressed, they feel more in need of the substance. The same mechanism may occur in cocaine addiction, in which there is depression and irritability following the euphoria, a depression that is best relieved by more cocaine or the addition of alcohol, sedatives, or opiates. Mello feels that any stimulus change may be important whether it is positive or negative and that aversive consequences may also reinforce drug use.[31]

The link between affective illness and addiction may not be direct but may relate through intervening variables such as unemployment, divorce, or other environmental variables. In 1951, Amark, in a study of psychiatric morbidity in male alcoholics and their relatives, found an increased risk of psychopathy and psychogenic psychoses that today would be considered among the affective disorders. The risk of alcoholism and criminality was found to be higher among brothers and fathers but not among sisters.[32]

Winokur studied the families of patients with affective disorders.[33] Among the parents of affectively ill probands, fathers demonstrated a higher incidence of alcoholism (9.5%) than mothers (1.1%), an incidence higher than that found in a control group (1.7% and 0%, respectively). Affective illness was more common in female relatives, and alcoholism and sociopathy were more common in male relatives. If one combined the prevalence of alcoholism and affective disorder in male relatives of affectively disordered patients, the total would approximate the combined prevalence of the same disorders in female relatives. Whether one looks at affective disorder or primary alcoholism in women under 40, a pattern of high incidence of affective disorder among the female relatives and alcoholism and sociopathy among the male relatives is sustained. Late-onset female depressives were found to represent a separate group compared to early onset females and more similar to late-onset male depressives, in which there was a higher incidence of affective disorder but not alcoholism or sociopathy. In 1974 Winokur concluded that depression includes subtypes, one of which he designated depression spectrum disease characterized by early onset, predominantly in females with alcoholic and antisocial male relatives and high numbers of first-degree female relatives with depression. His findings have received some support from Mendlewicz and Baron, who partially replicated data on morbid risk for alcoholism, sociopathy, and depression in the families of depressed patients.[34] This suggests the possibility of a broad-based genetic vulnerability to certain forms of mental illness with different phenotypic expressions in men and women.

In a study of the Amish, Egeland and Hostetter found that in this culturally and genetically homogeneous population without alcoholism and sociopathy, the rates of unipolar depression were equal for men and women.[35] Cloninger and co-workers argue that if alcoholism is more frequent in the families of nondepressed alcoholics than in the families of primary depressives with alcoholism, this phenomenon argues against the same underlying familial predisposition.[36] Cloninger believes

that alcoholism, sociopathy, and depression are genetically distinct and overlap as a result of intervening environmental variables. Goodwin agrees that, based on his adoption studies, the inheritance of alcoholism is separate from that of other disorders.[30] Sons of alcoholics reared away from home demonstrated an increase in alcoholism but not in antisocial personality or affective disorder. Goodwin also did not find an excess of depression in the daughters of alcoholics reared away from home and believes that it may very well be that living in a household with an alcoholic father may account for some of Winokur's findings. He believes that depression may be increased in the daughters and sisters of alcoholics through environmental variables. It is also possible that assortative mating, with depressives and alcoholics frequently marrying, leads to offspring at risk for both illnesses.

Another link between affective disorder and addiction is the finding that four fifths of successful suicides are associated with one or both of these disorders. In most of the substance-abuse cases, depression was considered to be secondary to the alcoholism, and only 8% had primary affective disorder with secondary alcoholism. Of Murphy's sample, 26% had experienced a major loss within the last 6 weeks; of those with uncomplicated alcoholism, 45% had experienced a recent major loss, and 64% had had a loss within the past year. The suicide risk for alcoholics has been estimated to be 30 times that of the general population.[37]

INTERACTIONS WITH ANXIETY DISORDERS

Anxiety and anxiety disorders can be primary or secondary to substance-use disorders. The way in which substance use interacts with anxiety and anxiety disorders is not yet well understood. Weissman found generalized anxiety disorder in 9% and phobias in 3% of alcoholics.[38] Rounsaville, in an inpatient population of addicts, found generalized anxiety disorder in 11%, phobic disorder in 5%, panic disorder in 3%, and obsessive compulsive personality disorder in 4%.[21]

Previously labeled as anxiety neurosis, panic disorder is marked by discrete panic attacks with multiple autonomic signs including hyperventilation and tremulousness, with an onset in the teens and twenties and a prevalence of 1% to 2% in the general population. An early history of separation anxiety and school phobias is found in many of these patients. The illness shows a familial pattern, and there may be a genetic vulnerability. In the *DSM-III* the condition is distinguished from generalized anxiety disorder. It is unclear from the existing literature whether the frequency of panic disorder is increased in the addicted population. There is a high familial prevalence of panic disorder and an increased prevalence of alcoholism among the male relatives of probands with panic disorder. Crowe found that 15% of those with panic disorder manifested alcohol abuse or dependence, compared with 4% of controls.[39]

Posttraumatic stress disorder (PTSD) is marked by the reexperiencing of the traumatic event, numbing of responsiveness to or reduced involvement with the external world, and a variety of autonomic and cognitive symptoms including hyperalertness, exaggerated startle response, insomnia, and dysphoria. These symptoms occur with latency of months or years. In the *DSM-III,* substance-use disorders have been listed as a complication of PTSD.

It is still controversial whether PTSD is associated with substance abuse. Archibald and associates first reported the persistence of symptoms in combat-fatigue patients in 1965.[40] There was an increase in symptomatology in their sample over time. They did not find an increase in alcoholism among their combat patients compared with their noncombat patients.

There were reports of heavy use of drugs and alcohol during the Vietnam war, a period during which there was a high degree of stress and substance availability.[41] Many of the veterans who returned home gave up drugs and only a very small percentage remained addicted. Egendorf has reported on the feelings of betrayal and alienation and the high incidence of arrest and alcoholism among Vietnam veterans. Sierles reported that 64% of 25 veterans with PTSD were alcoholics and 20% were drug dependent. Boscarino also found a higher incidence of alcohol use and binge drinking in those veterans who served actively in Vietnam. However, Roy postulates a bias in assignment to combat duty. The question can still be raised as to whether alcohol use is related directly to the stress response or whether those who developed alcoholism would have been vulnerable anyway.

INTERACTIONS WITH ORGANIC CONDITIONS

Alcoholism and drug addiction have long been associated with a variety of organic conditions. Organic psychoses were described by Kraepelin, and there is a large body of literature describing more subtle neuropsychological impairment and pathologic findings in addicts.[18] Begleiter, Wender, Tarter, and others have looked for neuropsychological impairment that might predispose to development of addiction or explain individual variation.[16,42,43]

Minimal brain dysfunction (MBD) in children and its persistence as ADD, residual type in adults has been found by several authors to be associated with alcoholism. MBD affects approximately 3% of prepubertal children. Often the diagnosis is suggested by teachers who note that in the classroom there is inattention, distractibility, overactivity, impulsivity, mood lability, and low frustration tolerance. Only in 5% of the cases will there be a clear associated neurologic disorder and, in a higher percentage, there may be soft neurologic signs. Attention problems may persist into late adolescence and early adulthood and, at that point, the condition is associated with an increased risk of sociopathy and drug and alcohol abuse.[42,43]

Mendelson and co-workers, in a prospective study of children between the ages of 12 and 16, found that a high percentage (59%) had had contact with the police, 18% had gone before the juvenile court, 15% were drinking excessively, 15% were setting fires, and 13% were enuretic.[44] A high percentage of the children with antisocial personality problems had parents with drinking problems. Wender reports that among those with adult psychiatric disorders, including early onset of alcoholism, there is a higher incidence of signs and symptoms of childhood hyperactivity.[42]

Tarter found that primary alcoholics had more symptoms of MBD than secondary alcoholics, who did not differ from normal controls.[43] The primary alcoholics had a younger age of onset of drinking, were younger at the time of the study, and had lower MMPI scales than the other groups with the exception of scale 9 (Ma). High scores for MBD were correlated with essential alcoholism. Essential alcoholics are described as dependent, passive, and psychosexually immature persons who begin drinking early in life without specific precipitating cause. Tarter suggests that hyperactivity or MBD may contribute to disturbed developmental history observed in essential alcoholics. It therefore is possible that some of the characteristics of essential alcoholics, which resemble those of familial alcoholics, could be due to MBD.

Hale and others have found high rates of MBD in childhood and combinations of hyperactivity, alcoholism, and sociopathy in the relatives of hyperactive children.[45] Goodwin's Danish study of male adoptees in 1975 found that half the alcoholics had demonstrated antisocial behavior and half were hyperactive as children.[30] Wender's group has reported the successful treatment of adults with ADD, residual type with methylphenidate and pemoline.[42] In summary, MBD or ADD in some form may persist into adulthood and is marked in these patients by a tendency to increased substance abuse in prospective studies through adolescence but not necessarily into adulthood. This may represent a small but significant population at risk.

Patients with substance-use disorders who are developmentally disabled with an IQ of 60 to 85 are concrete, easily manipulated, and have difficulty learning from experience. They may find the neighborhood bar to be a warm, nonjudgmental place where they feel accepted and part of a group. Since deinstitutionalization, many mentally retarded people who are living in the community and lacking necessary skills for positive socialization turn to alcohol and substance abuse as an easy solution. It is hard for them to learn about alcohol in programs with a strong emphasis on education, and they therefore need special support and help as well as a great deal of acceptance, warmth, and emotional support.

INTERACTIONS WITH PERSONALITY DISORDERS

In the *DSM III*, the diagnosis of personality disorder is to be made when a personality disorder has preceded the onset of substance-use disorders. It is also possible to list personality traits. There is a category of organically induced personality disorders that can be, but is not, widely used to represent personality problems that may develop as a result of organic effects of toxic substances. Currently, there is no good way to take into account the chronic toxic, organic, and psychosocial effects that long-term use of substances can have on personality. These effects may take a long time to resolve after abstinence. Our diagnostic system will some day need to find a better way to code interaction of Axis I disorders, such as substance dependency, with Axis II disorders, taking into account which disorder is primary.

Although many researchers have looked for a single addictive personality, no group of traits or single personality disorder has been found to be specific for addiction. However, addictive disorder may be overrepresented in a variety of personality disorders including antisocial personality, borderline personality, narcissistic personality, dependent personality, and passive aggressive personality. Using research diagnostic criteria, 10% to 20% of male and 5% to 10% of female alcoholics requiring admission can be diagnosed as antisocial personality. Narcotics addicts range from 20% in a mostly male population in a community inpatient service[21] to 73% of males and 61% of females in a court-referral service.[24] Schizotypal features have been found in 8%, borderline personality disorder in 3%, dependent personality in 2%, and Briquets syndrome in 0.7% of females and 0% of males.[21]

The prevalence of antisocial personality is also reflected in MMPI data. While some researchers concluded that there were no differences between alcoholics and comparable psychiatric patients, others described alcoholism as a distinct entity with special personality characteristics (Morey and Blashfield). High scorers on the McAndrew scale of the MMPI have been described as bold, uninhibited, self-confident, socially rebellious, and resentful of authority (McAndrew). Goldstein and Linden found two subtypes of pictures on the MMPI.[46] Type I is characterized by an elevated 4 (Pd) scale and is described as an emotionally unstable personality type exhibiting a trait disturbance marked by poorly controlled anger with temper tantrums and overt forms of emotional expression in response to frustration. This picture might be associated with psychopathic personality. Type II, having a 278 (D, Pt, and Sc) profile, is marked by the presence of either anxiety reaction or reactive depression with somatic complaints and suicidal ideation. These persons are described as psychoneurotic.

Subsequent studies have found a high 4 scale to be indicative of long-term heavy alcohol use with passive dependent personality style. The 278 cluster has been associated with the heaviest use of alcohol, more severe consequences, and severe psychopathology.[47,48] It has also been found that those with a 278 profile report a high degree of subjective distress while others deny heavy use and symptoms. Patients followed over long periods of time marked by either complete abstinence or occasional slips show improvement in their MMPIs.[9]

From the MMPI data, it appears that most of the pathology seen at the time of treatment reflects the course of the illness rather than premorbid characteristics. Subtypes on the MMPI have been used to try to select treatment and predict outcome.[5] Neurotic patients with elevated 2 scales have been found to have the best prognosis, while elevations of the 4 and 9 scales are associated with poor prognosis. Elevations of the 8 scale are correlated with the poorest pretreatment adjustment and failure to return during the follow-up period.

Conclusion

Patients with a substance-use disorder combined with other psychiatric disorders are among the most prevalent in psychiatric practice. Yet they are frequently underdiagnosed, undertreated, and more likely to meet exclusion criteria in studies than to be carefully researched. Although it is difficult to differentiate which disorder is primary and to separate out state–trait issues, such differentiation is critical for both clinical and research reasons. An abstinence approach that accepts the need of some patients for psychiatric medications is best for diagnostic and therapeutic success. Patients who present with substance abuse and psychopathology have a poorer prognosis than those who have a single substance disorder without accompanying psychiatric disorders; however, they respond to treatment better when the multiple problems are addressed in a treatment tailored to their needs. It is better to cut the shoes to fit the feet rather than the other way around.

REFERENCES

1. Robins LN, Helzer JE, Weissman MM et al: Lifetime prevalence of specific psychiatric disorders in three sites. Arch Gen Psychiatry 41:949–958, 1984

2. Myers JK, Weissman MM, Tischler GL et al: Six-month prevalence of psychiatric disorders in three communities. Arch Gen Psychiatry 41:958–967, 1984

3. Penick: Familial alcoholism and other psychiatric disorders, presented at APA in Dallas, abstract in APA Summary Syllabus, 1984, p. 173

4. Woody GE, McLellan AT, Luborsky L et al: Severity of psychiatric symptoms as a predictor of benefits from psychotherapy: the Veterans Administration-Penn study. Am J Psychiatry 141:1172–1177, 1984

5. Frances RJ, Bucky S, Alexopoulos GS: Outcome study of familial and nonfamilial alcoholism. Am J Psychiatry 141(11):1469–1471, 1984

6. Frances RJ, Alexopoulos G: The inpatient treatment of the alcoholic patient. Psychiatr Ann 12(4):386–391, 1982

7. McCord W, McCord J: Origins of alcoholism. Stanford, Stanford University Press, 1960

8. Vaillant GE: The course of alcoholism and lessons for treatment. In Grinspoon L (ed): Psychiatry Update, 3, pp 311–319. Washington, DC, American Psychiatric Association, 1984

9. Pettinati HN, Sugerman A, Maurer HS: 4 year MMPI changes in abstinent and drinking alcoholics. Alcoholism: Clinical and Experimental Research 6:487–494, 1982

10. Khantzian EJ, Khantzian NJ: Cocaine addiction: Is there a psychological predisposition? Psychiatr Ann 4:10, 1984

11. Minkoff K II: A map of chronic mental patients. In Talbott J (ed): The Chronic Mental Patient, pp 11–37. Washington, DC, American Psychiatric Association, 1978

12. The unconstitutionalized generation: A new breed of psychiatric patients. In Pepper B, Ryglervicz H, Kirshner MC (eds): New Directions for Mental Health Services (14): The Young Adult Chronic Patient, pp 3–14. San Francisco, Jossey-Bass, 1984

13. Salzman B: Problems with inadequate medication, response and adverse drug response often are related to other substance misuse and drug interactions: Opiates and severely disturbed patients. Am NY Acad Soc 398:58–64, 1982

14. Saxon S: Drug abuse and suicide. In Smith D et al (eds): A Multicenter View of Drug Abuse, pp 165–170. Cambridge, Hall/Schenkman, 1978

15. Alexopoulos GS, Lieberman W, Frances RJ: Platelet MAO activity in alcoholic patients and their first-degree relatives. Am J Psychiatry 140(11):1501–1504, 1983

16. Porjesz B, Begleiter H: Human evoked brain potentials and alcohol. Alcoholism: Clinical and Experimental Research 5:304–316, 1981

17. Kaij L: Studies on the etiology and sequels of abuse of alcohol. Thesis, University of Lund, Sweden, 1960

18. Kraepelin E: Lectures on clinical psychiatry. In Johnstone T (ed): Chronic Alcoholism, pp 171–179. New York, Hafner Publishing, 1968

19. Rado S: The psychoanalysis of pharmacothymia. Psychoanal Q 2:1–23, 1932

20. Keeler MH, Taylor CI, Miller WC: Are all recently detoxified alcoholics depressed? Am J Psychiatry 136:586–588, 1979

21. Rounsaville BJ, Rosenberger P, Wilber C et al: A comparison of the SADS/RDC and the DSM-III. J Nervous Mental Disease 168:90–97, 1980

22. Schuckit MA: Alcoholism and other psychiatric disorders. Hosp Community Psychiatry 34:1022–1026, 1983

23. Woodruff RA, Guze SB, Clayton PJ et al: Alcoholism and depression. Arch Gen Psychiatry 28:97–100, 1973

24. Croughan JL, Miller P, Wagelin D et al: Psychiatric illness in male and female narcotic addicts. J Clin Psychiatry 43:225–228, 1982

25. Cassidy WL, Flanagan MB, Spellman BA et al: Clinical observations in manic-depressive disease. JAMA 164:1535–1546, 1957

26. Mayfield DG: Alcohol and affect: Experimental studies. In Goodwin DW, Erickson CK (eds): Alcoholism and Affective Disorders: Clinical, Genetic, and Biochemical Studies. Jamaica, NY, Spectrum Publications, 1979

27. Reich LH, Davies RK, Himmelhock JN: Excessive alcohol use in manic-depressive illness. Am J Psychiatry 131:83–86, 1974

28. Winokur GA, Clayton PJ, Reich T: Manic Depressive Illness. St Louis, CV Mosby, 1969

29. Morrison JR: Bipolar affective disorder and alcoholism. Am J Psychiatry 131:1130–1133, 1974

30. Goodwin DW, Erickson CK (eds): Alcoholism and Affective Disorder. Jamaica, NY, Spectrum Publications, 1979

31. Mello NK: Control of drug self-administration: The role of adversive consequences. In Petersen RC, Stillman RC (eds): Phencyclidine (PCP) Abuse: An Appraisal, pp 289–308. National Institute on Drug Abuse Research Monograph 21. Washington, DC, Government Printing Office, 1978

32. Amark C: A study in alcoholism. Acta Psychiatrica Scand (suppl) 70:1–283, 1951

33. Winokur GA, Cadoret R, Dorzab JA et al: The division of depressive illness into depression spectrum disease and pure depressive disease. Int Pharmacopsychiatry 9:5–13, 1974

34. Mendelwicz J, Baron M: Morbidity risk in subtypes of unipolar depressive illness. Br J Psychiatry 139:463–466, 1981

35. Egeland JA, Hostetter AM: Amish study I: Affective disorders among the Amish. Am J Psychiatry 140:56–61, 1983

36. Cloninger RC, Reich T, Wetzel R: Alcoholism and affective disorders: Familial associations and genetic models. In Goodwin DW, Erickson CK (eds): Alcoholism and Affective Disorders, pp 57–86. Jamaica, NY, Spectrum Publications, 1979

37. Murphy GE, Armstrong JW, Hermele SL et al: Suicide in alcoholism. Arch Gen Psychiatry 36:65–68, 1979

38. Weissman MM, Myers JJ, Harding PS: Prevalence and psychiatric heterogeneity of alcoholism in a U.S. urban community. Journal of Studies on Alcohol 41:672–681, 1980

39. Crowe RR, Pauls PL, Slymen DJ et al: A family study of anxiety neurosis: Morbidity risk in families of patients with or without mitral valve prolapse. Arch Gen Psychiatry 37:77–79, 1980

40. Archibald HC, Tuddenham RD: Persistent stress reaction after combat. Arch Gen Psychiatry 12:475–481, 1965

41. Roy RE: Alcohol misuse and post-traumatic stress disorder (delayed): An alternative interpretation of the data. Journal of Studies on Alcohol 44:198–202, 1983

42. Wender PH, Reimherr FW, Wood DR: Attention deficit disorder (minimal brain dysfunction) in adults: A replication study of diagnosis in drug treatment. Arch Gen Psychiatry 38:449–456, 1981

43. Tarter RE: Psychosocial history in minimal brain dysfunction in differential drinking patterns of male alcoholics. J Clin Psychology 38:867–873, 1982

44. Mendelson W, Johnson N, Steward MA: Hyperactive children as teenagers: A follow-up study. J Nerv Ment Dis 153:273–279, 1971

45. Hale MS, Hesselbrock M, Hesselbrock V: Childhood deviance in sociopathy and alcoholism. J Psychiatr Treat Eval 4:33–36, 1982

46. Goldstein SG, Linden JD: Multivariate classification of alcoholics by means of the MMPI. J Abnorm Psychol 74:661–669, 1969

47. Donovan DM, Chaney EF, O'Leary MR: Alcohol MMPI subtypes: Relationship to drinking styles, benefits and consequences. J Nerv Ment Dis 166:553–561, 1978

48. Eshbaugh TM, Dick KV, Tosi DJ: Typological analysis of MMPI personality patterns of drug dependent females. J Personal Assess 46:488–494, 1982

Normal Sexuality and Introduction to Sexual Disorders

Human Sexual Response

Human sexual response may best be understood from a biopsychosocial perspective.[1] The investigation of the psychophysiology of human response was initiated by Masters and Johnson.[2] These investigators studied 382 women and 312 men in a laboratory setting. Since they later wrote a well-known book on sexual inadequacy, it is important to emphasize that their findings about the sexual response cycle were not based on observations of patients receiving treatment. Their classic observations were carried out with research volunteers engaged in a variety of types of sexual activities, usually culminating in orgasm. Subjects ranged in age from 18 to 89 years, and thousands of complete cycles were studied. The specific aspects of the sexual response cycle will be described in greater detail elsewhere in this text. It is important, however, to stress a few basic findings. Knowledge about sex differences in human sexual response took a great leap forward as a result of Masters and Johnson's data. They noted that the patterns with which the phases unfolded were more variable in females than in males. Perhaps even more important, Masters and Johnson documented the presence of a so-called "refractory" period following orgasm in males but not in females. Thus, males will not become immediately excited following an orgasm and progress to have another orgasm without delay, whereas females may do so. Another observa-

tion that clarified much confusion was that the physiology of orgasm was the same, regardless of the type of stimulation by which it was achieved. That is, whether orgasm occurred in a setting of masturbation or coitus or by vaginal or clitoral stimulation, its basic physiology was the same.

This point requires additional commentary since the so-called dual-orgasm theory, proposed by Freud, had been extremely influential until Masters and Johnson's work. The dual-orgasm theory involved a model of female sexual development as well as a model of the psychophysiology of sexual response. Freud assumed that the child first experiences the clitoris as the primary site of sexual excitement. However, in his view optimal psychological development required a shift from clitoral to vaginal erogenous zones. The healthy woman, therefore, should be able to achieve "vaginal orgasm" during coitus and excessive dependence on the clitoris was regarded as a sign of immaturity or psychopathology.[3] Kinsey, and others, had earlier observed that the clitoris is usually much more sensitive to stimulation than the vagina and had questioned Freud's model. Masters and Johnson's psychophysiologic studies, however, put the dual-orgasm theory to rest.

In addition to numerous changes in the sex organs during the sexual response cycle, other physiologic changes occur throughout the body. These include skin flushing, generalized myotonia, hyperventilation, tachycardia, and increased blood pressure. During orgasm sinus tachycardia occurs and systolic and diastolic blood pressure elevations are manifested in both sexes. It has been estimated that the total energy cost of one complete sexual response cycle is roughly similar to climbing one or two flights of stairs.[4]

It is important to emphasize that changes occur in the central nervous system and in the mind that parallel peripheral psychophysiologic events. In one well-known investigation, for example, Heath reported on a man and a woman who had multiple electrodes implanted in cortical and deep areas of their brain in order to study and treat intractable seizure disorders. It was possible to stimulate these individuals and also to record their electroencephalographic (EEG) responses. Not only were complete sexual response cycles observed, but the psychophysiologic changes of the cycle were produced by direct chemical stimulation of the brain (by microinjection of acetylcholine and levarterenol). Characteristic EEG findings of spike and slow wave in the septal region occurred with orgasm.[5] Such data as these, further supported by primate studies in which the central nervous system pathways for sexual response were meticulously mapped, attest to the role of the brain in the sexual response cycle. Associated with brain responses are those of the mind. These include feelings that are explicitly sexual or lustful and fantasies or images that are associated with sexual excitement. In addition, unconscious aspects of mental functioning are involved in sexual response and may enhance or inhibit the sequential changes of the sexual response cycle.

All studies of human sexual behavior attest to its great variability. This is true between individuals and social groups and within individuals. One reason for this variability is that the meaning attributed to sexuality depends on a person's state of mind. Thus, how a person feels in general influences and is influenced by his or her sexual behavior. The psychophysiologic studies of human sexual behavior, therefore, must be interpreted with respect for the central concept of behavioral variability. Consider the dual-orgasm theory previously described. A particular woman may find vaginal containment of the penis so pleasureful, within the context of lovemaking, that for her "vaginal" and "clitoral" orgasms seem truly different. Her partner might feel similarly about their lovemaking, and for him "masturbatory" versus "coital" orgasms might also seem different. These differences are, of course, due to the interpretation of the sexual act within its greater overall context. Individuals provide meaning to physiologic change by interpreting it within its psychosocial context and from the perspective of their past histories.

Psychoneuroendocrine Associations in the Adult

Sexuality appears to be dependent on androgens in both males and females. The evidence for this comes from a number of sources. Castration in males produces decreased sexuality, as does administration of antiandrogenic hormones. Other androgen-deficiency states are also associated with hyposexuality. In women, androgen is largely secreted by the adrenal gland. Removal of the adrenals appears to be associated with diminished sexuality, whereas removal of the ovaries does not. Administration of androgen to females appears to increase sexual desire, as does administration of androgen to hypogonadal men.[6]

It is also apparent that associations exist between the menstrual cycle and sexuality. Models of sexual behavior, therefore, must take into account the concept of cyclicity as opposed to tonicity. The research by Benedek[7] illustrates how complex naturalistically occurring behavior–hormone interactions may be. Benedek carried out an unusually ambitious and detailed longitudinal study of women who were psychoanalyzed. It was possible to predict cycle phase, independently determined, by analyzing the content (*e.g.,* free associations, dreams) of psychoanalytic sessions. Benedek reported systematic fluctuations in mental activity closely associated with menstrual cycle phase. Affects fluctuated along a pleasure/displeasure continuum, and certain specific types of negative affects, namely irritability, anxiety, and depression, constituted dysphoria when present. Sexual feelings also fluctuated in intensity, and the fantasies associated with sexual desire were different during different phases of the cycle. The luteal phase appeared to be associated with procreational fantasies in contrast to the stimulatory erotic fantasies of the follicular phase.

Many subsequent studies indicate that the menstrual cycle may influence sexuality.[8] A postmenstrual peak in activity is the most firmly established finding. Data are suggestive, however, that midcycle and premenstrual phases may be associated with increased sexual activity. The biopsychosocial mechanisms that determine these effects remain to be fully described.

After cessation of menses, the quality of sexuality is highly variable. Barring somatic complications of reduced hormones, such as atrophic vaginitis, it has not been demonstrated that the physical effects of menopause lead directly to diminished sexuality. Sexuality shows similar type of change with subsequent aging, as do other psychophysiological functions. Space does not allow discussion of this area here, and the topic has been recently reviewed by Mobarak and Shamoian.[9]

Prenatal Psychoneuroendocrine Considerations

The preceding discussion has focussed on hormone–behavior interactions of adults. A different type of hormonal effect occurs prenatally. During a critical period of embryologic life, testosterone must be present in order for the reproductive structures to differentiate as male. Absence of testosterone leads to differentiation as female. Moreover, androgen present during a critical phase of intrauterine life not only determines genital morphology but also influences the structure of the central nervous system. The effects of prenatal androgen on the brain are generally acknowledged to influence human behavior (as will be discussed more substantially below). Until the mid 1970s, however, the best available data seemed to indicate that the basic enduring sense of being male or female, the individual's core gender identity, resulted from postnatal psychosocial influences rather than prenatal hormonal ones. The conclusion that core gender identity differentiates as a result of learning (except in transsexuals) was reached through elaborate studies, primarily carried out at Johns Hopkins University by Money and collaborators.[10] These studies capitalized on errors of nature in which hermaphrodites with identical biological defects were raised as boys in some circumstances and as girls in others. Other situations were studied in which attempts had been made to change core gender identity at varying points in the life cycle. Study of individuals with rare chromosomal anomalies and other types of pathology (*i.e.*, absent genitalia, receptor insensitivity to effects of androgen, precocious puberty, and many other conditions) led to the central concepts of gender identity differentiation. According to these concepts, gender identity is not determined by chromosomal or gonadal sex but differentiates according to sex of rearing. Furthermore, gender identity may be changed during the early years of life, before the age at which it differentiates and becomes part of the ''core'' self-concept.

Questions were recently raised about the above model, however, by the research of Imperato-McGinley and colleagues.[11] In 1974, Imperato-McGinley and colleagues reported on a unique subgroup of male pseudohermaphrodites with 5α-reductase deficiency, an autosomal recessive genetic anomaly. In this unique condition, the prenatal and neonatal exposure of the brain to testosterone is that of the normal male. The enzyme deficiency produces ambiguous external genitalia, and many individuals are assigned as females at birth and raised as girls. However, these children then undergo a masculinizing puberty, with voice deepening, growth of the previously clitoral-like phallus, development of a rugated, hyperpigmented scrotum, full descent of testes, and a muscular habitus. Sexual histories were obtainable from 18 of these pseudohermaphrodites. Sixteen changed gender identity from female to male during the years following puberty, and one additional subject developed a severe gender identity disorder. This person dressed as a female but manifested extremely masculine mannerisms and had sex with women. Only one of these individuals continued to maintain female gender identity following puberty. Imperato-McGinley and colleagues noted that in most cases, when gender identity is concordant with rearing but discordant with chromosomal and gonadal sex, castration and sex hormone therapy has been initiated to coincide with sex of rearing. In the exceptional situation she described, postpubertal effects of testosterone on a prenatally masculinized brain appeared to override sex of rearing. Imperato-McGinley and colleagues have challenged the hypothesis that gender identity becomes fixed by 18 months to 4 years of age. She has pointed out that a good deal of the data on matched pairs discordant for sex or rearing but concordant for biological sex was derived from pseudohermaphrodites who were functionally testosterone deficient prenatally. Whether the view expressed by Imperato-McGinley and colleagues is accurate, in general, or not, the importance of the experiment in nature she and her group described is great. Thus, the conditions that determine core gender identity differentiation would appear *not* to be definitively established at this time.

Other behavioral effects of prenatal androgen have not been definitively established in the human. Effects on nonsexual behavior and also on sexual behavior are likely, however. With regard to nonsexual behavior there is considerable evidence that prenatal testosterone plays a role in sex differences in aggression. The fact that such sex differences exist is indisputable. ''Aggression'' actually refers to many types of behavior, and for detailed discussion of classificatory schemes, the reader is referred to the work of Moyer.[12] In all mammalian species, males are more aggressive than females. This is also true of all human societies and has always characterized human behavior throughout recorded history.[13] It is worthy of emphasis that the predisposition toward aggressivity does not simply result from grossly observable phenomena, such as the increased size and muscle mass of men compared with women, or the fact that the erect male phallus has the capacity to penetrate whereas females have no comparable organ. The psychobiological effect probably results from differences in central nervous system structure and function as a consequence of prenatal androgen influence. Maccoby and Jacklin[14] have pointed out that sex differences in aggression are formed early in life prior to the time when differential socialization is likely; that similar sex differences are formed in humans and subhuman primates and can similarly be influenced by experimental administration of sex hormones. The differences can be demonstrated across cultures, during childhood, and do not depend on specific definitions of aggression used in studies. The finding is valid regardless of how aggression is defined or measured. The principle of individual variability certainly applies here, and there are many individual exceptions to the general tendency. Be that as it may, the case for biological predisposition to sex-related aggressivity appears overwhelming.

Interestingly, Ehrhardt and Baker, in studies of children with congenital adrenal hyperplasia, found that girls in whom this condition was treated during early childhood manifested subsequent high energy levels, increased interest in rough and tumble activities, and tomboyism.[15] Follow-up studies of other girls who had progestin-induced hermaphroditism (*i.e.*, prenatal masculinizing of the brain) revealed similar findings. The latter two groups of patients were not hyperaggressive; however, their prenatal androgen excess was not comparable to the hormonal environment of normal males. The follow-up studies of girls with increased androgenization occurring prenatally are in fact comparable with the hypothesis about the biological basis for sex differences in aggression. Before leaving this topic, one notes that the differences between males and females with regard to aggression generally is even more pronounced with regard to sex-related aggression (*i.e.*, conditions in which sexual excitement and hyperaggressivity coexist). It may well be that prenatal androgen influ-

ences the likelihood of postpubertal sexual aggression in the human.

The other behavioral area about which there has been increasing interest in the role of prenatal androgens is that of sexual orientation. This effect is included in the discussion of homosexuality that follows.

Homosexuality

Many investigators and clinicians have attempted to define *homosexuality*, but no single definition of the term has gained universal acceptance. The most commonly used definitions have been erotic attraction to members of the same sex during adulthood and/or repetitive erotic activity with members of the same sex during adulthood and/or self-designation as "homosexual."[16,17] Kinsey's method of reporting homosexual and heterosexual behavior provided an innovative approach to the problem of defining homosexuality. Kinsey did not describe persons in terms of being homosexual or heterosexual. Instead, persons were placed on a hypothetical continuum with regard to their subjective behavior and their activity with others. Whereas a large group were exclusively heterosexual and a small group were exclusively homosexual, many were both heterosexual and homosexual to some degree in interest and/or activity.[18] In general, the term *homosexual* has been used in the scientific, clinical, and popular literature to connote an individual's sexual behavior, sexual fantasy life, sense of inner identity, and social role. These four parameters may be congruent or incongruent in any particular individual. For instance, a man may fantasize about sex with men, engage exclusively in homoerotic acts, feel that his inner identity is homosexual, and publicly live a homosexual role. Alternatively, an individual may fantasize exclusively about males but engage in erotic activity to orgasm with both sexes. He may feel that his inner identity is homosexual but may live publicly (either single or married) as a heterosexual.

For many years homosexual acts and feelings were, of course, regarded as pathologic by mental health professionals. The *Diagnostic and Statistical Manual of Mental Disorders* (*DSM-I*), published by the American Psychiatric Association in 1952, lists homosexuality in the sexual deviation category, which in turn is listed under sociopathic personality disturbances. The prevailing psychiatric opinion at that time suggested an intrinsic relationship between a person's sexual object preference and conscience structure, and homosexual activity was thought to be associated with superego defects. In the *DSM-II,* published in 1968, homosexuality was no longer placed in the sociopathic category but was still considered a mental disorder and an example of sexual deviation. Heterosexual intercourse was taken as a standard for sexual health at this time. Eight specific disorders are named in the sexual deviation section of the *DSM-II.* Homosexuality leads the list, followed by fetishism, pedophilia, transvestism, exhibitionism, voyeurism, sadism, and masochism. Shortly after the publication of the *DSM-II,* the idea that homosexuality *per se* should be considered a form of psychopathology came under widespread criticism. A series of dramatic and astonishing events occurred, including acrimonious debates between proponents and opponents of the pathologic view of homosexuality, a poll of members of the American Psychiatric Association about this concept, and disruption of scientific meetings by gay activists. In the *DSM-III,* (1980) homosexuality is deleted as a mental disorder. The category "Ego Dystonic Homosexuality" is reserved for individuals who have unwanted distressing sexual arousal to homosexual stimuli and who wish to desire or increase heterosexual arousal. This judgment about the pathologic significance of homosexual behavior marks one of the more dramatic reversals by authorities about a health–illness issue in the history of medicine.[19]

The deletion of homosexuality from the *DSM-III* resulted in good measure from an appreciation that many individuals who are predominately homosexual in subjective experience and/or activity are not impaired in their capacity to work, love, or play, or, for that matter, in any way at all. In one pioneering study, for example, Hooker demonstrated that projective tests did not distinguish homosexuals from heterosexuals.[20] Studies comparing homosexuals to heterosexuals are difficult to evaluate *in toto* because of differences in design. However, one is more impressed with similarities than differences between homosexuals and heterosexuals (however defined) with regard to most categories of psychopathology.[16,17]

Two additional concepts are helpful in discussing sexual orientation—the concept of the sexprint and the concept of secondary homosexuality. The term *sexprint,* originally coined by Person, indicates consciously perceived erotic fantasies that are structured and relatively unchanging from the early years of life (an "erotic signature"). I have used the term *secondary homosexuality* to refer to

some form of homosexual behavior (*i.e.,* sex print or erotic fantasies, sense of identity, sexual activity with others or social role) that occurs in association with a so-called primary or major syndrome of psychopathology such as, for example, schizophrenia.[21] Regardless of one's view about the pathologic significance of the homosexual sex print *per se,* it is important to stress that persons with primary basic psychopathology (Axis I and Axis II disorders in *DSM-III* terms) may use homosexual phenomena in a manner that is pathologic by any standard. In most instances homosexual phenomena are selected as symptoms precisely because homosexuality and heterosexuality have different meanings to the person. In our culture, homosexual imagery may symbolically express conflict in many areas. Psychopathologic disorders may organize homosexual behaviors and may be organized by them in a way that is not comparable to heterosexual behaviors. On the one hand, there is no evidence that homosexual phenomena cause or are caused by any of these Axis I or Axis II disorders as a general rule. On the other hand, an individual patient may process homosexual phenomena symbolically in a way that is personally meaningful and not analogous to heterosexuality. This illustrates the necessity for clinicians to work with people rather than with behaviors taken out of context. The range of homosexual phenomena routinely seen by practitioners (sex print or erotic fantasies, sense of identity, activity with others, social role) may have meaning in the mental apparatus that appears integrally linked with the symptoms of the primary major disorder, whatever that may be. For example, the conscious experience of a homosexual identity may be used to cope with identity diffusion in a borderline patient. Despite the fact that the meaning of homosexual identity in this type of case may be clearly pathologic by any standard, nonetheless, it is not the "homosexual identity" itself that is pathologic but rather it is the *patient* who uses the symptolic meaning of homosexual phenomena in a pathologic manner. Parallelism with heterosexuality in a situation such as that described previously makes no sense.

A religious Catholic patient with moderate childhood effeminacy developed a personality type that was predominantly paranoid. Prepubertal sex print was homosexual and also heterosexual. Postpubertally he manifested severe guilt about his homosexual fantasies and, to a lesser degree, his heterosexual fantasies. Reality testing was grossly more or less intact, but identity diffusion was severe. Preoccupied with the question "Am I homosexual or heterosexual," he finally made a suicide attempt and was hospitalized.

In this boy's case, his effeminacy, paranoid traits, and homosexual fantasies and identity diffusion obviously exerted reciprocal pathosynergistic effects. Conditions such as described previously, however, cannot be assumed to be models for the role of the homosexual sex print in the mental life of a reasonably well-integrated person. Homosexuality in any form, as far as we know, is not associated with any syndrome of psychopathology more than any other. It has not been demonstrated, for example, either that exclusive homosexual sex printing or so-called obligatory homosexuality actually occurs in a disproportionate frequency in any pathologic condition, including the borderline syndromes. Although some psychoanalysts would differ, my reading of the available data suggests that a large group of adults with homosexual sex print and sense of identity do not manifest significant character pathology as adults more frequently than heterosexuals do.[16,17] In adopting this view as a psychoanalyst, it is obviously with awareness that certain types of character pathology may initially present in a subtle manner, yet actually be severe. Patients with pathologic narcissism, for example, have been used as an illustration of this point.[22]

In contrast to the patient previously presented, consider the following history of an individual whom I believe to be reasonably well-integrated.

A 40-year-old engineer with homosexual sex print and identity was seen in a research and educational context. He had never experienced an erection in association with a consciously perceived heterosexual fantasy nor could he recall ever having heterosexual dreams. Homosexual dreams with orgasm had occurred from time to time during his life. From mid-adolescence to young adulthood he dated girls, hoping to become sexually aroused by them. Sexual activity was attempted a few times but never could proceed because of an absence of a feeling of sexual desire or any of the changes of the sexual response cycle. This man's sex print emerged prepubertally, years before he knew what a homosexual was. His first sexual activity with another person occurred during young adulthood, more or less coincident with the recognition that he "must" be homosexual. Some people in this person's interpersonal network knew of his homosexuality, and some did not, depending on his assessment of their attitudes and values. He had regular sexual activity with a few different partners but never "cruised," nor did he visit any bars or baths. He did not belong to a gay organization. As an adult, this man had a stable, productive work history. He had loyal, caring, durable friendships with men and

women and found pleasure in many aspects of his life. He had demonstrated the capacity for appropriate grief and appropriate feelings of depression during his life.

Consideration of the relationship between psychopathology and homosexuality is further complicated by the fact that there does seem to be a specific relationship between childhood gender role identity disturbances and the occurrence of a homosexual (or bisexual) sex print. It may be hypothesized that preadolescent gender role identity disturbances facilitate the emergence of a homosexual sex print. Absence of such disorders diminish the likelihood of a homosexual sex print. The evidence for this is as follows. In adult males, effeminacy would appear to be more common among homosexuals than heterosexuals (transvestites excluded). Follow-up data are limited but (tentatively) indicate that most effeminate children ultimately move toward homosexuality later in life.[23] Effeminate homosexuality is often considered a specific subset of "Gender Identity Disorders." An additional type of gender role identity disturbance also occurs with some frequency in the backgrounds of a different group of men "homosexual" by some standard. During oedipal and post-oedipal phases, these boys are fearful of physical injury, athletically awkward, and temperamentally unassertive, particularly in male peer aggressive-competitive situations. Prior to adolescence (and often subsequently as well), they manifest a dread of male peer aggression and an aversion to rough and tumble activities. These youngsters, to their shame, are unable to develop behaviors acceptable to male peers and as a result have extremely low peer group status; they feel unmasculine.[24] It should be noted that there are many boys whose gender role identity disturbance has features of both groups described above: the effeminate boy and the unmasculine boy.[25] Studies of identical twins, discordant for homosexuality and heterosexuality, also support the association between gender role identity disturbance and homosexual sex printing. Furthermore, in every single such study, aversion to rough and tumble activities has been noted in the prehomosexual twin and usually not in the preheterosexual twin.[26]

The etiology of the homosexual sex print must be considered unknown at this time. Two types of theories of etiology have currency in the scientific community: a biological theory and a psychoanalytic theory. Space does not allow for more than a cursory mention of either. However, it is important to emphasize that Freud's views regarding the origins of sexual object choice heavily emphasized biological predisposition.[27] Freud may have been receptive to the theory put forth by Dorner and co-workers,[28] MacCulloch and colleagues,[29] and others that a deficit of hypothalamic exposure to androgens during a critical period prenatally leads to homosexuality in males. According to this theory, the androgen deficit occurs such that the reproductive organs are unaffected and does not influence hypothalamic-testosterone relationships at puberty. However, an abnormal response of luteinizing hormone to estrogen infusion can be demonstrated during adulthood. Furthermore, Money has observed that a surprisingly large number of girls with early corrected congenital adrenal hyperplasia are on long-term follow up developing homosexual or bisexual sex printing, suggesting an androgen-dependent prenatal process in females as well.

It should be noted that whereas the psychoanalytic and psychobiologic theories of the etiology of homosexual phenomena are often presented as if they were competing points of view, this is not necessarily always the case. The psychoanalytic theories all share the idea that childhood traumata led to anxieties that ultimately result in homosexual sex printing. The psychoanalytic theories involve behavior during the postoedipal and oedipal phases. (For example, a boy identifies with his controlling seductive mother rather than his indifferent father. He experiences the identification and the wish to be loved by his father as his mother would, in the form of homosexual erotic imagery.) Since the time frames involved in the two types of theories (i.e., biological and psychoanalytic) are *sequential*, one can readily imagine subgroups of children, moving along a hypothetic pathway from prenatal predisposition to preoedipal, oedipal, and postoedipal phases characterized by the psychodynamic and psychosocial deviant patterns emphasized in the psychoanalytic literature about homosexuality.[30] This need not always occur, however. There should be room in models of etiology for direct biological disposition toward homosexuality on the one hand and predominant psychodynamic influence on the other. The relationship between childhood gender role identity disorders requires additional study. However, it would appear that many individuals do outgrow, as it were, earlier gender role identity disturbances. In other cases, gender role identity disorders persist in a variety of forms.

Prior to leaving the discussion of homosexuality, an observation about immutability versus plasticity of sex printing is in order. Many individuals appear to behave as if their sex print was a fully differentiated mental structure. Perhaps unfortunately, one cannot avoid recognition of the fact that others seem to manifest plasticity of sex printing during adulthood. This is most anxiety provoking for investigators who search for unitary theories of sex printing. Although many clinicians privately acknowledge that sex printing appears immutable in some people and plastic in others, clinical theories have tended not to dwell on the meaning of this variability. Many analysts apparently have clinical experience with patients in whom the homosexual sex print has all of the characteristics of a classic neurotic symptom. This phenomenon, however, only occurs in some subgroups of males (possibly a minority of those who manifest homosexual phenomena).

Conclusions

Five frames of reference provide the context for most discussions of normalcy: (1) statistical, (2) ethical, (3) religious, (4) legal, and (5) medical. Obviously these categories are not mutually exclusive. Ideally, the value system that influences medical judgment should prescribe an integral relationship between medicine and science. It is from the application of the scientific method that facts can be collected, which can then be applied to relieve the suffering of illness. The degree to which medicine has leaned, not on science, but on other frames of reference in making judgments about sexual normalcy and deviancy has at times been extreme.

The boundary between social values and constructs used by mental health professionals to diagnose illness has been the subject of progressively critical scrutiny in recent years. The impact of this criticism, taken in conjunction with the modern studies of sexual behavior, has led to substantial revision of once commonly accepted models of sexual development and sexual pathology. The initial social response to sex research has usually not been sanguine. Those whose findings have diverged from prescriptive norms have faced an outraged society. Dysphoric social reactions to new observations illustrate the important organizing function served by myths about sexuality. In these myths, idealized fantasies are treated as the actual behavior of most people on the one hand and as the optimal standard of sexual health on the other. The anxiety and anger mobilized by reports to the contrary may be likened to the effect of interpretation carried out during psychotherapy with a patient whose ego-integrative mechanisms are fragile.

The subsequent chapters on sexual disorders are yet another instance of the widespread usefulness of the biopsychosocial model as explicated by Engel. Interactionism, an open systems approach, and a development perspective are all components of this model.[1] The orientation taken toward diagnosis of sexual disorders in the *DSM-III* is highly specific. The categorical, criteria-based method of diagnosis is used for the sexual disorders as it is for all other disorders in the *DSM-III*. This highly specific framework is quite different from the extremely broad, open-ended orientation required by the biopsychosocial developmental model. The modern clinician must demonstrate flexibility in shifting frames of reference between the narrow approach required for the reliable diagnosis of sexual disorders, on the one hand, and that required for a more general understanding of sexual behavior, on the other.

REFERENCES

1. Engel GL: The need for a new medical model: A challenge for biomedicine. Science 196:129, 1977

2. Masters WH, Johnson VE: Human Sexual Response. Boston, Little, Brown & Co, 1966

3. Fisher S: The Female Orgasm. New York, Basic Books, 1973

4. Hellerstein HK, Friedman EH: Sexual activity and the post-coronary patient. Arch Intern Med 125:987, 1970

5. Heath RG: Pleasure and brain activity in man. J Nerv Ment Dis 154:3, 1972

6. Rose RM: The psychological effects of androgens and estrogens: A review. In Shader RI (ed): Psychiatric Complications of Medical Drugs, pp 251–295. New York, Raven Press, 1972

7. Benedek T: Studies in Psychosomatic Medicine: Psychosexual Functions in Women. New York, Ronald Press, 1952

8. Adams DB, Gold AR, Burt AD: Rise in female-initiated sexual activity at ovulation and its suppression by oral contraceptives. N Engl J Med 229:1145–50, 1978

9. Mobarak A, Shamoian C: Aging and Sexuality. In DeFries Z, Friedman RC, Corn R (eds): Sexuality: New Perspectives. Westport, CT, Greenwood Press (in press)

10. Money J, Ehrhardt AA: Man and Woman, Boy and Girl. Baltimore, Johns Hopkins University Press, 1972

11. Imperato-McGinley J, Peterson RE, Gautier T et al: The impact of androgens on the evolution of male gender identity. In Kogan SJ, Hafez ESE (eds): Pediatric Andrology, pp 99–108. Boston, Martinus Nijhoff Publishers, 1981. Reprinted in DeFries Z, Friedman RC, Corn R (eds): Sexuality: New Perspectives. Westport, CT, Greenwood Press (in press)

12. Moyer KI: Psychology of Aggression and Implications for Control. New York, Raven Press, 1976

13. Moyer KE: Sex differences in aggression. In Friedman RC, Richart RM, VandeWiele RL (eds): Sex Differences in Behavior. New York, John Wiley & Sons, 1974

14. Maccoby EE, Jacklin C: The Psychology of Sex Differences. Stanford, CA, Stanford University Press, 1974

15. Ehrhardt AA, Baker SW: Fetal androgens, human central nervous system differentiation and behavior sex differences. In Friedman RC, Richart RM, VandeWiele RL (eds): Sex Differences in Behavior, pp 33–53. New York, John Wiley & Sons, 1974

16. Saghir MT, Robins E: Male and Female Homosexuality. Baltimore, Williams & Wilkins, 1973

17. Marmor J: Homosexual Behavior: A Modern Reappraisal. New York, Basic Books, 1980

18. Kinsey AC, Pomeroy WB, Martin CE: Sexual Behavior in the Human Male. Philadelphia, WB Saunders, 1948

19. Bayer R: Homosexuality and American Psychiatry. New York, Basic Books, 1981

20. Hooker E: Male Homosexuality. Rorschach J Projective Techniques 22(1):33–54, 1958

21. Friedman RC: Male homosexuality: On the need for a multiaxial developmental model. Presented at the panel "Toward a Further Understanding of Homosexual Men," American Psychoanalytic Association, New York, 1983. Reprinted in DeFries Z, Friedman RC, Corn R (eds): Sexuality: New Perspectives. Westport, CT, Greenwood Press (in press)

22. Kernberg O: Borderline Conditions and Pathological Narcissism. New York, Jason Aronson, 1975

23. Money J, Russo AJ: Homosexual outcome of discordant gender identity role in childhood: Longitudinal followup. J Pediatr Psychol 4:29–41, 1979

24. Friedman RC, Stern LO: Juvenile aggressivity and sissiness in homosexual and heterosexual males. J Am Acad Psychoanal 8:427–440, 1980

25. Zuger B (reply by Friedman R): Letter to the editor. J Am Acad Psychoanal 9:485–487, 1981

26. Zuger B: Monozygotic twins discordant for homosexuality: Report of a pair and significance of the phenomenon. Compr Psychiatry 17:661–669, 1976

27. Freud S: Three Essays on the Theory of Sexuality. Strachey J (trans-ed). New York, Avon Books, 1962

28. Dorner G, Rohde W, Stahl F et al: A neuroendocrine predisposition for homosexuality in men. Arch Sex Behav 4:1–8, 1975

29. MacCulloch MJ, Waddington JL: Neuroendocrine mechanisms and the aetiology of male and female homosexuality. Br J Psychiatry 139:341, 1981

30. Socardies CW: Homosexuality. New York, Jason Aronson, 1978

Paraphilias and Gender Identity Disorders

The paraphilias and the gender identity disorders, although both relatively rare, have claimed more attention than sheer numbers warrant. The study of each has peaked at different historical moments in psychology and provides examples of how the study of apparently marginal phenomena sometimes opens up new vistas of knowledge. The study of the paraphilias (then designated as perversions) was decisive in Freud's formulations of normal psychosexual development and culminated in his publication of "Three Essays on the Theory of Sexuality."[1] The study of the gender identity disorders, particularly transsexualism, plays the same pivotal role in contemporary conceptualizations of gender.

The paraphilias are a group of disorders in which sexual excitement is contingent on the presence of an unusual (even bizarre) fantasy or behavior. They include transvestism, fetishism, sadism and masochism, exhibitionism and voyeurism, pedophilia, and some other rarer entities. The gender identity disorders are characterized by the ambiguity or reversal of core gender in the absence of any biological abnormality, the primary example being transsexualism. Although there are invariably distortions of sex and gender in both groups, the predominant disturbance in the paraphilias is sexual and one of gender in the gender identity disorders.

Although both are classified in the 1980 American Psychiatric Association's *Diagnostic and Statistical Manual of Mental Disorders* (*DSM-III*)[2] as psychosexual disorders, it would be more accurate to designate them psychological "disorders of sexuality and gender." Such a classification would reflect the most important new concept in the broad field of sexology in the past 2 decades: sexuality and gender, while interrelated, are two different aspects of personality organization and must be regarded as the culmination of closely interrelated, although separate, developmental lines. To designate both as "psychosexual" reflects an outdated schema of development in which gender was simply viewed as a by-product of sexual development.

Definitions of Sexuality and Gender

In order to fully understand the clinical presentation in each group, the fundamental definitions and conceptualizations of sexuality and gender and their interrelation must be considered:

Sex refers to biological sexuality and is defined by six component parts: chromosomes, gonads, internal genitalia, external genitalia, sex hormones, and secondary sexual characteristics.

Sexuality, in contrast to biological sex, refers to erotic excitement, genital arousal, and orgasm. It is expressed in fantasy and behavior, object choice, preferred activities, subjective desire, arousal, and actual orgasmic discharge. Each individual develops a characteristic pattern of sexual expression—his or her "sex print."[3]

The *sex print* is a person's erotic signature. The sex print signifies that the individual's sexual potential has been progressively narrowed between infancy and adulthood, and it possesses definitive characteristics. It conveys more than just preference for a particular sexual object and activity; it also indicates that an individualized script, whether conscious or unconscious, most reliably elicits erotic desire. From the subjective point of view, it is almost always thought of as deep rooted and stemming from one's nature rather than as chosen or conditioned by experience. Consequently it often forms part of the individual's conscious identity or sense of self and as such, may be regarded as sexual identity. In short, the sex print refers to objective patterns of sexuality, while *sexual identity* refers to the internal experience of sexual arousal patterns and self-labeling.

Sexuality remains fluid for some years, consolidating only after the biological changes of puberty take place, and it can then be fully established only within the context of definite sexual patterns and practices. Therefore, although sexuality begins with the genital sensations of infancy and early childhood and is patterned during the oedipal phase, the sex print and sexual identity only take their definitive shape following puberty, when fantasy and desire can be melded to physical sexuality. In some instances, the consolidation of sexuality may occur much later; in others, it may never occur.

Core-gender identity, the female–male polarity, reflects a self-image of biological sex and can be defined as an individual's self-designation as being female or male. As a general rule, core gender is clearly defined and corresponds to biological sex. However, in certain pseudohermaphroditic conditions, core gender is not clearly defined but may be ambiguous. This is also true in the gender identity disorders, or cross-gender disorders as they are commonly called.

Gender-role behavior and *gender-role identity* refer to the objective and subjective manifestations of masculinity and femininity. Gender-role behavior encompasses nonsexual attributes and behavior that are nonetheless gender dichotomous. These include characteristics such as physical appearance, dress, mannerisms, speech and emotional responsiveness, aggressiveness, and countless others.

In contrast, gender-role identity reflects a psychological self-image and can be defined loosely as an individual's self-evaluation of psychological maleness or femaleness—the belief that "I am feminine" or "I am masculine." Gender-role identity, necessarily, reflects gender assignment and therefore includes core gender identity. However, it is a much more complicated self-representation than the latter. Gender-role identity continues to develop well into adulthood and fluctuates throughout life. It is a dynamic, or functional, self-representation, an appraisal of one's own feelings as well as one's behavior and performance.

It must be emphasized that although an aberrant core-gender identity is invariably reflected in gender-role identity, it does not always affect gender-role behavior. When core gender is normal, gender-role identity is simply one's self-appraisal of masculinity or femininity, and it generally varies with the person's capacity to behave in accordance with the culturally prescribed gender role. Self-confidence and self-esteem ebb and flow with this process, as the person fails or succeeds in meeting role requirements. However, when core gender is ambiguous, feelings about gender adequacy are invariably affected, even when behavior is gender "appropriate." In other words, there may be doubts about the desirability or adequacy of masculinity or femininity even when gender-role behavior is unremarkable. For example, a transvestite, who self-identifies as both male and female, almost always appears to be masculine when dressed as a man.

Although paraphilias are predominantly disorders of sexuality, they are generally associated with some compromise in gender-role identity, just as aberrant or inhibited sexuality is commonly found in the gender identity disorders. The diagnosis of either sexual disorder or gender disorder depends on whether the predominant disturbance is sexual or gender. However, it is obvious that the paraphilias and gender identity disorders frequently exist on a continuum. For example, a transvestite may cross-dress fetishistically (paraphilia) or to relieve anxiety (cross-gender disorder).

Paraphilias

Sexual symptoms fall readily into two groups, and the sexual disorders can be classified accordingly: (1) pleasure inhibitors and (2) pleasure facilitators.[4] In the first group, called the sexual dysfunctions, there is an impairment, most often an inhibition, in initiation of the sexual cycle or in arousal or discharge. In other words, there is impairment of either desire or the sexual response itself. In the second group, the paraphilias (formerly labeled perversions or deviations) the sexual response is preserved but the symptom, either a deviation in either erotic stimuli or activity, becomes the precondition for sexual excitement and orgasm.

DEFINITION

Unlike those disorders in which the symptom is painful, in the paraphilias the symptom facilitates sexual pleasure. The paraphilias are defined, then, by the invariable invocation of unusual and unvarying imagery or behavior in order to achieve sexual excitement. Conversely, sexual excitement and arousal are impaired by the absence of the accompanying paraphiliac fantasies or behaviors.

Freud originally described perversion as presenting a distortion in sexual aim. This definition has been broadened to include distortions of object as well. Such distortions in either object or aim constitute a paraphilia only when they are prerequisite to the sexual act, when they are obligatory and not elective. Thus, if a man's sexual excitement were dependent on a sheep as an object (in fantasy or actuality), his sexuality would be considered perverse. In contrast, the sexual behavior of a herdsman who resorts to intercourse with a sheep in the absence of an "appropriate" object might be considered a sexual variation but not a paraphilia. Even so, since masturbation is always present as a sexual outlet, the choice of an animal object would raise the question of some predilection or minor perverse strain.

CHANGING CONCEPTS

In the *DSM-I*[5] (1952) sexual deviations were grouped with psychopathic personality disturbances. Such a classification reflected the fact that the enactments of certain paraphilias are legal offenses (*e.g.*, pedophilia and exhibitionism), but the classification also suggests the possibility that there were pejorative attitudes toward all the perversions. At that time homosexuality was also included among the sexual deviations. In the *DSM-II*[6] (1968) the sexual deviations were classified with the personality disorders. By 1980, with the publication of the *DSM-III*, the term *paraphilia* was substituted for perversion. In part, the name change was made because the new term is descriptive. As noted in the *DSM-III*, "The deviation (para) is in that to which the individual is attracted (philia)." The group was also reclassified under the category of psychosexual disorders, which also includes gender identity disorders, psychosexual dysfunctions, and ego-dystonic homosexuality. Both changes reflect a shift in attitude among psychiatrists and the general public as well—the unwillingness to stigmatize a patient for symptoms beyond his control, particularly since most of the paraphilias do not come within the purview of current law.

That homosexuality has now disappeared from the list of paraphilias reconfirms Freud's original distinction between inversion and perversion. He asserted the normality of homosexuals, declaring that inverts "strike the observer as a collection of individuals who may be quite sound in other respects." The argument regarding the normality of homosexuality, its status as variation rather than perversion, has now evolved into a complex argument about the overall mental health of homosexuals. I share the conviction that homosexuality *per se* does not constitute a paraphilia. (The reasons why will be discussed in the section on differential diagnosis.)

However, the exemption of homosexuality as a paraphilia raises some question about the validity of the classification in general. Paraphilias, unlike neurotic symptoms, provide pleasure of the highest order and may often be ego-syntonic. Many individuals with paraphilias, as is the case with homosexuals, do not regard themselves as ill. The question must then arise as to why their fantasies and behaviors are considered as pathologic rather than simply different. In fact, some liberation groups, such as S-M Lib (based on the model of gay liberation), have raised the question of whether the psychiatric profession is labeling some sexual behaviors perverse or deviant on moral grounds in the guise of medical ones.

Although one must share in the outrage against prejudices that attach to any psychiatric disorder, one must also evaluate the validity of maintaining the classification based on the best available information. Its legitimacy must rest on objective findings. Insofar as the symptoms may not be painful and may be ego syntonic, the justification for the diagnosis must then rest on the existence of some disability or impairment that attaches to them.

RATIONALE FOR THE CLASSIFICATION

Clearly, an evolutionary value system cannot be adhered to in which sexuality must be tied to reproduction to be considered normal and all other sexuality is considered suspect. However, there are grounds for preserving the concept and classification of paraphilias without invoking an evolutionary imperative. Two lines of argument can be used to demonstrate the legitimacy of this classification, one philosophic and the other psychiatric.

Nagel,[7] writing from the philosophic perspective, suggests that there is "something to be learned about sex from the fact that we possess a concept of sexual perversion." As he points out, social disapproval has never been sufficient to label something as perverse. For example, adultery has, at times, been viewed as a moral outrage, but adultery has never been viewed as a perversion. Nagel makes the point that, consequently, paraphilias must convey something unnatural rather than immoral. However, distinguishing what is natural and unnatural is the problem itself. Some sexual activities, such as shoe fetishism, are clearly paraphilias if anything is; others, such as heterosexual intercourse, are clearly not. Still other sexual behaviors are somewhere in between. However, Nagel ultimately fails to argue the essence of perversion adequately. He suggests it reflects an incomplete expression of sexuality, insofar as he insists that ''desire that one's partner be aroused by the recognition of one's desire that he or she be aroused'' is integral to normal sexuality. However, this predicates an interpersonal connotation to sexuality that is untenable. No one suggests that masturbation is perverse.

The argument in the *DSM-III*, similar to Nagel's, is that there is often an impairment in paraphilias for reciprocal affectionate sexual activity. Such an observation, however, is permeated with value biases. Why must sex be associated with affection? Furthermore, the criterion is not universally applied. Promiscuity is not listed among the paraphilias, and neither are loveless marriages.

Instead, the validity of the classification of paraphilias must rest on the ability of psychiatrists not only to elicit evidence for ''unnatural'' or ''bizarre'' sexuality but also to demonstrate that the perverse fantasy or activity permeates mental life to an excessive degree, that its suppression yields high-level anxiety or dysphoric affect, or that it is connected with some other personality dysfunction. This is the position that virtually all psychiatrists and psychoanalysts advance. In the more overt cases, those usually seen in clinical practice, these claims appear to be adequately demonstrated. However, there are many instances in which perverse elements are subsumed into sexuality in such a minor way that such a diagnosis is not warranted. Furthermore, the boundary between perverse and ''normal'' sexuality is not always clear-cut.

Above all, the major limitation to any absolute claim of ''abnormality'' is the failure of psychiatrists to study large groups of nonpatients who exhibit these behaviors. There are, however, certain exceptions. For example, Ovesey's and Person's study[8,9] of nonpatient transvestites supports the contention that, at least in the full-blown transvestitic syndrome there is associated disability and impairment that warrants the designation of disorder. However, comparable studies have not yet been carried out with respect to most of the other sexual deviations.

EPIDEMIOLOGY

Prevalence

Insofar as the perversion yields pleasure, many individuals do not seek psychiatric intervention. Even those persons in anguish may avoid confiding in a doctor out of profound shame. Therefore, very little is known about the incidence and distribution of the paraphilias.

Still, the paraphilias appear to be rare. Some are more common than others. In an individual psychiatric practice, masochism and fetishism are probably the most common, while the excretory perversions are rarely seen. Because some paraphilias depend on the ''participation'' of nonconsenting individuals and come to the attention of the courts (*e.g.*, pedophilia and exhibitionism), they may be overrepresented in attempts to determine relative frequencies.

Among the paraphilias, most recent attention has focused on transvestism. Although the growing interest in gender has stimulated interest in all the cross-gender disorders, the existence of a transvestitic subculture makes access to research subjects relatively easy.

Sex Ratio

One characteristic feature of the distribution of the paraphilias is remarkable: the enormous predominance of paraphilias in males. Except for sadism and masochism, almost all the reported cases are male. This preponderance in males is characteristic not just of the paraphilias but also of the gender disorders. Any attempt to explain this discrepancy must be related to our understanding of the etiology of the paraphilias. Insofar as etiology has not been conclusively demonstrated, the explanations can only be tentative and must be discussed in connection with a discussion of etiology.

Predisposing Factors

There is some evidence, based on case reports in the literature, that there may be an inclination to paraphilia or atypical gender identity in a parent of a paraphiliac patient. In one study of boys displaying femininity (considered at risk for atypical gender development including transvestism), of a sample of 20, two fathers were transvestites and two mothers were lesbians.[10]

CLINICAL DESCRIPTION

The term *paraphilia* denotes the presence of an obligatory behavior or fantasy that is deviant in respect either of the *object* of the sexual instinct or its *aim*. The *DSM-III* emphasizes that the perverse imagery and acts are unusual or bizarre. It describes the nature of the deviance as falling within three types: (1) "preference for use of a non-human object for sexual arousal," (2) "repetitive sexual activity with humans involving real or simulated suffering or humiliation," and (3) "repetitive sexual activity with nonconsenting partners."[2] In essence, then, sexuality is ritualized and relies on inanimate objects or partners viewed as demeaned or dehumanized.

The diagnosis of the specific paraphilia depends on the nature of the deviant fantasy, imagery, and behavior. The overt clinical syndrome most often begins shortly after puberty and follows a chronic course. In the paraphilias, by definition, the deviant fantasy and behavior must be the precondition for orgasmic discharge. Therefore, it is obvious that the diagnosis can only be made in adolescence or later. Even though there is evidence for antecedent psychological maladjustments or affective discomfort during childhood, these are not specific to or pathognomonic for the paraphilia and are therefore not predictive.

Syndromes

Each of the subclassifications of paraphilias or any specific paraphilia is distinguished by the central imagery and fantasy. Although there are many theories that attempt to explain the meaning of each perversion, the following sections will be limited to an exposition of the clinical features that are descriptive of each. Their "symbolic" meanings will be discussed as theories in the section on etiology.

TRANSVESTISM. *Transvestism* literally means cross-dressing. In psychiatry, however, the term is used not only phenomenologically but also diagnostically. It is defined as heterosexual cross-dressing in which the clothing is used fetishistically for sexual arousal. The cross-dressing may be used to promote sexual excitement that can lead to either masturbation or heterosexual intercourse. Although cross-dressing may begin in childhood, it usually becomes sexualized in adolescence. In the predominant pattern, the child spontaneously cross-dresses, using the garments of the mother or sister, and the activity most often remains surreptitious. In some instances, it is reported to have been initiated by the mother or mother surrogate. Cross-dressing can start with a desire to promote a sense of well-being and then become sexualized, or it can be erotic from the outset. It is sporadic at first and in most transvestites remains so. In some, however, it becomes a daily occurrence.

Transvestites are invariably preferential heterosexuals. Fetishistic arousal can be intense, but interpersonal sexuality is almost always attenuated. It is typical of a transvestite to report his entire sexual experience as limited to one or two partners.

In adulthood, the transvestite's behavior is masculine in male clothes, effeminate in female clothes. Many transvestites are employed in hypermasculine professions (*e.g.*, race car driving, munitions experts). Some transvestites carry photographs of themselves dressed as women; others habitually wear hidden female undergarments. These are mini-symbols of cross-dressing and enhance the illusion of being a woman even while dressed as a man.

Initiation fantasies permeate the collective fantasy life of transvestites. In their pornography, the initiation into cross-dressing is usually forced on the novice by either a dominant big-breasted, corseted, booted "phallic" woman who enslaves him or by a kindly protective woman who does so to save his life.

FETISHISM. In the case of fetishism, either an inanimate object (*e.g.*, shoe or a handkerchief) or a part-object (*e.g.*, a foot or a partner wearing high-heeled shoes) is required for sexual arousal. The fetish may itself be the sole object of sexual activity, in which case genital discharge is achieved through masturbation, or the fetish may be incorporated into sexual activity with a partner who either embodies the fetish or who wears the fetish. The fetish is most commonly associated in some way with humans or their bodily adornments, not something so far removed as furnishings or impersonal belongings. I saw a patient in whom urinals were used as fetishistic objects, but he was clearly in the psychotic range and the perversion, as such, merged with the excretory perversions. The fetish often has particular textural characteristics. Rubber, leather, and velvet are common fetishistic materials.

Fetishism has been reported only in males, both homosexual and heterosexual, and often exists in combination with other perversions. For example, some transvestites are easily aroused by wearing tightly bound rubber underpants or prefer leather clothing. Although some persons have single fetishes, others exhibit an interest in a number of them. In either case, the fetish or group of fetishes is most often favored for long periods of time.

SEXUAL MASOCHISM AND SEXUAL SADISM. Masochism and sadism are distinguished from the other paraphilias in two ways and are therefore of special interest. First, they are the only perversions that occur in both sexes and they occur among both heterosexuals and homosexuals. Second, they merge more perceptibly into aspects of normal sexuality. Indeed, in the *DSM-III* it is suggested that "the diagnosis of sexual masochism is made only if the individual engages in masochistic sexual acts, not merely fantasies."[2] This exemption is not applied to the other paraphilias, including sadism. This may be indicative of just how widespread masochistic fantasies are and certainly indicates that the distinction between normal and deviant is not clearly defined.

Cases of sadism are not seen in psychiatric practice to the same extent as cases of sexual masochism. Much of the information on both sadistic and masochistic perversions comes from the reports of prostitutes, and this bias may incorrectly suggest greater prevalance among heterosexual men. Both perversions are found extensively among the male homosexual population, as well, and their existence, although to a lesser degree, is being reported with greater frequency in the lesbian community.

Beginning with Freud, it has been recognized that masochism and sadism are often linked. Although an individual is usually preferentially a masochist or a sadist, he or she can occasionally enact the other role. This observation suggests that the masochist/sadist identifies with the S-M transaction, not exclusively with one role. The fantasy, often enacted, may involve degradation, humiliation, suffering, or injury, even to the point of murder. Typical examples of masochism include the desire to be bound, the transvestitic impersonation as a maid, and the desire to be beaten on the buttocks; typical sadistic fantasies are reciprocal to these masochistic ones. Masochistic elaborations of other paraphilias are common; for example, the erotic preference for being straddled and urinated upon is a combination of both an excretory and masochistic perversion.

Although it is commonly believed that masochism predominates among women, in fact, the case reports vary considerably. For example, almost all of Krafft-Ebing's reported cases were male.[11] Freud paradoxically derived the concept of feminine masochism from analyzing the masochistic perversion in men.[12] The enacted perversion or enacted fantasy may well be more common in men, although it is still an open question as to whether obligatory fantasies predominate in one sex or the other.

In some individuals, the need for an escalation in sadistic behavior prevails and may result in lust murder. Far more common, however, is the clinical finding (in men) that sexuality is inhibited because

an individual is reluctant to engage either in the sadistic fantasy or enactment that is requisite to arousal. These individuals give up sexuality rather than run the risk of indulging either the fantasy or the behavior. It might be argued that these patients are not perverse because they do not engage in any sadistic behavior and suppress the fantasy when possible. Nonetheless, in terms of personality organization and preoccupation, they are related to those persons who exhibit the overt syndrome.

EXHIBITIONISM. Sexual arousal is produced by exposure of the genitals to an unknown woman or girl, usually in a public place. Exposure is usually accompanied by masturbation. It is the compulsive character of the behavior and the individual's experience of it as an irresistible impulse that defines it as pathologic. Exhibitionism is reported only in men, some of whom may be married and have regular sexual contact with their wives. Obscene phone calls accompanied by masturbation, as a sexual outlet, constitute a related perversion.

VOYEURISM. Sexual arousal is achieved by looking at strange women in situations that are construed as sexual (*e.g.,* spying on a woman who is undressing, the proverbial Peeping Tom). Voyeurism is defined as a preference for masturbating while observing nude women (who are unaware of being seen) over heterosexual intercourse. Voyeurs do not otherwise accost the women observed. Excitement may sometimes be purely psychic. Voyeurism has only been reported in males.

PEDOPHILIA. In pedophilia, the preferred route to sexual excitement is fantasied or enacted sex with prepubescent children. The activity includes exposure of genitals, self-masturbation with or without the child's awareness or participation, manual manipulation of the child, or penetration. It may involve enticement or seduction of the child into masturbating the adult. Pedophilia has been reported in both heterosexual and homosexual males, more frequently among heterosexuals.

ZOOPHILIA. Although sporadic sexual relationships with animals can be elicited by history, it is very rare that this is the preferential route of sexual discharge. Some authors distinguish zoophilia (sexual excitement experienced with stroking or fondling animals) from bestiality (a sex act between an individual and an animal).

ATYPICAL PARAPHILIAS. Many of these atypical paraphilias are associated with excretory function or excretion (*e.g.,* coprophilia or urolagnia) or behaviors viewed as derivative (*e.g.*, the compulsive use of lewd language during sexual activity).

Essential Characteristics

The following features are essential for the diagnosis of the paraphilias and common to them all.[5,13]

The deviation appears fixed. Unusual fantasies or behaviors are persistent, repetitive, and permeate mental life. They are ritualized and stereotypic.

The deviant impulse must be both imperative and insistent. Perverse behavior appears driven and is pronounced.

The deviation must be the predominant mode of sexual gratification. However, the diagnosis should not be eliminated if the individual occasionally achieves sexual gratification without use of the deviant strategy. It is commonly observed that for married individuals, acting out the paraphilia will most often occur in the extramarital sexual situation, although the perverse fantasy may fuel the marital sexual encounter. Excitement is invariably greater with the deviant enactment.

Perverse behavior usually occurs in two distinct phases. The perverse activity is usually followed by a heterosexual or homosexual encounter or by masturbation. Sexual excitement and potency appear to be "facilitated" by the preceding perverse behavior. Therefore, most perverse behavior terminates with genital orgasm. It must be emphasized that neither the perverse behavior nor the sexual act necessarily require another person. For example, transvestism and fetishism are considered perversions even when the deviant activity is solitary and the genital activity is masturbation.

The deviation may be either ego-syntonic or ego-dystonic. When the individual is under the pressure of seeking orgasmic release, it will be most often experienced as ego-syntonic. However, there may be a marked ego-dystonic reaction after the enactment of the perverse activity. There may also be long periods in which the individual makes the attempt at disavowal of the perverse symptomatology.

Suppression of the perverse behavior is difficult if not impossible. When effected, it results in anxiety, depression, or the feeling of profound emptiness.

The question arises as to whether the presence of pervasive perverse fantasies, not acted out, is adequate for the diagnosis of paraphilias. In my view it is, insofar as the fantasies are requisite to sexual performance. Thus, although the behavioral manifestations of sexuality may appear normal, the patient is aware, if not alarmed, by the obligatory and sometimes obsessive nature of his fantasy life. However, if the perverse fantasies are incidental or occasional, they can be understood as part of "normal" sexuality and not of decisive psychological significance.

Associated Features

In addition to the central characteristics common to all the paraphilias, certain observations have been made about personality integration, associated pathology, and overall adaptation. Again, it must be emphasized that, by and large, such observations have only been made on the basis of a patient population. Therefore, their validity as regards a nonpatient population is by no means certain.

In some instances, the perverse activity tends to escalate over time. This seems particularly true of transvestism and sadism.

Aside from the perverse fantasy, other sexual fantasies and nonsexual fantasies appear impoverished. Among those who seek treatment, dreaming is relatively rare.

These individuals may regard their behavior as essentially normal, although they know that their preferences are unusual. Despite their claims of normality, they most often feel humiliation, guilt, and shame as well as a fear of legal entanglement. Insofar as they wish to suppress their perverse behaviors, they suffer dysphoric affects if they are successful and a feeling of lack of control if they are not.

Paraphilias are not invariably mutually exclusive. For example, one may see combinations of transvestism and sexual masochism. The paraphilias frequently coexist with sexual dysfunctions.

Although perversion is often associated with a borderline personality organization, most contemporary theorists emphasize that there may be higher and lower levels of personality integration. Of those patients who do fall within the borderline range, some are closer to a neurotic integration, others to a psychotic one. In the higher levels of integration, the perversion serves primarily to permit sexual functioning. It is among these individuals that perverse fantasies, rather than enactment, may suffice to facilitate potency. In the lower ranges, the additional function of the perversion is to maintain ego boundaries and sense of self and to bind aggression, not merely to promote pleasurable sexual function.

The nature of the paraphilia is not indicative of the kind of personality integration. Sometimes it has been assumed that certain paraphilias must be associated intrinsically with greater ego disturbance than others. Therefore, it is sometimes stated that to the extent the object is a part-object or denigrated, the overall personality is more primitive. Yet this is not so. Each syndrome comprises individuals exhibiting a wide diversity of personality integrations.

Although the *DSM-III* calls attention to the fact that there is "often impairment in the capacity for reciprocal affectionate sexual activity,"[2] this is variable. Within the higher levels of personality organization, the individual is more often able to approach reciprocal affectionate sexual relationships and maintain meaningful nonsexual relations.

The patients are depression prone; the depression often takes the form of an ongoing empty depression. Alcoholism or drug-addiction is widely observed and may represent a maladaptive attempt at self-medication of the depression.

Perverse behavior often entails interpersonal complications that themselves become the source of depression and anxiety; for example, it often is the source of discord in a marriage or relationship and in certain perverse behaviors with nonconsenting individuals may lead to legal entanglements.

ETIOLOGY

The etiology of the paraphilias is not definitively known. Some theorists have posited a biological predisposition, although, more commonly, allusion is made to the presence of unconscious conflict. There has been little evidence substantiating the presence of biological abnormalities however; at least one report of 17 cases suggests "an unusually high frequency of genetic, hormonal, or neurological abnormalities."[14]

Even if some biological predisposition is ultimately implicated, its influence would be mediated in interaction with cognitive, affective, and experiential development. Indeed, what specific biological abnormality could be suggested to account for the pleasure a masochist takes in being bound? Even in heterosexual or homosexual object choice the argument for an exclusive biological causality is difficult to support. Kinsey and colleagues[15] argued that the biological interpretation of homosexuality cannot account for the facts that there are no replicable distinguishing data (such as hormone assays)

and that homosexuality and heterosexuality are not mutually exclusive but may coexist in all combinations. Even when the etiology of preferential heterosexual object choice is considered, the best data indicate that it is largely the result of postnatal experience.[16] This is not to say that the specificity of the experiential or psychogenic causation of heterosexuality, homosexuality, or the paraphilias is known. It may certainly be that some sexual or nonsexual vulnerability or predisposition facilitates a pattern of variant psychosexual development.

However, it is possible to reconstruct the psychodynamics in the paraphilias and to assess the role of early childhood experiences in the construction of the perverse fantasy. Psychodynamic formulations are crucial to understanding the structure and meaning of the perverse fantasy but do not, in and of themselves, establish etiology.

Freud originally postulated that neuroses and perversions were inversely related, with neuroses representing symbolic displacement from perverse fixations while perversions were direct expressions of pre-oedipal psychosexual fixations. Most psychoanalysts have revised this early formulation and now regard perversion, too, as a defensive compromise.

Early psychoanalytic formulations suggested that the perversion served primarily as a defense against castration anxiety by symbolizing an illusory female phallus. The fetish was viewed as the prototypical perversion and was literally equated with the illusory female phallus.[17] It was thought to deny the sexual distinction and thereby the fear of castration anxiety. Freud made no effort to explain why castration anxiety sometimes led to perversion, at other times to homosexuality, but most commonly was resolved with no untoward influence.

More recent formulations have addressed the problem of the predisposition to experiencing unusual degrees of castration anxiety and, consequently, have investigated factors occurring earlier in development.[13,19] Problems in the separation-individuation phase seem to form the matrix within which perverse formation becomes more likely. These include the development of a poorly defined and unstable body image and the twin fears of engulfment and abandonment by the mother, usually with some oscillation between them. As a defensive maneuver against separation anxiety, the boy invokes a compensatory identification with his mother. The sight of the maternal genital then becomes frightening because it serves to emphasize the difference between the boy and his mother. At the same time, the feminine identification leaves the child vulnerable to an exaggerated threat of castration anxiety in the oedipal period, since he already doubts his masculinity. In this formulation, the fetish would be viewed as a bridge to the mother (a symbolic representation of her) that allays separation anxiety and not simply as a representation of the female phallus.

There is general agreement that the function of the paraphilia often goes beyond the facilitation of sexual potency. It may stabilize personality, either in helping to patch over flaws in reality testing or in warding off psychoses.[20] Aggressive wishes, deriving from the traumatic experiences of the pre-oedipal period, are bound and controlled in the perverse structure. Some authors go too far in emphasizing the perverse solution as playful, imaginative, and creative. They ignore the fact that the various perversions are not original creations but are stereotypic and constricting solutions to intrapsychic problems that concomitantly limit ego development.

To date, no psychodynamic formulation fully addresses the question of why one particular perverse fantasy is selected over another. Several theories have been suggested to account for the choice of the perversion, but none has been confirmed. The perverse fantasy or act is frequently described as a scenario in which the perverse "script" symbolizes the sexualization of, and triumph over, a real or imagined trauma of childhood.[21] Thus, the perversion is believed to undo an actual trauma from an early childhood period, often using actual occurrences. Some analysts have suggested that a spectrum of early experiences are common in the histories of patients with particular paraphilias and appeared to be actually or symbolically repeated in the perverse fantasy. (For example, it has been suggested that the transvestite's mother dressed him in girls' clothes or that the sadist was beaten.) However, the question has not been settled as to whether such histories reflect "real" events, retrospective and unconscious falsification, or a childhood misperception.

DIAGNOSIS AND DIFFERENTIAL DIAGNOSIS

Accurate diagnosis depends on eliciting the paraphiliac fantasy and ritualized behavior. The achievement of sexual excitement must depend on either the mental elaboration or behavioral enactment of the deviant fantasy. However, there are certain behaviors that some experts classify as paraphilias, while others do not. One example is rape. In my opinion, rape does not generally constitute a perversion. For most rapists, rape is neither the preferred sexual activity nor his fantasy preoccupation, and these remain the hallmarks requisite to the diagnoses.

Differential diagnosis is usually relatively easy. Occasionally there will be some confusion with the gender identity disorders or psychoses. The gender identity disorders are distinguished by an impairment of core gender. Occasionally the question will arise as to whether there is simply an obsessive fantasy in an otherwise neurotic patient. In the neurotic, although perverse fantasies are elicited in the course of in-depth therapy, they do not invade conscious life to the same degree as in the paraphilias.

Homosexuality cannot be classified as a paraphilia for the following reasons. First, the central imagery is not usually bizarre. Second, the homosexual impulse, like the heterosexual one (but unlike the deviant one), may or may not be driven. Third, the homosexual behavior need not be ritualized or stereotypic in the way that the paraphilias invariably are. Fourth, fantasy life is not impoverished. Fifth, and most important, it has not been demonstrated that homosexual ideation invariably permeates mental life to an excessive degree, that the suppression of homosexual behavior yields high-level anxiety or dysphoric affect, or that it is always connected to personality dysfunction. Furthermore, many observers, including myself, do not believe that homosexuality is a single entity at all but rather that it is more accurate to speak of the homosexualities.

TREATMENT

Treatment is extremely difficult, not only because the symptom yields pleasure and is therefore hard to relinquish but also because of the commonly associated borderline problem. This group of patients is subject to many kinds of secondary crises, including depressions, which can be very successfully treated by a variety of means. However, the primary method of treating the paraphilia itself is a psychoanalytically oriented therapy or psychoanalysis. But even this kind of intensive intervention is no guarantee of success. Although there are case reports of good results, there are no long-term follow-up studies. However, few therapists would claim a high percentage of positive results in patients with full-blown perverse syndromes. The patient's overall adaptation may well improve, but permanent change in the perverse structure is more problematic. Outcome will depend on the underlying personality organization. Insofar as the major function of the perversion is to facilitate sexual excitement, not to preserve the ego, there will be a greater opportunity for a successful treatment intervention. To the degree that borderline features are more prominent, the outcome is generally less favorable.

Aversion therapy and treatment with antiandrogenic medication have been attempted both with sex offenders and with patients with paraphilias. The studies have not been systematic nor are the results encouraging. Short-term control is easier to obtain than fundamental long-term change.[14,22] The limitation to the therapy is often the patient's noncompliance in taking medication. The main limitation to antiandrogenic medication is, in fact, its mode of operation; it acts by reducing sexual desire, not by selectively inhibiting deviant impulses. Over several years, patients may be unwilling to give up sexual pleasure. (An analogous problem is seen in some manic-depressives who are unwilling to forego manic bursts of energy.)

Cross-Gender Disorders (Gender Identity Disorders)

Disturbances of gender-role identity are widespread in psychopathology. This is so for both sexual and nonsexual disorders. In contrast, disturbances of core-gender identity are very limited in number and, with one exception, occur only when biological sex is defective. The single exception is transsexualism. In transsexualism, core-gender identity is aberrant. In all the other sexual disorders, core-gender identity remains intact. Thus, for example, effeminate male homosexuals may believe their masculinity is impaired but they do not doubt their intrinsic maleness. The same can be said for exhibitionists, fetishists, and so on. Their gender-role identity may be disturbed, but their core-gender identity is normal.

DEFINITION

Transsexualism can be defined operationally as the wish in biologically normal persons for hormonal and surgical sex reassignment. The wish may be transient and fluctuating or insistent and progressive. In the latter case, the wish forms the nucleus of the transsexual syndrome; it becomes an obsessive preoccupation and can assume fanatic proportions, so that it overshadows all other aspects of the patient's life. In such instances, the patient usually does not rest until he achieves his goal of sex reassignment.

Objections can legitimately be raised to this definition. This is the only syndrome in which the patient's insistence on a particular therapeutic intervention is the pivotal finding in establishing a diagnosis. Some students of transsexualism have suggested the term *transsexualism* be replaced by *gender dysphoria*. The latter term emphasizes the patient's subjective difficulties in establishing clear, unambiguous gender identifications. *Gender dysphoric syndrome,* as proposed by Meyer,[23] is the more inclusive term, but for clinical usefulness it must be modified in terms of "the primary features of the clinical presentation." Precisely because it includes so many more patients, it does not eliminate the necessity for a category restricted to those patients who insist on sex transformation, hence the usefulness in retaining the diagnosis of transsexualism.

For the sake of clarity, since both clinical descriptions and psychodynamics differ, male and female cross-gender disorders will be discussed separately. The male gender disorders that predominate and about which more is known will be discussed first. In addition, gender identity disorders of childhood will be briefly discussed.

MALE TRANSSEXUALISM

The transsexual syndrome in males is not a unitary disorder but a final common pathway for patients who otherwise differ markedly in clinical course, developmental history, and personality structure.[4,24,25] Some classification is required to account for this variation, and different attempts have been made. If those patients who are psychotic or delusional are excluded, and these are in the minority, there are three prototypic histories. Transsexuals can be classified in accordance with these prototypes: Primary transsexuals are transsexual throughout the course of their development. They are essentially asexual and progress toward a transsexual resolution of their gender and sexual problems without a significant history of either heterosexuality or homosexuality. Secondary transsexuals derive from two subgroups: (1) cross-dressing, masculine heterosexuals, commonly known as transvestites, and (2) cross-dressing, effeminate homosexuals. These latter two groups gravitate toward transsexualism only after sustained periods of either active transvestism or homosexuality. These subgroups are designated as transvestitic transsexuals and homosexual transsexuals.

Epidemiology

Homosexual transsexuals make up the largest group. In one sample, homosexual transsexuals represented 52% of the total, with primary transsexuals and transvestitic transsexuals each 18%, while 12% were unclassified.[26] The median age of primary and homosexual transsexuals at the time of presentation was in their early 20s, and for transvestitic transsexuals it was age 40.

Clinical Description

The key clinical characteristics and the differences between the three types of transsexuals can be summarized under the following headings:

CLINICAL COURSE. In primary transsexuals, the course is progressive from childhood. The disorder is evident as a syndrome, never a symptom. In both transvestites and homosexuals, however, the transsexual impulse can be transient and fluctuating, appearing symptomatically when the transvestitic and homosexual defenses fail under stress. In the transvestite this might occur when masculinity or dependency is severely threatened, for example, under the impact of job failure or after a competitive defeat, broken marriage, or birth of a child. In the homosexual, the impulse most often arises when dependent security is threatened in the homosexual adaptation, for example, rejection by a lover or the inability to find sexual partners. Under sustained stress the transient impulse may crystallize out into the full syndrome.

CORE-GENDER IDENTITY (SENSE OF MALENESS OR FEMALENESS). It is often reported that male transsexuals have a female core-gender identity, but this only appears to be true. The presenting complaint of transsexuals, both primary and secondary, is a variant of the complaint, ''I am a female soul trapped in a male body.'' The patient inevitably claims this is a life-long conviction, but the cross-gender fantasies of childhood and adolescence do not support this claim. The early fantasies are cast in the form of a wish, not a conviction; that is, ''I would like to be a girl,'' not ''I am a girl.'' Clinically, transsexuals appear confused about gender identity and their conviction of femaleness is an attempt to resolve this confusion. It is more accurate to describe their core-gender identity as flawed

or ambiguous, rather than female. The conviction of femaleness is, therefore, an evolutionary resolution in the search for gender certainty.

In the primary transsexual, ambiguity is marked and he has undiluted gender discomfort that becomes progressively more severe as he grows older. The ''conviction'' of femaleness crystallizes out rather abruptly in late adolescence or early adulthood when the patient learns of the existence of transsexualism. Only then does he appear to resolve the ambiguity through the assumption of a transsexual identity and, ultimately, sex reassignment. For many, ambiguity continues in the female role even after sex change, as evidenced by their endless quests for feminine perfection (facial surgery, removal of the Adam's apple, voice lessons, and so on).

The secondary transsexuals, on the other hand, are more successful in alleviating gender ambiguity and the consequent discomfort. Homosexual or transvestitic defenses tip the ambiguity toward a male core gender and, as long as these defenses work, male identity remains firm.

GENDER-ROLE BEHAVIOR. The primary transsexual's overt behavior in childhood is masculine. Only in adulthood, when he begins to live as a woman, does he adopt feminine mannerisms to coincide with his new role. The transvestite's behavior is masculine in male clothes, effeminate in female clothes. The homosexual transsexual is effeminate at all times, both in childhood and adulthood, although, of course, he is more so when cross-dressed.

CROSS-DRESSING. In the primary transsexual, cross-dressing is nonfetishistic and is used solely to relieve gender discomfort, that is, to make the patient feel more comfortable and less anxious. The clothing is conservative, and there is little interest in display. The patient wishes mainly to blend into the society inconspicuously as a woman.

In transvestism, cross-dressing, as already discussed, is fetishistic. In the effeminate homosexual, cross-dressing begins in childhood, usually well before puberty. It is occasionally reported to cause relaxation, but more typically the clothes are used to dramatize fantasies, never fetishistically. The theatrical potential of impersonation is realized early and cross-gender fantasies are frequently tied to movie actresses.

SEXUALITY, OBJECT-CHOICE, AND SEXUAL IDENTITY. The primary transsexual before sex reassignment is relatively asexual. To whatever extent he participates in sexual activity, either overtly or in fantasy, he prefers male objects. In such encounters, he views himself as female and therefore identifies himself as psychologically female and heterosexual. The transvestite prefers females and identifies himself as heterosexual. It is among the postoperative transvestitic transsexuals that one sees the famous "lesbian" syndrome, in which husband and wife may remain together as two women. The homosexual prefers males and identifies himself as homosexual.

EROTIC PLEASURE IN THE PENIS AND ATTITUDES TOWARD CASTRATION.

Erotic pleasure is almost nonexistent in the primary transsexual, but it is intense in both transvestites and homosexuals. The primary transsexual is never comfortable with his maleness. He loathes his penis and is eager to part with it. The transvestite and the homosexual have severe castration anxiety and under ordinary circumstances have no wish to part with their penises. Indeed, their symptoms allay castration anxiety and hence preserve both their erotic pleasure and their sense of maleness. They develop transsexual impulses only under stress when they regressively consider sacrificing their penises to the overriding need of dependent security.

THE WISH FOR CASTRATION.

The loathing of the insignia of one's masculinity is crucial to the development of transsexualism; the willingness, or rather eagerness, to part with the penis is the *sine qua non* of transsexualism. Not only is the transsexual impulse progressive, but the actual loathing of the male insignia is, itself, a progressive phenomenon. In part this is because the male insignia tend to block the credibility of womanhood. In part, willingness to part with the penis may be facilitated by a defectively schematized mental representation of the male genitalia. Although the transsexual may know he has a penis (hence the claim he is not delusional or psychotic), he attaches no symbolic meaning to it; in other words, the penis does not signify.

The actual mutilation that occurs from the conversion operation appears to have reference to an ambiguously conceptualized genital that is detached from the self-image. Transsexual patients anticipate surgery calmly (a true *la belle indifférence*). They may focus on the results of surgery, that is, on the good facsimile to female genitalia that they hope for. In general, they have no anxiety about mutilation, castration, or possible death, at least manifestly. The same patient, unconcerned about conversion surgery, may have appropriate anxiety for a relatively benign operative procedure. The near complete split between self-image and ambiguously conceptualized genitalia is reflected in the surprisingly benign psychological reactions after surgery. Contrary to expectation, in view of the theoretic emphasis usually placed on castration anxiety, psychotic and depressive reactions to castration and/or penectomy are relatively rare.

UNDERLYING DIAGNOSIS.

Transsexualism *per se* is not a psychotic disorder, although the desire for sex change is seen in some delusional states. Diagnostically, transsexuals, both primary and secondary, as well as transvestites and cross-dressing effeminate homosexuals, most often fall within the borderline range of psychopathology.

Etiology

The etiology of transsexualism, while much disputed, remains unknown (for a review of competing theories, see the work of Meyer[27]). Some investigators propose a genetic or fetal hormonal etiology despite the absence of any known laboratory tests that show transsexuals as a group to be different chromosomally, hormonally, or morphologically from a randomly sampled group. Although early life experiences have been postulated in the etiology of the phenomenon, there are very few detailed psychological studies in the literature.

As regards family constellations, familial or matrigenic theories of etiology are less than compelling. There are several predominant trends in family dynamics, but not one, by itself, accounts for any of these disorders. The three types of transsexuals may all develop in a variety of family settings.

Money and Gaskin,[28] attempting to integrate the concept of predisposition with that of early experience suggest that "The most likely etiological explanation in the majority of cases of transsexualism, on the basis of today's knowledge, is that transsexualism is an extremely tenacious and critical-period effect in the gender-identity differentiation of a child with a particular, but as yet unspecifiable, vulnerability." However, they raise the critical objection to this formulation, that is, that some transsexuals say their symptoms first appeared under stress in adolescence and some even in adulthood.

Stoller has described an extremely small group of male transsexuals that he claims are characterized by "a very rare coincidence of a number of factors, each of which is essential." These are a bisexual depressed mother who keeps her especially beautiful infant son too close to her body too long, creating a blissful, unending symbiosis that endures for several years and a psychologically absent father who does not interrupt this excessive symbiosis. This results in imprinting of femininity "upon the malleable infant's unresisting protopsyche and unfinished CNS," resulting in a female core-gender identity. Stoller regards this process as conflict free.

Stoller's formulation has not achieved widespread acceptance. First, most psychiatrists have not found transsexualism to be nonconflictual. Second, some theorists have raised doubts that such excessive symbiosis could be anything but conflictual. Third, the whole concept of imprinting as the theoretic underpinning for the acquisition of femininity has been challenged. Fourth, Stoller's explanation, even if it were to be verified for a minuscule number of patients, does not address the source of the transsexual wish in the vast majority of patients who seek sex conversion.

Essentially the etiology is unknown. The following formulation is psychodynamic, *not* etiologic, for reasons that will become clear. It has the advantage that it can account for the transsexual wish in the wide range of patients among whom it appears. It is based on the key observation that core gender in transsexuals is ambiguous, *not* female. To acknowledge core gender as ambiguous and fluctuant at once mediates against the theory of imprinting in transsexualism. Imprinting by definition implies a fixed, unchanging "femininity." It is the presence of an ambiguous core gender that suggests a conflictual, psychological development.

The suggestion that transsexual development is conflictual is reinforced by several different sets of clinical observations. First, it is important to note that the transsexual syndrome is not an isolated pathology. Patients suffering from cross-gender disorders fall within the borderline range of pathology, as characterized by identity diffusion and an empty depression. Second, by history, one elicits a report of many symptomatic behaviors suggestive of pervasive anxieties in childhood, for example, pronounced thumbsucking, enuresis, night terrors, behavior disorders, eating disorders, and prolonged attachment to transitional objects. Third, the request for surgery is frequently precipitated by a clear-cut psychological crisis in the transsexual's life. This is particularly striking in the case of secondary transsexuals.

Transsexualism is best thought of as a developmental disorder originating as a defense against unresolved separation anxiety or fears of annihila-

tion. Frequently the source of separation anxiety is clear-cut. In many patients, separation anxiety is triggered by actual separation. This is most usually accompanied by cumulative trauma in the mother–infant/toddler dyad that would itself engender massive infantile anxiety.

In order to counter the separation anxiety, the child invokes various mechanisms of defense in order to maintain the tie to his mother. First, he attempts to avoid separation anxiety by reestablishing symbiosis; if unsuccessful in assuaging the anxiety in reality, he may resort to a refusion of the mental representation of self and mother. In his unconscious mind he literally becomes the mother, and core gender is tilted toward femaleness in correspondence with this fantasy. This merger fantasy, magically reparative in its intent, appears to be the psychodynamic basis for transsexualism. The transsexual phenomenon can be understood clinically as an attempt to actualize psychic fusion by achieving physical femaleness. This formulation can account not only for those patients who have a lifelong "transsexual" history but also for those in whom the impulse occurs later in life and for those in whom it is fluctuant. Finally, in support of the hypothesis that the fusion fantasy is the central reparative maneuver, one observes the almost invariable memory attached to the first experience of cross-dressing in mother's clothes: "I felt very warm, very comfortable. I had company; I felt wanted." The mother's clothes appear to be a symbolic representation of the pregenital mother. Wearing them, the boy is imaginatively brought once more into an intimately developing relationship with her.

This formulation ought not to be construed as proposing a matrigenic etiology. Deficient mothering is certainly not the only agent responsible for separation anxiety, which may arise from actual trauma or individual predisposition. The focus here is on the role of separation anxiety, which seems to be a necessary, but not sufficient, antecedent in the genesis of transsexualism.

Separation anxiety and fusion fantasies are hardly specific to transsexualism. They occur intermittently as normal phenomena during the separation-individuation phase of infantile development, and they are widespread findings in many psychiatric disorders, particularly in the borderline ranges of psychopathology. To explain transsexualism etiologically, one would have to explain why in transsexuals, as distinct from these other patients, separation anxiety and fusion fantasies lead to ambiguous core gender and the wish for sex reassignment. Maternal devaluation of masculinity and disturbances in maternal gender identity are sometimes proposed as contributing factors.

Diagnosis and Differential Diagnosis

Even in cases of boyhood femininity, the diagnosis of transsexualism cannot be made. It may ultimately result in transsexualism but more frequently it precedes homosexuality or may disappear without consequence. Consequently, one cannot make an accurate diagnosis of transsexualism prior to adolescence and sometimes adulthood. Furthermore, in many instances of transsexualism, there are no manifest disturbances in gender behavior in childhood.

Because secondary transsexuals are diagnostically first either transvestites or cross-dressing effeminate homosexuals, the differential diagnosis is essentially a differentiation between primary transsexuals, on the one hand, and transvestites and cross-dressing effeminate homosexuals, on the other.

Treatment

Because some psychiatrists view transsexualism as an encapsulated psychosis, sex conversion is deemed, by them, equivalent to entering the patient's delusional world or, at best, similar to "stabilizing" an addict by administering narcotics. Others take the position that hormonal and surgical sex reassignment is warranted because there is no efficacious mode of psychological intervention in the adult transsexual. This argument, in turn, is countered by the charge that there have been no adequate trials of psychotherapy.

The major limitation of psychotherapy is the unwillingness of the patient to participate. This unwillingness, whatever its motivation, is intensified by the ready availability of sex reassignment. The problem of treatment is compounded by the propensity of some of these patients to attempt suicide or self-mutilation of the genitalia when sex conversion is denied.

At the same time, sex conversion is hazardous. It is both radical and irreversible. Most important, even the proponents of surgical treatment acknowledge it is essentially palliative and the underlying psychopathology remains unchanged.[29] Furthermore, it has gained acceptance as an appropriate mode of treatment despite the lack of rigorous long-term studies. The problem that has impeded the assessment of outcome is the notori-

ous tendency of these patients to disappear before follow-up.

Two studies have shed light on the benefits and limitations of surgical intervention.[29,30] What they demonstrate is that the patient appraises the results better than objective measures might indicate. However, some objective improvement is cited in both studies. The discrepancy between subjective (patient) and objective (physician) ratings tends to intensify the disputes about the appropriateness and efficacy of sex conversion. What is reflected in the dispute is not just an argument about outcome, but one about more fundamental values. Those who place a high premium on the alleviation of anxiety *per se* and who are sympathetic to the demand for medical self-determination (and bodily self-determination) will be more likely to support transsexual surgery.

Because of the nature of the psychopathology, there is a risk of suicide with or without treatment, whether it is psychotherapy, sex conversion, or both. Despite the limitation of both types of treatment one is forced to formulate a treatment plan for the individual patient. Every patient, at minimum, should receive an extensive psychiatric evaluation and a trial of psychotherapy. If this fails to stabilize the patient, sex conversion cannot be ruled out, but neither should it be recommended unless the patient meets certain rigid criteria. I favor those criteria suggested by Hunt and Hampson.[29] Conversion therapy can only be recommended with the full knowledge that the treatment is still experimental, may ultimately fall into disrepute, and deals at best with the superficial adjustment of the patient, not with the underlying pathology. In selected cases, it is the treatment of last resort, not a panacea.

The classification of transsexuals is crucial to formulating a treatment plan. The primary transsexual should theoretically make the best candidate for sex reassignment. He is transsexual from the beginning. He dislikes his penis and gets little or no erotic pleasure from it. In his case, surgery would be ego-syntonic and have the best chance for success. Those with a history of a protracted homosexual or transvestitic adjustment ought to be referred for conversion therapy with extreme caution, if ever. They are primarily transvestites and homosexuals and develop transsexualism only under stress. They value their penises and enjoy sex. Instead of being transformed into bonafide transsexuals, these patients could end up simply as castrated transvestites and homosexuals. The goal with these patients should be to relieve stress and foster a return to the original homosexual or transvestitic adaptation.

FEMALE TRANSSEXUALISM

Like male transsexualism, female transsexualism is either primary or secondary. However, the secondary transsexualism is always homosexual since among women, there are no transvestites. The vast majority of female transsexuals are homosexual transsexuals. The primary transsexual, like the male, is relatively asexual but, unlike the male, shows life-long cross-gender behavioral characteristics. Usually, female transsexuals report extreme masculine development beginning very early in life but, in some instances, identity may be subjectively perceived as masculine, while objective behavior is unremarkably feminine.

Clinical Course

Extreme masculine characteristics are usually present from early childhood. Typically, the girl expresses a daily wish to be a boy, prefers to play only with boys, has remarkably few relationships with girls, and only wishes to wear boys' clothes or unisex clothing. There may be a transitional period during which the girl will sometimes wear female clothing but it is frequently noted that, if something bothers her, she will take off the female clothing and begin to act and dress like a boy again. This "flipping" has also been reported in histories of male transsexuals and is also observed in the cross-gender disorders of childhood. Frequently these girls prefer to be called by a boy's name, and some girls stuff toilet paper in their underpants in order to mimic a penis. The girls express wishes to grow up to be boys, to urinate standing, and to have their hair cut as a boy. However, there is no confusion as to the biologic fact of their femaleness.

In the majority of the cases, sexuality, as it emerges in adolescence, is homosexual, although it may be regarded by the patient as "heterosexual" insofar as the female transsexual claims to be a male trapped in a female body. It is in the minority of cases, the female equivalent of the primary transsexual, that the sexual urge seems relatively absent.

Male impersonation can begin in adolescence. As soon as the patient takes male hormones, the public impersonation is more successful than that of the average male transsexual dressing as female. This is almost ensured by beard growth, since casual observers hardly ever suspect that the posses-sor of a beard or mustache is not male. In the female, impersonation is better when clothed, but obviously lacking when unclothed. Exactly the opposite is true of most male transsexuals. Typically the transsexual female avoids contact to her vagina during sexual encounters; masturbation is clitoral. In interpersonal sexuality, there is frequently a shared fantasy with her female partner that her clitoris is a small penis.

There are variants to the predominant clinical course just described. In one variant, feminine behavior is manifested behaviorally and appears unremarkable until some trauma. The abrupt appearance of masculine behavior may occur after adolescence or even in adulthood. In some of these cases, the female transsexual has engaged in heterosexual activity with males and, in some few instances, has been married and given birth to children before the overt homosexual and transsexual adaptations. These patients claim that they always felt inwardly estranged despite the fact of the gender "appropriate" behavior that was manifest for many years.

Etiology

There are no reports in the literature of a biological predisposition, and the cause is not known. The transsexual resolution seems to be related dynamically to the dynamics of certain extreme cases of masculine female homosexuality or what is commonly called "butch" homosexuality. However the etiology of female homosexuality is itself not fully understood. These patients very often take a protective attitude toward their mothers. Although the patient has eschewed an identification with females and made an apparent identification with the father, the affectionate bond to the mother is not lost. Even when the patient was mistreated at the hands of the mother, she still perceives the mother as good and loving, although weak and passive. Frequently, the mothers are viewed as exploited by men. In a series of female transsexuals I have seen there is a high incidence of physical and emotional trauma in the early years, much as one sees in the lives of the male homosexual. However, one sees some female transsexuals whose personality organization appears integrated at a much higher level than one is apt to see with male transsexuals.

Treatment

Since most cases can be regarded as secondary homosexual transsexualism, the conservative goal is to stabilize the patient in a homosexual adaptation.

If the patient demands hormonal and surgical conversion, the physician must insist on the same kind of rigorous preparation already recommended with regard to male transsexuals.

GENDER IDENTITY DISORDERS OF CHILDHOOD

In recent years there has been an increasing interest in children who display cross-gender behavior, fantasies, and preferences. This interest finds expression in the first-time listing of the "Gender Identity Disorders of Childhood" as a diagnostic category in the *DSM-III*.

Definition

The diagnosis is made when boys exhibit extreme feminine behaviors, interests, and identifications expressed in the wish to be girls or when girls exhibit extreme masculine behaviors, interests, and identifications expressed in the wish to be boys.

For boys, the *DSM-III* criteria necessary to make the diagnosis are as follow:

A. Strongly and persistently stated desire to be a girl, or insistence that he is a girl
B. Either 1 or 2 below
   1. Persistent repudiation of male anatomical structures as manifested by at least one of the following assertions:
      a. That he will grow up to become a woman (not merely in role)
      b. That his penis or testes are disgusting or will disappear
      c. That it would be better not to have a penis or testes
   2. Preoccupation with female stereotypical activities as manifested by a preference for either cross-dressing or simulating female attire, or a compelling desire to participate in the game and pastimes of girls
C. Onset of disturbance before puberty.

For girls the criteria are essentially parallel, only in reverse.

This section will deal predominantly with boyhood femininity, not with girlhood masculinity, because the former almost always has ramifications for future development, whereas "tomboyism" frequently disappears in adolescence without sequelae. Moreover, there are many more studies in the literature pertaining to boyhood femininity.

Epidemiology

There is no adequate base rate for the incidence of boyhood femininity. One study estimates its incidence as approximately 1 in 200,000.[31]

Green, who has conducted the most extensive demographic study of feminine boys to date (60 boys), found that boyhood femininity was unrelated to ethnic background, to religion, to the educational level of either parent, to the age of parents at the time of referral, or to the age of the parents at the time they gave birth to their son. It was also unrelated to the number of children in the family, to the birth order of the son, or to the age difference between the next oldest or youngest sibling.[32,33]

Clinical Description

Boys commonly express the wish to be a girl or wish to grow up to be a girl; have an intense interest in cross-dressing in female clothes; have an intense interest in female stereotypical activity such as playing with dolls, playing house, or play-acting the role of mother; display a preference for female peers over male ones; display female mannerisms; and avoid rough-and-tumble play.[32–38] Both clinical observations and parental interviews confirm the boys' interest in scarves, high-heeled shoes, dresses, jewelry, and cosmetics; their preferences for dolls and games such as playing house and jumping rope; their interests in the mother's makeup and clothes; and the large amount of time spent play-acting and impersonating females. Some boys express direct dislike of their male anatomy, stating they dislike their penises or find them disgusting. Some boys urinate sitting down, pretending to be girls. They do not, however, believe themselves anatomically to be female.

In Green's 1974 study,[32] all 50 boys displayed a compelling interest in dressing in women's clothes by the age of 6. In the Roosevelt Gender Project Study,[10] 16 of 20 boys showed an intense interest in their mothers' clothes before the age of 2. In addition to observable behavior, femininity appears in the psychological testing of these children. The boys avoid other boys and, if they are not loners, prefer the company of females. In addition, clinicians and researchers who have worked with these boys report severe disruption in peer relations. They are taunted by their peers, are ridiculed, are rejected, and become scapegoats.

The Roosevelt Hospital Gender Identity Project has recorded concomitant psychopathology in the form of severe separation anxiety, manifested by shadowing their mothers and inability to leave their mother to go into the treatment sessions; 75%

meet the criterion for *DSM-III* separation-anxiety disorders. Of that group, 60% were also school avoidant. Further evidence of psychopathology was manifested by social withdrawal, depression, and aggression. However, there was no indication either of gross impairment of reality testing or psychotic functioning.

As already noted, masculine or tomboyish girls have not been as well studied as feminine boys. In part, this is simply because tomboyishness or masculinity does not have the same predictive value for psychopathology later in life. Masculine girls eschew skirts and feminine clothing, prefer boy's clothing, prefer boys as playmates, prefer body-contact sports, and show a marked interest in trucks and guns. Some state that they would prefer to be males.

Clinical Course

It should not be assumed that the adult outcome of this childhood entity, whether treated or not, can be predicted. Researchers have sometimes erroneously assumed that the gender identity disorders of childhood are continuous with transsexualism. However, the few long-term follow-ups of effeminate boys indicate that they may grow up to be heterosexual, although the predominant outcome appears to be either bisexual or homosexual. Only a very small number will evolve into transsexuals or transvestites. From the studies in the literature,[39–41] it seems clear that boyhood femininity is related to a high incidence of homosexual object choice and/or atypical gender behavior in later life. However, one is unable to predict the outcome in any given patient.

Masculinity in girls, while more common than femininity among boys, appears to have less consequence for adult development. However, one elicits retrospective histories of tomboyism and masculinity in girlhood among adult female homosexuals and transsexuals. Thus, it appears in certain instances that girlhood masculinity is continuous with homosexual or atypical gender behavior in adulthood. However, the correlation is not of the same magnitude as the correlation between boyhood femininity and male homosexuality.

Etiology

There are essentially three major theories of etiology: (1) biological, (2) reinforcement (social-conditioning), and (3) conflictual. Although these differ in focus, they are by no means incompatible or mutually exclusive.

Some girls who present tomboyish behavior may have a history of exposure to androgenlike hormones, for example, those girls with the androgenital syndromes described by Ehrhardt and Baker.[42] Typically these girls show more interest in rough-and-tumble play and are less interested in playing with dolls than age-mated normals. Such studies point to the probable neuroendocrine background of certain gender behaviors. However, these girls have not been diagnosed as having a childhood identity disorder.

Green[32] is the major proponent of the reinforcement theory. He views social reinforcement as the major factor in boyhood femininity and cites the critical variable as "no discouragement . . . by the child's principal caretaker."

The conflictual theory implicates some disturbance in the family milieu and concomitant evidence of psychological impairment in the effeminate boys. Preliminary findings from the Roosevelt Hospital Gender Identity Project indicate that there are significant disturbances in the family milieu. A large number of the mothers were themselves depressed during the first years of the child's life and suffered from a number of dramatically traumatic events. Green[33] reported that 22% of his sample had been hospitalized in the early years of life. In the Roosevelt Hospital study 20% of the children and 48% of the mothers had been hospitalized. In Green's sample, 34% of the boys had been separated from their fathers by divorce, abandonment, and death. In the Roosevelt Hospital study there were absent fathers and also fathers who described themselves as remote, violent, or sometimes alternately remote and violent. Maternal overprotectiveness of the boy, particularly from the physical environment, may coincide with emotional insensitivity. Many of the mothers also used harsh and authoritarian forms of disciplines and some were full of rage. Some mothers encouraged their sons to become the mother's helper.

The development of boyhood femininity appears to require the convergence of multiple forces. It almost always develops in a family matrix of severe psychological disruption, although why early abandonment, separation, and trauma are associated with the development of boyhood femininity is unclear. Social reinforcement and parental gender confusion may both prove to be contributing factors. Although biological abnormalities have not been found in effeminate boys, the possibility that some biological compliance not yet identifiable may contribute to the child's behavioral characteristics cannot be ruled out. One does not yet know the necessary or sufficient biological and/or experiential factors or the different clusters of factors that are necessary to produce boyhood femininity.

However, it does seem clear that boyhood femininity does not present as a symptom in isolation. It almost always coexists with a separation anxiety disorder and other behavioral disturbances.[10]

Differential Diagnosis

All the criteria suggested in the *DSM-III* are crucial to make this diagnosis. It is important not to make the diagnosis indiscriminantly when a child expresses an occasional cross-gender interest or displays an occasional cross-gender behavior. There is a great deal of normal variability among boys and girls.

Treatment

In view of the fact that boyhood femininity is seldom an isolated phenomena and nearly always has ramifications in terms of adult development, treatment intervention is recommended. Psychotherapy, using psychoanalytically oriented intervention is the treatment of choice. This should be conducted in conjunction with treatment of other family members. All the therapists involved should consult jointly in order to coordinate the therapy plan.

REFERENCES

1. Freud S: Three essays on the theory of sexuality. In Strachey J (ed): The Standard Edition of the Complete Works of Sigmund Freud, vol 7. London, Hogarth Press, 1905

2. Diagnostic and Statistical Manual of Mental Disorders (DSM-III). Washington, DC, American Psychiatric Association, 1980

3. Person ES: Sexuality as the mainstay of identity: Psychoanalytic perspectives. In Stimpson CR, Person ES (eds): Women: Sex and Sexuality. Chicago, University of Chicago Press, 1980

4. Ovesey L, Person E: Gender identity and sexual psychopathology in men: A psychodynamic analysis of homosexuality, transsexualism and transvestism. J Am Acad Psychoanal 1:53–72, 1973

5. Diagnostic and Statistical Manual of Mental Disorders (DSM-I). Washington, DC, American Psychiatric Association, 1952

6. Diagnostic and Statistical Manual of Mental Disorders (DSM-II). Washington, DC, American Psychiatric Association, 1968

7. Nagel T: Sexual perversion. J Philosophy 66(1):5–17, 1969. Reprinted in Brake M (ed): Human Sexual Relations: Towards a Redefinition of Sexual Politics. New York, Pantheon Books, 1982

8. Ovesey L, Person E: Transvestism: A disorder of the sense of self. Int J Psychoanal Psychother 5:219–236, 1976

9. Person E, Ovesey L: Transvestism: New perspectives. J Am Acad Psychoanal 6:301–323, 1978

10. Coates S, Person E: Boyhood femininity: Behavioral correlates and family matrix. Unpublished manuscript, 1983

11. Krafft-Ebing R: Psychopathia Sexualis, Translated from the 12 German Edition by Klaf SS. New York, Stein & Day, 1965

12. Freud S: The economic problem of masochism. In Strachey J (ed): The Standard Edition of the Complete Works of Sigmund Freud, vol 19. London, Hogarth Press, 1961

13. Ostow M: Sexual Deviation: Psychoanalytic Insights. New York, Quadrangle, 1974

14. Berlin FS, Meinecke CF: Treatment of sex offenders with antiandrogenic medication: Conceptualization, review of treatment modalities, and preliminary findings. Am J Psychiatry 138:601–607, 1981

15. Kinsey A, Pomeroy W, Martin CE: Sexual Behavior in the Human Male. Philadelphia, WB Saunders, 1948

16. Baker SW: Biological influences on human sex and gender. In Stimpson CR, Person ES (eds): Women: Sex and Sexuality, pp 175–191. Chicago, University of Chicago Press, 1980

17. Bak R: Fetishism. J Am Psychoanal Assoc 1:285–298, 1953

18. Bak R: The phallic woman: The ubiquitous fantasy in perversions. Psychoanal Study Child 23:15–36, 1968

19. Greenacre P: Perversions: General considerations concerning their genetic and dynamic background. In Emotional Growth, vol 1, pp 300–314. New York, International Universities Press, 1968

20. Glover E: The relation of perversion formation to the development of reality sense. Int J Psychoanal 14:486–504, 1953

21. Stoller RJ: Perversion: The Erotic Form of Hatred. New York, Pantheon Books, 1975

22. Abel GG, Levis DJ, Clancy J: Aversion therapy applied to taped sequence of deviant behavior in exhibitionism and other sexual deviations: A preliminary report. J Behav Ther Exp Psychiatry 1:59–66, 1970

23. Meyer JK: Clinical variants among applicants for sex reassignment. Arch Gen Psychiatry 3:527–528, 1974

24. Person E, Ovesey L: The transsexual syndrome in males: I. Primary transsexualism. Am J Psychother 28:4–20, 1974

25. Person E, Ovesey L: The transsexual syndrome in males: II. Secondary transsexualism. Am J Psychother 28:174–193, 1974

26. Sulcov M: Transsexualism: Its solid reality, unpublished doctoral thesis. Indiana University, 1973

27. Meyer JK: The theory of gender identity disorders. J Am Psychoanal Assoc 30:381–418, 1982

28. Money J, Gaskin RJ: Sex reassignment. Int J Psychiatry 9:249–282, 1970

29. Hunt DD, Hampson JL: Follow-up of 17 biologic male transsexuals after sex-reassignment surgery. Am J Psychiatry 137:432–438, 1980

30. Meyer JK, Reter DJ: Sex reassignment. Arch Gen Psychiatry 36:1010–1018, 1979

31. Rekers GA, Rosen AC, Lovaas OI et al: Sex-role stereotypy and professional intervention for childhood gender disturbance. Professional Psychol 9:127–136, 1978

32. Green R: Sexual Identity Conflict in Children and Adults. New York, Basic Books, 1974

33. Green R: One hundred ten feminine and masculine boys: Behavioral contrasts and demographic similarities. Arch Sex Behav 5:425–446, 1976

34. Bates JE, Bentler PM, Thompson SK: Measurement of devi-

ant gender development in boys. Child Dev 44:591–598, 1973

35. Bates JE, Skilbeck WM, Smith DVR et al: Gender role abnormalities in boys: An analysis of clinical ratings. J Abnorm Child Psychol 2:1–16, 1974

36. Bentler PM, Rekers GA, Rosen AC: Congruence of childhood sex-role identity and behavior disturbances. Child Care Health Dev 5:267–283, 1979

37. Zucker KG: Childhood gender disturbance: Diagnostic issues. J Am Acad Child Psychiatry 21:274–280, 1982

38. Zucker KJ, Doering RW, Bradley S et al: Sex-typed play in gender-disturbed children: A comparison to sibling and psychiatric controls. Arch Sex Behav 2:309–321, 1982

39. Money J, Russo AJ: Homosexual outcome of discordant gender identity/role in childhood: Longitudinal follow-up. J Pediatr Psychol 4:29–41, 1979

40. Green R: Childhood cross-gender behavior and subsequent sexual preference. Am J Psychiatry 36:106–108, 1979

41. Zuger B: Effeminate behavior in boys from childhood: Ten additional years of follow-up. Compr Psychiatry 19:363–369, 1978

42. Ehrhardt A, Baker SW: Fetal androgens, human central nervous systems differentiation, and behavior sex differences. In Friedman RC, Richart RM, Vande Wiele RL (eds): Sex Differences in Behavior, pp 33–51. New York, John Wiley & Sons, 1974

SUGGESTED READING

Bak R: Aggression and perversion. In Lorand S, Balint M (eds): Perversions: Psychodynamics. New York, Random House, 1956

Benjamin H: The Transsexual Phenomenon. New York, Julian Press, 1966

Coen SJ: Sexualization as a predominant mode of defense. J Am Psychoanal Assoc 29:893–920, 1981

Gillespie W: Notes on the analysis of sexual perversion. Int J Psychoanal 33:397–402, 1952

Gillespie W: The general theory of sexual perversion. Int J Psychoanal 37:396–403, 1956

Goy RW: Role of androgens and the establishment and regulation of behavioral sex differences in mammals. J Animal Sci 25:21–35, 1966

Green R, Money J (eds): Transsexualism and Sex Reassignment. Baltimore, Johns Hopkins University Press, 1969

Khan MMR: The function of intimacy and acting out in perversions. In Slovenko R (ed): Sexual Behavior and the Law, pp 397–412. Springfield, IL, Charles C Thomas, 1965

MacDougall J: Plea for a Measure of Abnormality. New York, International Universities Press, 1980

Person E: Some new observations on the origins of femininity. In Strouse J (ed): Women and Analysis: Dialogues on Psychoanalytic Views of Femininity, pp 250–261. New York, Grossman, 1974

Person E, Ovesy L: The psychodynamics of male transsexualism. In Friedman RC, Richart R, Vande Wiele R (eds): Sex Differences in Behavior, pp 315–325. New York, John Wiley & Sons, 1974

Person E, Ovesy L: Psychoanalytic theories of gender identity. J Am Acad Psychoanal 11:2, 1983

Person E, Ovesy L: Homosexual Cross-Dressers. J Am Acad Psychoanal 12:167–186, 1984

Rekers GA, Crandall BF, Rosen AC et al: Genetic and physical studies of male children with psychological gender disturbances. Psychol Med 9:373–375, 1979

Stoller RJ: Sex and Gender. New York, Science House, 1968

Stoller RJ: Facts and fancies: An examination of Freud's concept of bisexuality. In Strouse J (ed): Women and Analysis: Dialogues on Psychoanalytic Views of Femininity, pp 343–364. New York, Grossman, 1973

Stoller RJ: Parental influences on the earliest development of masculinity in baby boys. Psychoanal Forum 5:232–262, 1975

Stoller RJ: Sex and Gender, vol 2, The Transsexual Experiment. New York, Jason Aronson, 1975

Stoller RJ: Primary femininity. J Am Psychoanal Assoc 24:59–78, 1976

Stoller RJ: Sexual excitement: Dynamics of Erotic Life. New York, Pantheon, 1979

36
Helen S. Kaplan

Psychosexual Dysfunctions

The last 15 years have witnessed profound changes in our views of sexual disorders and also significant improvement in assessment and treatment methods. This chapter is an overview of current concepts of the psychosexual dysfunctions and of the clinical techniques employed in the management of these syndromes.

Definition

In the past the human sexual response was seen as a single psychophysiologic entity and all psychosexual disorders were subsumed under the labels frigidity or impotence. One of the significant advances of the last decade was the recognition that the sexual response cycle of men and women consists of three neurophysiologically separate phases—desire, excitement, and orgasm, and that there are actually at least seven different psychosexual syndromes. These are produced when a single phase is impaired, while the other aspects of the sexual response cycle are spared. It is clinically significant that each psychosexual disorder has a distinctive set of causes and responds to different therapeutic interventions and also carries its own prognosis.

The classification system used in *Diagnostic and Statistical Manual of Mental Disorders,* 3rd ed (*DSM-III*) (American Psychiatric Association, 1980) is based on this tri-phasic concept and describes the essential feature of the *psychosexual dysfunctions* as "an inhibition of the appetitive or psy-chophysiological phases that characterize the sexual response cycle."[1] Impairment of the orgasm phase produces inhibited female orgasm, retarded ejaculation and premature ejaculation, whereas inhibited female excitement and impotence result from impairment of the female and male excitement phases. *Inhibited sexual desire* (ISD) denotes the clinical syndrome associated with impaired sexual desire in both genders. Psychosexual disorders associated with painful spasms of the genital muscles as well as sexual phobias and avoidances can also be considered as belonging in the general category of the psychosexual dysfunctions. Although these syndromes are not associated with a specific phase like the disorders mentioned above, they too are the product of sexual anxieties and respond to similar treatment strategies.

Epidemiology

Although no accurate data on the incidence of sexual disorders in the general population are available as of this writing, Masters and Johnson estimate that 50% of all Americans suffer from a sexual problem some time during their life.[2] Clinical experience suggests that mild forms of these disorders, which are likely to respond to brief therapeutic interventions, are far more prevalent than the sexual symptoms that are associated with more severe psychopathologic processes which require more complex and lengthy treatment methods.

Clinical Descriptions*

ORGASM PHASE DISORDERS: INHIBITED FEMALE ORGASM, RETARDED EJACULATION, PREMATURE EJACULATION

Inhibited Female Orgasm

DSM-III describes the following diagnostic criteria for impaired female orgasm (302.73) when it is due to psychological inhibition: "Recurrent and persistent inhibition of the female orgasm as manifested by a delay in or absence of orgasm following a normal sexual excitement phase during the sexual activity that is judged by the clinician to be adequate in focus, intensity, and duration" (p 279).[1]

Patients in this diagnostic category are not "frigid" in any sense of that outdated term. They may be loving, care about men, be interested in sex, and have the capacity for erotic pleasure. During loveplay, they may feel aroused and may lubricate. In other words, the desire and excitement phases of the sexual response are intact and their chief complaint is only that orgasm is delayed or absent.

The female orgasm threshold is distributed along a continuum.[4] At one extreme are those rare women who can have an orgasm without any physical contact with the clitoral area, merely by engaging in erotic fantasies, kissing, or stimulation of the breasts. Then there are the approximately 20% to 30% who are able to achieve orgasm through coitus alone without direct clitoral stimulation. Next on the continuum are women who can climax together with their partner but only if coitus is assisted by clitoral stimulation. Women who fall into the next segment of the distribution cannot reach orgasm in the presence of a partner, even if they receive clitoral stimulation. They can, however, stimulate themselves to orgasm when they are alone and employing erotic fantasies. At the pathologic extreme of the orgasm threshold continuum are the totally anorgastic women who have never had an orgasm at all. These constitute approximately 8% of the United States female population.[5]

The demarcation between normalcy and pathology is controversial. There is little disagreement that the last two response patterns are clearly path-

* The descriptions of the clinical features of the psychosexual dysfunctions are quoted in part from Kaplan HS: The Evaluation of Sexual Disorders: Psychological and Medical Aspects. New York, Brunner/Mazel, 1983.

ologic and that treatment should be recommended for such patients. But lesser degrees of inhibition are not easily classified as to their normalcy and the appropriate of these is a matter of dispute. Some psychoanalytically oriented clinicians feel that all women who cannot reach a climax on penetration unless assisted by additional clitoral stimulation are abnormal and in need of treatment, even if they are orgastic with a partner. However, it is the consensus of current professional opinion that such a response pattern constitutes a normal variation of the female sexual response.[1]

It has been my experience that some coitally anorgastic women can acquire an orgastic response to penetration and a couple should be given the opportunity for treatment if they request this. However, most often it makes more sense to counsel the couple to accept and enjoy clitoral erotism as a normal sexual response pattern.

The reaction of women and their partners to orgasm dysfunction varies widely. In contrast to males, who are always distressed when sexual excitement does not lead to ejaculation, some women are perfectly content about not having orgasms and do not seem to suffer from tension or discomfort after sexual stimulation. In some cases this constitutes denial, but there really are women who simply find sex gratifying even if they do not experience a climax, and this is not necessarily a sign of pathologic passivity. It is my feeling that the person's point of view should be respected and that such women should not be pressured into treatment by husbands or by well meaning therapists. However, other anorgasmic women are desperate about their situation, sometimes to the point of obsession. They complain of tension, physical pelvic discomfort, and anger at their partner when the sex act always ends with a climax for him but never for her.

Some men are more concerned about their wife's orgasm than she is. Others are unaware or uncaring. But partner reaction is always an important diagnostic issue because, even though he may not have caused the patient's problem, his negative or pressuring response may create an obstacle to her cure, while his cooperation and support are invaluable for the success of sex therapy.

RETARDED EJACULATION OR INHIBITED MALE ORGASM

DSM-III describes the following criteria for inhibited male orgasm (302.74): "Recurrent and persistent inhibition of the male orgasm as manifested by a delay in or absence of ejaculation following an adequate phase of sexual excitement" (p. 280).[1] This syndrome is analogous to inhibited female orgasm and the severity of the inhibition also ranges from very mild situational delays of ejaculation to total anorgasmia.

Patients who suffer from the most severe forms of retarded ejaculation (RE) complain that they have never experienced ejaculation in their lives. Some are even able to inhibit themselves when they sense an impending nocturnal emission during sleep. Fortunately, this severe form is rare. Milder situational forms of RE are more common. Some of these men can ejaculate only on masturbation when they are alone and immersed in erotic fantasy. Those with still milder inhibitions can reach orgasm by self-manipulation in the presence of a partner or by manual and oral stimulation. They are unable, however, to reach orgasm inside the vagina. The mildest forms of retarded ejaculation are characterized by excessively long periods of intravaginal thrusting. Some men with a tendency towards ejaculatory inhibition experience a delay of orgasm only when they sense that their partner is not responsive or welcoming.

Desire and excitement are usually not impaired in this syndrome. Retarded ejaculators may have high sex drive and usually have no difficulties with erection. In these respects they are like anorgastic females. Only their orgasm is blocked or difficult to achieve.

Patients with RE describe their problem in terms similar to those used by women with inhibited orgasm, although males are more likely to be distressed by this problem. Some males with this syndrome simulate orgasm and the wife may be completely unaware of her spouse's problem. When she knows, however, she is usually distressed and may feel rejected by her partner's inability to ejaculate in her vagina. The partner's response is always important in the dynamics and treatment of sexual dysfunction and should be carefully investigated during the evaluation. In rare instances a patient experiences retardation of his ejaculation only on masturbation or oral sex but is able to ejaculate intravaginally. This pattern of inhibition presents a clinical problem only in the absence of a partner or when illness in the patient or his partner precludes intromission and requires that the patient ejaculate in response to oral or manual stimulation.

Partially Retarded Ejaculation

In this rare clinical variation of retarded ejaculation the emission phase of the ejaculatory reflex is normal but the pleasurable ejaculatory phase is inhibited.[4] This is analogous to female "missed" orgasm, which is characterized by muscular contractions without pleasure.

Patients with this syndrome have normal erections. They say that after a period of stimulation and arousal, they feel a sense of "release" but they experience no real orgastic pleasure and no contractions and do not feel gratified after sex. Ejaculation in this patient population is characterized by a quiet "seepage" and not a pulsating "squirting" of semen from the penis. One of my patients has described this experience as "peeing" in contrast to a true orgasm. Another clinical characteristic of diagnostic impotence is that the penis remains firm and erect for a fairly long time (5 to 10 minutes) after the seepage of emission in contrast to the more rapid resolution of the excitement phase when ejaculation is normal.

This syndrome is fascinating because selective inhibition separates the emission from the ejaculatory phase of the male orgasm. From a psychodynamic vantage it is interesting that the nonpleasurable reproductive aspect is not disturbed but erotic pleasure and gratification are lost. The examiner should be alert to general pleasure inhibitions when evaluating these patients.

Premature Ejaculation (Inadequate Ejaculatory Control)

DSM-III describes the following criteria for premature ejaculation (PE)(302.75): "Ejaculation occurs before the individual wishes it, because of recurrent and persistent absence of reasonable voluntary control of ejaculation and orgasm during sexual activity. The judgment of 'reasonable control' is made by the clinician's taking into account factors that affect duration of the excitement phase, such as age, novelty of the sexual partner, and frequency and duration of coitus" (p 280).[1]

The presenting complaint of the premature ejaculator is typical. He says that he loves sex, he is attracted to his partner, he has no problem obtaining an erection (in fact, premature ejaculators often have a strong sex drive). But as soon as he reaches a certain point of excitement, he ejaculates reflexively and rapidly.

Usually PE occurs with all partners because the man simply has not learned voluntary control over his ejaculatory reflexes. Sometimes control problems are situational and the symptom is more severe with a specific partner or a specific type of partner. Often control is better on masturbation, but the patient has not realized this. The examiner can test the patient's capacity for insight by asking him for his explanation of why he climaxes more rapidly when he is with a partner.

Premature ejaculators and their partners have diverse reactions to this problem. Some are unconcerned and are able to develop mutually enjoyable lovemaking patterns despite lacking control. The man may bring his partner to orgasm before intromission or after he has ejaculated. Very young men may compensate by making love several times. Such men experience distress only when the aging process begins to impair the ability to experience multiple orgasms. On the other end of the spectrum of reactions one sees very distressed couples. The wife may feel rejected and desperately unhappy because she (erroneously) concludes that her husband is hostile to her and wishes to deprive her of pleasure. Or the partner of a premature ejaculator may become obsessed with the desire for coital orgasm which she fears will elude her forever because of her husband's rapid ejaculation. Such wives feel deprived and rejected, misinterpreting the rapid ejaculation as a sign of the husband's indifference, while he feels guilty and pressured, which does little to improve the situation.

In our society many males are very much invested in the duration of their excitement phase and feel like sexual failures because they cannot exert voluntary control. They are often obsessed about their rapid climax. They may develop a secondary pattern of sexual avoidance.

EXCITEMENT PHASE DISORDERS: IMPOTENCE AND IMPAIRED FEMALE EXCITEMENT

Sexual excitement in both males and females is caused by reflex vasodilation and congestion of the genital organs. This influx of blood changes them from the quiescent state and prepares them for their reproductive functioning. The excitement phase in males is marked by penile erection and in females by vaginal lubrication and swelling.

Impotence (Impaired Male Excitement, Inhibited Sexual Excitement in the Male)

DSM-III describes the following diagnostic criteria for psychogenic impotence or inhibited sexual excitement of the male (302.72): "Recurrent and per-

sistent inhibition of sexual excitement during sexual activity manifested by . . . partial or complete failure to attain or maintain erection until completion of the sexual act" (p 279).[1]

Impotent men retain their interest in sex and often can ejaculate with a flaccid penis. It is only the erectile aspect of the sexual response system that is impaired. However, some of these men develop a secondary avoidance of sex so that it may look as though they are completely asexual. There are few other symptoms that are as threatening to the male.

Careful and meticulous questioning is often necessary to elicit the precise and detailed information about the specific circumstances under which the erectile difficulty appears that is needed to differentiate between organic and psychogenic impotence and also to formulate treatment strategies for psychologically impotent men. Some patients have morning erections, or can masturbate without difficulty when they are alone, but are impotent with a partner. Some complain they cannot attain an erection. Others lose it when they take their clothes off, when they are about to penetrate, when they are inside the vagina, when there is a demand for performance, when they are with certain types of women, or when they are in an intimate or committed situation. Still others complain that their erections are not completely firm. The partners reports are frequently helpful in clarifying these important diagnostic issues.

Women vary greatly in their reaction to their partner's impotence. Some are marvelously supportive and convey to the man the message that he—not his erect penis—is important to her. Such loving attitudes rule out partner pressure as an etiologic factor and are invaluable assets for sex therapy. At the other extreme are partners who are sexually demanding and critical and carry on when their man does not perform to their satisfaction. Some women insist on penetration as their only means of gratification. Some create additional problems by objecting to their partner's attempts to help himself with erotica, or oral and manual genital stimulation. The pressure created for a man when he knows that his partner expects him to attain an erection rapidly and maintain it until she is satisfied heightens his performance anxiety and is likely to create or aggravate his potency problem. It should be noted, however, that the notion that the aggressive "new liberated woman" is causing an increase in impotence has no basis in reality. In fact, most partners of impotent men, if anything, are excessively passive sexually.[4]

Impaired Female Excitement (Frigidity, Inhibited Sexual Excitement in Females)

DSM-III describes the following criteria for psychogenically impaired or inhibited sexual excitement in females (302.72): "A recurrent and persistent inhibition of sexual excitement during sexual activity, manifested by . . . partial or complete failure to attain or maintain the lubrication-swelling response of sexual excitement until completion of the sexual act. (p 279).[1]

Women who meet the criteria for this syndrome feel the desire for sex and like lovemaking. Frequently, they can have orgasms, especially when stimulated intensely with a vibrator. However, they remain dry when they are stimulated in a manner that would be adequate for most women. Penetration without normal lubrication and swelling can result in painful and uncomfortable intercourse. This may result in secondary problems such as dyspareunia, vaginismus, and loss of sexual desire. Partners of such patients often feel rejected and upset by what they take to be a personal sexual rejection or evidence that they are poor lovers. Others are oblivious.

DESIRE PHASE DISORDERS: INHIBITED SEXUAL DESIRE OF MALES AND FEMALES

DSM-III describes the following diagnostic criteria for deficient sexual desire when this is psychogenic: "Persistent and pervasive inhibition of sexual desire. The judgment of inhibition is made by the clinician's taking into account factors that affect sexual desire such as age, sex, health, intensity and frequency of sexual desire, and the context of the individual's life" (p 278).[1] In other words, low sexual desire with an unsuitable person or in the absence of an attractive erotic situation is not to be regarded as a sexual disorder. It makes sense to use the term *impaired sexual desire* to designate a deficient sex drive before the differentiation between psychogenic inhibition and organic deficit has been made.

When the sex drive is inhibited because of psychological causes, desire tends to be blocked for a specific partner or situation only, while interest in others, in masturbation, in fantasy, *etc.* is retained. When a person lacks sexual interest for a clearly destructive or inappropriate partner, one can hardly speak of a dysfunction. However, patients with this syndrome feel no sexual interest even when the partner is consciously perceived as desirable and beloved and may be puzzled by their lack of arousal.

Psychological inhibition can also occur in a global form so that the patient loses his erotic interest entirely. This variety of ISD is clinically indistinguishable from low libido caused by certain drugs, such as beta adrenegic blocking agents, or disease states such as those associated with testosterone deficiency. Patients with a global libido deficit say that they do not desire sex with their partner and that they have also lost their sexual appetite for all the situations which had evoked arousal in the past.

Patients with a low sex drive can often force themselves to function physically, but do with little pleasure or gratification. Often they must use intensive fantasies to overcome the sexual avoidance. Sometimes the inhibited patient continues to enjoy the nongenital aspects of sexuality—kissing, cuddling, caressing—although these activities do not result in erotic arousal. Others develop an aversion to all physical contact. Some manage to "get through" the sex act, but feel compelled to leave the partner immediately afterwards and cleanse themselves. In more severe cases any contemplation of sex is abhorrent and such patients may develop elaborate and ingenious avoidance rituals. They get a headache, get busy, get depressed, or get lost. They bring work home from the office, avoid intimacy, start arguments at bedtime, *etc.*

Sexual avoidance that is secondary to loss of desire, must be differentiated from sexual avoidance that is associated with sexual phobia and avoidance, and also from the low frequency which occurs because a partner is deliberately withholding sex from the other.

Some persons are not disturbed about their asexuality and would not seek treatment were it not for their partner's insistence. Others are deeply distressed and fear that their lowered sex drive signals the end of potency and the approach of old age.

Partners also react in diverse ways. Some, with sexual problems of their own, may be relieved by cessation of sexual demands. But others feel threatened and abandoned. When the ISD patient's partner has unresolved problems from infancy and childhood that involve fears of parental abandonment and sibling or oedipal rivalry, he or she may be unable to deal with the sexual rejection in a rational manner. When such partners obsessively pressure the inhibited patient for sex, sexual avoidance becomes intensified.

SEXUAL PAIN AND DISORDERS ASSOCIATED WITH GENITAL MUSCLE SPASM: DYSPAREUNIA, VAGINISMUS, AND EJACULATORY PAIN

The classification of this group of sexual disorders can be confusing. *DSM-III* places vaginismus and functional dyspareunia into two separate diagnostic categories. But from a clinical, as well as theoretical, point of view vaginismus belongs with a group of sexual symptoms that are caused by involuntary spasm of genital muscles, which can be painful, while other kinds of sexual pain are produced by different psychic mechanisms.

In the following discussion, *dyspareunia* includes all types of sexual pain with the exception of syndromes that are caused by painful spasms of the genital muscles. These are described under vaginismus and ejaculatory pain due to genital muscle spasm.

Dyspareunia

DSM-III restricts functional dyspareunia (302.76) to pain on coitus and gives the following criteria: "recurrent and persistent genital pain, in either the male or the female" (p 280).[1] Actually, it makes more sense to use the term to designate pain associated with orgasm and sexual excitement, as well as with intercourse, because the causes and treatment of all of these are similar.

Sex should not hurt and when it does something is wrong. Chronic sexual pain often has a deleterious effect on a couple's sex life and may affect the entire relationship adversely.

Vaginismus (306.51)

According to *DSM-III*, vaginismus is defined as follows: "There is a history of recurrent and persistent involuntary spasm of the musculature of the outer third of the vagina that interferes with coitus" (p 280).[1]

Ordinarily, when a woman is sexually aroused, the vaginal muscles relax and the introitus opens. But in vaginismic women the muscles snap together so tightly that penetration may be impossible. The husband will tell you, "I just can't get in, there is a block, an obstruction." When the vaginal muscle spasm is somewhat less severe, entry may be forcibly attained but the experience is painful for the woman. The patient has no voluntary control over her response, and on a conscious level vaginismic patients are often extremely distressed by their inability to have intercourse and children.

It is interesting to note that while some patients with this disorder also have other sexual problems, many have normal sexual desire, lubricate, and are orgasmic. In fact, some vaginismic women are capable of having multiple orgasms. It is only penetration that is difficult, painful, or impossible.

In most cases, the vaginal muscles go into spasm in response to any attempt at vaginal penetration, so that the patient cannot use tampons and has great difficulty in undergoing a pelvic examination. Sometimes anesthesia is required for this purpose. A few patients have a specific vaginismus that only occurs during coital attempts and not at other attempts at vaginal penetrations. These patients can be examined without difficulty and this situational pattern rules out organic obstruction.

Ejaculatory Pain due to Muscle Spasm of the Male Genitals

This rather rare syndrome is analogous to vaginismus in the sense that it is caused by a painful and involuntary spasm of the muscles of the reproductive and sexual organs. In the male the cremasteric muscles or the smooth muscles of the internal male reproductive organs or the perineal muscles react with painful spasm as the man ejaculates or immediately thereafter. Patients typically experience a sharp cramplike pain immediately on ejaculation. This may be mild but can be excruciating and disabling. The pain is experienced in the perineum and in the shaft of the penis. It may be transient or last for hours and even days. The urologic and physical examination is normal between episodes and there may be no physical signs while the patient is in pain. Sometimes, however, the scrotum and perineum is red, swollen, tender, and tense during an attack.

Patients tend to be extremely distressed by this symptom and develop a fear of and an avoidance of orgasm, which creates an intense conflict when they feel sexual tension. Some patients always experience the pain whenever they ejaculate, that is, with masturbation as well as with a partner. In other cases the symptom is situational and is experienced only when they are ambivalent about ejaculating.

SEXUAL PHOBIA AND AVOIDANCE

The avoidance of sex because of irrational fears and panic is not strictly speaking a sexual dysfunction. This topic has been included in this context because many patients and couples with sexual complaints are actually suffering from a phobic avoidance of sex, and also this condition is often amenable to sex therapy methods with or without the addition of antipanic drugs.

Actually, there is a phobic element in almost all sexual complaints. This must be detected and treated before the actual dysfunction can be addressed. Thus, for example, it would be impossible to treat a vaginismic patient with gradual vaginal dilatation if she phobically avoids all genital contact. However, in true sexual phobia and avoidance the patient is able to function physically when not panicked and the avoidance of sex is the central therapeutic issue.

Applying the *DSM-III* criteria for *phobia* to sex yields the following definition: The essential feature of a sexual phobia is the persistent and irrational fear of and compelling desire to avoid sexual feelings and/or experiences. The fear is recognized by the individual as excessive and unreasonable.

Sexually phobic patients may avoid all aspects of sexuality or they may be phobic of specific situations only, such as, for example, intercourse, sexual failure, fantasy, orgasm, pregnancy, nudity, the genitals, *etc.* Fear and avoidance of sex is highly distracting in itself and may also seriously impair the person's psychosexual development, the capacity for romantic relationships, marriage with family, and may be extremely damaging to self-esteem. The life of patients who avoid sex may become progressively restricted as a result of their avoidance. Some patients with sexual phobias remain virgins all of their lives, many do not marry, and some become socially isolated. Other phobic patients manage to marry despite their phobias, but their lives are never easy. It is important to gain an understanding of the emotional damage that has resulted from a patient's phobic avoidance of sex, and this usually requires specific therapeutic intervention apart from the sexual phobia.

A typical phobic experience is as follows: "By the afternoon I already start to worry. It is hard for me to keep my attention on my work because I know that when I get home she will expect me to have intercourse with her. Sometimes I'll stop at a bar before I get home. I'll make any excuse. I'll bring a briefcase full of work home. I'll busy myself on the phone. I'll fix the sink, the window, anything else. I'll knock myself out with another drink, anything to avoid that pressure." When a patient is trapped in a situation where sex can no longer be avoided because of the risk of losing a valued partner or feeling guilty about hurting a beloved one, the experience is extremely unpleasant, so the patients report that they feel panic or revulsion and sometimes rage during sex. A common experience is "trying to get it over with as quickly as possible."

Some partners of phobic patients are amazingly supportive; others are furious and threatened and try to manipulate and pressure the phobic patient for sex. The partner's reaction is a significant variable in planning therapy and in estimating the prognosis because the cooperation of a gentle, nonthreatening partner is extremely helpful in treatment.

Sexual phobias should be differentiated from other kinds of problems that result in sexual avoidance. Some patients with ISD avoid sex because it gives them no pleasure. Others with anxiety about their sexual performance are afraid to face this humiliation, frustration, and failure. Still other patients avoid intercourse because it is physically painful or uncomfortable, while some deliberately withhold sex to punish their partner.

Of special importance is the differentiation between patients who have a generally normal anxiety level and whose sexual phobia is specifically related to an unconscious sexual conflict, and those patients who have a generalized panic disorder that puts them at high risk of developing multiple phobias. Patients in the former category, with "simple" sexual phobias, can be treated successfully with psychosexual therapy alone, whereas all patients with panic disorder require the addition of antipanic medication.[6]

Etiology and Evaluation

Identical sexual symptoms can stem from either organic or a wide range of psychological causes. Because of the multidetermined nature of these disorders evaluation is perhaps the single most important function of the clinician who deals with sexual complaints. A successful treatment outcome depends on accurate and clinically relevant assessment of the causes of the patient's sexual problem. Incorrect or inadequate diagnosis leads to inappropriate treatment, and many treatment failures can be traced to faulty evaluation procedures.

DIFFERENTIATING BETWEEN ORGANIC AND PSYCHOLOGICAL CAUSES

Before anything else, the evaluation of each patient with a sexual complaint requires that sexual symptoms caused by biological stressors—depression, certain drugs, endocrine disorders and other disease states, be ruled out. Traditional medical evaluation procedures were not originally designed to assess sexual problems and many subtle drug and disease related disorders are still not likely to be detected by routine medical examinations.[7,8] New diagnostic methods have recently become available which have greatly improved the accuracy of the differential diagnosis between the subtler organic and psychogenic sexual symptoms. Among the most useful of these are the nocturnal penile tumescence (NPT) monitor which provides a record of reflexive sleep erections, penile blood flow studies using the doppler effect to measure small vessel circulatory changes which can impair the erectile mechanism, cavernosograms to detect occult uteriovenous leakages, which also cause this difficulty, and sophisticated endocrine measures for detecting early pituitary and gonadal abnormalities, which may have no other signs and symptoms apart from sexual deficiency. The clinician who undertakes the care of sexually dysfunctional patient's should familiarize himself with the sexual symptoms that are associated with disease states and the diagnostic techniques used to rule these out, as well as with the sexual side-effects of many commonly prescribed medications in order to ensure that patients with subtle medical problems are not erroneously treated with psychotherapy.

ANALYSIS OF THE PSYCHOLOGICAL CAUSES

By the same token, the standard psychiatric examination was developed before sexual disorders were fully understood and by itself this procedure does not provide sufficient data for the proper management of sexual disorders. Special assessment methods are needed for this patient population.

The two main objectives of the psychological aspect of the evaluation of patients or couples with sexual complaints are to analyze the psychological causes that have produced the sexual symptom in detail and in depth, and also to select the appropriate treatment modality.

The therapeutic requirements of patients with psychosexual disorders vary widely and it is important to choose the correct treatment modality from a wide therapeutic armamentarium that includes psychoanalysis, psychotherapy, couple therapy, behavior therapy, medication, sex therapy, and sexual rehabilitation for patients with partial organic deficits. This requires, first, that patients with

serious or treatable psychopathology be identified. Included in this category are patients whose sexual complaints are secondary to major psychiatric disorders including depression, panic states, schizophrenia, and the severe borderline and narcissistic personality disorders. Patients with such pathologic conditions are not suitable candidates for brief sex therapy and require psychiatric management of their primary psychiatric illness first. For these reasons, a brief mental status examination and psychiatric history should be conducted for all symptomatic patients and their partners as well as an integral part of the evaluation.

The treatment of sexual disorders is highly individualized to fit the specific dynamic requirements which vary with each case. The basically healthy patient whose erectile difficulty is primarily due to performance anxiety requires a different treatment approach that the immature, neurotic man who makes a "mother" out of his current sexual partner, while still another tactic is needed to help the couple who are having difficulty because the wife is excerting pressure on her husband with her excessive and unreasonable sexual demands.

Because so many different dynamics can produce sexual symptoms, a detailed and in depth analysis of the intrapsychic and dyadic causes is necessary to formulate an effective treatment plan and should precede commencement of treatment in each case.

The psychodynamic aspect of the evaluation can be organized around behavior analysis, psychodynamic analysis, and analysis of the couple's interactions.

Behavioral Analysis

What is the immediate antecedent or cause of the sexual symptom? In other words, it is important to assess precisely what defenses against sexuality are currently operating. Is the patient excessively anxious about his sexual performance? Does he flood himself with negative images when she approaches him? Does she obsessively observe and judge his sexual response? A detailed examination of the patient's current sexual experience, his "sexual status," which includes his physical responses as well as the mental and emotional state during love making yield this information. A detailed analysis of the contingencies of the patient's current sexual experience is essential for planning the behavioral aspect of sex therapy.

Psychodynamic Analysis

Sometimes the sexual symptom is solely the product of the kind of "minor" consciously perceived anxieties mentioned above.[2] In other cases deeper intrapsychic sexual conflict or more serious problems in the couple's relationship which may be beyond the patient's conscious awareness are associated with the sexual symptom. A brief family and psychosexual history of both partners is necessary to obtain this information. It is important to investigate the deeper dynamics of a patient's or a couple's sexual complaint in order to understand the problem from a historic perspective. Unconscious sexual conflicts and neurotic processes may mobilize anxieties and resistances to the behavioral aspects of the treatment process, and therefore the extent and the focus of the psychotherapeutic aspects of psychosexual therapy depend on the nature of the dynamic infrastructure of the sexual problem.

Analysis of the Couple's Interactions

Finally, the couple's relationship must be assessed from the vantage of their current experience with each other and also in depth. Is the sexual problem specific to this couple or would the symptomatic patient experience difficulty with any partner no matter how loving and attractive? What specific point of difficulty are operative between these two individuals? Is their problem simply a matter of poor communication in an otherwise compatible and loving relationship, or are deeper issues involved? Neurotic interactions that are commonly seen in this patient population include mutual parental transferences and serious power struggles. The dyadic aspect of the treatment is designed to resolve those problems in the couple's relationship that impair their sexual gratification and functioning. Sex therapy is not likely to succeed unless critical aspects of a couple's sexual and emotional interactions can be improved within the therapeutic context.

Treatment

All the treatment methods mentioned in the previous section have a place in the management of psychosexual disorders. It is the current consensus of professional opinion that sexual problems that are associated with severe psychopathology should be treated with long-term reconstructive psychotherapy. Included in this category are patients with severe borderline and narcissistic personality disorders and those with profound and deepseated neurotic conflicts about sexuality. In the same vein, many sexual complaints are secondary to serious relationship problems which require resolution of the destructive dynamics of the couple's system. Such couples cannot be expected to improve with any sort of short-term intervention. But psychosexual difficulties frequently arise from relatively mild and moderate sexual anxieties, culturally engendered antisexual attitudes, and also from minor struggles in otherwise sound relationships. Many authorities believe that the brief sex therapies are the treatment of choice for such patients, both from the standpoint of effectiveness and the relative rapidity and economy of treatment.

Lief has estimated that in 30% to 40% of cases symptomatic improvement will occur without major psychodynamic changes. He divides the remaining 60% as follows: 10% need long-term individual therapy, 20% need marital therapy, setting aside sex therapy until much later, and 30% need a combination of sex and marital therapy.[9] Our own experience is similar to his, with the addition that approximately 25% of our patients receive psychoactive medication for depression or panic disorder concomitantly with sex therapy.

CURRENT CONCEPTS OF SEX THERAPY

Two features distinguish sex therapy from other forms of psychotherapy. The first is that the objective of treatment is the relief of the sexual symptoms apart from any other emotional problems that the patient or couple may have, except as these constitute an obstacle to improve sexual functioning. Second, modern sex therapy uses a combination of behavioral and psychotherapeutic interventions. The behavioral task consists of a series of structured erotic interactions that are conducted by the patient or the couple in the privacy of their home. These are integrated with psychotherapeutic sessions with the therapist in his office, either with the individual patient or conjointly with the couple.

Masters and Johnson's original protocol called for a two-week intensive treatment program that was conducted by a dual sex therapy team and only couples ("marital units") were accepted for treatment. Currently clinicians tend to apply the principles of sex therapy in a more flexible manner. Single patients as well as couples are treated, solo therapists of either gender are common, sessions may be conducted on a weekly basis, and treatment varies from one session to more than 20.

When the patient's anxieties are relatively mild

and the couple enjoy a cooperative and caring relationship, sexual symptoms can often be relieved without any basic changes in the symptomatic patient's psychic structure or in the couples marriage. However, even though the focus of sex therapy is on relief of the sexual symptom, couples frequently gain greater intimacy and emotional gratification as a result of the treatment process.

INTEGRATED TREATMENT

The basic treatment strategy of the new sex therapies is to attempt to modify the immediate defense against sexual functioning by means of behavioral interventions and to handle resistances to the treatment process with various psychotherapeutic techniques. Common immediate or currently operating causes found in sexually dysfunctional patients include such consciously perceived defenses as anxiety about sexual failure, obsessive self-judgements, "spectatoring," an emphasis on performance to the detriment of pleasure, the tendency to "turn oneself off" by focusing on negative thoughts or "antifantasies."[10] At the same time, the therapist must be prepared to deal with unconscious intrapsychic neurotic processes, and deeper dyadic problems which are frequently associated with sexual disorders and which may be expected to generate resistances to the rapid improvement of long standing sexual disabilities. Unless these deeper conflicts can be resolved to the point where the patient accepts himself as a functional sexual person, treatment is not likely to be successful.

It may be speculated that the integration of behavioral and psychodynamic methods is the key to the success of the new sex therapies and also to their advantage over both insight and behavioral methods alone. Insight therapy both in the form of individual and conjoint psychodynamically oriented treatment direct their efforts at resolving deeper and unconscious sexual conflicts, but neglect the crucial details of the patient's currently operating defenses against sexual adequacy and the destructive contingencies that operate in the "here and now" that cause and maintain the patient's symptoms.

On the other hand, the strictly behavioral approaches that are excellent in recognizing and modifying the immediate causes and antecedents of sexual symptoms generally do not deal adequately with the deeper unconscious conflicts and neurotic processes which are often crucial in these cases. Many treatment failures of the strictly behavioral approaches can be attributed to the neglect of deeper emotional issues.

An analysis of the various techniques that have reported successes in the treatment of psychosexual dysfunctions has led to the speculation that in order to cure a sexual symptom, it is necessary to modify its immediate psychological cause or antecedent.[10] This seems to be the necessary condition of cure. If the immediate psychological antecedent is not modified, the symptom may very well persist even if the patient gains insight into the remote or deeper sexual anxieties and conflicts that are ultimately responsible for the genesis of the disorder. This construct is useful in providing the conceptual structure for planning treatment and also explains those puzzling cases where insight therapy is successful in providing the patient with a deeper understanding of himself and improving the quality of his life while at the same time his sexual symptom persists. Such patients frequently improve rapidly when they are specifically treated for their anorgasmia, prematurity, or impotence. On the other hand, sexual functioning can be expected to improve if the immediate currently operating cause can be modified. Moreover, symptom relief is relatively independent of whether the patient or the couple actually suffer from an underlying sexual or relationship conflict. As long as the currently operating cause that has given rise to the sexual symptoms can be rectified, it does not seem to matter whether such deep and intrapsychic or dyadic conflicts do in fact exist or whether these are "bypassed" in the course of sexual therapy. Thus, it is not unusual to find that while the anxious neurotic woman who had been anorgastic or the inmature impotent man with the demanding wife becomes sexually functional as a result of sex therapy, they are at the end of treatment just as neurotic or inmature or miserable with their marriages as they had been before. It should be noted, however, that while brief sex therapy obviously can not be expected to cure long-standing neuroses or incompatible marriages, many patients do, in fact, receive benefits that extend beyond the relief of their symptom of sexual inadequacy. The "ripple effect" of successful sex therapy can include increased self-esteem, the gain of insights and coping strategies for other problems, and improvement in the nonsexual aspects of the couples relationship.

THE BEHAVIORAL ASPECT OF SEX THERAPY

The structured erotic and intimate tasks that are assigned to the patient or couple and other behavioral techniques such as training in communication skills and sexual assertiveness are designed to modify the specific and immediate currently operating causes of the sexual symptoms. It has been found that these immediate causes are highly specific for each different dysfunction. This has led to the development of highly specific and different behavioral protocols for each disorder.[4,10] Thus, the homework assigned to anorgasmic women is different from the sequence of erotic tasks described for couples who suffer from inhibited sexual desire, while the patient with inadequate ejaculatory control and his partner receive yet another set of behavioral instructions. It is beyond the scope of this chapter to describe the specific and immediate defenses that are associated with each of the different psychosexual disorders or the specific behavioral program that has been developed for each disorder. This information is widely available for the clinician interested in acquiring expertise in treating psychosexual disorders.[2–4,10] It should be emphasized in this context that the behavioral interventions are not likely to be effective except in the simplest cases if they are applied in a "cookbook" fashion. The best results are achieved and the therapeutic process is most gratifying when the behavioral interventions are applied in a flexible and creative manner that fits the individual dynamic requirements of each case.

THE PSYCHOTHERAPEUTIC ASPECT OF SEX THERAPY

This emphasis on the behavioral aspect of treatment should not be taken to mean that insight and the resolution of unconscious conflicts have no place in the modern treatment of psychosexual dysfunctions. To the contrary, the skillful resolution of unconscious intrapsychic conflicts that give rise to existence of sexual inadequacy and the improvement of the destructive dynamics in the relationship is the true art of sex therapy, and for most cases the key to successful treatment. When the sexual symptom is the result of very mild performance anxieties and lack of communication, the rapid improvement of sexual dysfunctions often occurs in response to behavioral interventions alone without significant psychotherapeutic intervention. Thus, it is by no means unusual to see a patient gain relief of his prematurity or impotence without any appreciable insight into the underlying sexual conflict. But in the majority of cases the sexual symptom is related to unconscious conflictual processes and the rapid improvement of sexual gratification evokes anxieties in a symptomatic patient, and even more so in the partner. The intrapsychic equilibrium of the patient and the equilib-

rium of the previously stable dyadic system is disturbed both by the outcome and the process of sex therapy. Therefore, astute psychotherapeutic intervention in the intrapsychic conflict and in the couple's problematic system is of the utmost importance to the success of these techniques.

The therapeutic sessions are used to instruct, clarify and encourage the couple in their quest for sexual adequacy and improvement of their relationship. But, except in the simplest cases, the therapist's task extends well beyond these "coaching" functions. The couple often needs to be confronted with their anxieties about and resistances to sexual gratification and success in their love relationship. Some of the active techniques used in other forms of brief treatment are very useful in sex therapy. Thus, for example, the tactic of "joining the resistance" is often helpful to heighten a patient's awareness of his sabotage of his own sexual pleasure and of his destructive behavior toward a valued relationship. Sometimes creating a crisis can effectively move a stalled treatment forward.[4] Such active confrontations and maneuvers need to be balanced with sensitive and genuine support of each partner's sexuality and capacity for pleasure and intimacy. A couple's positive feeling for each other and the importance of their commitment to their relationship often needs reinforcement and encouragement.

Sometimes mere confrontation is not sufficient to foster therapeutic progress and clarification and interpretation of unconscious sexual conflict is required. Common underlying psychological obstacles to sexual adequacy of a deeper, more complex nature which are common in this patient population include neurotic conflicts about sexuality and love that originate in early family problems, culturally engendered guilt about sexual pleasure and mutual parental transferences between the couple that taint their current sexual experience with incestuous overtones. Such issues frequently arise within the context of psychosexual therapy and the therapist may use dreams, memories, role playing, and other insight-producing techniques in order to resolve these.

In our experience interpretations and confrontations regarding the unconscious acting out of "loser roles" assigned to the patient by his family, unconscious success and competition conflicts with their self-destructive sequellae, and regressive infantile attitudes towards the partner are useful issues that can be dealt with in the context of brief sex therapy. Interpretation of this kind of material is usually ego syntonic and does not tend to mobilize undue resistances. However, attempts to deal with more primitive and threatening oedipal and pre-oedipal material, even when this is relevant to a particular case, is generally inappropriate and ineffective within the context of brief treatment.

Treatment Outcome and Prognosis

The results of the two most impressive outcome studies in this field indicate that brief sex therapy is considerably more effective than the long-term psychodynamically oriented psychotherapies in treating sexual dysfunctions. In 1972, O'Connor and Stern reported a cure rate of 25% for female and 57% for male patients treated for functional sexual disorders with psychoanalysis and long-term psychotherapy at the Columbia Psychoanalytic Institute in New York City. The study reported the results of 96 patients who were treated 2 to 4 times a week for at least 2 years. No follow-up studies were reported.[11] In contrast, Masters and Johnson reported an overall success rate that exceeded 80% in response to their two-week intensive sex therapy program. In all, 733 cases were treated over an 11 year period at the Masters and Johnson Institute in St. Louis.[2] The relapse rate after 5 years was only 5.1%.

Despite recent criticism regarding some inadequacies in Masters and Johnson's outcome criteria, these results have never been effectively challenged, and the vast clinical experience that has been accumulated in the past decade tends to confirm the efficacy of the brief sex therapies.

However, two variables must be considered in interpreting these as well as other outcome studies in this area—the specific diagnosis and the severity of the associated psychopathology. For one, the different psychosexual syndromes vary significantly in their response to treatment and it makes little sense to lump them together for the purpose of predicting outcome. In our experience, the orgasm phase dysfunctions, especially PE and inhibited female orgasm, and the psychosexual disorders associated with painful genital muscle spasm, vaginismus, and male functional ejaculatory pain have an excellent prognosis with brief sex therapy, with successes that fall in the 80% to 90% range.[2] In our experience with these syndromes this high cure rate is relatively independent of other psychological variables. Next are the excitement phase disorders, more specifically impotency, which has a more variable success rate. We have found that the prognosis for erectile dysfunction is more dependent on the severity of associated intrapsychic and

marital problems. Psychogenic impairment of the desire phase is, in our experience, the most difficult problem to treat with sex therapy and has the least favorable outcome, with results being comparable to those reported by the Columbia Psychoanalytic Institute for all the sexual dysfunctions.[11] Finally, the prognosis for patients with sexual phobias seems to depend on whether or not antipanic medication is included in the treatment regimen. It may be speculated that the results of treatment are similar to those with phobias not related to sex.[6]

Perhaps the greatest difficulty in evaluating the effectiveness of treatment is the great variability of the severity of the psychodynamic and relationship problems that can be associated with identical sexual symptoms. Treatment results may be expected to vary with the degree of psychopathology in the sample, and it may be possible that, apart from the technical superiority of sex therapy over long-term psychotherapy for these complaints, one of the reasons for the striking discrepancy between the treatment outcomes reported by O'Connor and Stern versus those of Masters and Johnson was that the patients seen in New York were sicker than the ones treated in St. Louis. The foregoing considerations underscore the vital need to define and refine clinical criteria and to develop specific protocols for the treatment of sexual dysfunctions.

Training

At this point in the development of the field, a variety of approaches have been developed, which all report successes in the treatment of psychosexual disorders. In the light of this diversity, the clinician who is interested in working with this patient population cannot be wedded to any one particular approach. He needs to acquire skills in a broad spectrum of therapy—sex therapy, the psychodynamic therapies, behavior therapy, pharmacotherapy, and brief as well as long-term couples therapy—so that he can apply these when appropriate in a individualistic and creative manner. Education and training in human sexuality ought to reflect this need for a broad and flexible approach, and should equip the students with a wide range of diagnostic and therapeutic skills.

REFERENCES

1. American Psychiatric Association: Diagnostic and Statistical Manual, Third Edition. (DSM-III) Washington, DC, American Psychiatric Association Press, 1980

2. Masters WH, Johnson V: Human Sexual Inadequacy. Boston, Little Brown, 1970

3. Kaplan HS: The Evaluation of Sexual Disorders: Psychological and Medical Aspects. New York, Brunner/Mazel, 1983

4. Kaplan HS: The New Sex Therapy. New York, Brunner/Mazel, 1974

5. Fisher S: The Female Orgasm. New York Basic Books, 1973

6. Klein DF: Anxiety reconceptualized. Klein Rabkin (eds) In Anxiety: New Research and Changing Concepts. pp 235–241. New York, Raven Press, 1980

7. Schiavi RC: Androgens and male sexual function: A review of human studies. J Sex Marital Ther, 1976

8. Spark RF, White RA, Connoly PB: Impotence is not always psychogenic: Hypothalamic-pituitary gonadal dysfunction. JAMA, 243:750–755, 1980

9. Lief HI: Sexual Problems in Medical Practice. Monroe, WI, American Medical Association, 1981

10. Kaplan HS: Disorders of Sexual Desire. New York, Brunner/Mazel, 1979

11. O'Connor JF, Stern LO: Results of treatment in functional sexual disorders. NY State J Med 1972, 1927, 1934.

Subject Index

INDEX